BARBARA O'NEILL NATURAL HERBAL REMEDIES COMPLETE COLLECTION

30 in 1: The Lost Book of Self-Healing Recipes and Secrets for Holistic Health and Optimal Well-Being

Fiona Wren

GET YOUR BONUSES NOW!

The BONUSES below are **100% FREE**, and all you need
to get them is a name and an email address. **It's super simple!**

BONUS 1
BARBARA O'NEILL EXCLUSIVE VIDEOS

BONUS 2
1000 DR. BARBARA NATURAL REMEDIES

BONUS 3
DR. BARBARA SELF-HEALING COOKBOOK

TO GET THEM SCAN
THE QR CODE BELOW OR GO TO

bonusbookshelf.com/fiona-wren-hc

TABLE OF CONTENTS

PART 1: DR. BARBARA'S HOLISTIC HEALTH OVERVIEW

D r. Barbara's holistic health approach is a comprehensive journey into the interconnectedness of the mind, body, and spirit, emphasizing the importance of natural healing and plant-based nutrition. At the core of her philosophy lies the belief that the body possesses an inherent ability to heal itself, given the right conditions and support.

This approach advocates for a balanced lifestyle that harmonizes nutritional choices, physical activities, and mental well-being to foster overall health and prevent diseases.

Central to Dr. Barbara's method is the understanding that every individual is unique, requiring personalized strategies for optimal health.

She emphasizes the role of nutrition as medicine, advocating for a diet rich in whole, unprocessed foods that nourish the body and support its natural detoxification processes.

The mind-body-spirit connection is another pillar of her philosophy, highlighting the impact of psychological and emotional well-being on physical health.

Dr. Barbara introduces the concept of natural healing through the use of herbal remedies, essential for supporting the body's self-healing mechanism.

These remedies, rooted in ancient wisdom and validated by modern science, offer gentle yet effective alternatives to conventional treatments, minimizing the risk of side effects.

This holistic health approach extends beyond the individual, encouraging a sustainable lifestyle that respects and protects our planet's natural resources.

By choosing plant-based nutrition and natural remedies, individuals contribute to a healthier environment, reducing their ecological footprint.

Dr. Barbara's holistic health approach is not just a set of guidelines but a transformative journey towards self-awareness, empowerment, and harmony with nature.

It invites readers of all ages and backgrounds to explore the healing power within themselves and the natural world, promising a path to wellness that is both nurturing and life-affirming.

Dr. Barbara's holistic health approach represents a profound and comprehensive journey that delves into the deep interconnectedness of the mind, body, and spirit.

Her philosophy revolves around the concept that true health and well-being stem from a harmonious balance of these elements, where each supports the other to create a resilient and thriving individual.

This approach emphasizes the importance of natural healing, plant-based nutrition, and a lifestyle that aligns with the rhythms of nature.

- **The Body's Inherent Ability to Heal**

At the core of Dr. Barbara's philosophy is the belief that the body has an inherent capacity to heal itself when provided with the right conditions. She advocates for creating an environment—both internally and externally—that supports the body's natural healing mechanisms.

This involves nourishing the body with wholesome, nutrient-rich foods, engaging in regular physical activity, managing stress, and utilizing natural remedies to enhance the body's ability to recover from illness and maintain optimal health.

- **Nutrition as Medicine**

A key pillar of Dr. Barbara's approach is her focus on nutrition as a form of medicine.

She promotes a diet that prioritizes whole, unprocessed foods, particularly those derived from plants, as these are rich in the vitamins, minerals, and antioxidants necessary for supporting the body's natural detoxification processes and overall vitality.

Dr. Barbara highlights the importance of plant-based nutrition not only for physical health but also for its positive impact on mental and emotional well-being. She encourages the consumption of nutrient-dense foods that work synergistically with the body to prevent disease and promote longevity.

- **Personalized Health Strategies**

Recognizing the uniqueness of each individual, Dr. Barbara emphasizes the need for personalized health strategies. She understands that there is no one-size-fits-all solution to well-being.

Each person's body, mind, and spirit are distinct, requiring tailored approaches that consider individual needs, preferences, and life circumstances. Her holistic methods are adaptable, offering flexibility in finding the right balance that works for each individual. This personalized approach fosters a deeper understanding of one's body and empowers individuals to take control of their own health journey.

- **The Mind-Body-Spirit Connection**

Central to Dr. Barbara's holistic philosophy is the mind-body-spirit connection, which highlights how psychological and emotional well-being can directly influence physical health.

Stress, anxiety, and emotional imbalances can manifest in the body as physical symptoms, leading to illness and disease. Dr. Barbara advocates for practices such as meditation, mindfulness, and self-reflection to cultivate mental clarity and emotional stability.

By nurturing the mind and spirit, individuals can enhance their overall health and foster a more balanced and harmonious life.

- **Natural Healing with Herbal Remedies**

Dr. Barbara introduces the concept of natural healing through the use of herbal remedies, which she sees as essential for supporting the body's self-healing capabilities.

These remedies are rooted in ancient wisdom and traditions but are also validated by modern scientific research. She emphasizes that herbal treatments offer gentle, effective alternatives to conventional medicine, helping to restore balance and vitality without the harsh side effects often associated with synthetic drugs. This approach aligns with her belief in the power of nature to heal and rejuvenate the body.

- **Sustainable Living and Environmental Consciousness**

Dr. Barbara's holistic health philosophy extends beyond personal well-being, advocating for a lifestyle that is sustainable and environmentally conscious. She encourages choices that respect and protect the Earth's natural resources, such as opting for plant-based nutrition and utilizing natural, eco-friendly products. By living in harmony with the planet, individuals not only enhance their own health but also contribute to the well-being of the environment. This sustainable approach reduces the ecological footprint and promotes a healthier, more balanced world for future generations.

- **A Transformative Journey**

Dr. Barbara's holistic health approach is more than just a set of guidelines; it is a transformative journey that invites individuals to explore the healing power within themselves and the natural world. It is a path of self-awareness, empowerment, and connection with nature, offering a nurturing and life-affirming way to achieve wellness. Her philosophy encourages readers of all ages and backgrounds to embrace holistic living as a means of achieving lasting health, happiness, and harmony.

CHAPTER 1: UNDERSTANDING HOLISTIC HEALTH

Holistic health is a comprehensive approach that goes beyond merely treating symptoms to address the root causes of illness and promote overall well-being. It recognizes the body as an interconnected system where physical, mental, and spiritual health are fundamentally linked. This means that a disturbance in one aspect of health can affect the others, highlighting the importance of a balanced lifestyle that nurtures all parts of the individual. At the heart of holistic health is the belief that the body has an innate ability to heal itself when supported with the right environment and resources. This includes nourishing foods, regular physical activity, adequate rest, and a positive mental state. Nutrition plays a pivotal role in this model, with a focus on whole, unprocessed foods that provide essential nutrients to support the body's natural healing processes. These dietary choices are not just about preventing or managing illness but are also about thriving and achieving optimal health.

The mind-body-spirit connection is another key element of holistic health, emphasizing the impact of psychological well-being and emotional balance on physical health. Stress, for instance, can lead to a host of physical problems, including heart disease, digestive issues, and weakened immune function. Conversely, physical ailments can affect mental health, leading to anxiety or depression. Recognizing these connections, holistic health practices often incorporate stress-reduction techniques such as meditation, yoga, and deep-breathing exercises to support overall well-being.

Holistic health also encourages individuals to take an active role in their health care, advocating for self-awareness and self-care practices that empower people to make informed choices about their health. This includes understanding how lifestyle factors such as sleep patterns, exercise habits, and social connections can influence well-being and making adjustments to foster a healthier life. In embracing a holistic approach to health, there is also a recognition of the individual's unique needs and circumstances. What works for one person may not work for another, underscoring the importance of personalized health plans that consider the whole person, including their life experiences, environment, and genetic makeup. This individualized approach ensures that health strategies are tailored to meet the specific needs and goals of each person, offering a more effective and sustainable path to health and wellness.

Holistic health is not just about avoiding illness but about living in a way that promotes vitality, happiness, and longevity. It invites us to look beyond the physical symptoms and explore deeper aspects of our health, encouraging a proactive and preventive approach to well-being that integrates the best of natural healing with conventional medicine when necessary. By focusing on the whole person and the interconnectedness of various aspects of health, holistic health offers a comprehensive framework for living a balanced and fulfilling life.

Holistic health also places a significant emphasis on the environment and its impact on our well-being. The quality of the air we breathe, the water we drink, and the food we consume are all critical factors that can contribute to our health or detract from it. This approach advocates for a sustainable lifestyle that minimizes exposure to toxins and environmental pollutants, recognizing that a healthy environment is essential for a healthy body and mind. It encourages choices that not only benefit personal health but also the health of our planet, such as opting for organic produce, reducing plastic use, and supporting eco-friendly initiatives.

Another cornerstone of holistic health is the power of relationships and social connections in influencing health outcomes. Positive interactions with family, friends, and the community can provide emotional support, reduce stress, and promote a sense of belonging and happiness. On the other hand, isolation and negative social interactions can lead to deteriorations in mental and physical health. Holistic health practices thus often include building and maintaining healthy relationships as a key component of overall well-being.

The role of spirituality in holistic health cannot be overstated. Whether through organized religion, personal belief systems, or a connection with nature, spirituality offers a way to find meaning, purpose, and connection in life. It can provide comfort in times of illness, strength in times of difficulty, and a sense of peace and well-being. Holistic health recognizes the importance of nurturing the spirit alongside the body and mind, offering a comprehensive approach to health that honors the full spectrum of human experience. Education and knowledge are also vital elements of holistic health. Empowering individuals with the information they need to make informed decisions about their health care, understand the principles of nutrition and exercise, and recognize the signs of imbalance in their bodies is crucial. Holistic health advocates for continuous learning and growth, encouraging individuals to explore various healing modalities, understand the science behind health recommendations, and stay informed about advances in health care.

In summary, holistic health is a dynamic and integrative approach to well-being that recognizes the complexity of the human body and the multiple factors that contribute to health. It combines the wisdom of traditional healing practices with the insights of modern science, offering a path to health that is personalized, proactive, and rooted in the principles of natural living and sustainability. By embracing holistic health, individuals can embark on a journey toward not just surviving but thriving, achieving a state of health that encompasses the body, mind, and spirit in harmony with the world around them.

DR. BARBARA'S PHILOSOPHY ON HEALTH

Dr. Barbara's philosophy on health is deeply rooted in the belief that true wellness encompasses not only the physical body but also the mind and spirit. She posits that health is not merely the absence of disease but a state of complete physical, mental, and social well-being.

Central to her philosophy is the conviction that our bodies have a remarkable capacity for self-healing, a process that can be significantly enhanced through natural means and lifestyle choices that support the body's intrinsic healing mechanisms. Key to this philosophy is the emphasis on preventive care rather than reactive treatment. Dr. Barbara advocates for a proactive approach to health, encouraging individuals to adopt lifestyle habits that support their well-being before the onset of illness. This includes a diet rich in whole, plant-based foods, regular physical activity, adequate rest, and stress management practices. She underscores the importance of listening to our bodies and responding to its signals with care and attention, fostering a harmonious relationship between the body and its environment.

Nutrition holds a place of paramount importance in Dr. Barbara's approach to health. She emphasizes that food should be seen as medicine, with the power to heal, nourish, and revitalize our bodies. By choosing foods that are as close to their natural state as possible, we can ensure that we are providing our bodies with the nutrients needed to function optimally.

This philosophy extends to the rejection of processed foods and substances that can harm the body, advocating instead for organic and sustainably sourced ingredients that support not only individual health but also the health of the planet.

Dr. Barbara also highlights the significance of the mind-body-spirit connection, advocating for practices that nurture all aspects of our being. She believes that mental and emotional well-being is just as crucial as physical health, and that spiritual practices, whether they be in the form of meditation, prayer, or connection with nature, can provide a foundation for a balanced and healthy life. Through this holistic approach, Dr. Barbara aims to empower individuals to take control of their health, leading lives that are not just free from illness but are vibrant, joyful, and deeply fulfilling.

MIND-BODY-SPIRIT CONNECTION

The mind-body-spirit connection is a fundamental aspect of holistic health, underscoring the intricate interplay between our psychological state, physical health, and spiritual well-being. This triad forms the cornerstone of Dr. Barbara's holistic health approach, emphasizing that true wellness can only be achieved when all three components are in harmony.

The concept is not new; it has roots in ancient healing traditions worldwide, which understood health to be the result of a balanced life, not merely the absence of disease.

At the heart of the mind-body-spirit connection is the understanding that our thoughts, feelings, and beliefs have a profound impact on our physical health. The body's physiological responses to stress, such as increased heart rate, elevated cortisol levels, and a weakened immune system, are clear indicators of how closely our mental state is linked to our physical well-being. Conversely, physical ailments can lead to psychological distress, creating a cycle that can only be broken by addressing both aspects simultaneously.

Spirituality, whether it involves organized religion, personal belief systems, or a deep connection with nature, plays a crucial role in this holistic model. It offers a sense of purpose and meaning, providing a solid foundation for both mental and physical health. Spiritual practices such as meditation, prayer, or simply spending time in nature can foster a sense of peace and well-being, reducing stress and promoting healing. Dr. Barbara advocates for a holistic approach to health care that incorporates strategies for nurturing the mind, body, and spirit.

This includes adopting a diet rich in whole, unprocessed foods to nourish the body, engaging in regular physical activity to strengthen and revitalize the body, and practicing mindfulness or meditation to calm the mind. Additionally, fostering spiritual connections and pursuing activities that bring joy and fulfillment are essential for maintaining emotional and psychological health.

Understanding the mind-body-spirit connection also involves recognizing the signals our bodies send us. Symptoms of discomfort or disease are often the body's way of communicating imbalances that may have psychological or spiritual roots.

By tuning into these messages and responding with appropriate self-care practices, individuals can initiate their journey towards holistic healing.

The integration of the mind-body-spirit connection into daily life can be transformative, leading to improved health outcomes, increased happiness, and a deeper sense of connection with oneself and the world. It invites us to view health not as a static state but as a dynamic process of continuous growth and self-discovery. Through this lens, challenges become opportunities for learning and growth, guiding us towards a more balanced and fulfilling life.

As we delve deeper into the nuances of the mind-body-spirit connection, it becomes evident that this holistic approach offers a powerful framework for understanding health and wellness. It challenges the conventional medical model by proposing a more comprehensive, integrative approach that honors the complexity of the human experience. By embracing this interconnectedness, individuals can unlock their healing potential and embark on a path towards true wellness.

Harnessing the power of the mind-body-spirit connection requires a conscious effort to cultivate practices that nurture each aspect of our being. For the mind, this might involve engaging in activities that stimulate mental clarity and emotional resilience, such as journaling, cognitive behavioral techniques, or engaging in meaningful conversations that challenge and expand our perspectives. The body benefits from not only physical exercise and proper nutrition but also from adequate rest and relaxation, allowing for regeneration and healing. Spiritually, finding what uniquely speaks to each individual—be it through meditation, connecting with community, or exploring nature—can significantly enhance one's sense of belonging and purpose in the world.

The symbiotic relationship between the mind, body, and spirit also emphasizes the importance of a supportive environment that fosters growth and well-being. Surrounding ourselves with positive influences, whether through relationships that uplift us, choosing work that inspires us, or creating a living space that reflects our values and needs, can profoundly impact our health journey. It's about making choices that align with our deepest selves, thereby enhancing our overall harmony and balance.

Moreover, the practice of gratitude and positive thinking plays a pivotal role in the mind-body-spirit connection. Cultivating an attitude of gratitude can shift our focus from what we lack to the abundance we possess, promoting a state of well-being that permeates our entire being.

Positive thinking doesn't mean ignoring life's challenges but rather approaching them with a mindset that favors resilience and growth.

This outlook can mitigate the impact of stress and anxiety on our physical health, demonstrating the profound power our thoughts and attitudes have on our bodily state.

Another crucial aspect of nurturing the mind-body-spirit connection is learning to listen to our intuition. Our bodies are incredibly wise, often knowing what we need before we consciously realize it. Tuning into this inner guidance can help us make healthier choices, seek out healing practices that resonate with us, and ultimately lead us towards a more authentic and fulfilling life. In integrating these practices into our lives, it's essential to remember that the journey towards holistic health is personal and unique. What works for one person may not work for another, and the key is to explore different practices and modalities to discover what truly helps us thrive.

By honoring our individuality and listening to our bodies, we can navigate the path to wellness with wisdom and grace.

The mind-body-spirit connection, therefore, is not merely a concept but a lived experience that encompasses every aspect of our lives. It invites us to view health as a holistic endeavor, where nurturing our mental, physical, and spiritual well-being leads to a richer, more vibrant life. By embracing this interconnectedness, we open ourselves to a world of healing possibilities, empowering us to live our lives to the fullest. Through this holistic lens, we see that every aspect of our existence holds the potential for healing and growth, guiding us towards a state of balance and harmony that radiates from the inside out.

THE ROLE OF NUTRITION IN HOLISTIC HEALTH

The role of nutrition in holistic health cannot be overstated as it forms the foundation upon which our physical well-being is built. Nutrition, in the context of holistic health, transcends the simple act of eating to fill an empty stomach. It involves selecting foods that are vibrant, full of life, and capable of nourishing the body at the deepest levels. Each food choice we make can either support our body's natural healing processes or hinder them, making it crucial to choose wisely and with intention.

Whole, unprocessed foods are the cornerstone of a diet that promotes holistic health. These foods are minimally altered from their natural state, retaining their nutritional integrity and the life energy they contain. Fruits, vegetables, whole grains, nuts, seeds, and legumes are all examples of whole foods that provide a symphony of nutrients essential for maintaining and restoring health. These nutrients include vitamins, minerals, antioxidants, fiber, and phytochemicals, each playing a unique role in supporting bodily functions and promoting resilience against disease.

The concept of food as medicine is central to understanding the role of nutrition in holistic health. This ancient idea, embraced by cultures around the world, recognizes that certain foods have the power to prevent, alleviate, or even cure illness. For instance, the anti-inflammatory properties of turmeric, the heart-healthy fats found in avocados, and the immune-boosting vitamin C in citrus fruits all exemplify how food can act as medicine. By incorporating a diverse range of nutrient-dense foods into our diet, we equip our body with the tools it needs to heal itself and maintain optimal health. Moreover, the way we eat is just as important as what we eat. Mindful eating practices, such as taking the time to chew food thoroughly, eating without distractions, and listening to our body's hunger and fullness cues, enhance our connection to food and improve digestion and nutrient absorption. This mindful approach to eating encourages a deeper appreciation for the nourishment food provides and fosters a harmonious relationship with food that is often lost in today's fast-paced world.

Hydration also plays a pivotal role in holistic nutrition. Water is essential for virtually every bodily function, including digestion, absorption, circulation, and detoxification. Drinking sufficient amounts of clean, pure water daily supports health and vitality, yet is often overlooked in discussions about nutrition. Herbal teas and infusions can also be beneficial, offering hydration along with the therapeutic properties of herbs.

In the realm of holistic health, nutrition is not only about feeding the body but also about supporting the mind and spirit. Foods that are rich in omega-3 fatty acids, for example, are not only good for the heart but also support cognitive function and mental well-being. Similarly, foods that are vibrant and alive can uplift our spirits and enhance our connection to the natural world. As we delve deeper into the intricacies of nutrition in holistic health, it becomes clear that our dietary choices have far-reaching implications for our overall well-being. The foods we choose to consume can either support our journey towards health and harmony or detract from it. By embracing a holistic approach to nutrition, we acknowledge the profound impact that food has on our physical, mental, and spiritual health, and take an important step towards achieving a balanced and vibrant life.

Emphasizing the quality of the foods we eat, organic and locally sourced produce plays a significant role in holistic nutrition. These foods are grown without harmful pesticides and chemicals, ensuring that what we consume supports not just our health but also the health of the environment. The act of choosing organic and local foods is a commitment to a sustainable food system that respects the earth and its ecosystems. This choice aligns with the holistic health principle of living in harmony with nature, recognizing that our health is deeply interconnected with the health of our planet.

Seasonal eating further enhances the nutritional value of our diet. Foods grown and consumed during their appropriate seasons are more nutritionally dense and energetically aligned with our body's needs. For example, the abundance of fruits and vegetables in the summer provides the perfect hydration and nutrients necessary for that season, while the root vegetables and hearty greens available in the winter offer warmth and sustenance. Seasonal eating not only supports our body's natural rhythms but also encourages a varied diet, which is essential for providing a wide range of nutrients.

The concept of bioindividuality is another important aspect of nutrition in holistic health. It acknowledges that no single diet works for everyone and that each person has unique dietary needs based on factors such as age, genetics, environment, and health status. This personalized approach to nutrition empowers individuals to discover what foods best support their health and well-being, rather than following one-size-fits-all dietary guidelines. It encourages experimentation and attunement to one's own body to identify foods that enhance vitality and those that may not be as beneficial.

Combining foods for optimal nutrition and digestion, known as food combining, is also considered in holistic nutrition. This practice is based on the understanding that certain food combinations can enhance nutrient absorption and improve digestive health, while others may hinder these processes. For instance, combining iron-rich plant foods with vitamin C-rich foods can enhance iron absorption, beneficial for those focusing on plant-based nutrition.

Detoxification through diet is another principle of holistic nutrition, emphasizing foods that support the body's natural detox pathways. Incorporating foods rich in antioxidants, fiber, and essential nutrients helps to facilitate the elimination of toxins and promotes liver health. Regular consumption of leafy greens, cruciferous vegetables, fresh herbs, and fruits can support detoxification processes and contribute to overall vitality.

Finally, the role of nutrition in holistic health extends beyond the physical to include emotional and spiritual nourishment. Foods prepared with intention and consumed with gratitude can have a profound impact on our well-being. The act of cooking and sharing meals can serve as a form of self-care and an opportunity to connect with others, nourishing the soul as well as the body.

In embracing a holistic approach to nutrition, we recognize the profound impact that our dietary choices have on our overall well-being. By choosing whole, unprocessed foods, paying attention to the quality and source of our food, eating seasonally, respecting our body's unique needs, practicing mindful eating, and acknowledging the emotional and spiritual aspects of food, we support our health in the most comprehensive sense. This approach to nutrition not only fosters physical health but also contributes to a balanced and fulfilling life, where food is celebrated as a key element of a holistic health journey.

CHAPTER 2: CORE PRINCIPLES OF NATURAL HEALING

The core principles of natural healing revolve around the understanding that the body is a self-healing organism, capable of regenerating and repairing itself when given the right conditions. This belief is rooted in the idea that by aligning with nature and its inherent wisdom, we can foster optimal health and well-being. The first principle central to natural healing is the power of prevention. Rather than waiting for disease to manifest, natural healing emphasizes the importance of maintaining balance and harmony within the body and mind to prevent illness. This involves adopting a lifestyle that supports health through nutrition, exercise, stress management, and avoiding toxins.

Another fundamental principle is the holistic approach to health, which considers the individual as a whole, integrating the physical, mental, emotional, and spiritual aspects of well-being.

This perspective recognizes that symptoms of disease are often manifestations of imbalances in one or more of these areas. Therefore, healing practices under this principle aim to address the root causes of illness, not just the symptoms. This may involve a combination of dietary changes, herbal remedies, physical activities, and mindfulness practices tailored to the individual's unique needs and circumstances. Nutrition plays a pivotal role in natural healing, based on the principle that food is medicine. This concept dates back to ancient times and is a cornerstone of many traditional healing systems. A diet rich in whole, unprocessed foods provides the body with essential nutrients that support its natural healing processes. Foods that are vibrant and alive can significantly influence our physical health and emotional well-being. Incorporating a variety of fruits, vegetables, whole grains, nuts, seeds, and legumes into the diet ensures a broad spectrum of vitamins, minerals, antioxidants, and phytochemicals that work synergistically to promote health.

Detoxification is another key principle of natural healing, emphasizing the body's need to periodically cleanse itself of toxins and waste products.

This can be supported through specific foods, fasting, herbal teas, hydrotherapy, and other practices that stimulate the body's detoxification pathways. By assisting the body in eliminating toxins, we can help prevent the accumulation of substances that may contribute to disease. The principle of the healing power of nature, or vis medicatrix naturae, suggests that the body inherently knows how to heal itself and strives to maintain balance. Natural healing practices aim to support this innate wisdom through methods that enhance the body's own healing capabilities. This might include exposure to natural sunlight for vitamin D synthesis, breathing fresh air for improved oxygenation, and grounding or earthing practices to reduce inflammation and improve sleep.

Herbal medicine, a cornerstone of natural healing, utilizes the therapeutic properties of plants to treat and prevent illness. Each herb has unique properties that can support healing in various ways, such as boosting the immune system, calming the nervous system, or improving digestive function. Herbal remedies are chosen based on the individual's specific needs, taking into account the holistic nature of their health. The principle of do no harm, or primum non nocere, is central to natural healing. This means choosing the most gentle and non-invasive methods necessary to facilitate healing, minimizing the risk of side effects or harm. Natural healing practices prioritize interventions that work in harmony with the body's natural processes, often using the least force necessary to stimulate healing.

Lastly, the principle of the therapeutic order guides the approach to natural healing, starting with the most foundational aspects of health, such as diet and lifestyle, and moving towards more specific interventions only as needed. This ensures that the simplest and most natural methods are employed first, reserving more invasive measures for when they are truly necessary. These core principles of natural healing underscore the importance of living in harmony with nature and recognizing the body's capacity for self-repair. By adopting practices that support the body's natural healing processes, individuals can enhance their health and vitality, paving the way for a balanced and holistic approach to well-being.

Understanding the body's unique language and responding to its signals is essential in natural healing. This involves tuning into the subtle cues our bodies give us, such as changes in energy levels, mood swings, and physical symptoms, to identify imbalances early on.

By paying attention to these signals, we can take proactive steps to address issues before they escalate into more serious conditions. This principle emphasizes the importance of self-awareness and mindfulness in maintaining health and preventing disease.

The role of emotional and mental well-being in natural healing cannot be overstated. Stress, anxiety, and negative emotions can have a profound impact on physical health, contributing to the development of chronic diseases and hindering the body's healing processes. Natural healing practices, therefore, incorporate techniques for managing stress and promoting mental and emotional balance, such as meditation, yoga, deep breathing exercises, and spending time in nature.

These practices not only improve mental health but also facilitate physical healing by reducing stress-related hormones and inflammation in the body.

Another critical principle is the importance of community and social connections in healing. Humans are inherently social beings, and our relationships with others can significantly influence our health. Positive social interactions and a supportive community can enhance well-being, boost immunity, and increase longevity. Natural healing recognizes the therapeutic value of community and encourages individuals to cultivate meaningful relationships and social networks that provide support, love, and connection. The principle of education and empowerment is fundamental to natural healing. It advocates for individuals to take an active role in their health by learning about their bodies, understanding the principles of healthy living, and making informed choices about their care. This includes educating oneself about the benefits and uses of different healing modalities, understanding the nutritional value of foods, and learning how to listen to and interpret the body's signals.

By empowering individuals with knowledge, natural healing fosters a sense of autonomy and confidence in managing one's health. Finally, the principle of integration and balance underscores the idea that true healing involves balancing all aspects of the individual—physical, emotional, mental, and spiritual. This holistic approach recognizes that each aspect of our being is interconnected and that imbalances in one area can affect the others.

Natural healing practices aim to restore balance and harmony within the individual, leading to holistic well-being and vitality. This may involve integrating various healing modalities, such as combining dietary changes with herbal remedies and mindfulness practices, to address the needs of the whole person. By embracing these core principles, natural healing offers a comprehensive and holistic approach to health that empowers individuals to nurture their well-being in harmony with nature's wisdom. It encourages a proactive and preventive stance towards health, emphasizing the importance of listening to the body, fostering emotional and mental balance, building supportive communities, educating oneself, and seeking balance and integration in all aspects of life. Through this holistic lens, natural healing provides a path to vibrant health and well-being, rooted in the profound connection between the individual and the natural world.

CHAPTER 3: NUTRITION AS MEDICINE

The transformative power of nutrition as medicine is rooted in the understanding that the foods we consume go beyond mere sustenance; they are potent tools for healing and wellness. This concept, deeply embedded in Dr. Barbara's holistic health approach, emphasizes the critical role of diet in preventing, managing, and sometimes even reversing chronic diseases. By selecting foods rich in vitamins, minerals, antioxidants, and other essential nutrients, we can support the body's natural defense mechanisms, promote detoxification, and enhance our overall health.

At the heart of using nutrition as medicine is the principle of bioindividuality, which acknowledges that each person's body is unique, with specific nutritional needs and responses to food. This personalized approach to diet allows for the customization of nutritional plans that cater to individual health conditions, preferences, and goals. It involves a deep understanding of how different foods can affect bodily functions and the importance of adjusting dietary habits to align with one's health journey.

Incorporating whole, unprocessed foods into the diet is a cornerstone of nutritional medicine. These foods are minimally altered from their natural state, ensuring that they retain their nutritional integrity and life energy. Fruits, vegetables, whole grains, nuts, seeds, and legumes are packed with a symphony of nutrients that work synergistically to nourish the body at the cellular level.

These nutrient-dense foods provide the building blocks for health, supporting the body's healing processes and promoting vitality. The anti-inflammatory diet is a prime example of using nutrition as medicine. Chronic inflammation is a root cause of many diseases, including heart disease, diabetes, and autoimmune conditions. By focusing on foods that naturally combat inflammation, such as leafy greens, berries, fatty fish, and nuts, while avoiding pro-inflammatory foods like processed meats, refined carbs, and sugary beverages, individuals can significantly reduce inflammation and its harmful effects on the body.

Gut health is another area where nutrition plays a medicinal role. The gut microbiome, consisting of trillions of bacteria, is integral to digestion, immunity, and even mental health. A diet rich in prebiotic and probiotic foods, such as garlic, onions, asparagus, yogurt, and kefir, can help maintain a healthy balance of gut bacteria, promoting digestive health and enhancing immune function. Detoxification through diet is also a key aspect of nutritional medicine. Certain foods, such as cruciferous vegetables, berries, garlic, and green tea, have been shown to support the body's detox pathways, helping to eliminate toxins and reduce the burden on the liver. Regular consumption of these foods can aid in the prevention of toxin-related diseases and contribute to overall well-being.

In addition to these specific dietary strategies, the practice of mindful eating is an essential component of nutrition as medicine. This involves being fully present during meals, savoring each bite, and listening to the body's hunger and fullness cues. Mindful eating can enhance the digestive process, improve nutrient absorption, and foster a healthier relationship with food. As we continue to explore the vast potential of nutrition as medicine, it's clear that our dietary choices have profound implications for our health. By embracing a diet centered on whole, nutrient-dense foods, tailored to our individual needs, we can harness the healing power of nutrition to support our body's natural ability to heal and thrive.

The role of specific nutrients in preventing and managing chronic conditions underscores the medicinal value of nutrition. Essential fatty acids, for instance, found in flaxseeds, chia seeds, and walnuts, play a crucial role in brain health, reducing inflammation, and supporting heart health. Antioxidant-rich foods like berries, dark chocolate, and spices such as turmeric and cinnamon help combat oxidative stress, a key factor in aging and many chronic diseases. By focusing on these nutrient-dense foods, individuals can protect their cells from damage and support the body's repair mechanisms.

The concept of food synergy is also vital in understanding how nutrition functions as medicine. It's not just about individual nutrients but how they work together to enhance their healing effects.

For example, the combination of vitamin C-rich foods with iron-rich plant sources can significantly improve iron absorption, crucial for those at risk of anemia. Similarly, the fat-soluble vitamins A, D, E, and K require the presence of dietary fat for optimal absorption, highlighting the importance of a balanced diet that includes healthy fats.

Addressing dietary deficiencies is another way nutrition serves as medicine. Deficiencies in vitamins and minerals can lead to a range of health issues, from anemia and fatigue to weakened immunity and poor bone health. By ensuring a diet rich in a variety of fruits, vegetables, whole grains, and lean proteins, individuals can meet their nutritional needs and prevent these deficiencies. For those unable to meet their nutritional requirements through diet alone, supplementation may be necessary, emphasizing the need for a personalized approach to nutrition.

The therapeutic potential of dietary patterns is also evident in the success of diets such as the Mediterranean diet, known for its heart-healthy benefits, and the DASH diet, designed to combat high blood pressure. These diets emphasize whole foods, lean proteins, and healthy fats, demonstrating how a holistic dietary approach can manage and even reverse specific health conditions.

Furthermore, the role of nutrition in mental health cannot be overlooked. Emerging research suggests a strong link between diet and mental health, with certain dietary patterns associated with reduced risk of depression and anxiety.

Foods rich in omega-3 fatty acids, B vitamins, and antioxidants are particularly beneficial for brain health, offering a natural means of supporting mental well-being.

The integration of nutrition into medical treatment plans signifies a shift towards a more holistic approach to health care. By recognizing the role of diet in disease prevention and management, health professionals can provide comprehensive care that addresses the root causes of illness rather than merely treating symptoms.

This approach not only enhances the efficacy of medical treatments but also empowers individuals to take an active role in their health journey. In conclusion, the medicinal power of nutrition is a testament to the complex and dynamic relationship between diet and health. By embracing a holistic approach to eating, focused on whole, nutrient-dense foods and personalized dietary strategies, individuals can harness the healing power of nutrition to enhance their health and vitality. As we continue to uncover the intricate ways in which diet influences our well-being, the adage "let food be thy medicine" has never been more relevant, offering a foundation for a life of optimal health and wellness.

THE BODY'S SELF-HEALING MECHANISM

The body's self-healing mechanism is a remarkable and complex system designed to protect and repair itself from the myriad of challenges it faces daily. At the heart of this system is the immune response, a sophisticated network of cells, tissues, and organs that work in concert to defend the body against pathogens, including bacteria, viruses, and parasites. This intricate defense system is capable of identifying and neutralizing foreign invaders, showcasing the body's inherent wisdom and capacity for self-preservation.

Central to the body's ability to heal itself is the process of inflammation, a natural response to injury or infection. While often perceived negatively, inflammation is actually a crucial part of the healing process. It signals the immune system to send white blood cells and nutrients to the affected area to fight off infections and begin the repair process. This initial inflammatory phase is a testament to the body's proactive measures to heal and protect itself.

Another key component of the body's self-healing mechanism is the ability to regenerate and repair damaged tissues. Cells in the human body have varying degrees of regenerative capacity. For example, liver cells can regenerate after injury, skin wounds heal through the proliferation of epidermal and dermal cells, and bones mend by the remodeling process, where new bone tissue replaces damaged tissue. This regenerative process underscores the body's remarkable resilience and adaptability. The role of the nervous system in the body's self-healing mechanism cannot be overstated. The nervous system controls various bodily functions, including the response to pain and the regulation of the healing process. Through the release of neurotransmitters and hormones, the nervous system communicates with the immune system, signaling the need for healing and repair.

This intricate communication underscores the interconnectedness of the body's systems and their collective role in maintaining health and well-being. Moreover, the body's self-healing mechanism is significantly influenced by psychological and emotional factors. Stress, for example, can suppress the immune response and hinder the healing process, while positive emotions and a calm mind can enhance immune function and promote healing. This connection between the mind and body highlights the importance of mental and emotional well-being in the context of physical health.

Nutrition also plays a critical role in supporting the body's self-healing mechanism. A diet rich in vitamins, minerals, and antioxidants can bolster the immune system, reduce inflammation, and facilitate tissue repair. Foods that are vibrant and alive with nutrients provide the essential building blocks for healing, emphasizing the adage that food is indeed medicine.

Hydration is another fundamental aspect of self-healing. Water is vital for all bodily functions, including the transport of nutrients to cells and the removal of toxins from the body. Adequate hydration ensures that the body's cells are well-nourished and that the organs function optimally, supporting the overall healing process.

The body's self-healing mechanism is a testament to its inherent wisdom and capacity for regeneration and repair. By understanding and supporting this natural process through healthy lifestyle choices, individuals can enhance their resilience and vitality.

The interplay between the immune system, inflammation, tissue regeneration, the nervous system, psychological well-being, nutrition, and hydration illustrates the complexity and efficiency of the body's self-healing mechanism, a process that continues to fascinate and inspire those seeking to live in harmony with their body's natural rhythms and capabilities.

Sleep is another crucial factor that significantly impacts the body's self-healing capabilities. During sleep, the body undergoes numerous restorative processes, including muscle repair, protein synthesis, and the release of growth hormones essential for tissue growth and repair.

This rest period allows the immune system to recalibrate and strengthen, preparing the body to fight off infections and continue the healing process. The quality and quantity of sleep directly influence the efficiency of these healing mechanisms, highlighting the importance of adequate rest in maintaining health and facilitating recovery.

Exercise, too, plays a vital role in supporting the body's self-healing mechanism. Regular physical activity can boost the immune system, help manage inflammation, and promote healthy circulation, ensuring that nutrients and oxygen are efficiently delivered to cells in need of repair. Furthermore, exercise stimulates the release of endorphins, "feel-good" hormones that reduce pain and enhance mood, further supporting the healing process.

The body's ability to detoxify itself is another testament to its self-healing prowess. The liver, kidneys, lungs, lymphatic system, and skin all work in tandem to remove toxins and waste products from the body, preventing them from causing damage and disease. Supporting these detoxification pathways through hydration, nutrition, and lifestyle choices can bolster the body's natural defenses and healing capabilities.

Environmental factors also play a significant role in the body's self-healing mechanism. Exposure to natural sunlight, for instance, can boost vitamin D production, essential for immune function and bone health. Meanwhile, clean air and a toxin-free environment reduce the body's toxic burden, allowing it to focus its energy on healing and maintenance rather than detoxification. The role of social connections and support in healing cannot be overlooked.

Positive relationships and a strong social support network have been shown to enhance immune function, reduce stress levels, and improve overall well-being, underscoring the significance of emotional and social health in the context of physical healing.

Finally, the practice of mindfulness and stress management techniques such as meditation, yoga, and deep breathing exercises can significantly impact the body's healing process. By reducing stress and promoting a state of calm, these practices can lower inflammation, enhance immune function, and support the body's natural regenerative processes.

THE POWER OF WHOLE, UNPROCESSED FOODS

Whole, unprocessed foods serve as the foundation for a nourishing diet, offering a plethora of health benefits that are pivotal for maintaining and enhancing the body's natural healing abilities. These foods, which include fruits, vegetables, whole grains, nuts, seeds, and legumes, are rich in essential nutrients such as vitamins, minerals, fiber, and antioxidants. By incorporating these foods into our daily diet, we support the body's various functions, including immune defense, detoxification, and tissue repair, thereby promoting overall health and well-being.

The consumption of whole, unprocessed foods plays a crucial role in preventing chronic diseases such as obesity, diabetes, heart disease, and certain types of cancer. The natural composition of these foods, with their high fiber content and low glycemic index, helps regulate blood sugar levels, reduce cholesterol, and maintain a healthy weight. The antioxidants found in colorful fruits and vegetables, such as beta-carotene, vitamin C, and flavonoids, combat oxidative stress and inflammation, which are underlying factors in many chronic conditions.

Digestive health is significantly enhanced by the intake of whole, unprocessed foods.

The fiber in these foods aids in digestion, promotes regular bowel movements, and serves as a prebiotic, feeding the beneficial bacteria in the gut microbiome. A healthy gut is essential for immune function, nutrient absorption, and even mental health, as it is closely linked to the brain through the gut-brain axis.

In addition to their physical health benefits, whole, unprocessed foods also have a positive impact on mental and emotional well-being. Nutrients such as omega-3 fatty acids, found in flaxseeds and walnuts, and magnesium, abundant in leafy greens and nuts, are known for their mood-stabilizing effects. Eating a diet rich in whole foods can improve cognitive function, reduce symptoms of depression and anxiety, and enhance overall mood.

Transitioning to a diet centered around whole, unprocessed foods also encourages a more mindful approach to eating. It invites individuals to connect with their food sources, appreciate the natural flavors and textures of foods, and make conscious choices that align with their health goals and ethical values.

This mindful eating practice can lead to a more satisfying and nourishing eating experience, fostering a healthy relationship with food. To incorporate more whole, unprocessed foods into the diet, start by making simple swaps such as choosing whole fruit instead of fruit juice, brown rice or quinoa instead of white rice, and snacking on raw nuts and seeds rather than processed snack foods. Experiment with a variety of fruits and vegetables, aiming to create a colorful plate that ensures a wide range of nutrients. Additionally, cooking from scratch allows for control over ingredients, enabling the avoidance of added sugars, salts, and unhealthy fats often found in processed foods.

THE ROLE OF NUTRIENTS IN HEALING

The role of nutrients in healing is a testament to the body's intricate design and its ability to utilize natural resources for restoration and balance. Nutrients, the compounds found in food, are the building blocks of health, playing pivotal roles in cellular function, energy production, and the maintenance of bodily systems. Each nutrient, from macronutrients like carbohydrates, proteins, and fats to micronutrients such as vitamins and minerals, contributes uniquely to the healing process, underscoring the importance of a varied and nutrient-dense diet.

Carbohydrates, often maligned in popular diet culture, serve as the primary energy source for the body, fueling all bodily activities including the healing process. Complex carbohydrates, found in whole grains, vegetables, and fruits, are particularly valuable, providing a steady release of energy alongside fiber, vitamins, and minerals that support gut health and toxin elimination. Proteins, composed of amino acids, are essential for the repair and regeneration of tissues. After an injury or during illness, the body's demand for protein increases to rebuild damaged cells and synthesize immune cells. Sources of high-quality protein include lean meats, fish, legumes, and dairy products, each offering a unique profile of essential amino acids.

Fats, especially those from unprocessed sources like avocados, nuts, seeds, and oily fish, play a crucial role in healing. Omega-3 fatty acids, a type of polyunsaturated fat, are renowned for their anti-inflammatory properties, aiding in the reduction of inflammation associated with many chronic conditions and facilitating the healing process. In addition to serving as a dense energy source, fats are vital for the absorption of fat-soluble vitamins—A, D, E, and K—which are crucial for immune function, cell regeneration, and bone health.

Vitamins and minerals, though required in smaller quantities than macronutrients, are indispensable to healing. Vitamin C, for example, is a potent antioxidant that also stimulates the production of collagen, a protein that is foundational to wound healing and tissue repair. The mineral zinc plays a critical role in immune function, protein synthesis, and cell division, all of which are essential during the healing process. Iron is another key mineral, essential for the transport of oxygen in the blood, supporting energy levels and aiding in the recovery from injuries or surgeries.

The synergistic effect of nutrients illustrates the complexity of the healing process and the necessity of a holistic approach to nutrition. For instance, vitamin C enhances iron absorption when consumed together, demonstrating the importance of combining nutrients to maximize their healing potential. Similarly, the anti-inflammatory effects of omega-3 fatty acids are complemented by the antioxidant properties of vitamins C and E, offering a multifaceted approach to reducing inflammation and promoting recovery.

Understanding the role of each nutrient in the healing process empowers individuals to make informed dietary choices that support their health and well-being. Incorporating a wide variety of whole foods into the diet ensures a comprehensive intake of these essential nutrients, laying the foundation for effective healing and long-term health. As we continue to explore the nuances of nutrition and its impact on the body, it becomes clear that food truly is medicine, offering natural and powerful means to support the body's healing capabilities.

Water-soluble vitamins like B-complex and vitamin C are also crucial in the healing journey, emphasizing the body's need for a continuous supply of these nutrients due to their limited storage capacity. B vitamins are particularly important for energy metabolism, playing a vital role in converting our food into energy, a process essential for repair and recovery. They also assist in the creation of new blood cells, which are crucial for delivering oxygen and nutrients to healing tissues. Vitamin C, beyond its role in collagen formation and immune support, acts as a powerful antioxidant, protecting cells from damage by free radicals, which are often elevated during times of physical stress or injury.

Minerals such as magnesium and selenium further contribute to the healing process. Magnesium, involved in over 300 biochemical reactions in the body, supports muscle and nerve function, maintains heart rhythm, and aids in bone health. It also plays a part in the body's stress-response system, helping to manage the physiological effects of stress.

Selenium functions as a component of antioxidant enzymes, guarding the body against oxidative stress and inflammation, which can impede the healing process. Its role in immune function is also critical, as it helps to prevent infection and promote recovery. The importance of hydration in healing cannot be overstressed. Water is essential for all forms of life and plays a key role in every healing phase. It aids in the transportation of nutrients and oxygen to cells, supports efficient cellular function, facilitates the removal of waste products, and helps maintain a stable environment for tissue repair. Adequate fluid intake is especially crucial during recovery, as the body's demand for water increases to support heightened metabolic activity and to replace fluids lost due to fever or inflammation.

Dietary fiber, while not a nutrient per se, is an essential component of a healing diet. Found in whole grains, fruits, vegetables, and legumes, fiber supports digestive health, ensuring the efficient elimination of toxins and waste products from the body.

It also plays a role in regulating blood sugar levels and supporting cardiovascular health by reducing cholesterol levels. The prebiotic nature of certain fibers fosters a healthy gut microbiome, which is essential for immune function and overall health.

Incorporating phytonutrients, bioactive compounds found in plants, adds another layer to the healing diet. These compounds, such as flavonoids, carotenoids, and polyphenols, offer a range of health benefits, including anti-inflammatory, antioxidant, and anti-carcinogenic properties. They work in synergy with vitamins, minerals, and other nutrients to enhance the body's resistance to disease and support recovery. Foods rich in phytonutrients, such as berries, green leafy vegetables, nuts, and seeds, not only add color and flavor to the diet but also provide powerful healing benefits.

The integration of these nutrients into a balanced and varied diet supports the body's natural healing mechanisms. It's not about focusing on single nutrients but rather the dietary pattern as a whole that emphasizes the consumption of a wide array of nutrient-dense foods. This approach ensures that the body receives the full spectrum of compounds it needs for recovery and health maintenance. Listening to the body's cues and responding with nutritional support is key to facilitating healing. Whether recovering from an illness, injury, or surgery, the body requires an increased supply of certain nutrients to repair itself. Tailoring one's diet to meet these increased needs, while also considering individual health conditions, preferences, and dietary restrictions, can significantly impact the healing process.

IMPORTANCE OF HYDRATION

Hydration plays a pivotal role in maintaining optimal health and facilitating the body's natural healing processes.

Water, the most essential nutrient, is fundamental for every cellular function in our bodies, from aiding digestion and absorption of nutrients to oxygen delivery and toxin removal. Proper hydration supports the mind and spirit by enhancing cognitive function, mood, and overall well-being. It lubricates joints, maintains skin health, and regulates body temperature, showcasing its critical role in our physiological processes.

The human body is composed of about 60% water, which underscores the importance of staying adequately hydrated. Dehydration, even in its mildest form, can lead to fatigue, headaches, decreased concentration, and impaired physical performance.

In the context of nutrition as medicine, water acts as a catalyst for the metabolic processes that convert food into energy, making it indispensable for optimizing health.

To ensure adequate hydration, it is recommended to consume at least 8-10 cups of water daily, though individual needs may vary based on factors such as age, weight, activity level, and environmental conditions. Incorporating foods with high water content, such as fruits and vegetables, can also contribute to overall fluid intake.

Herbal teas and infused waters offer therapeutic benefits and variety, making hydration more enjoyable while providing the body with antioxidants and other health-promoting compounds.

Understanding the signs of dehydration is crucial for preventing it. These signs can include thirst, dry mouth, dark-colored urine, and dizziness. By recognizing these early indicators, one can take immediate steps to increase fluid intake and avoid the adverse effects of dehydration on health.

In addition to drinking water, avoiding excessive caffeine and alcohol consumption is vital, as these can lead to increased fluid loss. Emphasizing the role of hydration in holistic health, it becomes clear that water is not just a mere component of our diet but a foundational element of a balanced lifestyle that supports healing, vitality, and longevity.

CHAPTER 4: 5 INTRODUCTORY HERBAL RECIPES

ELDERBERRY SYRUP

Beneficial effects

Elderberry syrup is renowned for its immune-boosting properties. It's packed with antioxidants and vitamins that can help fight off colds and flu. Studies suggest that elderberry can reduce the severity and duration of these illnesses, making it a go-to natural remedy during cold and flu season.

Portions

Makes approximately 16 ounces (about 475 milliliters) of syrup.

Preparation time

15 minutes

Cooking time

45 minutes to 1 hour

Ingredients

- 3/4 cup dried elderberries (about 4 ounces or 113 grams)
- 3 cups of water (about 710 milliliters)
- 1 teaspoon dried ginger (about 2 grams)
- 1/2 teaspoon cinnamon powder (about 1 gram)
- 1/4 teaspoon ground cloves (about 0.5 grams)
- 1 cup raw honey (about 340 grams or 8 ounces)

Instructions

1. Combine the dried elderberries, water, dried ginger, cinnamon powder, and ground cloves in a medium saucepan.

2. Bring the mixture to a boil, then reduce the heat and simmer, covered, for about 45 minutes to 1 hour, or until the liquid has reduced by almost half.

3. Remove from heat and let the mixture cool to room temperature.

4. Once cooled, mash the berries carefully using a spoon or a masher.

5. Pour the mixture through a fine mesh strainer or cheesecloth into a large bowl, pressing on the berries to extract all the liquid.

6. Discard the elderberries and let the liquid cool to lukewarm.

7. When the liquid is no longer hot, add the raw honey and stir well until fully incorporated.

8. Pour the syrup into a clean, airtight glass bottle or jar.

Variations

- For an extra immune boost, add 1 tablespoon of fresh grated ginger or turmeric to the recipe.

- If you prefer a vegan version, substitute the honey with maple syrup or agave nectar, though keep in mind this will alter the flavor slightly.

Storage tips

Store the elderberry syrup in the refrigerator. It will keep for up to two months. For longer storage, consider freezing the syrup in an ice cube tray and then transferring the cubes to a freezer bag for easy portioning.

Tips for allergens

If you're allergic to honey, using maple syrup or agave nectar as a substitute can be a safe alternative. Always ensure that you source your elderberries from a reputable supplier to avoid contamination with toxic varieties.

Scientific references

- "Randomized study of the efficacy and safety of oral elderberry extract in the treatment of influenza A and B virus infections" - Journal of International Medical Research.

- "Inhibitory effect of elderberry fruit extract on the inflammatory response in influenza virus-infected bronchial epithelial cells" - Phytochemistry Letters.

FIRE CIDER

Beneficial effects

Fire Cider is renowned for its ability to boost the immune system, aid in digestion, and warm the body on cold days. Its ingredients, rich in vitamins, antioxidants, and anti-inflammatory properties, work synergistically to support overall health and well-being.

Portions

Makes about 32 ounces

Preparation time

15 minutes

Cooking time

3 to 4 weeks for infusion

Ingredients

- 1/2 cup freshly grated organic ginger root
- 1/2 cup freshly grated organic horseradish root
- 1 medium organic onion, chopped
- 10 cloves of organic garlic, crushed or chopped
- 2 organic jalapeno peppers, chopped
- Zest and juice from 1 organic lemon
- 2 tablespoons dried rosemary leaves
- 1 tablespoon turmeric powder or 2 tablespoons freshly grated turmeric root
- 1/4 teaspoon cayenne powder
- Approximately 32 ounces raw apple cider vinegar
- 1/4 cup raw, local honey, or to taste

Instructions

1. In a clean, quart-sized glass jar, combine the ginger, horseradish, onion, garlic, jalapeno peppers, lemon zest and juice, rosemary, turmeric, and cayenne powder.

2. Pour the apple cider vinegar over the ingredients until they are completely submerged. Leave about an inch of space at the top of the jar.

3. Place a piece of parchment paper under the lid to prevent corrosion from the vinegar, then seal the jar tightly.

4. Store the jar in a cool, dark place for 3 to 4 weeks, shaking it daily to mix the ingredients.

5. After the infusion period, strain the mixture through a fine mesh sieve or cheesecloth into a clean jar. Squeeze or press the solids to extract as much liquid as possible.

6. Stir in the honey until well combined. Taste and adjust the sweetness if necessary.

7. Transfer the finished Fire Cider into smaller bottles, if desired, or keep it in the quart jar.

Variations

- Add fresh thyme, oregano, or other herbs for additional flavor and health benefits.

- Include a few tablespoons of fresh grated beetroot for color and sweetness.

- For a citrus twist, add the zest and juice of an orange.

Storage tips

Store Fire Cider in the refrigerator. It will keep for several months, and the flavor will continue to mature over time.

Tips for allergens

For those sensitive to spicy foods, reduce or omit the jalapeno peppers and cayenne powder. If honey allergies are a concern, substitute it with maple syrup or omit it entirely for a more potent tonic.

Scientific references

- "Antimicrobial properties of allicin from garlic," Microbes and Infection, 1999.

- "Ginger in gastrointestinal disorders: A systematic review of clinical trials," Food Science & Nutrition, 2019.

- "Curcumin: A Review of Its' Effects on Human Health," Foods, 2017.

- "Vinegar: Medicinal Uses and Antiglycemic Effect," MedGenMed, 2006.

ST. JOHN'S WORT OIL

Beneficial effects

St. John's Wort Oil is renowned for its anti-inflammatory and antibacterial properties, making it an excellent remedy for soothing skin irritations, wounds, and minor burns. It also has been used to alleviate symptoms of depression and anxiety when applied topically, as it's believed to help with nerve pain and inflammation.

Ingredients

- 1 cup of fresh St. John's Wort flowers

- 2 cups of olive oil or almond oil

Instructions

1. Harvest St. John's Wort flowers around midday when the oils are most potent.

2. Gently rinse the flowers to remove any dirt or insects, and let them dry completely to avoid mold growth in the oil.

3. Once dry, lightly crush the flowers with your hands to release the active compounds.

4. Place the crushed flowers in a clean, dry glass jar.

5. Pour the olive or almond oil over the flowers until they are completely submerged.

6. Seal the jar tightly and place it in a sunny spot for 4 to 6 weeks, shaking it gently every few days to mix the contents.

7. After the infusion period, strain the oil through a fine mesh sieve or cheesecloth into another clean, dry jar, pressing the flowers to extract as much oil as possible.

8. Discard the flowers and transfer the St. John's Wort Oil into a dark glass bottle for storage.

Variations

For an enhanced soothing blend, you can add a few drops of lavender or chamomile essential oil to the finished St. John's Wort Oil.

Storage tips

Store the oil in a cool, dark place. If stored properly, the oil can last for up to a year.

Tips for allergens

If you're allergic to olive or almond oil, consider using jojoba or coconut oil as a base for the infusion. Always perform a patch test on a small area of your skin before applying broadly, especially if you have sensitive skin.

Scientific references

Studies have shown that St. John's Wort possesses anti-inflammatory properties, which can aid in healing wounds and burns. Its antibacterial effects also make it beneficial for skin health. (Journal of Ethnopharmacology, 2016).

PEPPERMINT TINCTURE

Beneficial effects

Peppermint tincture is renowned for its ability to soothe digestive issues, relieve headaches, and reduce symptoms of anxiety. The menthol in peppermint acts as a natural muscle relaxant and pain reliever, making this tincture a versatile addition to your natural health toolkit.

Ingredients

- 1 cup fresh peppermint leaves, thoroughly washed
- 2 cups high-proof alcohol (vodka or brandy works well)
- A clean glass jar with a tight-fitting lid

Instructions

1. Finely chop or crush the fresh peppermint leaves to release their oils.

2. Place the chopped peppermint leaves into the clean glass jar.

3. Pour the high-proof alcohol over the peppermint leaves until they are completely submerged. Leave about an inch of space at the top of the jar.

4. Seal the jar tightly and label it with the date and contents.

5. Store the jar in a cool, dark place for 4 to 6 weeks. Shake the jar gently every few days to mix the contents.

6. After the infusion period, strain the tincture through a fine mesh sieve or cheesecloth into another clean glass jar or bottle. Press or squeeze the leaves to extract as much liquid as possible.

7. Label the container with the date and contents.

Variations

For a non-alcoholic version, vegetable glycerin can be used as a substitute for the alcohol, although the extraction process and preservation qualities may vary.

Storage tips

Store the finished tincture in a cool, dark place. When stored properly, it can last for several years.

Tips for allergens

Individuals with allergies to menthol or other compounds in peppermint should use caution and consult with a healthcare provider before using.

Scientific references

Studies have shown that peppermint oil, which shares many properties with peppermint tincture, can effectively relieve symptoms of irritable bowel syndrome (IBS) and reduce abdominal pain. (Gastroenterology, 2007 & Journal of Clinical Gastroenterology, 2014).

CHAMOMILE TEA

Beneficial effects

Chamomile tea is renowned for its calming properties, which can help reduce stress and promote a peaceful sleep. It's also used to aid digestion, alleviate menstrual pain, and reduce inflammation. The antioxidants present in chamomile can support skin health, boost immune function, and may play a role in preventing certain types of cancer.

Portions

1 serving

Preparation time

5 minutes

Cooking time

5-10 minutes

Ingredients

- 1-2 teaspoons of dried chamomile flowers or 1 chamomile tea bag

- 8 ounces of boiling water

- Honey or lemon (optional, for taste)

Instructions

1. Boil 8 ounces of water in a kettle or a pot.

2. Place the dried chamomile flowers or tea bag in a mug.

3. Pour the boiling water over the chamomile flowers or tea bag.

4. Cover the mug with a lid or a small plate and let it steep for 5-10 minutes. The longer it steeps, the stronger the tea.

5. Remove the chamomile flowers or tea bag from the mug. If using flowers, you can strain them out.

6. Optional: Add honey or lemon to taste.

7. Enjoy the tea while it's warm for the best experience.

Variations

- For a cooler, refreshing drink, let the chamomile tea cool to room temperature, then refrigerate to serve cold.

- Add a mint leaf or ginger for an additional flavor profile and digestive benefits.

- Mix chamomile tea with green tea for an antioxidant boost.

Storage tips

Dried chamomile flowers should be stored in an airtight container in a cool, dark place to preserve their quality and health benefits.

Tips for allergens

Individuals with allergies to plants in the daisy family should avoid chamomile as it may cause allergic reactions. Always consult with a healthcare provider if unsure.

Scientific references

- Srivastava, J. K., Shankar, E., & Gupta, S. (2010). Chamomile: A herbal medicine of the past with a bright future (Review). Molecular Medicine Reports, 3(6), 895–901. This study highlights the anti-inflammatory and anticancer properties of chamomile.

- Amsterdam, J. D., Li, Y., Soeller, I., Rockwell, K., Mao, J. J., & Shults, J. (2009). A randomized, double-blind, placebo-controlled trial of oral Matricaria recutita (chamomile) extract therapy for generalized anxiety disorder. Journal of Clinical Psychopharmacology, 29(4), 378–382. This trial demonstrates the effectiveness of chamomile in treating generalized anxiety disorder.

PART 2: PLANT-BASED NUTRITION

Embracing a plant-based diet is a cornerstone of holistic health, focusing on the consumption of whole, unprocessed foods derived from plants. This includes a wide variety of fruits, vegetables, grains, nuts, and seeds, all of which are rich in essential nutrients that our bodies need to thrive. A plant-based diet not only supports physical well-being but also aligns with sustainable environmental practices by reducing the carbon footprint associated with animal farming and processing.

The benefits of a plant-based diet are extensive, ranging from improved heart health due to lower cholesterol levels to a reduced risk of certain chronic diseases such as type 2 diabetes and certain cancers.

This dietary approach is rich in fiber, which aids in digestion and promotes a healthy gut microbiome, crucial for overall health and effective immune function. Additionally, plant-based foods are high in antioxidants and phytonutrients, compounds that protect the body against oxidative stress and inflammation, key factors in disease prevention and longevity.

Transitioning to a plant-based diet can be a rewarding journey, starting with small, manageable changes. Incorporating more fruits and vegetables into meals, experimenting with meat substitutes, and exploring the vast world of legumes and whole grains can make this transition enjoyable and sustainable. It's important to plan meals to ensure a balanced intake of all essential nutrients, including protein, iron, calcium, and vitamins B12 and D, which are commonly misconceived as difficult to obtain from a plant-based diet. However, with careful planning and a variety of food choices, these nutrients can be adequately sourced from plants and fortified foods.

Understanding the nutritional content of plant-based foods and learning how to combine them to create complete proteins is essential for maintaining muscle health and overall energy levels. Quinoa, buckwheat, soy products, and combining beans with rice or nuts with whole grains are examples of how to achieve a balanced amino acid profile, crucial for bodily functions and repair.

Hydration remains a key aspect of holistic health, with water-rich fruits and vegetables like cucumbers, tomatoes, oranges, and melons contributing to daily fluid intake, enhancing the body's natural detoxification processes through improved kidney function and skin health.

The role of herbs and spices in a plant-based diet extends beyond flavor enhancement; many possess medicinal properties that can support health in various ways, from boosting immunity to reducing inflammation. Incorporating herbs like turmeric, ginger, and cinnamon into meals not only adds depth and complexity to plant-based dishes but also leverages their health-promoting benefits.

As we delve deeper into the principles of plant-based nutrition, we will explore the practical aspects of meal planning, grocery shopping, and cooking techniques that maximize nutrient retention and bioavailability. This approach not only nurtures the body but also supports a lifestyle that is in harmony with the planet, promoting a sustainable and ethical way of living that benefits both individual health and the environment.

Meal planning is a crucial step in adopting a plant-based diet effectively. It involves selecting a variety of foods across all food groups to ensure a comprehensive intake of nutrients. Start by creating a weekly menu that includes a diverse range of fruits, vegetables, whole grains, legumes, nuts, and seeds. This not only helps in maintaining a balanced diet but also in reducing food waste by buying only what you need. For those new to plant-based eating, there are numerous resources available, including cookbooks and online platforms, offering recipes that cater to different tastes and preferences.

Grocery shopping for a plant-based diet emphasizes the importance of reading labels carefully to avoid products with hidden animal-based ingredients and excessive additives. Opting for organic and non-GMO products can further enhance the health benefits of a plant-based diet.

Farmers' markets and local health food stores often provide a wide selection of fresh, seasonal produce that supports local agriculture and reduces the environmental impact associated with long-distance food transportation.

Cooking techniques play a significant role in preserving the nutritional value of plant-based foods. Methods such as steaming, blanching, and sautéing in a small amount of healthy fat can help retain vitamins and minerals that might be lost during high-heat cooking processes.

Experimenting with raw food recipes is another way to enjoy the full nutritional benefits of fruits and vegetables. Smoothies, salads, and raw soups can be nutrient-packed options that are both easy to prepare and delicious.

Understanding the concept of bioavailability is also important in a plant-based diet. Certain nutrients, such as iron and zinc, are better absorbed by the body when paired with vitamin C-rich foods.

For instance, adding strawberries to a spinach salad or squeezing lemon juice over a lentil dish can enhance nutrient absorption. Similarly, soaking nuts, seeds, and legumes overnight can improve digestibility and nutrient availability by reducing phytic acid, a natural substance that can bind minerals and reduce their absorption.

Finally, embracing a plant-based diet is not just about food choices; it's a lifestyle that encourages mindfulness and sustainability. It's about making conscious decisions that benefit not only personal health but also the well-being of our planet. Reducing plastic use by opting for reusable bags and containers, minimizing food waste by composting, and supporting ethical and sustainable farming practices are all integral aspects of a holistic plant-based lifestyle.

By adopting these principles, individuals can enjoy a rich and varied diet that supports both their health and the environment. Whether you're a seasoned plant-based eater or just beginning your journey, the key is to approach this lifestyle with curiosity and openness, allowing yourself to explore new foods, flavors, and cooking methods. With each plant-based meal, you're contributing to a healthier body and a more sustainable world.

CHAPTER 1: THE FUNDAMENTALS OF PLANT-BASED EATING

A plant-based diet is centered around foods primarily from plants. This includes not only fruits and vegetables, but also nuts, seeds, oils, whole grains, legumes, and beans. It doesn't mean that you are vegetarian or vegan and never eat meat or dairy. Rather, you are proportionately choosing more of your foods from plant sources. What is fundamental to this diet is an emphasis on eating whole, unprocessed foods that are rich in nutrients. These foods are packed with vitamins, minerals, fiber, antioxidants, and phytochemicals, which work together to support overall health and well-being.

One of the key benefits of a plant-based diet is its impact on heart health. Studies have shown that eating a diet high in fruits, vegetables, whole grains, and nuts can reduce the risk of heart disease. This is partly due to the lower levels of saturated fats found in plant-based foods compared to animal products, which can contribute to higher cholesterol levels and increased risk of heart disease. Additionally, the high fiber content found in plant-based diets helps to lower cholesterol levels and improve blood sugar control, further protecting the heart.

Another significant advantage of adopting a plant-based diet is its potential for weight management. Plant-based foods are typically lower in calories and fat than animal products, while their high fiber content can help you feel full and satisfied, reducing the overall calorie intake. This can be particularly beneficial for those looking to lose weight or maintain a healthy weight.

The environmental benefits of a plant-based diet cannot be overlooked. Animal farming is a major contributor to greenhouse gas emissions, deforestation, and water use. By choosing more plant-based foods, you can help reduce the demand for animal products, thereby lessening your environmental footprint. This shift not only benefits your health but also contributes to a more sustainable and ethical food system.

Transitioning to a plant-based diet can be a gradual process. Start by incorporating more fruits and vegetables into your meals, replacing meat with plant-based protein sources like beans, lentils, and tofu, and choosing whole grains over refined grains. It's also important to vary your diet to ensure you're getting a wide range of nutrients. For example, dark leafy greens are rich in calcium, iron, and vitamin K, while berries are loaded with antioxidants and vitamin C.

As you embark on this journey, remember that balance and variety are key. A plant-based diet offers a plethora of flavors, textures, and nutrients that can not only support your physical health but also bring joy and satisfaction to your meals. Whether you're making a smoothie packed with fruits and vegetables for breakfast, enjoying a hearty lentil soup for lunch, or savoring a quinoa and vegetable stir-fry for dinner, the possibilities are endless.

Embracing a plant-based diet also means paying attention to protein sources. It's a common misconception that plant-based diets lack sufficient protein. However, many plant foods are rich in protein and can meet daily requirements when consumed in adequate quantities. Legumes, such as beans, lentils, and chickpeas, are excellent sources of protein and fiber. Nuts and seeds, including almonds, chia seeds, and hemp seeds, not only provide protein but also healthy fats and various vitamins and minerals. Quinoa and soy products like tofu and tempeh are also high in protein and versatile enough to be used in a multitude of dishes. By including a variety of these plant-based protein sources in your diet, you can ensure that your protein needs are met without relying on animal products.

Moreover, a plant-based diet can play a crucial role in reducing inflammation in the body. Chronic inflammation is linked to a host of health issues, including arthritis, heart disease, and certain cancers. Foods rich in antioxidants and phytonutrients, found abundantly in fruits, vegetables, nuts, and seeds, can help combat inflammation. Turmeric, ginger, and berries are just a few examples of foods known for their anti-inflammatory properties. Incorporating these foods into your diet can aid in reducing inflammation and promoting overall health.

Another aspect of a plant-based diet is the importance of healthy fats. While it's beneficial to reduce intake of saturated fats commonly found in animal products, your body still needs healthy fats for energy and to support cell growth and nutrient absorption. Avocados, olive oil, nuts, and seeds are great sources of monounsaturated and polyunsaturated fats, including omega-3 fatty acids, which are beneficial for heart health and brain function.

When it comes to carbohydrates, choosing complex carbs over simple carbs is key to maximizing the health benefits of a plant-based diet. Whole grains, legumes, and starchy vegetables provide slow-releasing energy, keeping you fuller for longer and helping to stabilize blood sugar levels. These foods are also packed with fiber, which is essential for digestive health and can help prevent constipation.

The diversity of plant-based foods offers an array of vitamins and minerals essential for health. For instance, vitamin C, found in citrus fruits and bell peppers, supports the immune system, while iron, abundant in leafy greens and legumes, is crucial for blood health.

Calcium, necessary for bone health, can be found in fortified plant milks and tofu. To ensure adequate intake of vitamin B12, which is naturally found in animal products, those following a plant-based diet should consider fortified foods or supplements.

Lastly, adopting a plant-based diet doesn't have to mean sacrificing flavor or satisfaction. There are countless ways to prepare and season plant-based dishes to make them delicious and fulfilling. Experimenting with different herbs, spices, and cooking techniques can elevate simple ingredients into flavorful and nutritious meals. From roasting vegetables to bring out their natural sweetness to blending soaked cashews for a creamy sauce, the options are endless.

By focusing on whole, unprocessed foods and incorporating a variety of fruits, vegetables, whole grains, legumes, nuts, and seeds, you can enjoy a nutritious and satisfying diet that supports long-term health and well-being. Remember, transitioning to a plant-based diet is a personal journey that should be tailored to your individual needs and preferences. With a little creativity and openness to trying new foods, embracing a plant-based lifestyle can be an enjoyable and rewarding experience.

DR. BARBARA'S NUTRITIONAL GUIDELINES

Dr. Barbara's nutritional guidelines are designed to empower individuals with the knowledge and tools needed to nourish their bodies optimally, promoting health and vitality through a plant-based diet. At the heart of these guidelines is the principle of consuming a variety of whole, unprocessed foods that provide a symphony of nutrients necessary for maintaining balance and wellness in the body. Emphasizing fruits, vegetables, whole grains, legumes, nuts, and seeds, these guidelines encourage a diet rich in fiber, vitamins, minerals, and phytonutrients, all of which play crucial roles in supporting the body's natural healing processes and preventing chronic diseases.

Key to Dr. Barbara's approach is the understanding that every individual's body is unique, with specific nutritional needs and preferences. Thus, while the foundation of the diet is plant-based, flexibility and personalization are encouraged to meet the diverse requirements of each person. This includes paying attention to one's own body signals and adjusting food choices accordingly to enhance energy levels, improve digestion, and support overall well-being.

Incorporating a wide array of colorful fruits and vegetables is paramount, as these foods are not only nutrient-dense but also contain antioxidants that combat oxidative stress and inflammation, underlying factors in many health conditions. Dr. Barbara advises making these plant-based foods the centerpiece of every meal, ensuring that a variety of colors and types are consumed throughout the day to maximize the range of beneficial compounds ingested.

Whole grains and legumes form another cornerstone of the diet, providing essential carbohydrates for energy, fiber for digestive health, and a host of vitamins and minerals. These foods, when consumed in their whole form, offer sustained energy release, helping to maintain stable blood sugar levels and a feeling of fullness, which can aid in weight management.

Nuts and seeds are highlighted for their healthy fats, including omega-3 fatty acids, which are vital for brain health, reducing inflammation, and supporting heart health. Dr. Barbara recommends incorporating a small portion of these nutrient powerhouses daily, either as snacks, added to salads, or blended into smoothies, to benefit from their wide range of nutrients.

Protein, often a concern when adopting a plant-based diet, is addressed through the inclusion of a variety of plant-based sources. Legumes, nuts, seeds, whole grains, and soy products like tofu and tempeh are excellent sources of protein that can easily meet and exceed daily requirements when consumed in adequate amounts. Dr. Barbara emphasizes the importance of combining different plant proteins to ensure a complete amino acid profile, supporting muscle repair, growth, and overall bodily functions.

Hydration is another critical aspect of the nutritional guidelines, with a focus on drinking plenty of water throughout the day to support cellular functions, digestion, and detoxification processes. Herbal teas and infused waters are also recommended for their additional health benefits and for adding variety to fluid intake.

Finally, Dr. Barbara encourages mindful eating practices, suggesting that individuals take the time to savor their food, eat without distractions, and listen to their hunger and fullness cues. This approach not only enhances the enjoyment of meals but also fosters a healthier relationship with food, promoting eating habits that are in tune with the body's needs.

By following these nutritional guidelines, individuals can embark on a journey towards improved health and vitality, embracing a plant-based diet that supports not only their own well-being but also the health of the planet.

MICRONUTRIENTS AND THEIR SOURCES

Micronutrients, essential vitamins and minerals required in small quantities, play pivotal roles in maintaining health and preventing disease. Unlike macronutrients, which provide the body with energy, micronutrients support various functions, including bone health, immune response, and blood clotting. A plant-based diet, rich in fruits, vegetables, nuts, seeds, and whole grains, provides a diverse array of these vital nutrients.

Vitamin C, a powerful antioxidant, aids in the repair of tissues, the absorption of iron, and the maintenance of immune health. Citrus fruits like oranges and lemons, strawberries, bell peppers, and dark leafy greens are excellent sources. Vitamin E, another antioxidant, supports immune function and skin health, found abundantly in almonds, sunflower seeds, and spinach.

B vitamins, including B12, folate, thiamine, and riboflavin, are crucial for energy production, nerve function, and the synthesis of DNA and red blood cells. While B12 is predominantly found in animal products, fortified plant milks, breakfast cereals, and nutritional yeast can provide this essential nutrient in a plant-based diet. Legumes, seeds, and green vegetables are rich in other B vitamins.

Vitamin D, vital for bone health and immune function, can be challenging to obtain from a plant-based diet alone. Fortified foods and sun exposure are primary sources, with mushrooms being one of the few plant-based foods providing vitamin D.

Minerals such as calcium, important for bone health and muscle function, can be found in fortified plant milks, tofu, and leafy greens. Iron, crucial for oxygen transport and energy production, is abundant in lentils, chickpeas, and spinach. Plant-based iron is non-heme, so consuming it with vitamin C-rich foods can enhance absorption.

Zinc supports immune function and wound healing, with nuts, seeds, and legumes as prime sources. Magnesium, involved in over 300 enzymatic reactions, is found in whole grains, nuts, and green leafy vegetables. Potassium, which aids in muscle contractions and heart function, is abundant in bananas, potatoes, and avocados.

Selenium, an antioxidant that plays roles in thyroid function and immune health, can be obtained from Brazil nuts, whole grains, and seeds. Iodine, essential for thyroid health, is found in seaweeds like nori, as well as in iodized salt and fortified foods.

For those adopting a plant-based diet, understanding the sources of these micronutrients ensures nutritional needs are met, supporting overall health and well-being. It's also beneficial to consider supplementation for nutrients like B12 and vitamin D, particularly in regions with limited sunlight. Regular blood tests can help identify any deficiencies, allowing dietary adjustments or supplementation as needed. By focusing on a varied and colorful diet, individuals can enjoy the full spectrum of micronutrients essential for optimal health.

BENEFITS OF A PLANT-BASED DIET

Adopting a plant-based diet brings a multitude of benefits that extend beyond personal health to include environmental sustainability and animal welfare. One of the most significant advantages is the reduction in risk for chronic diseases such as heart disease, hypertension, type 2 diabetes, and certain cancers. Plant-based diets are rich in fiber, vitamins, minerals, and antioxidants, which play a crucial role in maintaining health and preventing disease. The high fiber content found in fruits, vegetables, legumes, and whole grains aids in digestion, improves gut health, and contributes to a feeling of fullness, which can help in weight management and obesity prevention.

Another benefit is the positive impact on heart health. Diets high in fruits, vegetables, nuts, and seeds, and low in saturated fats and cholesterol, have been shown to reduce blood pressure, lower cholesterol levels, and improve overall heart function. This is particularly important considering heart disease remains one of the leading causes of death worldwide. Additionally, the antioxidants and phytonutrients found in plant-based foods can reduce inflammation, a key factor in chronic disease development.

From an environmental perspective, shifting towards a plant-based diet can significantly reduce one's carbon footprint. The production of plant-based foods generally requires less water, land, and energy compared to animal agriculture, and results in lower greenhouse gas emissions. By choosing plant-based options, individuals can contribute to a reduction in the demand for animal products, leading to less strain on natural resources and a decrease in biodiversity loss.

Moreover, a plant-based diet supports animal welfare by reducing the demand for animal farming, which often involves inhumane practices. By opting for plant-based foods, individuals can take a stand against animal cruelty and promote a more ethical treatment of animals.

Mental health benefits are also associated with a plant-based diet. Studies have suggested that the nutrients found in fruits, vegetables, and nuts can improve brain function and may lower the risk of developing mental health disorders such as depression and anxiety. The connection between diet and mental health highlights the importance of nutrition in maintaining not only physical but also mental well-being.

Furthermore, adopting a plant-based diet can lead to increased energy levels and better physical fitness. The nutrient-dense nature of plant-based foods provides the body with a steady supply of energy, improving stamina and reducing fatigue. Athletes and fitness enthusiasts may find that a plant-based diet supports quicker recovery times and enhances performance.

In terms of longevity, research has indicated that individuals who follow a plant-based diet tend to have a lower risk of mortality from all causes. This can be attributed to the diet's emphasis on whole, nutrient-rich foods that support the body's natural healing processes and promote longevity.

Lastly, transitioning to a plant-based diet can be an empowering experience, offering individuals the opportunity to explore a wide variety of foods and cuisines. It encourages creativity in the kitchen and can lead to a more mindful and appreciative approach to eating. By making conscious food choices, individuals can enjoy the health benefits of a plant-based diet while also contributing to a more sustainable and compassionate world.

BALANCING YOUR PLATE WITH WHOLE FOODS

Balancing your plate with whole foods is about creating meals that are not only delicious and satisfying but also rich in the nutrients your body needs to thrive. A balanced plate is visually divided into sections for vegetables, fruits, whole grains, and plant-based proteins, ensuring that you get a variety of nutrients from natural sources. This method simplifies meal planning and encourages eating a wide range of whole foods, which naturally leads to a diet high in fiber, vitamins, minerals, and phytonutrients.

Start by filling half of your plate with vegetables and fruits, emphasizing a variety of colors to maximize the intake of different antioxidants and phytonutrients.

Vegetables can be raw, steamed, roasted, or sautéed, while fruits can be fresh, frozen, or dried without added sugars. This not only makes your meals more appealing but also ensures you're getting a broad spectrum of health-promoting compounds.

A quarter of your plate should be dedicated to whole grains such as quinoa, brown rice, whole wheat, barley, or oats. These grains provide essential carbohydrates for energy, fiber for digestive health, and a host of B vitamins and minerals. Opting for whole grains over refined grains enhances satiety and supports stable blood sugar levels.

The remaining quarter of your plate should consist of plant-based protein sources. Legumes like beans, lentils, and chickpeas; tofu and tempeh; and a variety of nuts and seeds are excellent choices. These foods not only contribute protein but also fiber, healthy fats, and important minerals like iron and zinc. Incorporating a diverse range of plant proteins ensures you receive all essential amino acids necessary for muscle repair and growth.

Healthy fats are an integral part of a balanced plate, though they don't need a dedicated section. Including small amounts of avocados, nuts, seeds, and olive oil in your meals adds flavor, aids in the absorption of fat-soluble vitamins, and provides essential fatty acids that support brain health and reduce inflammation.

Hydration plays a crucial role in overall health, complementing a balanced plate. Water, herbal teas, and infused waters should be consumed throughout the day to support digestion, nutrient absorption, and detoxification processes. Limiting sugary drinks and high-caffeine beverages helps maintain optimal hydration levels and contributes to a balanced diet.

Mindful eating practices enhance the benefits of a balanced plate. Taking the time to chew thoroughly, savoring the flavors, and paying attention to hunger and fullness cues can improve digestion and prevent overeating.

This approach to eating encourages a deeper connection with food and its impact on health.

By focusing on whole foods and balancing your plate according to these guidelines, you can enjoy meals that are nourishing, satisfying, and supportive of your health goals. This simple yet effective method makes healthy eating accessible and enjoyable, promoting a lifestyle that is beneficial for both the individual and the environment.

CHAPTER 2: SUPERFOODS AND THEIR BENEFITS

Superfoods, though not a scientific term, have captured the attention of health enthusiasts and researchers alike for their nutrient density and potential health benefits. These foods are packed with vitamins, minerals, antioxidants, and other compounds beneficial to health, offering a powerful means to enhance diet quality and protect against chronic diseases. The benefits of incorporating superfoods into a plant-based diet are vast, ranging from improved heart health and enhanced immune function to reduced inflammation and better digestive health.

Leafy greens like kale, spinach, and Swiss chard are prime examples of superfoods, rich in vitamins A, C, K, and minerals like iron and calcium. These nutrients support bone health, protect against oxidative stress, and promote healthy skin and eyes. The high fiber content also aids in digestion and helps maintain a healthy gut microbiome.

Berries, including blueberries, strawberries, and raspberries, are another group of superfoods celebrated for their high antioxidant content, particularly vitamin C and flavonoids. These compounds combat oxidative stress and inflammation, reducing the risk of developing chronic diseases such as heart disease and cancer. Berries also contribute to brain health, improving cognitive function and possibly slowing age-related decline.

Seeds and nuts, such as chia seeds, flaxseeds, almonds, and walnuts, are packed with healthy fats, including omega-3 fatty acids, which are essential for brain health and reducing inflammation. They also provide protein, fiber, and various vitamins and minerals, supporting heart health and helping to manage weight by promoting satiety.

Quinoa and other whole grains offer a wealth of benefits, being high in fiber and protein compared to other grains. They contain all nine essential amino acids, making them a complete protein source, which is particularly valuable in a plant-based diet. These grains also supply B vitamins, magnesium, iron, and antioxidants.

Legumes, including beans, lentils, and chickpeas, are not only excellent protein sources but also rich in fiber, iron, folate, and potassium. They support heart health by improving cholesterol levels and blood pressure, and their high fiber content promotes digestive health and aids in weight management.

Cruciferous vegetables like broccoli, Brussels sprouts, and cauliflower are loaded with vitamins C, K, and E, fiber, and cancer-fighting compounds such as glucosinolates. These vegetables support detoxification processes in the liver and have been linked to a reduced risk of cancer.

Avocados are a unique fruit, offering a substantial amount of monounsaturated fats, which are heart-healthy fats. They're also an excellent source of fiber, potassium, and vitamins C, E, and K. Avocados contribute to heart health, help in maintaining healthy cholesterol levels, and can be beneficial for vision due to their lutein and zeaxanthin content.

Sweet potatoes and other colorful root vegetables are high in beta-carotene, a precursor to vitamin A, which is essential for immune function, eye health, and skin integrity. They also provide fiber, vitamins C and B6, and potassium.

Fermented foods like kimchi, sauerkraut, and kefir are rich in probiotics, beneficial bacteria that promote a healthy gut microbiome. A balanced gut microbiome supports digestion, immune function, and may even influence mood and mental health.

Incorporating these superfoods into a plant-based diet enhances nutrient intake and offers a range of health benefits. It's important to consume a variety of these foods to ensure a broad intake of nutrients. Superfoods can easily be included in meals and snacks throughout the day, from adding leafy greens and berries to smoothies, incorporating nuts and seeds into salads and yogurt, to enjoying legumes and whole grains as part of hearty, satisfying dishes.

While superfoods are powerful allies in maintaining health and preventing disease, it's crucial to remember that no single food can provide all the necessary nutrients for optimal health. A balanced, varied diet, rich in whole, plant-based foods, is the best approach to achieving and maintaining good health.

IDENTIFYING PLANT-BASED SUPERFOODS

Identifying plant-based superfoods involves recognizing foods that are exceptionally nutrient-dense and beneficial for health.

These superfoods are powerhouses of vitamins, minerals, antioxidants, and other health-promoting compounds that can significantly enhance a plant-based diet. To effectively incorporate these superfoods into your daily meals, it's essential to know what to look for and understand the unique benefits they offer.

Leafy greens such as kale, spinach, and arugula are among the most nutrient-rich foods available. They are packed with vitamins A, C, and K, calcium, and several phytonutrients that support a wide range of bodily functions, including vision, immune system, and bone health. Including a variety of leafy greens in your diet can help protect against chronic diseases and promote overall wellness.

Berries, including blueberries, strawberries, and blackberries, are celebrated for their high antioxidant content. These small but mighty fruits offer protection against inflammation, aging, and disease by neutralizing free radicals in the body. Their versatility makes them an easy addition to any meal, from breakfast cereals to salads and desserts.

Nuts and seeds, such as almonds, walnuts, chia seeds, and flaxseeds, are excellent sources of healthy fats, protein, and fiber. They also contain important minerals like magnesium, zinc, and selenium. Consuming a small portion of nuts and seeds daily can support heart health, aid in weight management, and provide sustained energy.

Quinoa, amaranth, and other whole grains are not only great sources of complex carbohydrates but also provide a complete protein, containing all nine essential amino acids. These grains are rich in fiber, B vitamins, and iron, making them a staple in any plant-based diet for their energy-boosting and health-sustaining properties.

Legumes, including beans, lentils, and chickpeas, are another category of plant-based superfoods. They are an excellent source of protein, fiber, iron, and folate, which support heart health, digestive health, and energy production. Legumes can be incorporated into a variety of dishes, from soups and stews to salads and spreads.

Cruciferous vegetables like broccoli, cauliflower, and Brussels sprouts are loaded with fiber, vitamins C, E, and K, and compounds that have been shown to protect against cancer. Their ability to support detoxification in the body makes them a valuable addition to a health-promoting diet.

Avocados are unique among fruits for their high content of monounsaturated fats, which are beneficial for heart health. They also provide fiber, potassium, and vitamins C, E, and K. Avocados can enhance the absorption of fat-soluble vitamins from other foods when eaten together, making them a perfect complement to vegetable-rich meals.

Sweet potatoes and other colorful root vegetables are rich in beta-carotene, which the body converts into vitamin A, essential for immune function and eye health. They also offer fiber, vitamins C and B6, and potassium, contributing to a well-rounded diet.

Fermented foods like sauerkraut, kimchi, and tempeh are valuable for their probiotic content, enhancing gut health and supporting immune function. Incorporating these foods into your diet can aid digestion and nutrient absorption.

To identify and include plant-based superfoods in your diet, focus on variety and color. Aim to fill your plate with a rainbow of fruits and vegetables, diverse grains and legumes, and a handful of nuts and seeds. This approach ensures a broad intake of the various nutrients these superfoods offer, promoting optimal health and well-being. Remember, while superfoods can significantly enhance your diet, balance and moderation are key. A diet based on a wide range of whole, plant-based foods will provide the most comprehensive health benefits.

GREENS AND SEA VEGETABLES

Greens and sea vegetables stand out as nutritional powerhouses in a plant-based diet, offering a wide array of health benefits that are essential for maintaining a balanced and holistic lifestyle. Rich in vitamins, minerals, and antioxidants, these foods contribute significantly to heart health, immune function, and overall well-being.

Leafy greens such as kale, spinach, and Swiss chard are loaded with vitamins A, C, E, and K, as well as calcium, iron, and potassium. These nutrients support bone health, aid in blood clotting, and help protect against oxidative stress. Incorporating a variety of greens into your diet can also enhance your intake of dietary fiber, which promotes digestive health and aids in weight management by keeping you feeling full longer.

Sea vegetables, including nori, kelp, and dulse, are unique in their rich iodine content, a mineral vital for thyroid function, which regulates metabolism.

They also offer a plant-based source of omega-3 fatty acids, particularly EPA, which is often found in fish. Omega-3s are crucial for brain health, reducing inflammation, and preventing chronic diseases. Furthermore, sea vegetables contain powerful compounds like fucoidans, which have been studied for their anti-inflammatory and anti-cancer properties.

To incorporate more greens and sea vegetables into your diet, consider adding spinach or kale to smoothies, salads, or soups.

Sea vegetables can be used in sushi rolls, as a garnish on salads, or added to broths to enhance flavor and nutritional content.

Experimenting with these ingredients can not only elevate the nutritional value of your meals but also introduce new textures and flavors to your diet.

Beneficial effects: Enhances bone health, supports thyroid function, boosts immune system, aids in weight management, and reduces inflammation.

Ingredients:

- 1 cup of fresh kale, chopped

- 1 cup of spinach, chopped

- 1/4 cup of dried nori, cut into strips

- 1/4 cup of kelp, chopped

- 2 tablespoons of olive oil

- Juice of 1 lemon

- Salt and pepper to taste

Instructions:

1. Wash and prepare the kale and spinach by chopping them into bite-sized pieces.

2. Rehydrate the kelp according to package instructions, then chop.

3. In a large bowl, combine the kale, spinach, nori, and kelp.

4. Drizzle with olive oil and lemon juice, then toss to coat evenly.

5. Season with salt and pepper to taste.

6. Serve as a nutritious side dish or add to your favorite grain bowl for a complete meal.

Variations: For an extra boost of protein, consider adding chickpeas, lentils, or quinoa to the salad. You can also incorporate other sea vegetables like dulse or arame for varied flavors and textures.

Storage tips: Store any leftover salad in an airtight container in the refrigerator for up to two days. It's best to dress the salad just before serving to prevent wilting.

Tips for allergens: For those with allergies to iodine or specific greens, always consult with a healthcare provider before introducing new items into your diet. Substitute any ingredients as necessary to accommodate dietary restrictions.

Incorporating greens and sea vegetables into your diet is a simple yet effective way to enhance your nutritional intake and support your holistic health journey. Their wide range of beneficial nutrients makes them an invaluable component of a balanced, plant-based diet.

INCORPORATING SUPERFOODS INTO DAILY MEALS

Incorporating superfoods into daily meals is a straightforward and effective strategy to enhance your diet with nutrient-dense foods that support overall health and well-being. Superfoods, rich in vitamins, minerals, antioxidants, and other essential nutrients, can be easily added to your favorite meals to boost their nutritional value without compromising on taste. Here are practical ways to include a variety of superfoods into your daily eating habits.

Beneficial effects: Boosts nutritional intake, supports immune system, enhances energy levels, aids in disease prevention, and promotes overall health.

Ingredients:

- Chia seeds

- Quinoa

- Blueberries

- Spinach

- Almonds

- Avocado

- Sweet potatoes

- Kale

- Garlic

- Ginger

Instructions:

1. **Start with Breakfast**: Mix chia seeds or ground flaxseeds into oatmeal, yogurt, or smoothies. These seeds are high in omega-3 fatty acids, fiber, and protein, making them a perfect start to your day.

2. **Upgrade Your Salads**: Toss in a handful of blueberries, sliced almonds, and chunks of avocado with your greens for a salad rich in antioxidants, healthy fats, and vitamins. Kale and spinach are excellent leafy choices for the base due to their nutrient profile, including iron, calcium, and vitamins A, C, and K.

3. **Supercharge Your Snacks**: Swap out processed snack foods for nutrient-rich alternatives like raw nuts, seeds, or homemade sweet potato chips. Almonds and walnuts are particularly beneficial for brain health and are a satisfying, crunchy snack.

4. **Enhance Main Dishes**: Incorporate quinoa or amaranth as a side dish or base for your meals. These grains are complete proteins, offering all nine essential amino acids, and are versatile enough to pair with a variety of flavors.

5. **Boost Soups and Stews**: Add garlic, ginger, and turmeric to soups and stews. These spices not only provide a burst of flavor but also have anti-inflammatory and immune-boosting properties.

6. **Desserts and Baking**: Use avocado as a butter substitute in baking for a healthier fat option. Incorporate pureed sweet potatoes or beets into baked goods to increase their fiber and antioxidant content without altering the taste significantly.

Variations: Experiment with different superfoods based on seasonal availability and personal preference. For example, swap blueberries for acai berries, or use pumpkin seeds instead of almonds for a change in texture and nutrients.

Storage tips: Most superfoods, like nuts, seeds, and grains, should be stored in airtight containers in a cool, dry place to maintain their freshness. Fresh fruits and vegetables are best kept in the refrigerator's crisper drawer to preserve their nutrients and flavor.

Tips for allergens: For those with nut allergies, seeds like chia or hemp can provide similar nutritional benefits without the risk. Always ensure to read labels carefully when purchasing processed superfoods to avoid hidden allergens.

By integrating these superfoods into your meals, you can effortlessly increase your intake of essential nutrients. This approach not only enhances your diet but also supports a holistic health lifestyle, aligning with Dr. Barbara's philosophy of nourishing the body with whole, unprocessed foods for optimal health.

CHAPTER 3: DETOX DIETS AND CLEANSING

Detox diets and cleansing have become popular methods for removing toxins from the body, improving health, and promoting weight loss. These diets typically involve a period of fasting, followed by a strict diet of fruits, vegetables, juices, and water. Some also include herbs, teas, supplements, and enemas or colon cleanses to empty the intestines. While the body is equipped with its own natural detoxification systems, such as the liver, kidneys, and colon, proponents of detox diets argue that today's polluted environment and poor dietary habits overload these systems, necessitating external detoxification methods.

Beneficial effects: Detox diets are believed to provide numerous health benefits, including improved energy levels, clearer skin, enhanced digestion, weight loss, and reduced inflammation. By eliminating processed foods, sugar, and other harmful substances from the diet, these programs can help reset the body's natural detoxification processes and promote a healthier lifestyle.

Ingredients:

- Fresh, organic fruits and vegetables

- Pure, filtered water

- Herbal detox teas

- Natural supplements (e.g., milk thistle, dandelion root)

- Freshly squeezed fruit and vegetable juices

Instructions:

1. **Preparation Phase**: Begin reducing your intake of sugar, caffeine, alcohol, and processed foods at least a week before starting the detox to minimize withdrawal symptoms and cravings.

2. **Fasting Phase**: For the first 1-3 days, consume only liquids such as water, herbal teas, and freshly squeezed fruit and vegetable juices to give your digestive system a rest.

3. **Reintroduction Phase**: Gradually reintroduce solid foods into your diet, starting with easily digestible items like fruits and vegetables. Over the next few days, you can add nuts, seeds, and legumes.

4. **Maintenance Phase**: After completing the detox, maintain a healthy diet rich in whole foods, and limit the intake of processed foods, caffeine, and alcohol to keep your body's detoxification systems running smoothly.

Variations: Depending on individual health goals and preferences, detox diets can be modified. For those who find it difficult to stick to a juice-only detox, incorporating smoothies and soups can offer more variety and sustenance. Adding protein sources like plant-based protein powders can also help maintain muscle mass and energy levels.

Storage tips: Fresh produce should be stored in the refrigerator to preserve its nutrients and freshness. Juices and smoothies are best consumed immediately after preparation, but they can be stored in the fridge for up to 24 hours if necessary.

Tips for allergens: For those with allergies or sensitivities, it's important to choose detox ingredients that do not trigger adverse reactions. Gluten, dairy, and nut-free options are available for most detox recipes. Always consult with a healthcare provider before starting a detox, especially if you have existing health conditions or are taking medication.

Detox diets and cleansing can offer a way to jumpstart a healthier lifestyle and may help some people feel more energetic and revitalized. However, it's important to approach detoxification with caution and to view it as part of a broader, balanced approach to health. Long-term health and wellness are best achieved through a diet rich in whole foods, regular physical activity, and adequate hydration, rather than periodic detoxes.

DR. BARBARA'S APPROACH TO DETOX

Dr. Barbara's approach to detoxification emphasizes the body's inherent wisdom and its capacity to heal and purify itself when given the right support. Recognizing the modern challenges that come with exposure to environmental toxins, processed foods, and stress, her method integrates gentle, nourishing practices designed to enhance the body's natural detox pathways rather than harsh or restrictive detox regimes.

Central to her philosophy is the belief that detoxification should not be an occasional intervention but a daily practice woven seamlessly into one's lifestyle to continuously support the body's detoxification processes.

At the heart of Dr. Barbara's detox approach is the focus on whole, plant-based foods rich in nutrients, antioxidants, and fiber. These foods act as natural detoxifiers, aiding the body in eliminating toxins through improved digestion and supporting liver function, the body's main detox organ. She advocates for a colorful diet filled with fruits, vegetables, herbs, and spices known for their detoxifying properties, such as leafy greens, beets, turmeric, and ginger.

These foods not only support the liver but also provide a wide range of health benefits, including reducing inflammation and boosting the immune system.

Hydration plays a crucial role in Dr. Barbara's detox plan. Drinking ample amounts of purified water throughout the day is encouraged to facilitate the removal of waste products through the kidneys. Additionally, herbal teas such as dandelion or milk thistle tea are recommended for their liver-supporting properties. These beverages offer a therapeutic approach to detoxification, enhancing the body's ability to cleanse itself naturally.

Mindful eating practices are also a key component of her detox methodology. Dr. Barbara stresses the importance of paying attention to the body's hunger and fullness signals, eating slowly, and choosing foods that are both nourishing and satisfying.

This mindfulness aspect helps to foster a deeper connection with food and its impact on the body, encouraging choices that support detoxification and overall well-being.

Another aspect of Dr. Barbara's approach includes reducing exposure to toxins in the environment. This involves choosing organic foods to minimize pesticide exposure, using natural cleaning and personal care products, and being mindful of air and water quality.

By reducing the toxin load from external sources, the body is better able to handle internal detoxification processes without being overwhelmed.

Incorporating regular physical activity into one's routine is also emphasized. Exercise boosts circulation and encourages sweating, another effective way the body eliminates toxins. Gentle, restorative movements such as yoga or walking are particularly recommended to support the body's natural detox pathways while also reducing stress, which can further hinder the detoxification process.

Dr. Barbara's detox approach is holistic, recognizing that detoxification is not just about removing toxins from the body but also about nourishing the mind and spirit. Stress reduction techniques such as meditation, deep breathing exercises, and spending time in nature are encouraged to support overall health and enhance the body's detoxification capabilities. This comprehensive approach ensures that detoxification is a balanced, integrated practice that supports the body's natural rhythms and healing processes, paving the way for sustained health and vitality.

Sleep is another critical element in Dr. Barbara's detoxification strategy, often overlooked in traditional detox programs.

Adequate rest is essential for the body to repair and regenerate, allowing the liver and other detox organs to function optimally. She advises establishing a calming bedtime routine to enhance sleep quality, which in turn supports the body's natural detoxification processes during the night. This might include practices such as turning off electronic devices an hour before bed, engaging in gentle stretching or meditation, and ensuring the sleeping environment is dark and quiet.

The use of specific detoxifying herbs and supplements under professional guidance is also part of Dr. Barbara's comprehensive approach. Supplements like spirulina, chlorella, and activated charcoal have properties that can bind to toxins and help in their excretion from the body. However, Dr. Barbara emphasizes the importance of individualized consultation with a healthcare provider before starting any supplement regimen, to ensure it's tailored to one's specific health needs and conditions.

Emotional detoxification is also a key aspect of her methodology. Dr. Barbara believes that emotional well-being is deeply connected to physical health, and holding onto negative emotions can hinder the body's detoxification efforts.

She encourages practices that support emotional release, such as journaling, counseling, and engaging in creative activities that bring joy and fulfillment. This holistic view recognizes that a healthy mind contributes to a healthy body, and vice versa.

Community and social connections are highlighted as vital components of a detox lifestyle. Being part of a supportive community can provide motivation, reduce stress, and encourage healthy lifestyle choices. Dr. Barbara suggests participating in group activities that align with detox goals, such as cooking classes, gardening clubs, or fitness groups, to foster a sense of belonging and shared purpose.

Finally, Dr. Barbara underscores the importance of patience and kindness towards oneself throughout the detox process. Detoxification is not about perfection or adhering to strict rules, but about making gradual, sustainable changes that honor the body's needs.

She advocates for celebrating small victories and learning from setbacks, viewing the detox journey as an ongoing process of learning and growth.

By integrating these principles into daily life, Dr. Barbara's approach to detoxification becomes a holistic practice that not only cleanses the body but also nurtures the mind and spirit, leading to lasting health and wellness.

SAFE AND EFFECTIVE CLEANSING TECHNIQUES

Safe and effective cleansing techniques focus on supporting the body's natural detoxification systems rather than imposing harsh regimens that can lead to nutrient deficiencies and stress on the body. These methods prioritize gentle, nourishing practices that enhance the body's ability to cleanse itself while maintaining nutritional balance and overall well-being.

Beneficial effects: Enhances the body's natural detoxification processes, supports liver and kidney function, improves digestion and elimination, boosts energy levels, and promotes a sense of overall health and vitality.

Ingredients:

- Fresh, organic fruits and vegetables
- Filtered or spring water
- Herbal teas (dandelion, milk thistle, green tea)
- Probiotic-rich foods (yogurt, kefir, sauerkraut)
- High-fiber foods (flaxseeds, chia seeds, legumes)
- Healthy fats (avocado, nuts, olive oil)

Instructions:

1. Start your day with a glass of warm lemon water to stimulate digestion and liver function.

2. Incorporate a smoothie for breakfast that includes leafy greens, a source of healthy fat (such as avocado or flaxseeds), and a high-quality protein (like plant-based protein powder). This combination provides fiber, antioxidants, and essential nutrients that support detoxification.

3. Throughout the day, drink at least 8-10 glasses of filtered water to help flush toxins through the kidneys.

4. Include at least one serving of probiotic-rich foods daily to support gut health, which is crucial for effective detoxification and elimination.

5. For lunch and dinner, focus on a plant-based plate with half of the meal consisting of vegetables, a quarter of high-quality plant-based protein, and a quarter of whole grains or starchy vegetables. Add a serving of healthy fats to support nutrient absorption.

6. Snack on whole fruits, nuts, and seeds to provide your body with energy and essential nutrients without overburdening the digestive system.

7. Sip on herbal teas such as dandelion or milk thistle throughout the day to support liver health and provide antioxidants.

8. Engage in at least 30 minutes of moderate exercise daily to boost circulation and encourage sweating, another detoxification pathway.

9. Practice deep breathing or meditation to reduce stress, which can negatively impact the body's detoxification systems.

10. Ensure 7-9 hours of quality sleep each night to allow your body to repair and regenerate, supporting effective detoxification.

Variations: Customize your detox plan based on personal preferences and dietary restrictions. For example, if you are allergic to nuts, substitute seeds such as hemp or pumpkin seeds for healthy fats. If you prefer not to consume soy, choose alternative plant-based proteins such as lentils or chickpeas.

Storage tips: Prepare fresh meals as much as possible to maximize nutrient intake. If you need to store leftovers, keep them in an airtight container in the refrigerator for up to two days to maintain freshness and prevent nutrient loss.

Tips for allergens: Always choose ingredients that do not trigger your allergies. For those sensitive to lactose, opt for lactose-free kefir or plant-based yogurt alternatives.

Gluten-sensitive individuals should select gluten-free grains like quinoa or brown rice.

By following these safe and effective cleansing techniques, you can support your body's natural detoxification processes without resorting to extreme diets or interventions. This approach ensures that you nourish your body with essential nutrients while gently encouraging the elimination of toxins, leading to improved health and vitality.

CLEANSING FOODS AND THEIR BENEFITS

Cleansing foods play a pivotal role in supporting the body's natural detoxification processes, providing essential nutrients that aid in eliminating toxins and promoting overall health. These foods are rich in antioxidants, fiber, vitamins, and minerals, which collectively enhance liver function, improve digestion, and boost the immune system. Incorporating a variety of cleansing foods into your diet can lead to numerous health benefits, including increased energy levels, improved mental clarity, and a stronger defense against disease.

Beneficial effects: Promotes liver health, supports digestion, enhances immune function, increases energy, and aids in the natural detoxification process.

Ingredients:

- Leafy greens (kale, spinach, dandelion greens)

- Cruciferous vegetables (broccoli, Brussels sprouts, cabbage)

- High-fiber fruits (apples, pears, berries)

- Citrus fruits (lemons, limes, oranges)

- Garlic and onions

- Beets

- Ginger and turmeric

- Green tea

- Nuts and seeds (flaxseeds, chia seeds, almonds)

- Legumes (lentils, chickpeas)

Instructions:

1. Begin your day with a glass of warm water with lemon to stimulate the liver and aid digestion.

2. For breakfast, prepare a smoothie with kale, spinach, and berries. Add a tablespoon of flaxseeds or chia seeds for an extra fiber boost.

3. Snack on a small handful of almonds or an apple to keep energy levels up and support detoxification with their high nutrient content.

4. Include a salad with lunch that features a variety of leafy greens, topped with slices of avocado for healthy fats and lemon juice for flavor and detox support.

5. Incorporate cruciferous vegetables like broccoli or Brussels sprouts into your dinner. These can be steamed, roasted, or stir-fried with garlic and onions, which contain sulfur compounds that support the liver.

6. Sip on green tea throughout the day for its antioxidant properties, which aid in liver function and the elimination of toxins.

7. Use herbs and spices such as ginger and turmeric in cooking to reduce inflammation and support digestion.

Variations: Customize your intake of cleansing foods based on personal taste preferences and seasonal availability. For example, swap out apples for pears, or use watercress instead of kale for variety in your salads. Experiment with adding different legumes to your meals for plant-based protein and fiber.

Storage tips: Store leafy greens and other vegetables in the crisper drawer of your refrigerator to maintain freshness. Keep nuts and seeds in airtight containers in a cool, dry place to preserve their natural oils and nutrients.

Tips for allergens: For those with nut allergies, focus on seeds like flaxseeds and chia seeds as alternatives. If you're sensitive to citrus, consider using apple cider vinegar as a substitute in dressings and recipes for its detoxifying properties.

By making these cleansing foods a regular part of your diet, you can support your body's natural detoxification systems, leading to improved health and vitality. Remember, the key to a successful detox is not just about what you remove from your diet, but also about what you include. These foods provide a powerful way to cleanse the body while nourishing it with essential nutrients for optimal health.

CHAPTER 4: 5 HERBAL DETOX RECIPES

DANDELION ROOT TEA

Beneficial effects

Dandelion Root Tea is celebrated for its detoxifying properties, supporting liver function, aiding digestion, and acting as a diuretic to help the body eliminate toxins. Rich in vitamins and minerals, it can also provide a gentle boost to the immune system.

Portions

1 serving

Preparation time

5 minutes

Cooking time

5-10 minutes

Ingredients

- 1 tablespoon dried dandelion root

- 8 ounces of water

- Honey or lemon (optional, for taste)

Instructions

1. Bring 8 ounces of water to a boil in a small pot.

2. Add 1 tablespoon of dried dandelion root to the boiling water.

3. Reduce heat and simmer for about 5-10 minutes, depending on how strong you prefer your tea.

4. Strain the tea into a cup, removing the dandelion root.

5. Optional: Add honey or lemon to taste for flavor enhancement.

6. Enjoy the tea warm for maximum benefits.

Variations

- For a more complex flavor, add a pinch of cinnamon or ginger to the tea while it simmers.

- Combine with peppermint leaves during the simmering process for a refreshing twist.

Storage tips

Store dried dandelion root in a cool, dry place, away from direct sunlight and moisture, to preserve its potency and freshness.

Tips for allergens

Individuals with allergies to ragweed and related plants should proceed with caution when trying dandelion root tea for the first time, as it may cause allergic reactions in sensitive individuals.

Scientific references

- Clare, B. A., Conroy, R. S., & Spelman, K. (2009). The diuretic effect in human subjects of an extract of Taraxacum officinale folium over a single day. Journal of Alternative and Complementary Medicine, 15(8), 929–934. This study supports the diuretic action of dandelion root.

- Wirngo, F. E., Lambert, M. N., & Jeppesen, P. B. (2016). The Physiological Effects of Dandelion (Taraxacum officinale) in Type 2 Diabetes. The Review of Diabetic Studies : RDS, 13(2-3), 113–131. This review highlights the potential benefits of dandelion root in managing type 2 diabetes and its role in modulating glucose metabolism.

BURDOCK ROOT INFUSION

Beneficial effects

Burdock Root Infusion is celebrated for its powerful detoxifying properties. It supports liver function, aids in purifying the blood, and can help clear skin issues such as acne and eczema. Burdock root contains inulin, a prebiotic that may improve gut health and digestion. Additionally, its antioxidant compounds help to fight free radicals, reducing inflammation and promoting overall health.

Portions

Makes about 4 cups

Preparation time

10 minutes

Cooking time

30 minutes

Ingredients

- 1 tablespoon dried burdock root

- 4 cups water

Instructions

1. Bring 4 cups of water to a boil in a medium-sized pot.

2. Add 1 tablespoon of dried burdock root to the boiling water.

3. Reduce the heat and simmer for about 30 minutes.

4. After 30 minutes, remove the pot from the heat and let it cool slightly.

5. Strain the infusion through a fine mesh sieve or cheesecloth into a large pitcher or jar, discarding the solid pieces of burdock root.

6. Serve the infusion warm, or let it cool completely and refrigerate for a cold beverage.

Variations

- For a sweeter taste, add a teaspoon of honey or maple syrup while the infusion is still warm.

- Enhance the detoxifying effects by adding a slice of fresh ginger or a few slices of lemon to the pot during simmering.

- Combine with dandelion root for an extra potent detox infusion.

Storage tips

Store any leftover burdock root infusion in the refrigerator for up to 5 days. Ensure it's in a sealed container to maintain freshness and prevent absorption of other flavors or odors.

Tips for allergens

Individuals with allergies to plants in the Asteraceae family, such as daisies, chrysanthemums, or ragweed, should proceed with caution when trying burdock root for the first time due to potential cross-reactivity. Always start with a small amount to test for any adverse reactions.

Scientific references

- "Antioxidative and in vitro antiproliferative activity of Arctium lappa root extracts" - BMC Complementary and Alternative Medicine. This study supports the antioxidant properties of burdock root, highlighting its potential health benefits.

- "Prebiotic effectiveness of inulin extracted from edible burdock" - Anaerobe. This research outlines the benefits of inulin, a component of burdock root, on gut health and digestion.

MILK THISTLE SMOOTHIE

Beneficial effects

Milk Thistle Smoothie is designed to support liver health and detoxification. Milk thistle contains silymarin, a group of compounds said to have antioxidant and anti-inflammatory effects, which can help rejuvenate liver cells and protect against damage. Incorporating this smoothie into your diet may aid in digestion, improve skin health, and support overall detoxification processes in the body.

Portions

1 serving

Preparation time

5 minutes

Ingredients

- 1 cup unsweetened almond milk

- 1 ripe banana

- 1 tablespoon milk thistle powder

- 1/2 cup fresh or frozen mixed berries (such as blueberries, raspberries, and strawberries)

- 1 tablespoon chia seeds

- 1 handful of fresh spinach leaves

- Ice cubes (optional, for a colder smoothie)

Instructions

1. In a blender, combine the unsweetened almond milk and ripe banana. Blend these together until smooth.

2. Add the milk thistle powder, mixed berries, chia seeds, and fresh spinach leaves to the blender.

3. If you prefer a colder smoothie, add a few ice cubes.

4. Blend all the ingredients together until the mixture is smooth and creamy. Ensure there are no chunks or unblended seeds.

5. Once fully blended, pour the smoothie into a glass and enjoy immediately for the best taste and health benefits.

Variations

- For added protein, include a scoop of your favorite plant-based protein powder.

- Substitute almond milk with coconut water or another non-dairy milk of your choice for different flavors and nutritional profiles.

- Add a tablespoon of flaxseed oil or a handful of nuts for healthy fats that support liver health.

Storage tips

It's best to consume the Milk Thistle Smoothie immediately after preparation to enjoy its full nutritional benefits. However, if you need to store it, keep the smoothie in an airtight container in the refrigerator for up to 24 hours. Shake well before drinking if separation occurs.

Tips for allergens

For those with nut allergies, substitute almond milk with oat milk, rice milk, or soy milk. Always ensure that any added ingredients, such as protein powders or supplements, are free from allergens that may affect you.

Scientific references

- "Silymarin, the Antioxidant Component and Silybum marianum Extracts Prevent Liver Damage." Food and Chemical Toxicology, 2010. This study discusses the antioxidant properties of silymarin in milk thistle and its effects on liver health.

- "The Use of Silymarin in the Treatment of Liver Diseases." Drugs, 2001. This review highlights the therapeutic potential of silymarin in treating various liver diseases, supporting the inclusion of milk thistle in detoxification diets.

GINGER AND TURMERIC DETOX DRINK

Beneficial effects

Ginger and Turmeric Detox Drink harnesses the powerful anti-inflammatory and antioxidant properties of its two main ingredients. Ginger is known for its ability to soothe digestion, reduce nausea, and fight the flu and common cold. Turmeric, on the other hand, contains curcumin, a compound with strong anti-inflammatory effects that can help detoxify the body and support liver health. Together, they create a potent detox drink that not only cleanses the body but also boosts the immune system and improves overall health.

Portions

2 servings

Preparation time

5 minutes

Cooking time

10 minutes

Ingredients

- 1 tablespoon fresh grated ginger

- 1 tablespoon fresh grated turmeric (or 1 teaspoon turmeric powder if fresh is unavailable)

- 4 cups of water

- Juice of 1/2 lemon

- 1 tablespoon honey (optional, for sweetness)

- A pinch of black pepper (to enhance curcumin absorption)

Instructions

1. Bring the water to a boil in a medium saucepan.

2. Add the freshly grated ginger and turmeric to the boiling water. If using turmeric powder, ensure it's completely dissolved.

3. Reduce the heat and let the mixture simmer for about 10 minutes.

4. Remove from heat and let it cool slightly.

5. Strain the mixture into mugs or a large container, removing the solid pieces.

6. Add the fresh lemon juice and honey to taste, stirring until the honey dissolves.

7. Sprinkle a pinch of black pepper into the drink and stir well.

Variations

- For a cold version, let the drink cool completely and then refrigerate. Serve over ice for a refreshing detox beverage.

- Add a cinnamon stick during the simmering process for additional flavor and blood sugar regulation benefits.

- For an extra immune boost, include a clove of garlic in the simmering process. Remove it before serving.

Storage tips

If you have leftovers or prefer to prepare in advance, store the ginger and turmeric detox drink in the refrigerator for up to 5 days. Reheat gently on the stove or enjoy cold.

Tips for allergens

For those with honey allergies or following a vegan diet, substitute honey with maple syrup or simply omit the sweetener. If allergic to citrus, omit the lemon juice or replace it with a splash of apple cider vinegar for a similar zesty flavor.

Scientific references

- "Anti-Oxidative and Anti-Inflammatory Effects of Ginger in Health and Physical Activity: Review of Current Evidence" - International Journal of Preventive Medicine, 2013.

- "Curcumin: A Review of Its' Effects on Human Health" - Foods, 2017. This study highlights turmeric's curcumin compound for its anti-inflammatory and antioxidant properties, supporting detoxification and overall health.

LEMON AND CAYENNE PEPPER CLEANSE

Beneficial effects

The Lemon and Cayenne Pepper Cleanse is designed to kickstart your digestive system, boost your metabolism, and help in detoxifying your body. Lemon juice acts as a natural antioxidant and aids in digestion, while cayenne pepper can stimulate the circulatory system and encourage the body to purge toxins. This combination is also believed to support weight loss efforts by enhancing metabolic rates.

Ingredients

- 2 tablespoons of freshly squeezed lemon juice

- 1/10 teaspoon of cayenne pepper

- 8-10 ounces of purified or spring water

- 1-2 teaspoons of organic maple syrup (optional, for sweetness)

Instructions

1. Warm the water to a comfortable drinking temperature, not too hot or cold.

2. Squeeze the lemon to get about 2 tablespoons of juice and add it to the water.

3. Add the cayenne pepper to the lemon-water mixture.

4. If desired, add organic maple syrup to taste for sweetness.

5. Stir the mixture thoroughly until all the ingredients are well combined.

6. Drink this cleanse first thing in the morning on an empty stomach, and wait at least 30 minutes before eating breakfast.

Variations

- For an extra detox boost, add a tablespoon of apple cider vinegar to the mix.

- Increase or decrease the amount of cayenne pepper according to your tolerance level.

- Substitute lemon juice with lime juice for a different flavor profile.

Storage tips

It's best to prepare the Lemon and Cayenne Pepper Cleanse fresh each morning to ensure potency and effectiveness. However, if you need to prepare it in advance, store it in a glass jar in the refrigerator for up to 24 hours. Shake well before drinking.

Tips for allergens

Individuals with citrus allergies can substitute lemon juice with a small amount of apple cider vinegar for similar detoxifying benefits. If you're sensitive to spicy foods, start with a tiny pinch of cayenne pepper and gradually increase to tolerance.

Scientific references

- "Effects of capsaicin, green tea and CH-19 sweet pepper on appetite and energy intake in humans in negative and positive energy balance." Clinical Nutrition, 2009.

- "Lemon detox diet reduced body fat, insulin resistance, and serum hs-CRP level without hematological changes in overweight Korean women." Nutrition Research, 2015.

PART 3: GUT HEALTH AND DIGESTION

Gut health and digestion are foundational elements of holistic health, emphasizing the critical role the gastrointestinal (GI) tract plays in overall wellness. The gut is not only responsible for the digestion and absorption of nutrients but also serves as a key player in the immune system, the production of certain vitamins, and the regulation of hormones. A healthy gut microbiome, which is the community of beneficial bacteria residing in the GI tract, is essential for maintaining the integrity of the intestinal barrier, synthesizing essential nutrients, and protecting against pathogens.

The gut-brain connection highlights the intricate communication network between the gut and the brain, mediated through neural, hormonal, and immunological pathways. This connection underscores the impact of gut health on mental well-being, illustrating how imbalances in the gut microbiota can influence mood, cognitive functions, and susceptibility to stress. Therefore, nurturing gut health is a critical component of a holistic approach to health, with dietary choices playing a pivotal role.

Incorporating a diverse range of whole, unprocessed foods is key to supporting a healthy gut. Foods rich in fiber, such as fruits, vegetables, whole grains, and legumes, act as prebiotics, feeding beneficial gut bacteria and promoting their growth. Fermented foods like yogurt, kefir, sauerkraut, and kombucha introduce probiotics, which are live beneficial bacteria that can enhance the diversity and functionality of the gut microbiome.

These dietary practices not only support the structure and function of the gut barrier but also contribute to the production of short-chain fatty acids (SCFAs), which have anti-inflammatory effects and play a role in maintaining the health of the colon.

Hydration is another crucial aspect of supporting gut health and digestion. Adequate fluid intake ensures the proper function of the GI tract, facilitating the digestion of food and the absorption of nutrients while preventing constipation by maintaining stool softness and regularity. Herbal teas, in addition to water, can be beneficial, with certain herbs offering soothing properties that can alleviate digestive discomfort and support gut health.

Mindful eating practices further enhance gut health by encouraging slower eating, better chewing, and reduced stress during meals, which can improve digestion and nutrient absorption. Paying attention to the body's hunger and satiety cues helps to avoid overeating, which can strain the digestive system and disrupt gut microbiota balance.

Addressing food sensitivities and intolerances by eliminating or reducing certain foods from the diet can also be instrumental in maintaining gut health.

Common irritants include gluten, dairy, and highly processed foods, which can contribute to inflammation, digestive issues, and alterations in gut microbiota composition. An elimination diet, followed by a careful reintroduction of foods, can help identify sensitivities and tailor a dietary approach that supports individual gut health needs.

The role of diet in gut health extends beyond the simple act of nourishment. It involves a comprehensive strategy that supports the microbiome, enhances digestive function, and contributes to the body's overall well-being. By embracing a diet rich in whole foods, prioritizing hydration, and adopting mindful eating practices, individuals can foster a healthy gut environment that supports not only their digestive health but their holistic health journey.

Regular physical activity is another pillar supporting optimal gut health and digestion.

Exercise not only improves the efficiency of the digestive tract but also positively influences the composition of the gut microbiota. Physical activity encourages the growth of beneficial bacterial species that can enhance barrier function, reduce inflammation, and even improve mood and cognitive function through the gut-brain axis. Incorporating a mix of aerobic exercises, strength training, and flexibility workouts can stimulate gut motility, helping to prevent constipation and promote regular bowel movements.

Stress management is equally crucial for maintaining a healthy gut.

Chronic stress can disrupt the microbiome balance and intestinal barrier integrity, leading to a range of digestive issues. Techniques such as yoga, meditation, deep breathing, and spending time in nature can reduce stress levels and mitigate its negative effects on gut health. These practices not only soothe the nervous system but also enhance the immune response and support the overall function of the digestive system.

The importance of sleep cannot be overstated in the context of gut health.

Quality sleep contributes to the regulation of gut function and the maintenance of microbiome balance.

Disruptions in sleep patterns can affect the production of appetite-regulating hormones, leading to changes in food preferences and eating behaviors that may negatively impact gut health. Establishing a consistent sleep schedule and creating a restful environment free from electronic distractions can promote restorative sleep and support digestive health.

In addition to these lifestyle factors, certain supplements may also support gut health. Prebiotics and probiotics can supplement dietary intake, especially in individuals struggling to consume a varied diet rich in fiber and fermented foods. Omega-3 fatty acids, found in fish oil supplements, have been shown to reduce intestinal inflammation and support the health of the gut lining. However, it's important to consult with a healthcare provider before starting any supplement regimen to ensure it's appropriate for your specific health needs and conditions.

Finally, regular medical check-ups and screenings can play a pivotal role in maintaining gut health and early detection of potential issues. Conditions such as irritable bowel syndrome (IBS), inflammatory bowel disease (IBD), and gastroesophageal reflux disease (GERD) require medical diagnosis and management. Working with healthcare professionals to develop a personalized approach to diet, lifestyle, and treatment can help manage these conditions effectively and support overall gut health.

In conclusion, gut health and digestion are central to holistic health, requiring a multifaceted approach that includes a balanced diet, regular physical activity, stress management, adequate sleep, and appropriate medical care.

By adopting these practices, individuals can support their gut health and contribute to their overall well-being, demonstrating the interconnectedness of the body's systems and the importance of a comprehensive approach to health.

CHAPTER 1: DR. BARBARA'S APPROACH TO GUT HEALTH

D r. Barbara emphasizes the importance of a healthy gut as the cornerstone of overall health, recognizing its role not only in digestion and nutrient absorption but also in immune function, mental health, and chronic disease prevention. Her approach to gut health is rooted in the belief that a balanced and diverse microbiome is key to maintaining the integrity of the gut barrier and optimizing gut function. To achieve this, she advocates for a diet rich in a variety of whole, plant-based foods that provide the necessary nutrients and fibers to nourish and support a healthy gut flora.

Fermented foods are a staple in Dr. Barbara's gut health strategy, offering a natural source of probiotics that help to increase the diversity and abundance of beneficial bacteria in the gut. She encourages the inclusion of foods like yogurt, kefir, sauerkraut, kimchi, and kombucha in daily diets to help replenish and maintain a healthy microbial balance. These probiotic-rich foods are complemented by prebiotic foods such as garlic, onions, bananas, asparagus, and whole grains that feed the beneficial bacteria, promoting their growth and activity.

Understanding the gut-brain axis, Dr. Barbara highlights the impact of gut health on mental well-being, noting that an imbalance in gut flora can contribute to mood disorders, anxiety, and stress. She suggests incorporating stress reduction techniques and mindfulness practices as part of a holistic approach to gut health, recognizing the bidirectional relationship between the gut and the brain.

Practices such as meditation, yoga, and deep breathing exercises are recommended to manage stress, which in turn can help mitigate its negative effects on gut health.

Hydration is another critical component of Dr. Barbara's approach, with a focus on drinking ample amounts of water throughout the day to support digestive health and facilitate the removal of waste and toxins from the body. Herbal teas, particularly those with digestive soothing properties like peppermint, ginger, and chamomile, are also recommended to aid digestion and alleviate discomfort.

Physical activity is encouraged as a means to enhance gut health, with regular exercise shown to improve gut motility, reduce inflammation, and positively influence the composition of the gut microbiome.

Dr. Barbara advises incorporating a mix of cardiovascular, strength, and flexibility exercises into weekly routines to support overall digestive health and well-being.

In addressing food sensitivities and intolerances, Dr. Barbara underscores the importance of listening to the body and identifying foods that may trigger digestive issues. An elimination diet, followed by gradual reintroduction, can be an effective way to pinpoint specific food sensitivities, allowing for a personalized dietary plan that avoids triggers and supports gut health.

Supplementation with prebiotics, probiotics, and other gut-supportive nutrients like omega-3 fatty acids may be considered, especially for individuals needing additional support or those with specific health conditions affecting gut health.

However, Dr. Barbara emphasizes the importance of consulting with a healthcare provider before starting any supplement regimen to ensure it aligns with individual health needs and goals.

By adopting these practices, individuals can support their gut health and contribute to their overall health and wellness.

Dr. Barbara's approach to gut health is integrative and personalized, recognizing the unique needs of each individual and the critical role of the gut in achieving and maintaining optimal health.

GUT-BRAIN CONNECTION

The gut-brain connection is a fundamental aspect of understanding how our digestive system not only influences but also communicates with our mental state, affecting mood, cognitive functions, and overall mental health.

This intricate relationship is primarily facilitated through the vagus nerve, one of the largest nerves connecting the gut and the brain. It serves as a two-way communication highway, with signals flowing from the gut to the brain and vice versa. This connection explains why our gut health can have a profound impact on our mental well-being and conversely, how our brain can affect gastrointestinal health.

Beneficial effects: Enhancing the gut-brain connection can lead to improved mental clarity, reduced symptoms of anxiety and depression, better stress management, and a more robust immune response. A healthy gut microbiome can also influence the production and regulation of key neurotransmitters like serotonin, which is predominantly produced in the gut, and dopamine, both of which play a crucial role in regulating mood and emotions.

Ingredients:
- High-fiber foods (e.g., legumes, whole grains, vegetables, fruits)
- Fermented foods (e.g., yogurt, kefir, sauerkraut, kimchi)
- Omega-3 fatty acids (e.g., flaxseeds, chia seeds, walnuts, fatty fish)
- Polyphenol-rich foods (e.g., berries, nuts, green tea, dark chocolate)
- Prebiotic foods (e.g., garlic, onions, bananas, asparagus)

Instructions:

1. Incorporate a variety of high-fiber foods into your diet to feed beneficial gut bacteria and promote their growth. Aim for at least 25-30 grams of fiber per day.

2. Include fermented foods in your daily meals to introduce probiotics into your gut, enhancing the diversity of your microbiome.

3. Consume omega-3 fatty acids regularly to reduce inflammation in the brain and body, supporting cognitive function and mental health.

4. Add polyphenol-rich foods to your diet to protect the gut lining and promote the growth of beneficial gut bacteria.

5. Eat prebiotic foods to provide the necessary nutrients that feed healthy microbiota, fostering a balanced and thriving gut environment.

Variations: To accommodate different dietary preferences or restrictions, plant-based sources of omega-3s and probiotics can be used. For those with sensitivities to dairy, lactose-free kefir or plant-based yogurt alternatives can be excellent probiotic sources. Gluten-free grains can be substituted for whole grains if gluten sensitivity is a concern.

Storage tips: Keep fermented foods refrigerated to maintain the viability of probiotic cultures. Store nuts and seeds in a cool, dry place to preserve their omega-3 fatty acids. Fresh produce should be stored properly to retain fiber content and nutritional value, with most vegetables and fruits kept in the refrigerator's crisper drawer.

Tips for allergens: For individuals with food allergies or sensitivities, always check labels on fermented foods for potential allergens. Substitute nuts or seeds with allergies in mind, opting for hemp seeds or flaxseeds as alternatives. Ensure any supplements used, such as omega-3 or probiotic capsules, are free from allergenic fillers or coatings.

By nurturing the gut-brain connection through these dietary practices, individuals can support their mental and physical health simultaneously. This holistic approach underscores the importance of a balanced, nutrient-rich diet in maintaining the delicate balance between our gut and brain, ultimately contributing to our overall well-being and quality of life.

THE IMPACT OF DIET ON GUT HEALTH

The foods we consume play a pivotal role in the health and function of our gut. A diet rich in whole, plant-based foods provides the necessary fiber, vitamins, and minerals that support a healthy microbiome, the community of beneficial bacteria residing in our gut. These microorganisms are crucial for digestion, absorption of nutrients, and the synthesis of certain vitamins. Fiber acts as a prebiotic, feeding these beneficial bacteria and promoting their growth, leading to a balanced gut flora which is essential for overall health.

Conversely, a diet high in processed foods, sugar, and saturated fats can disrupt this delicate balance, leading to an overgrowth of harmful bacteria. This imbalance can contribute to a range of digestive issues, including bloating, gas, constipation, and irritable bowel syndrome (IBS). Furthermore, the integrity of the gut lining can be compromised, potentially leading to leaky gut syndrome, where toxins and undigested food particles escape into the bloodstream, triggering inflammation and immune responses that can affect the body system-wide.

Incorporating a variety of fruits, vegetables, whole grains, nuts, and seeds can enhance gut health by providing a broad spectrum of nutrients and antioxidants that protect the gut lining and support the immune system. Fermented foods such as yogurt, kefir, sauerkraut, and kombucha are also beneficial, as they introduce probiotics, live bacteria that can help restore the gut microbiome to a healthy state.

Hydration is another key aspect of maintaining gut health, as water is essential for the digestion of food and the absorption of nutrients. It also helps to keep the digestive system moving and prevent constipation.

By understanding the impact of diet on gut health and making mindful choices about what we eat, we can support our gut microbiome and enhance our overall health and well-being.

THE ROLE OF DIET IN GUT HEALTH

The foods we choose to eat have a profound impact on the health and functionality of our gut. A diet that emphasizes whole, plant-based foods is rich in fiber, vitamins, and minerals, all of which are essential for nurturing a healthy microbiome. The microbiome, a complex community of beneficial bacteria within our gut, plays a critical role in digestion, nutrient absorption, and even the synthesis of certain vitamins. Fiber, particularly, serves as a prebiotic, fueling these beneficial bacteria and fostering a balanced gut flora, which is crucial for overall health.

On the flip side, diets laden with processed foods, excessive sugars, and saturated fats can throw this delicate microbial balance off-kilter. Such dietary patterns can promote the overgrowth of harmful bacteria, leading to a slew of digestive woes including bloating, gas, constipation, and irritable bowel syndrome (IBS). Moreover, the disruption of this balance can compromise the integrity of the gut lining, potentially leading to leaky gut syndrome. This condition allows toxins and partially digested food particles to escape into the bloodstream, inciting inflammation and immune responses that can have widespread effects on the body.

To support gut health, incorporating a diverse array of fruits, vegetables, whole grains, nuts, and seeds is advisable. These foods offer a spectrum of nutrients and antioxidants that safeguard the gut lining and bolster the immune system. Additionally, fermented foods like yogurt, kefir, sauerkraut, and kombucha are invaluable for their probiotic content, introducing live bacteria that aid in restoring and maintaining a healthy gut microbiome.

Hydration plays a pivotal role in gut health as well. Water is not only essential for the digestion of food and absorption of nutrients but also for maintaining the movement of the digestive system and preventing constipation. Ensuring adequate fluid intake is a simple yet effective way to support gut health.

By making informed dietary choices, we can significantly influence the health of our gut microbiome. This, in turn, enhances our overall health and well-being, underscoring the importance of diet in maintaining gut health.

SIGNS OF POOR GUT HEALTH

Recognizing signs of poor gut health is crucial for taking timely action to restore balance and ensure overall well-being. Common indicators include persistent digestive issues such as bloating, gas, diarrhea, constipation, and heartburn. These symptoms can signal an imbalance in the gut microbiome or issues with gut motility and function. Unexplained fatigue and sluggishness are also signs, as a healthy gut is essential for energy production and nutrient absorption. Skin conditions like eczema, acne, and psoriasis may reflect gut health problems due to the gut-skin connection, where inflammation in the gut can manifest on the skin.

Frequent infections and illnesses can be a red flag, indicating a compromised gut microbiome's role in immune function. A healthy gut contributes to a strong immune system, so recurrent colds or infections might suggest gut dysbiosis or a weakened gut barrier. Mood swings, depression, and anxiety are increasingly linked to gut health, given the gut-brain axis. The gut produces a significant amount of neurotransmitters, and an imbalanced microbiome can affect mood and cognitive functions.

Unexpected weight changes without a change in diet or exercise habits can indicate gut health issues. Weight gain may result from impaired nutrient absorption or insulin resistance, while weight loss might occur due to malabsorption or an overgrowth of certain bacteria. Food intolerances and sensitivities are often signs of poor gut health, as a compromised gut can have difficulty processing certain foods, leading to symptoms like nausea, abdominal pain, and headaches.

Addressing these signs involves dietary changes, stress management, adequate sleep, and possibly probiotics or other supplements to support gut health and restore balance. Recognizing and responding to these signs early can prevent more serious health issues and support long-term health and vitality.

CHAPTER 2: FOODS THAT SUPPORT GUT HEALTH

Foods that support gut health are foundational to maintaining a balanced microbiome, crucial for overall wellness. A diet rich in diverse, plant-based foods fuels beneficial gut bacteria, promoting digestion, nutrient absorption, and immune function. Key components include high-fiber foods, fermented products, and polyphenol-rich items, each playing a unique role in gut health.

High-fiber foods are indispensable for a healthy gut. Sources such as legumes, beans, peas, oats, bananas, berries, asparagus, and leeks provide soluble and insoluble fibers. Soluble fiber dissolves in water, forming a gel-like substance that helps regulate blood sugar and lower cholesterol. Insoluble fiber adds bulk to the stool and aids in food's movement through the digestive system, preventing constipation. These fibers also act as prebiotics, nourishing the beneficial bacteria in the gut.

Fermented foods are another cornerstone of gut health, introducing probiotics—live beneficial bacteria—into the digestive system. Yogurt, kefir, sauerkraut, kimchi, miso, and kombucha are excellent sources. These foods help restore the balance of gut flora, essential for digestion, synthesizing certain vitamins, and bolstering the immune system. Regular consumption of fermented foods can enhance the diversity of gut bacteria, linked to improved health outcomes.

Polyphenol-rich foods, found in items like dark chocolate, red wine, green tea, almonds, onions, blueberries, and broccoli, offer potent antioxidant properties. Polyphenols can promote the growth of beneficial gut bacteria while inhibiting harmful ones. These compounds also reduce inflammation and are linked to a lower risk of various diseases.

Incorporating a variety of these foods into daily meals can significantly impact gut health positively. For instance, starting the day with a high-fiber breakfast of oats topped with berries, transitioning to a lunch featuring a quinoa and legume salad, and enjoying fermented vegetables as a side for dinner. Snacks could include almonds or slices of apple, both high in fiber and polyphenols.

Hydration, too, plays a critical role in maintaining gut health.

Water aids digestion, helps dissolve fibers and nutrients, making them more accessible to the body, and ensures the smooth passage of waste through the digestive system. Aim for at least 8 cups of water daily, adjusting based on activity level and climate.

By focusing on these key dietary components, individuals can support their gut health, contributing to a stronger immune system, improved mood and cognitive function, and a lower risk of chronic diseases. Remember, diversity in the diet is crucial; a wide range of plant-based foods ensures a broad spectrum of nutrients and compounds beneficial for the gut microbiome.

PROBIOTIC FOODS FOR A HEALTHY GUT

Probiotic foods are essential for maintaining a healthy gut as they introduce beneficial bacteria that support the digestive system and enhance the immune function.

These live microorganisms, found in fermented foods, help balance the gut microbiome, crucial for overall health. Regular consumption of probiotic-rich foods can alleviate digestive disorders, reduce inflammation, and even improve mental health due to the gut-brain connection.

Yogurt is one of the most well-known sources of probiotics, containing strains such as Lactobacillus and Bifidobacterium. It's important to choose yogurts with live or active cultures and minimal added sugars for maximum benefits. Kefir, a fermented milk drink, offers a wider variety of bacterial cultures compared to yogurt and can be a good option for those who are lactose intolerant, as the fermentation process breaks down much of the lactose found in milk.

Sauerkraut, made from fermented cabbage, is not only a probiotic powerhouse but also rich in vitamins C and K, potassium, and fiber. It's vital to select unpasteurized sauerkraut because pasteurization kills the live and active bacteria. Similarly, kimchi, a spicy Korean side dish made from fermented vegetables, combines probiotics with antioxidants and vitamins.

For a non-dairy option, kombucha, a fermented tea, provides a unique blend of bacteria and yeast. Its tangy flavor can vary based on the fermentation time and the types of tea and sugar used. Miso, a Japanese seasoning produced by fermenting soybeans with salt and koji, adds a rich flavor to dishes and offers the gut health benefits of probiotics.

Incorporating a variety of these probiotic foods into your diet can contribute to a robust and diverse gut microbiome. Start with small portions to see how your body reacts, as some individuals may experience bloating or gas initially. Over time, these foods can help improve gut health, leading to better overall wellness.

FERMENTED FOODS AND THEIR BENEFITS

Fermented foods have been a staple in human diets for thousands of years, offering a range of health benefits due to their unique process of lacto-fermentation. During this process, natural bacteria feed on the sugar and starch in the food, creating lactic acid.

This not only preserves the foods but also promotes the growth of beneficial probiotics. These probiotics are key to improving gut health, enhancing digestion, and boosting the immune system. Regular consumption of fermented foods can lead to an increase in the diversity of gut bacteria, which is linked to improved digestion and a reduced risk of many chronic diseases.

Beyond their probiotic content, fermented foods are also rich in vitamins, particularly B vitamins, and minerals.

They can aid in the absorption of nutrients from our diet, making the vitamins and minerals more available to the body. This is particularly beneficial for those looking to improve their overall nutrient intake without significantly changing their diet. Fermented foods like sauerkraut, kimchi, and kefir are also known for their detoxifying properties, as they can help to flush out toxins and heavy metals from the body.

Incorporating fermented foods into the diet can be simple and delicious. Adding a spoonful of sauerkraut to a salad, enjoying a glass of kombucha during lunch, or incorporating kefir into a morning smoothie are easy ways to enjoy these foods daily.

It's important to start with small servings and gradually increase the amount to allow the gut to adjust, minimizing potential discomfort such as bloating or gas.

The benefits of fermented foods extend beyond gut health, potentially impacting mental health, skin clarity, and even weight management. The connection between the gut and brain, often referred to as the gut-brain axis, means that a healthy gut can contribute to a healthier mind, reducing symptoms of anxiety and depression. With their complex flavors and health-promoting properties, fermented foods are a valuable addition to a holistic health approach, offering a simple yet powerful way to support the body's natural healing processes.

FOODS TO AVOID FOR BETTER GUT HEALTH

For better gut health, it's crucial to be mindful of consuming certain foods that can disrupt the delicate balance of the gut microbiome. Highly processed foods, rich in additives and preservatives, can harm beneficial gut bacteria, leading to dysbiosis and digestive issues. These foods often contain high levels of refined sugars, which feed harmful bacteria and yeasts, promoting their overgrowth and contributing to conditions like candidiasis.

Artificial sweeteners, found in many diet products, have been shown to negatively affect gut bacteria and potentially lead to glucose intolerance. Similarly, trans fats, present in many fried and baked goods, can promote inflammation and negatively impact gut health.

Reducing intake of these fats is advisable for maintaining a healthy gut lining and overall well-being.

Excessive alcohol consumption can damage the gut lining, leading to increased permeability, often referred to as leaky gut syndrome. This condition allows toxins and undigested food particles to enter the bloodstream, triggering inflammation and immune responses. Limiting alcohol intake can help preserve gut integrity and support the growth of beneficial bacteria.

Foods high in sulfites, such as dried fruits, wines, and some processed meats, can trigger digestive discomfort in sensitive individuals by disrupting the balance of gut bacteria.

Additionally, gluten, found in wheat, barley, and rye, can be problematic for those with gluten sensitivity or celiac disease, leading to inflammation and gut health issues.

For individuals with lactose intolerance, consuming dairy products can lead to digestive distress, including bloating, gas, and diarrhea, as their bodies lack the enzyme needed to break down lactose.

Opting for lactose-free or plant-based alternatives can alleviate these symptoms and support gut health.

By avoiding or limiting these foods, individuals can support their gut microbiome, reduce inflammation, and promote overall digestive wellness. Emphasizing a diet rich in whole, unprocessed foods, with plenty of fiber, healthy fats, and fermented products, can enhance gut health and contribute to a balanced and thriving microbiome.

DR. BARBARA'S GUT-FRIENDLY MEAL SUGGESTIONS

Creating meals that support gut health doesn't have to be complicated or bland. Dr. Barbara suggests incorporating a variety of whole, plant-based foods that are rich in fiber, probiotics, and prebiotics to nourish the gut microbiome and promote overall digestive wellness. Here are some gut-friendly meal suggestions that are not only nutritious but also delicious and easy to prepare.

Beneficial effects: These meals are designed to support a healthy gut microbiome, enhance digestion, reduce inflammation, and provide a balanced array of nutrients. They are rich in fiber, which acts as a prebiotic to feed beneficial gut bacteria, and include sources of probiotics to help maintain a healthy balance of gut flora.

Breakfast: Probiotic Yogurt Bowl

- **Portions**: 1

- **Preparation time**: 5 minutes

Ingredients:

- 1 cup plain, unsweetened probiotic yogurt (or a plant-based alternative)

- ½ cup fresh berries (blueberries, strawberries, or raspberries)

- 1 tablespoon chia seeds

- 1 tablespoon ground flaxseed

- A drizzle of honey or maple syrup (optional)

- A handful of almonds or walnuts

- **Instructions**:

1. In a bowl, combine the yogurt with fresh berries.

2. Sprinkle chia seeds and ground flaxseed on top for added fiber and omega-3 fatty acids.

3. Add a drizzle of honey or maple syrup for a touch of sweetness if desired.

4. Top with almonds or walnuts for a crunchy texture and a dose of healthy fats.

- **Variations:** Swap out the berries for other fruits like sliced banana or kiwi. Use any nuts or seeds you prefer for different textures and nutritional benefits.

- **Storage tips:** Best enjoyed immediately. However, you can mix the seeds with yogurt and refrigerate overnight for a thicker texture.

- **Tips for allergens:** For a dairy-free version, use coconut, almond, or soy-based yogurt. Ensure nuts are suitable for those with nut allergies or substitute with pumpkin seeds or hemp seeds.

Lunch: Quinoa and Roasted Vegetable Salad

- **Portions**: 2

- **Preparation time**: 15 minutes

- **Cooking time**: 20 minutes

Ingredients:

- 1 cup quinoa

- 2 cups water

- 2 cups mixed vegetables (bell peppers, zucchini, carrots, and broccoli)

- 2 tablespoons olive oil

- Salt and pepper to taste

- 1 avocado, sliced

- 2 tablespoons lemon juice

- A handful of fresh spinach or kale

- **Instructions**:

1. Rinse quinoa under cold water and drain.

2. In a medium saucepan, bring quinoa and water to a boil. Reduce heat, cover, and simmer for 15 minutes or until water is absorbed.

3. While quinoa cooks, toss vegetables in olive oil, salt, and pepper. Spread on a baking sheet and roast in a preheated oven at 400°F for 20 minutes or until tender.

4. Combine cooked quinoa and roasted vegetables in a large bowl. Add sliced avocado and fresh greens.

5. Drizzle with lemon juice and toss to combine.

- **Variations:** Include any seasonal vegetables you enjoy. For added protein, mix in chickpeas or black beans.

- **Storage tips:** Store in an airtight container in the refrigerator for up to 3 days.

- **Tips for allergens:** Ensure the dish is gluten-free by using certified gluten-free quinoa. For those sensitive to citrus, substitute lemon juice with a balsamic vinaigrette.

Dinner: Lentil Soup with Fermented Vegetables

- **Portions**: 4
- **Preparation time**: 10 minutes
- **Cooking time**: 30 minutes

Ingredients:

- 1 tablespoon olive oil
- 1 onion, diced
- 2 garlic cloves, minced
- 1 carrot, diced
- 1 stalk celery, diced
- 1 cup lentils, rinsed
- 4 cups vegetable broth
- 1 teaspoon ground turmeric
- Salt and pepper to taste
- ½ cup sauerkraut or kimchi for serving

- **Instructions**:

1. In a large pot, heat olive oil over medium heat. Add onion and garlic, sautéing until translucent.

2. Add carrot and celery, cooking for a few more minutes until softened.

3. Stir in lentils, vegetable broth, and turmeric. Season with salt and pepper.

4. Bring to a boil, then reduce heat and simmer for 25-30 minutes, or until lentils are tender.

5. Serve hot, topped with a spoonful of sauerkraut or kimchi for a probiotic boost.

- **Variations:** Add spinach or kale in the last few minutes of cooking for extra greens. Spice it up with cumin or chili flakes.

- **Storage tips:** Cool completely and store in an airtight container in the refrigerator for up to 5 days or freeze for up to 3 months.

- **Tips for allergens:** For a nightshade-free version, omit the sauerkraut or kimchi and add a splash of apple cider vinegar for tanginess.

These meal suggestions are designed to be adaptable to individual dietary needs and preferences while providing a foundation for gut health through balanced, nutrient-rich ingredients.

CHAPTER 3: NATURAL REMEDIES FOR DIGESTIVE ISSUES

Digestive issues can range from occasional discomfort to chronic conditions, significantly impacting quality of life. Natural remedies offer a gentle yet effective approach to managing these issues, focusing on supporting the body's healing processes and maintaining digestive health. Here, we explore several herbal and natural solutions known for their beneficial effects on digestion.

Beneficial effects: These remedies aim to soothe digestive discomfort, enhance gut health, and promote the healing of the digestive tract. They can help alleviate symptoms such as bloating, gas, indigestion, and irregular bowel movements. Incorporating these into your daily routine can support the body's natural digestive processes and contribute to overall well-being.

Ginger Tea for Nausea and Indigestion

- **Portions**: 1

- **Preparation time**: 5 minutes

Ingredients:

- 1 inch fresh ginger root, thinly sliced

- 1 cup boiling water

- **Instructions**:

1. Place ginger slices in a mug.

2. Pour boiling water over the ginger and cover the mug. Let it steep for 5 minutes.

3. Strain the tea and drink warm.

- **Variations:** Add a teaspoon of honey or a slice of lemon for additional flavor and benefits.

- **Storage tips:** Best consumed fresh but can be stored in the refrigerator for up to 24 hours.

- **Tips for allergens:** Suitable for most individuals, including those with common food allergies.

Peppermint Oil Capsules for IBS

Beneficial effects: Peppermint oil has antispasmodic properties that can help relax the muscles of the digestive tract, reducing symptoms of irritable bowel syndrome (IBS) such as cramping and bloating.

- **Portions**: Follow manufacturer's dosage recommendations.

- **Preparation time**: Not applicable.

Ingredients:

- Peppermint oil capsules (available at health food stores)

- **Instructions**:

1. Take one capsule with water, 20-30 minutes before meals, up to three times a day.

- **Variations:** Some may prefer peppermint tea as a milder option.

- **Storage tips:** Keep in a cool, dry place as per the product's instructions.

- **Tips for allergens:** Check the label for any potential allergens, especially if the capsules contain additional ingredients.

Fennel Seeds for Bloating and Gas

- **Portions**: 1
- **Preparation time**: 5 minutes

Ingredients:

- 1 teaspoon of fennel seeds
- 1 cup boiling water
- **Instructions**:

1. Crush the fennel seeds lightly to release their oil.

2. Place the crushed seeds in a mug and cover with boiling water.

3. Cover the mug and let it steep for 10 minutes.

4. Strain and drink the tea warm.

- **Variations:** Combine with peppermint or ginger tea for added digestive benefits.

- **Storage tips:** Fennel seeds should be stored in a cool, dry place to maintain their potency.

- **Tips for allergens:** Fennel is generally well-tolerated, but those with plant-based allergies should proceed with caution.

Aloe Vera Juice for Gut Healing

Beneficial effects: Aloe vera is known for its anti-inflammatory and healing properties, making it beneficial for soothing and repairing the gut lining.

- **Portions**: 2-4 ounces

- **Preparation time**: Not applicable unless extracting juice directly from the plant.

Ingredients:

- Pure aloe vera juice (commercially prepared)
- **Instructions**:

1. Consume 2-4 ounces of aloe vera juice, either on its own or diluted in water, in the morning on an empty stomach.

- **Variations:** Mix with another juice, such as apple or carrot, for improved taste.

- **Storage tips:** Follow the storage instructions on the bottle. Usually, it should be refrigerated after opening.

- **Tips for allergens:** Pure aloe vera juice is generally free from common allergens, but check labels for additives.

Probiotic-Rich Foods for Gut Flora Balance

Beneficial effects: Probiotics help maintain a healthy balance of gut flora, essential for proper digestion and immune function.

- **Portions**: Varies by food type.

- **Preparation time**: Varies by recipe.

Ingredients:

- Yogurt, kefir, sauerkraut, kimchi, miso, tempeh
- **Instructions**:

1. Incorporate a serving of probiotic-rich food into your diet daily, such as adding yogurt to breakfast or sauerkraut to a salad.

- **Variations:** Choose dairy-free options like coconut yogurt or water kefir for those with dairy sensitivities.

- **Storage tips:** Most probiotic-rich foods should be stored in the refrigerator to preserve their live cultures.

- **Tips for allergens:** Always check labels for potential allergens, especially in commercially prepared fermented foods.

Incorporating these natural remedies into your daily routine can significantly improve digestive health and alleviate common digestive issues. Remember, it's essential to listen to your body and adjust accordingly, as individual responses to these remedies can vary. For persistent or severe symptoms, consulting with a healthcare professional is recommended.

HERBAL REMEDIES FOR BLOATING

Beneficial effects: Herbal remedies for bloating offer natural, gentle relief from discomfort, aiding in digestion and reducing gas buildup. These remedies can soothe the digestive tract, promote the expulsion of gas, and help maintain a healthy balance of gut flora, contributing to overall digestive wellness.

Caraway Seeds Digestive Tea

- **Portions**: 1

- **Preparation time**: 5 minutes

Ingredients:

- 1 teaspoon of caraway seeds

- 1 cup of boiling water

- **Instructions**:

1. Crush the caraway seeds slightly to release their volatile oils.

2. Place the crushed seeds in a cup and pour boiling water over them.

3. Cover and let steep for 10 minutes.

4. Strain the tea and drink warm to relieve bloating.

- **Variations:** Mix with fennel seeds for enhanced digestive benefits.

- **Storage tips:** Caraway seeds should be stored in a cool, dry place to maintain their potency.

- **Tips for allergens:** Generally well-tolerated; however, those with specific seed allergies should proceed with caution.

Peppermint Tea for Quick Relief

- **Portions**: 1

- **Preparation time**: 5 minutes

Ingredients:

- 1 peppermint tea bag or 1 tablespoon of dried peppermint leaves

- 1 cup of boiling water

- **Instructions**:

1. If using dried leaves, place them in a tea infuser.

2. Pour boiling water over the tea bag or infuser in a cup.

3. Let steep for 5-7 minutes.

4. Remove the tea bag or infuser and drink the tea warm.

- **Variations:** Add a slice of ginger for additional anti-inflammatory benefits.

- **Storage tips:** Store dried peppermint leaves in a sealed container in a cool, dark place.

- **Tips for allergens:** Peppermint is generally safe, but those with GERD should consult a healthcare provider as it can exacerbate symptoms.

Ginger and Lemon Digestive Aid

- **Portions**: 1

- **Preparation time**: 10 minutes

Ingredients:

- ½ inch piece of fresh ginger, peeled and sliced

- 1 cup of water

- Juice of ½ lemon

- Honey to taste (optional)

- **Instructions**:

1. Boil water and add sliced ginger.

2. Simmer for 5 minutes.

3. Remove from heat and add lemon juice.

4. Strain into a cup and add honey if desired.

5. Drink warm to alleviate bloating and stimulate digestion.

- **Variations:** Include a pinch of cayenne pepper for additional metabolism-boosting properties.

- **Storage tips:** Fresh ginger can be stored in the refrigerator; lemon should also be refrigerated.

- **Tips for allergens:** Suitable for most, but those with citrus allergies can omit the lemon.

Dandelion Root Tea for Digestive Support

- **Portions**: 1

- **Preparation time**: 5 minutes

Ingredients:

- 1 teaspoon of dried dandelion root

- 1 cup of boiling water

- **Instructions**:

1. Place dandelion root in a tea infuser or directly in a cup.

2. Pour boiling water over the root and cover.

3. Let steep for 10 minutes.

4. Strain and drink warm to support digestion and reduce bloating.

- **Variations:** Blend with peppermint or chamomile for a soothing, flavorful mix.

- **Storage tips:** Store dried dandelion root in a cool, dry place away from direct sunlight.

- **Tips for allergens:** Dandelion is generally safe, but those with ragweed allergies or gallbladder issues should consult with a healthcare provider before use.

Incorporating these herbal remedies into your routine can provide natural and effective relief from bloating. Always listen to your body and adjust as needed, and consult with a healthcare professional for persistent or severe symptoms.

MANAGING IBS NATURALLY

Irritable Bowel Syndrome (IBS) is a common condition that affects the large intestine, leading to symptoms such as cramping, abdominal pain, bloating, gas, and diarrhea or constipation. Managing IBS naturally involves a holistic approach focusing on diet, stress management, and natural remedies to alleviate symptoms and improve gut health.

Beneficial effects: A natural approach to managing IBS aims to reduce inflammation, balance gut flora, and alleviate symptoms without the need for pharmaceuticals. By incorporating specific foods, herbs, and lifestyle changes, individuals can see improvements in digestive function, reduced stress levels, and overall enhanced well-being.

Aloe Vera Juice for Gut Healing

- **Portions**: 1

- **Preparation time**: 5 minutes

Ingredients:

- ¼ cup of pure aloe vera juice

- ¾ cup of water or any non-citrus juice

- **Instructions**:

1. Mix the aloe vera juice with water or your choice of non-citrus juice to dilute its potency.

2. Drink this mixture on an empty stomach in the morning to soothe the digestive tract and promote healing.

- **Variations:** For added flavor and benefits, mix with cucumber juice or ginger tea.

- **Storage tips:** Store aloe vera juice in the refrigerator after opening to maintain freshness.

- **Tips for allergens:** Aloe vera is generally safe but start with a small dose to ensure no allergic reaction.

Peppermint Oil Capsules for Reducing Spasms

- **Portions**: Depends on the dosage recommended on the product.

- **Preparation time**: Not applicable.

Ingredients:

- Peppermint oil capsules (purchased from a health store)

- **Instructions**:

1. Take one capsule 20-30 minutes before meals, or as directed on the package, to help relax the muscles of the intestines.

- **Variations:** Some may prefer peppermint tea if capsules are not available.

- **Storage tips:** Keep the capsules in a cool, dry place.

- **Tips for allergens:** Peppermint is generally well-tolerated, but those with GERD or a hiatal hernia should avoid it as it can exacerbate symptoms.

High-Fiber Diet Adjustment

- **Portions**: Varies according to individual dietary needs.

- **Preparation time**: Varies based on meal preparation.

Ingredients:

- A variety of high-fiber foods such as oats, flaxseeds, chia seeds, berries, and vegetables.

- **Instructions**:

1. Gradually increase fiber intake to avoid gas and bloating.

2. Include soluble fiber sources like oats and flaxseeds which are gentler on the gut.

3. Drink plenty of water to help fiber move through the digestive system.

- **Variations:** Adjust fiber types and amounts based on personal tolerance.

- **Storage tips:** Store dry fiber-rich foods in airtight containers in a cool, dry place.

- **Tips for allergens:** Be mindful of any food sensitivities or allergies when selecting high-fiber foods.

Stress Management Techniques

Beneficial effects: Reducing stress through mindfulness, yoga, or meditation can significantly improve IBS symptoms by lowering the body's stress response, which is often a trigger for flare-ups.

- **Instructions**:

1. Practice mindfulness or meditation daily, aiming for at least 10-15 minutes.

2. Engage in gentle yoga, focusing on poses that support digestion.

3. Consider deep-breathing exercises to manage acute stress and relax the digestive tract.

Scientific references:

- Studies have shown that peppermint oil can significantly improve IBS symptoms by relaxing the smooth muscles of the colon, which helps to reduce pain and bloating.

- Aloe vera juice has been found to have anti-inflammatory properties that can help soothe the digestive tract and reduce IBS symptoms.

- Research supports the role of stress management in alleviating IBS symptoms, highlighting the importance of a holistic approach to treatment.

By incorporating these natural remedies and lifestyle changes, individuals with IBS can manage their symptoms more effectively and improve their quality of life. Always consult with a healthcare professional before starting any new treatment regimen, especially when dealing with chronic conditions like IBS.

HEALING LEAKY GUT

Leaky gut syndrome, characterized by an increase in intestinal permeability, has been linked to a variety of health issues ranging from digestive disturbances to systemic conditions such as autoimmune diseases. The integrity of the gut lining plays a crucial role in overall health, acting as a barrier that selectively allows nutrients to pass into the bloodstream while keeping harmful substances out. When this barrier is compromised, undigested food particles, toxins, and bacteria can leak through the intestinal wall, triggering inflammation and immune responses. Healing leaky gut focuses on restoring the health of the gut lining through dietary changes, supplementation, and lifestyle modifications.

Beneficial effects: Addressing leaky gut can lead to improved digestion, reduced inflammation, enhanced nutrient absorption, and a decrease in the occurrence of autoimmune reactions and other health issues related to increased intestinal permeability.

Bone Broth for Gut Lining Repair

- **Portions**: 4-6

- **Preparation time**: 24 hours

Ingredients:

- 2 pounds of mixed organic bones (chicken, beef, or fish)

- 2 carrots, chopped

- 1 onion, chopped

- 2 stalks of celery, chopped

- 2 tablespoons of apple cider vinegar

- 1 teaspoon of sea salt

- 1 teaspoon of black peppercorns

- Enough water to cover the bones

- **Instructions**:

1. Place all ingredients in a large stockpot or slow cooker.

2. Add water until bones are fully submerged.

3. Bring to a boil, then reduce heat to simmer.

4. Simmer for 24 hours, skimming off any foam that forms on the surface.

5. Strain the broth, discarding the solids.

6. Cool the broth and store it in the refrigerator for up to 5 days or freeze for longer storage.

Fermented Foods for Gut Flora Balance

- **Portions**: Varies

- **Preparation time**: Varies by recipe

Ingredients:

- Various, depending on the fermented food (e.g., cabbage for sauerkraut, milk for kefir)

- **Instructions**:

1. For sauerkraut, thinly slice cabbage and mix with salt. Pack tightly into a jar until the liquid covers the cabbage. Seal and let it ferment at room temperature for at least 2 weeks.

2. For kefir, mix kefir grains with milk in a jar. Cover with a cloth and let it ferment at room temperature for 24 hours.

3. Consume fermented foods daily to support gut flora balance.

L-Glutamine Supplement for Intestinal Repair

- **Portions**: As recommended by a healthcare provider

- **Preparation time**: Not applicable

Ingredients:

- L-Glutamine powder or capsules

- **Instructions**:

1. Take L-Glutamine according to the product instructions or a healthcare provider's recommendation, typically on an empty stomach for better absorption.

2. Gradually increase the dose as tolerated, up to the recommended daily intake.

Anti-Inflammatory Diet for Reducing Gut Inflammation

- **Portions**: Varies

- **Preparation time**: Varies based on meal preparation

Ingredients:

- A variety of anti-inflammatory foods such as leafy greens, berries, nuts, seeds, and fatty fish

- **Instructions**:

1. Incorporate a wide range of anti-inflammatory foods into daily meals.

2. Focus on whole, unprocessed foods to reduce intake of inflammatory additives and sugars.

3. Stay hydrated and avoid known food allergens and irritants.

Stress Reduction Techniques for Gut Health

Beneficial effects: Managing stress is vital for healing leaky gut as stress can exacerbate gut permeability and inflammation.

- **Instructions**:

1. Practice daily mindfulness or meditation to reduce stress levels.

2. Engage in regular, gentle exercise like walking or yoga.

3. Ensure adequate sleep and adopt a bedtime routine to improve sleep quality.

Scientific references:

- Research indicates that bone broth contains collagen, glutamine, and other compounds that can support the repair of the intestinal lining.

- Studies have shown that fermented foods enhance the diversity and health of the gut microbiome, which is crucial for gut barrier integrity.

- L-Glutamine supplementation has been documented to promote the regeneration of the gut lining and reduce intestinal permeability.

- An anti-inflammatory diet has been associated with reduced markers of inflammation and may help in managing conditions related to leaky gut syndrome.

Incorporating these strategies into a comprehensive approach can significantly contribute to healing leaky gut, improving not only digestive health but also overall well-being. Always consult with a healthcare professional before making significant changes to your diet or starting new supplements, especially if you have existing health conditions or are taking medication.

CHAPTER 4: 5 HERBAL RECIPES FOR GUT HEALTH

SLIPPERY ELM PORRIDGE

Beneficial effects

Slippery Elm Porridge is a soothing, nutritious recipe designed to support gut health and digestion. The mucilage properties of slippery elm can help coat and protect the digestive tract, easing inflammation, and providing relief from conditions such as acid reflux, gastritis, and irritable bowel syndrome (IBS). It's also rich in fiber, which can aid in regular bowel movements and overall digestive health.

Portions

2 servings

Preparation time

5 minutes

Cooking time

10 minutes

Ingredients

- 2 cups water or almond milk

- 1 cup rolled oats

- 2 tablespoons slippery elm bark powder

- 1 tablespoon maple syrup or honey (optional, for sweetness)

- 1/2 teaspoon cinnamon (optional, for flavor)

- Fresh fruit or nuts for topping (optional)

Instructions

1. In a medium saucepan, bring the water or almond milk to a boil.

2. Reduce the heat to medium and stir in the rolled oats. Cook for about 5 minutes, stirring occasionally.

3. Reduce the heat to low and mix in the slippery elm bark powder, stirring continuously to prevent clumps.

4. Add the maple syrup or honey and cinnamon, if using, and stir until well combined.

5. Cook for an additional 5 minutes on low heat, or until the porridge reaches your desired consistency.

6. Remove from heat and let it sit for a couple of minutes to thicken further.

7. Serve warm, topped with fresh fruit or nuts if desired.

Variations

- For a vegan version, ensure to use almond milk and maple syrup instead of honey.

- Incorporate a tablespoon of ground flaxseed or chia seeds for extra fiber and omega-3 fatty acids.

- Spice up the porridge with a pinch of nutmeg or cardamom for additional flavor complexity.

Storage tips

Store any leftover porridge in an airtight container in the refrigerator for up to 2 days. Reheat on the stove or in the microwave, adding a little water or almond milk to adjust consistency if necessary.

Tips for allergens

For those with gluten sensitivities, ensure to use certified gluten-free oats. If allergic to nuts, avoid using almond milk and opt for water or a non-nut-based milk alternative like oat milk or rice milk.

Scientific references

- "Slippery Elm, its Biochemistry, and use as a Complementary and Alternative Treatment for Laryngeal Irritation." Journal of Investigational Biochemistry, 2012. This study discusses the mucilage content of slippery elm and its beneficial effects on the digestive and respiratory tracts.

- "Dietary Fiber and Prebiotics and the Gastrointestinal Microbiota." Gut Microbes, 2017. This article highlights the importance of fiber for gut health and how it supports the growth of beneficial gut bacteria.

MARSHMALLOW ROOT TEA

Beneficial effects

Marshmallow Root Tea is known for its soothing properties, particularly for the digestive system. It can help relieve irritation and inflammation in the gut lining, making it beneficial for those with digestive issues such as gastritis, indigestion, and acid reflux. The mucilage content of marshmallow root forms a protective layer on the digestive tract, promoting healing and reducing discomfort.

Portions

1 serving

Preparation time

15 minutes

Cooking time

5 minutes

Ingredients

- 2 tablespoons dried marshmallow root

- 8 ounces of filtered water

- Honey or lemon (optional, for taste)

Instructions

1. Boil 8 ounces of water in a small pot.

2. Remove from heat and add 2 tablespoons of dried marshmallow root to the hot water.

3. Cover the pot and allow it to steep for about 10 to 15 minutes. This long steeping time allows the mucilage properties of the marshmallow root to be fully released.

4. Strain the tea into a cup, removing the marshmallow root.

5. Optional: Add honey or lemon to taste for flavor enhancement.

6. Enjoy the tea while warm for the best soothing effect on the digestive system.

Variations

- For a cold remedy, add a slice of fresh ginger during the steeping process to enhance the tea's soothing properties.

- Combine with chamomile tea for additional relaxation and digestive benefits.

Storage tips

Dried marshmallow root should be stored in a cool, dry place, away from direct sunlight and moisture, to maintain its potency and freshness.

Tips for allergens

For those with specific plant allergies, it's important to ensure that marshmallow root does not trigger a similar reaction. Always start with a small amount to test for any adverse effects.

Scientific references

- "The effect of herbal teas on the relief of irritable bowel syndrome: A systematic review," Journal of Ethnopharmacology, 2020. This review highlights the effectiveness of herbal teas, including marshmallow root, in managing symptoms of IBS due to their anti-inflammatory and soothing properties.

LICORICE ROOT DECOCTION

Beneficial effects

Licorice Root Decoction is known for its soothing properties that can help alleviate various digestive issues, including heartburn, stomach ulcers, and gastritis. It has anti-inflammatory and immune-boosting effects, which contribute to healing the gut lining and reducing irritation. Additionally, licorice root can help in managing symptoms of acid reflux and improving overall gut health.

Portions

Makes about 4 cups

Preparation time

5 minutes

Cooking time

15 minutes

Ingredients

- 1 tablespoon dried licorice root

- 4 cups water

Instructions

1. Combine 4 cups of water and 1 tablespoon of dried licorice root in a medium-sized pot.

2. Bring the mixture to a boil over high heat.

3. Once boiling, reduce the heat to low and let it simmer for about 15 minutes.

4. After simmering, remove the pot from the heat and allow it to cool slightly.

5. Strain the decoction through a fine mesh sieve or cheesecloth into a large pitcher or jar, discarding the solid pieces of licorice root.

6. Serve the decoction warm, or allow it to cool completely for a refreshing cold drink.

Variations

- For a sweeter taste, add a teaspoon of honey or maple syrup while the decoction is still warm.

- Enhance the digestive benefits by adding a slice of fresh ginger or a cinnamon stick during the simmering process.

- Combine with chamomile tea for additional soothing and relaxing effects on the digestive system.

Storage tips

Store any leftover licorice root decoction in the refrigerator for up to 48 hours. Ensure it's in a sealed container to maintain freshness and prevent absorption of other flavors or odors.

Tips for allergens

Individuals with hypertension should be cautious with licorice root consumption, as it can affect blood pressure levels. For those with concerns about licorice root's potential effects on health, consider consulting with a healthcare provider before incorporating it into your regimen.

Scientific references

- "The effect of deglycyrrhizinated licorice on peptic ulcer: Systematic review and meta-analysis" - Journal of Ethnopharmacology, 2018. This study highlights the beneficial effects of licorice root, particularly its deglycyrrhizinated form, on peptic ulcers and overall digestive health.

ALOE VERA JUICE

Beneficial effects

Aloe Vera Juice is renowned for its soothing and healing properties, especially for the digestive tract. It can help to reduce inflammation in the gut, promote regularity, and enhance the absorption of nutrients. Aloe Vera is also known for its hydrating properties, making it beneficial for skin health and overall hydration.

Portions

2 servings

Preparation time

10 minutes

Ingredients

- 1 large Aloe Vera leaf (approximately 1/2 cup of Aloe Vera gel)
- 2 cups of water or coconut water
- 1 tablespoon of honey or agave syrup (optional, for sweetness)
- Juice of 1 lemon or lime (optional, for flavor)

Instructions

1. Carefully slice off the serrated edges of the Aloe Vera leaf.

2. Split the leaf open with a knife and use a spoon to scoop out the clear gel inside.

3. Rinse the gel with cold water to remove any remaining aloin (a laxative compound in the latex).

4. Place the Aloe Vera gel into a blender.

5. Add 2 cups of water or coconut water to the blender.

6. If desired, add honey or agave syrup for sweetness and lemon or lime juice for flavor.

7. Blend on high speed for about 30 seconds or until completely smooth.

8. Strain the mixture using a fine mesh sieve or cheesecloth to remove any pulp or residue.

9. Serve the Aloe Vera Juice immediately or chill in the refrigerator before serving.

Variations

- For a refreshing twist, add a handful of fresh mint leaves or a piece of ginger to the blender before mixing.
- Incorporate a cup of your favorite fresh fruit, such as strawberries or mango, for added flavor and nutrients.
- For an extra health boost, add a scoop of protein powder or a teaspoon of spirulina powder to the blend.

Storage tips

Store any leftover Aloe Vera Juice in an airtight container in the refrigerator for up to 24 hours. Shake well before consuming if separation occurs.

Tips for allergens

Individuals with sensitivity to Aloe Vera should start with a small amount to ensure no adverse reactions occur. For those with allergies to honey or agave, the sweetener can be omitted or replaced with a suitable alternative like stevia.

Scientific references

- "Aloe Vera: A Short Review" - Indian Journal of Dermatology. This review discusses the moisturizing, anti-inflammatory, and healing effects of Aloe Vera, particularly in the context of skin and digestive health.

- "Effect of Aloe Vera juice on growth and activities of Lactobacilli in-vitro" - Acta Poloniae Pharmaceutica. This study highlights the potential of Aloe Vera juice to support the growth of beneficial gut bacteria, contributing to healthy digestion.

FENNEL SEED INFUSION

Beneficial effects

Fennel Seed Infusion is known for its ability to soothe the digestive system, reduce bloating, and alleviate gas pains. It's rich in volatile oils that contribute to its antispasmodic properties, helping to relax the gastrointestinal tract muscles. This infusion can also aid in improving nutrient absorption and promoting a healthy appetite.

Portions

2 servings

Preparation time

5 minutes

Cooking time

5-10 minutes

Ingredients

- 2 teaspoons of fennel seeds
- 2 cups of boiling water
- Honey or lemon (optional, for taste)

Instructions

1. Crush the fennel seeds lightly with a mortar and pestle to release their oil.

2. Place the crushed fennel seeds in a teapot or a heat-resistant glass container.

3. Pour 2 cups of boiling water over the fennel seeds.

4. Cover and let the infusion steep for 5-10 minutes, depending on your preferred strength.

5. Strain the infusion into cups, discarding the fennel seeds.

6. If desired, add honey or lemon to taste before serving.

Variations

- For a refreshing twist, add a slice of fresh ginger or a few mint leaves to the infusion while steeping.

- Combine with chamomile flowers for a more relaxing and sleep-promoting beverage.

- For a cooler drink, allow the infusion to cool down and serve it over ice.

Storage tips

It's best to enjoy the Fennel Seed Infusion fresh. However, if you have leftovers, you can store them in a sealed container in the refrigerator for up to 2 days. Reheat gently or enjoy cold.

Tips for allergens

If you're sensitive to pollen or have a known allergy to carrots or celery, as fennel belongs to the same botanical family, start with a small amount to ensure no adverse reactions occur.

Scientific references

- "The effect of fennel (Foeniculum Vulgare) seed oil emulsion in infantile colic: a randomized, placebo-controlled study" published in Alternative Therapies in Health and Medicine, 2003. This study supports the antispasmodic and gas-relieving effects of fennel on the digestive system.

PART 4: IMMUNE SYSTEM SUPPORT

Supporting the immune system is a cornerstone of maintaining health and well-being, a fact that underscores the importance of adopting a holistic approach to health care. The immune system, a complex network of cells, tissues, and organs, works tirelessly to protect the body from pathogens, including bacteria, viruses, and fungi. A strong immune system relies on a balanced and nutritious diet, regular physical activity, adequate rest, and effective stress management techniques. Herbal remedies, known for their immune-boosting properties, play a significant role in supporting and enhancing the body's natural defense mechanisms.

Echinacea, for example, is widely recognized for its ability to enhance the immune response. This herb stimulates the activity of immune system cells, such as macrophages and T-cells, which play critical roles in fighting off infections. Incorporating echinacea into your wellness routine can be as simple as enjoying it in a tea or taking it as a supplement during cold and flu season to help ward off illnesses.

Another powerful immune-supportive herb is elderberry. Rich in antioxidants and vitamins that can boost the immune system, elderberry has been shown to reduce the duration and severity of colds and flu. Elderberry syrups and extracts are popular ways to take this herb, providing a tasty and beneficial addition to one's health regimen.

Astragalus root, a staple in traditional Chinese medicine, is revered for its immune-boosting and antiviral properties. It's believed to increase the body's production of white blood cells, which are crucial for fighting off infections. Astragalus can be taken as a supplement, added to soups, or brewed as a tea, making it a versatile option for enhancing immune health.

Garlic, with its potent antiviral and antibacterial properties, is another simple yet powerful way to support the immune system. Regular consumption of garlic can help prevent colds and other infections, thanks to its active compound allicin. Adding garlic to meals not only boosts flavor but also provides significant health benefits.

Maintaining hydration is essential for overall health, including the immune system. Water plays a key role in the production of lymph, which carries white blood cells and other immune system cells through the body. Proper hydration ensures that the immune system operates efficiently, and incorporating herbal teas can provide additional immune support.

Stress management is also crucial for immune health, as chronic stress can suppress the immune response. Techniques such as meditation, yoga, and deep breathing exercises can help reduce stress levels, thereby supporting the immune system. Incorporating these practices into daily life can enhance overall well-being and provide the body with the resilience it needs to fend off illnesses.

In addition to these strategies, regular physical activity and adequate sleep are foundational elements of a strong immune system. Exercise promotes circulation, which allows immune cells to move through the body more effectively, while sleep provides the body with the opportunity to repair and regenerate immune cells.

By embracing a holistic approach to health that includes a balanced diet, herbal remedies, hydration, stress management, physical activity, and rest, individuals can support their immune system and enhance their body's natural defenses against disease. This comprehensive strategy not only contributes to a robust immune system but also to a vibrant, healthy life.

Optimizing gut health is another essential aspect of supporting the immune system, as a significant portion of the immune system is located in the gut. Probiotics, beneficial bacteria found in fermented foods like yogurt, kefir, sauerkraut, and kombucha, help maintain a healthy balance of gut flora, which in turn supports immune function. These probiotics can enhance the intestinal barrier, inhibit the growth of harmful bacteria, and stimulate the body's production of natural antibodies.

Vitamin D plays a pivotal role in immune health as well, with studies showing that it can modulate the immune response. Vitamin D deficiency has been linked to an increased susceptibility to infection. While sunlight is the best natural source of vitamin D, supplements can also be beneficial, especially in regions with limited sun exposure. Foods rich in vitamin D, such as fatty fish, egg yolks, and fortified foods, should also be included in the diet.

Zinc is a mineral critical for the development and function of immune cells. Incorporating zinc-rich foods like seeds, nuts, legumes, and whole grains into the diet can help ensure adequate zinc levels, which support immune response and healing processes.

Antioxidant-rich foods, such as fruits and vegetables, combat oxidative stress and inflammation, thereby supporting the immune system. Berries, leafy greens, nuts, and seeds are all excellent sources of antioxidants and should be consumed regularly to help protect the body against infections.

Herbal teas, beyond providing hydration, can offer various immune-boosting benefits depending on the herbs used. For instance, green tea is rich in antioxidants, while chamomile tea can help reduce stress and promote sleep, both of which are beneficial for immune health.

Maintaining a healthy weight is also important for immune function, as obesity has been linked to impaired immunity. A diet rich in whole, plant-based foods can support weight management and provide the nutrients necessary for optimal immune function.

Finally, minimizing toxin exposure by choosing organic foods when possible, using natural cleaning and personal care products, and avoiding smoking and excessive alcohol consumption can help reduce the burden on the immune system, allowing it to function more effectively.

By integrating these practices into daily life, individuals can create a comprehensive and natural strategy for bolstering the immune system. This holistic approach not only supports the body's ability to fend off infections but also promotes overall health and longevity, empowering individuals to lead vibrant, healthy lives.

CHAPTER 1: DR. BARBARA'S IMMUNE PRINCIPLES

D r. Barbara emphasizes the significance of nurturing the immune system as a fundamental aspect of achieving and maintaining optimal health. The immune system, a complex and dynamic network, defends the body against infections, diseases, and environmental aggressors. To support this vital system, Dr. Barbara advocates for a holistic approach that integrates nutrition, herbal remedies, lifestyle modifications, and mindful practices.

A cornerstone of Dr. Barbara's immune health principles is the incorporation of nutrient-dense, whole foods into the diet. Foods rich in vitamins C and E, beta-carotene, zinc, and selenium play pivotal roles in enhancing immune function. Citrus fruits, berries, nuts, seeds, leafy greens, and colorful vegetables are not only packed with essential nutrients but also antioxidants that help combat oxidative stress, a known immune suppressor.

Herbal remedies are another key component of Dr. Barbara's approach. Herbs such as echinacea, astragalus, and elderberry are celebrated for their immune-boosting properties. Echinacea is utilized for its ability to enhance the immune response, astragalus is known for its deep immune system support, especially in preventing colds and upper respiratory infections, and elderberry is prized for its antiviral effects against flu viruses. These herbs can be consumed in various forms, including teas, tinctures, and supplements, offering a natural and effective means to bolster the immune system.

Hydration is emphasized as essential for immune health. Water is crucial for the production of lymph, a fluid in the circulatory system that carries immune cells throughout the body. Adequate hydration ensures these cells can travel freely and function optimally. Herbal teas, such as green tea, are recommended for their additional antioxidant benefits and immune support.

Stress management is identified as a critical factor in immune health. Chronic stress can lead to elevated cortisol levels, which may suppress immune function. Dr. Barbara encourages practices such as meditation, yoga, and deep breathing exercises to help manage stress and support the immune system. These practices not only reduce stress but also improve overall well-being, creating a positive feedback loop that enhances immune function.

Physical activity is highlighted for its role in promoting a healthy immune system. Regular, moderate exercise can improve circulation, allowing immune cells to move more efficiently throughout the body. Exercise also helps to alleviate stress and improve sleep, both of which are beneficial for immune health.

Sleep quality is directly linked to immune function. Adequate rest allows the body to repair and regenerate immune cells, making sleep a priority for anyone looking to support their immune system. Dr. Barbara suggests establishing a calming bedtime routine and aiming for 7-9 hours of sleep per night to ensure the immune system has the resources it needs to protect the body effectively.

Lastly, Dr. Barbara underscores the importance of a supportive environment for immune health. This includes not only the physical environment, such as maintaining a clean and toxin-free living space but also the social and emotional environment. Positive relationships and a strong support network can have profound effects on stress levels and, by extension, immune health.

By following Dr. Barbara's immune health principles, individuals can empower themselves to support and enhance their immune system through natural, holistic means. This comprehensive approach not only fosters immune resilience but also promotes a lifestyle conducive to overall health and longevity.

FACTORS THAT WEAKEN IMMUNITY

Several factors can significantly weaken the immune system, leaving the body more susceptible to infections and diseases. Poor nutrition, characterized by a diet lacking in essential vitamins and minerals, undermines the body's ability to fight off pathogens. Vitamins A, C, D, E, and minerals such as zinc and selenium are crucial for maintaining robust immune function. A diet high in processed foods, sugars, and unhealthy fats can lead to deficiencies in these vital nutrients.

Chronic stress is another major culprit that impairs immune function. When stress is prolonged, it triggers the release of the hormone cortisol, which, in high levels, suppresses the effectiveness of the immune system. Similarly, inadequate sleep disrupts the production of infection-fighting antibodies and cells, making it harder for the body to combat infections.

Lack of physical activity contributes to a weakened immune system as well. Regular, moderate exercise boosts circulation, allowing immune cells to move through the body more efficiently. On the flip side, obesity has been linked to a decreased immune response due to inflammation and the potential for immune cell dysfunction.

Excessive alcohol consumption and smoking are known to compromise immune defense mechanisms. Alcohol disrupts immune pathways in complex ways, impairing the body's ability to defend against infection. Smoking damages the immune system by increasing the risk of bronchitis and pneumonia, among other diseases, and it reduces the levels of protective antioxidants in the blood.

Environmental toxins, including pollutants and chemicals found in everyday products, can also weaken the immune system by introducing substances that the body must detoxify, diverting the immune system's attention away from pathogens.

Finally, certain medications, especially those that suppress the immune system like corticosteroids and chemotherapy drugs, can reduce the body's ability to fight infections. While these medications are often necessary for treating specific conditions, they can leave the body more vulnerable to other diseases.

Addressing these factors through lifestyle changes, such as adopting a balanced diet, managing stress, getting adequate sleep, engaging in regular physical activity, and avoiding harmful substances, can significantly bolster the immune system's ability to protect the body.

SIGNS OF A COMPROMISED IMMUNE SYSTEM

Recognizing signs of a compromised immune system is crucial for taking proactive steps towards health and well-being. Frequent colds and infections indicate that the immune system may be struggling to fend off pathogens. Typically, adults might expect to get two to three colds a year; a higher frequency could suggest an immune deficiency. Another sign is prolonged recovery times, where even minor infections lead to extended periods of illness, indicating the immune system's response is not as robust as it should be.

Chronic fatigue, unlinked to changes in sleep patterns or physical exertion, often points to an underlying issue with immune function. The body may be expending extra energy to fight off viruses or bacteria, leading to persistent tiredness. Digestive issues like loss of appetite, diarrhea, and abdominal cramping can also signal immune distress, as a significant portion of the immune system is located in the gut. Disruptions in gut flora can impact overall immunity.

Wounds that are slow to heal suggest compromised skin integrity and an immune system struggling to perform its reparative function. The skin acts as a barrier against external pathogens, and when healing is delayed, it can indicate weakened immune defenses. Additionally, frequent infections such as pneumonia, bronchitis, or sinus infections can be a red flag, especially if they recur or become chronic.

An increase in autoimmune responses, where the body mistakenly attacks its cells, can also indicate an overburdened or malfunctioning immune system. Conditions such as rheumatoid arthritis or lupus are characterized by this misdirected immune response and can manifest in various symptoms across the body.

Lastly, experiencing severe reactions to common colds or viruses, where symptoms are disproportionately intense or lead to complications, can signal an immune system that is not adequately protecting the body. Recognizing these signs early and consulting with a healthcare professional can help address underlying issues, support immune health, and prevent more serious health problems.

STRENGTHENING IMMUNITY THROUGH LIFESTYLE CHOICES

Strengthening immunity through lifestyle choices involves adopting habits and practices that enhance the body's natural defenses against disease and infection. A balanced diet rich in fruits, vegetables, whole grains, lean proteins, and healthy fats provides the essential nutrients that the immune system needs to function optimally. These foods supply vitamins, minerals, antioxidants, and phytonutrients that support immune health, reduce inflammation, and protect against oxidative stress. Regular physical activity is another pillar of strong immunity. Exercise promotes circulation, helping immune cells to move more efficiently throughout the body to detect and combat pathogens. It also aids in reducing stress and improving sleep, both of which are crucial for maintaining a healthy immune response.

Adequate hydration is vital for immunity as water is necessary for the production of lymph, a fluid that carries white blood cells and other immune cells. Drinking plenty of water, herbal teas, and consuming water-rich fruits and vegetables helps to keep the lymphatic system working effectively. Managing stress through mindfulness practices, meditation, yoga, or deep breathing exercises helps to lower cortisol levels, a stress hormone that can suppress immune function when chronically elevated. Ensuring sufficient, quality sleep each night allows the body to repair and regenerate immune cells, making sleep a critical component of immune health.

Minimizing exposure to toxins by choosing organic foods when possible, using natural cleaning and personal care products, and avoiding smoking and excessive alcohol consumption reduces the burden on the immune system, allowing it to respond more effectively to pathogens. Additionally, fostering positive relationships and a supportive social network can influence immune health positively by reducing stress and promoting feelings of well-being.

Incorporating probiotics through fermented foods like yogurt, kefir, sauerkraut, and kombucha supports gut health, where a significant portion of the immune system resides. These beneficial bacteria help to balance the gut microbiome, enhancing the gut barrier function and the body's ability to fend off pathogens. Supplementation with vitamins and minerals such as vitamin D, zinc, and omega-3 fatty acids, when dietary intake is insufficient, can further support immune function. Vitamin D, for instance, modulates the immune response and has been linked to a lower risk of viral infections.

By integrating these lifestyle choices into daily routines, individuals can bolster their immune system, reduce their susceptibility to infections, and enhance their overall health and well-being. These practices, combined with regular healthcare check-ups and vaccinations as recommended, form a comprehensive approach to strengthening immunity and promoting a vibrant, healthy life.

DR. BARBARA'S IMMUNE-STRENGTHENING STRATEGIES

Dr. Barbara's immune-strengthening strategies focus on harnessing natural remedies and lifestyle adjustments to fortify the body's defenses. Central to her approach is the belief that certain herbs, when incorporated into daily routines, can significantly enhance immune function. Echinacea, known for its ability to stimulate the immune system, is recommended for regular use, especially during times when the body might be more susceptible to infections, such as the cold and flu seasons. A simple echinacea tea, made by steeping the dried herb in hot water, can be a comforting and effective way to ingest this powerful plant.

Astragalus root, another cornerstone of Dr. Barbara's strategy, offers deep immune support, particularly in bolstering the body's resistance to stress and infection. Incorporating astragalus into the diet through soups or teas can provide a steady foundation for immune health. Garlic, with its potent antimicrobial and antiviral properties, is advised for daily consumption. Its active compounds, including allicin, have been shown to fight off common pathogens, making garlic a simple yet powerful addition to meals.

Dr. Barbara also emphasizes the importance of vitamin D for immune strength. With many individuals lacking adequate exposure to sunlight, resulting in vitamin D deficiency, she suggests seeking out natural food sources of vitamin D, such as fatty fish and egg yolks, and considering supplementation as necessary. Regular, moderate exposure to sunlight, when possible, is also encouraged to naturally boost vitamin D levels, which in turn supports the immune system.

Zinc is highlighted for its critical role in immune cell function and signaling. A zinc-rich diet, including seeds, nuts, and whole grains, can help ensure the immune system operates at its best. For those who struggle to get enough zinc from food alone, Dr. Barbara recommends exploring zinc supplements, always adhering to the recommended daily allowances to avoid toxicity.

Probiotics play a pivotal role in Dr. Barbara's immune-strengthening strategies, given their influence on gut health and, by extension, the immune system. Regular consumption of fermented foods like yogurt, kefir, and sauerkraut can help maintain a healthy balance of gut flora, which is essential for immune function. For individuals who do not consume these foods regularly, probiotic supplements may be a beneficial alternative.

Hydration is underscored as a key element in maintaining immune health. Water not only transports nutrients to where they're needed but also removes toxins from the body, thus supporting the immune system's function. Herbal teas, particularly those made from immune-supporting herbs like green tea, ginger, and turmeric, offer additional benefits, including antioxidants and anti-inflammatory properties.

Finally, Dr. Barbara advocates for a holistic approach to stress management, recognizing the detrimental impact of chronic stress on immune function. Practices such as yoga, meditation, and deep breathing exercises are recommended to reduce stress and support overall well-being. By integrating these strategies into daily life, individuals can create a comprehensive and natural approach to enhancing their immune system, promoting resilience against infections and diseases, and supporting long-term health and vitality.

CHAPTER 2: NUTRITION FOR IMMUNE HEALTH

Focusing on nutrition for immune health involves incorporating foods rich in specific nutrients that are known to enhance the immune system's ability to fight off infections and diseases. A diet that supports immune health is diverse and includes a variety of fruits, vegetables, proteins, whole grains, and healthy fats, each playing a unique role in maintaining and boosting the body's natural defenses.

Vitamins A, C, and E are powerful antioxidants that help to combat oxidative stress, a condition that can weaken the immune response. Vitamin A can be found in sweet potatoes, carrots, and dark leafy greens, while citrus fruits, strawberries, and bell peppers are excellent sources of vitamin C. Vitamin E-rich foods include nuts, seeds, and spinach. These antioxidants support the immune system by protecting cells from damage and supporting the body's ability to fight off invading pathogens.

Zinc is a mineral crucial for the development and function of immune cells. Incorporating zinc-rich foods like beef, shellfish, hemp seeds, and pumpkin seeds into meals can help ensure the body has enough zinc to support healthy immune function.

Zinc acts directly on pathogens and supports the immune response, making it a critical nutrient for fighting infections.

Selenium is another essential mineral for immune health, playing a role in preventing cell damage and enhancing immunity. Foods high in selenium include Brazil nuts, seafood, and mushrooms. Just a few Brazil nuts can provide the daily recommended intake of selenium, supporting antioxidant activity and overall immune function.

Omega-3 fatty acids, found in fatty fish like salmon and mackerel, as well as in flaxseeds and walnuts, are known for their anti-inflammatory properties. Chronic inflammation can suppress the immune system, so incorporating omega-3s into the diet can help reduce inflammation and support immune health.

Probiotic foods like yogurt, kefir, sauerkraut, and kombucha support gut health, where a significant portion of the immune system is located.

These foods introduce beneficial bacteria to the digestive system, enhancing the gut microbiome and, in turn, supporting immune function. A healthy gut microbiome can improve the body's defense against harmful pathogens and support overall immune health.

Prebiotic foods, such as garlic, onions, asparagus, and bananas, provide nourishment for beneficial gut bacteria and help maintain a healthy gut microbiome. A diet rich in prebiotics can enhance the effectiveness of probiotics and, by extension, support immune health.

Hydration is essential for overall health and plays a critical role in supporting the immune system. Water helps in the production of lymph, which carries white blood cells and other immune cells throughout the body. Staying hydrated ensures that the immune system can function efficiently, and incorporating herbal teas can provide additional immune support with their antioxidant and anti-inflammatory properties.

Incorporating these nutrients and foods into a balanced diet can significantly support and enhance the immune system. Eating a variety of nutrient-rich foods ensures that the body receives the vitamins, minerals, and other compounds it needs to maintain a strong immune response, protect against illness, and promote overall health and well-being.

IMMUNE-BOOSTING FOODS

Eating a diet rich in immune-boosting foods is a powerful way to support your body's ability to fend off illnesses and maintain optimal health. These foods are packed with essential nutrients that strengthen the immune system's response to pathogens. Incorporating a variety of these foods into your daily diet can make a significant difference in how your body responds to external threats.

Sweet potatoes, carrots, and dark leafy greens are excellent sources of Vitamin A, an antioxidant that plays a critical role in enhancing immune function by maintaining the integrity of skin and mucosal cells, which are the body's first line of defense against pathogens. Citrus fruits, strawberries, and bell peppers, rich in Vitamin C, help stimulate the production and function of white blood cells, which are key players in fighting infections. Vitamin E, found in nuts, seeds, and spinach, acts as a powerful antioxidant that helps the body fight off infection.

Zinc is essential for immune cell development and communication and can be found in beef, shellfish, hemp seeds, and pumpkin seeds. It plays a vital role in the inflammatory response and significantly affects the outcome of health during illness. Selenium, another immune-essential mineral, supports the body's antioxidant defense system and can be found in Brazil nuts, seafood, and mushrooms. Just a small amount of selenium-rich foods can meet your daily requirement and aid in boosting your immune health.

Omega-3 fatty acids, known for their anti-inflammatory properties, are crucial for managing inflammation and maintaining a healthy immune system. Fatty fish like salmon and mackerel, as well as flaxseeds and walnuts, are rich sources of omega-3s. Chronic inflammation can suppress your immune system, so incorporating these foods into your diet is beneficial for immune support.

Probiotic foods such as yogurt, kefir, sauerkraut, and kombucha introduce beneficial bacteria to your gut, where a significant portion of the immune system resides. These foods enhance the gut microbiome, which in turn supports immune function. A healthy gut microbiome is essential for protecting the body against harmful pathogens.

Prebiotic foods like garlic, onions, asparagus, and bananas nourish the beneficial gut bacteria and help maintain a healthy gut environment, further supporting immune health.

Hydration plays a crucial role in immune health as well. Water aids in the production of lymph, which carries white blood cells and other immune cells throughout the body. Ensuring you stay hydrated allows your immune system to function more efficiently. Herbal teas can also offer additional immune support with their antioxidant and anti-inflammatory properties.

By incorporating these immune-boosting foods into a balanced diet, you provide your body with the necessary tools to maintain a strong immune response, protect against illness, and promote overall health and well-being. Remember, a diverse diet rich in vitamins, minerals, and other essential nutrients is key to supporting a healthy immune system.

THE ROLE OF ANTIOXIDANTS

Antioxidants play a crucial role in supporting the immune system by protecting the body against damage from free radicals, which are unstable molecules that can harm cellular structures. These free radicals are produced during normal metabolic processes but can increase dramatically during times of environmental stress, such as exposure to pollution, radiation, and toxins. The body's defense against free radicals involves a variety of antioxidants that can neutralize these harmful molecules, preventing them from causing cellular damage that can lead to chronic inflammation and various diseases.

Vitamins A, C, and E, along with minerals like selenium and compounds found in plants such as flavonoids and carotenoids, are potent antioxidants. Each of these antioxidants contributes uniquely to the immune defense. Vitamin C, for example, not only acts directly to neutralize free radicals but also helps to regenerate other antioxidants, including vitamin E, thereby enhancing the body's overall antioxidant defense system. Additionally, vitamin C supports the production and function of white blood cells, which are essential for fighting infections.

Selenium, a trace mineral, plays a role in the prevention of cellular damage from free radicals. Its antioxidant properties help in maintaining a healthy immune system by preventing the oxidative stress that can lead to inflammation and disease. Foods rich in selenium, such as Brazil nuts, seafood, and mushrooms, can provide this essential nutrient in significant amounts.

The body also produces its own antioxidants, such as glutathione, which is considered one of the most powerful antioxidants. Glutathione plays a key role in reducing oxidative stress and supporting the immune system. However, the body's ability to produce glutathione and other antioxidants can be affected by diet, lifestyle, and environmental factors.

Thus, consuming foods high in antioxidants is vital for maintaining optimal levels of these protective compounds.

Incorporating a variety of antioxidant-rich foods into the diet can enhance the body's ability to fight off infections and reduce the risk of chronic diseases. Fruits and vegetables are particularly high in antioxidants, with berries, leafy greens, nuts, and seeds being excellent sources. By focusing on a diet that includes these foods, individuals can support their immune health and protect against the damaging effects of free radicals.

Moreover, certain herbs and spices, such as turmeric, ginger, and cinnamon, have been recognized for their antioxidant properties. These can be easily incorporated into meals and beverages to boost the body's antioxidant intake. Green tea is another excellent source of antioxidants, specifically catechins, which have been shown to enhance immune function and protect against oxidative stress.

To maximize the benefits of antioxidants for immune health, it's important to consume a diverse range of these nutrients, as they work synergistically to protect the body. This means eating a wide variety of colorful fruits and vegetables, nuts, seeds, whole grains, and healthy fats, all of which contribute to a robust antioxidant defense system. By doing so, individuals can support their immune system, reduce inflammation, and promote overall health and well-being.

DR. BARBARA'S ANTI-INFLAMMATORY DIET TIPS

Adopting an anti-inflammatory diet is a cornerstone of enhancing immune health and overall well-being. Chronic inflammation is a root cause of many diseases, and by focusing on anti-inflammatory foods, you can significantly reduce your risk of health issues and support your body's natural defense system.

Dr. Barbara recommends incorporating a variety of foods rich in antioxidants, omega-3 fatty acids, and phytonutrients to combat inflammation and boost your immune system.

Start by increasing your intake of fruits and vegetables, aiming for a colorful plate at every meal. These foods are high in antioxidants, which neutralize harmful free radicals that can cause inflammation. Berries, leafy greens, and beets are particularly beneficial, offering a high concentration of vitamins, minerals, and flavonoids that support immune health and reduce inflammation.

Omega-3 fatty acids are another critical component of an anti-inflammatory diet. Fatty fish like salmon, mackerel, and sardines are excellent sources of omega-3s, which have been shown to reduce inflammation and support heart and brain health. For vegetarians or those who do not consume fish, flaxseeds, chia seeds, and walnuts are great plant-based sources of omega-3s.

Incorporating whole grains into your diet can also help reduce inflammation. Unlike refined grains, whole grains are rich in fiber, which has been shown to lower levels of C-reactive protein, a marker of inflammation in the blood. Choose quinoa, brown rice, oats, and barley to keep your digestive system healthy and reduce inflammation.

Spices and herbs are not only great for adding flavor to your dishes but also possess powerful anti-inflammatory properties. Turmeric, ginger, garlic, and cinnamon are some of the top anti-inflammatory spices that can easily be incorporated into your daily meals. Turmeric, for example, contains curcumin, a compound with strong anti-inflammatory and antioxidant effects.

Hydration is crucial for maintaining optimal health and reducing inflammation.

Water helps flush toxins from the body and ensures that your cells are functioning properly. Aim to drink at least eight glasses of water a day, and consider adding lemon or cucumber for extra flavor and health benefits.

Finally, it's important to limit the intake of foods that can cause inflammation.

Processed foods, sugary snacks, and fried foods are high in trans fats and sugars, which can trigger inflammation. Similarly, reducing the consumption of red meat and processed meats can also help lower inflammation levels in the body.

By following these anti-inflammatory diet tips from Dr. Barbara, you can support your immune system, reduce inflammation, and promote overall health and well-being. Remember, making small changes to your diet can have a significant impact on your health, so start incorporating these foods into your meals today and enjoy the benefits of a balanced, anti-inflammatory diet.

CHAPTER 3: NATURAL IMMUNE-BOOSTING PRACTICES

Daily practices to enhance immune function involve more than just the foods we eat. Engaging in regular physical activity, ensuring adequate sleep, managing stress effectively, and maintaining hygiene can profoundly impact our immune health. Physical activity, even moderate, can stimulate the circulation of immune cells, making it easier for the body to detect and defend against pathogens. Aim for at least 150 minutes of moderate exercise per week, such as brisk walking, cycling, or swimming. This not only aids in circulating immune cells but also reduces inflammation and supports overall well-being.

Adequate sleep is another pillar of strong immune health. During sleep, the body repairs itself, and immune functions are enhanced.

Adults should strive for 7-9 hours of quality sleep per night. Establishing a regular sleep schedule and creating a restful environment free from electronic devices can help improve sleep quality.

Stress management is crucial for immune health as chronic stress can suppress the immune response. Techniques such as meditation, deep breathing exercises, yoga, and mindfulness can reduce stress levels. Even dedicating a few minutes a day to these practices can make a significant difference in lowering stress hormones and boosting immune function.

Maintaining hygiene is fundamental to preventing the spread of pathogens. Regular hand washing with soap and water, especially before eating or touching the face, and after using the restroom or coming into contact with public surfaces, is essential.

Additionally, covering the mouth and nose with a tissue or the elbow when coughing or sneezing can prevent the spread of germs.

Incorporating herbal teas into daily routines can offer immune support due to their antioxidant, anti-inflammatory, and antimicrobial properties. Herbs such as echinacea, ginger, turmeric, and green tea can be brewed into teas and consumed regularly to support immune health. Echinacea is known for its ability to enhance the immune system, ginger and turmeric for their anti-inflammatory effects, and green tea for its high antioxidant content.

Beneficial effects: Enhances immune function, reduces inflammation, supports overall well-being, aids in stress management, and promotes hygiene to prevent the spread of pathogens.

Ingredients:

- Echinacea (1 teaspoon of dried herb or 1 tea bag)

- Ginger (1 inch, fresh or 1 teaspoon powdered)

- Turmeric (1 inch, fresh or 1 teaspoon powdered)

- Green tea (1 tea bag or 1 teaspoon of loose leaves)

Instructions:

1. Boil water in a kettle or pot.

2. If using fresh ginger and turmeric, grate them finely.

3. Place the echinacea, grated ginger, grated turmeric, and green tea in a teapot or large mug.

4. Pour boiling water over the ingredients and let steep for 5-10 minutes.

5. Strain the tea into a cup if using loose ingredients or remove the tea bags.

6. Optional: Add honey or lemon for taste.

Variations: Customize the tea by adding other immune-supporting herbs such as astragalus, lemon balm, or elderberry. Adjust the amount of each ingredient based on personal preference and desired strength.

Storage tips: Fresh ginger and turmeric can be stored in the refrigerator for longevity. Dried herbs and tea bags should be kept in a cool, dry place to preserve their potency.

Tips for allergens: Those with allergies to specific herbs should avoid them and can substitute with other non-allergenic herbs. Always consult with a healthcare provider before starting any new herbal regimen, especially for those with existing health conditions or who are pregnant or breastfeeding.

Scientific references: Studies have demonstrated the immune-boosting properties of echinacea, the anti-inflammatory effects of ginger and turmeric, and the antioxidant benefits of green tea, supporting their use in enhancing immune health.

DAILY PRACTICES TO ENHANCE IMMUNE FUNCTION

Engaging in daily practices that enhance immune function is a cornerstone of maintaining health and preventing illness. These practices, rooted in a holistic health approach, focus on nurturing the body's natural defense mechanisms through lifestyle choices that support physical, emotional, and mental well-being.

Regular physical activity plays a pivotal role in boosting immune function. Exercise promotes the circulation of immune cells, making it easier for the body to fight off infections. Aim to incorporate at least 30 minutes of moderate exercise into your daily routine, such as walking, cycling, or yoga, to stimulate your immune system.

Adequate sleep is essential for immune health, as it allows the body to repair and regenerate. Adults should aim for 7-9 hours of quality sleep each night. Establishing a consistent sleep schedule and creating a calming bedtime routine can significantly improve sleep quality. Avoiding screens and heavy meals before bedtime can also help in achieving restful sleep.

Stress management is crucial for maintaining a healthy immune system.

Chronic stress can suppress immune function, making the body more susceptible to infections. Incorporate stress-reduction techniques such as deep breathing exercises, meditation, and mindfulness into your daily life. Even a few minutes of these practices can lower stress levels and enhance immune function.

Hygiene practices are fundamental in preventing the spread of pathogens. Frequent hand washing with soap and water, especially before meals and after returning home, can reduce the risk of infection. Additionally, practicing good respiratory hygiene, such as covering your mouth and nose with your elbow or a tissue when coughing or sneezing, helps prevent the spread of germs.

Nutrition plays a critical role in supporting the immune system. Focus on a balanced diet rich in fruits, vegetables, whole grains, lean proteins, and healthy fats.

These foods provide essential nutrients, such as vitamins A, C, and E, zinc, and omega-3 fatty acids, that are vital for immune health. Incorporating probiotic-rich foods like yogurt, kefir, and fermented vegetables can also support gut health, which is closely linked to immune function.

Hydration is key to optimal health and immune function. Water supports all bodily functions, including the immune system. Aim to drink at least eight glasses of water a day to stay hydrated. Herbal teas, such as green tea, echinacea, and ginger tea, can also provide immune-boosting benefits.

Incorporating these daily practices into your lifestyle can significantly enhance immune function and contribute to overall health and well-being. Remember, consistency is key, and small, manageable changes can make a big difference in supporting your body's natural defenses.

STRESS MANAGEMENT FOR IMMUNE HEALTH

Managing stress effectively is a critical component of supporting immune health. Chronic stress can lead to an imbalance in immune cell function, making the body more susceptible to infections and diseases. The body's stress response, often referred to as the "fight or flight" response, can be beneficial in short bursts but detrimental to health when activated too frequently or for prolonged periods.

This response releases a flood of stress hormones, like cortisol, which can suppress the immune system's ability to fight off antigens, leaving us more vulnerable to infections.

The beneficial effects of stress management include reduced levels of stress hormones in the body, improved sleep quality, and a lower risk of chronic diseases. These benefits collectively enhance the body's immune function, making it more efficient at fighting off illnesses and maintaining overall well-being.

To manage stress and support immune health, consider incorporating the following practices into your daily routine:

1. **Mindfulness Meditation**: Mindfulness involves paying attention to the present moment without judgment. Regular mindfulness meditation has been shown to reduce stress levels and improve immune function. Start with just a few minutes a day, focusing on your breath or a mantra, and gradually increase the time as you become more comfortable with the practice.

2. **Deep Breathing Exercises**: Deep breathing helps activate the body's relaxation response, reducing stress and enhancing immune function. Practice deep breathing by inhaling slowly through your nose, holding the breath for a few seconds, and then exhaling slowly through your mouth. Repeat this process for several minutes whenever you feel stressed.

3. **Regular Physical Activity**: Exercise not only improves physical health but also reduces stress and boosts the immune system. Aim for at least 30 minutes of moderate exercise most days of the week. Activities like walking, cycling, yoga, or swimming can be particularly beneficial for stress reduction.

4. **Adequate Sleep**: Sleep is essential for immune health. Lack of sleep can increase stress and weaken the immune system. Ensure you get 7-9 hours of quality sleep each night by establishing a regular sleep schedule and creating a restful environment free from electronic devices before bedtime.

5. **Healthy Eating Habits**: A balanced diet rich in fruits, vegetables, whole grains, lean proteins, and healthy fats can support the immune system and reduce stress. Foods high in antioxidants and omega-3 fatty acids are particularly beneficial for combating stress and boosting immune function.

6. **Social Support**: Maintaining strong relationships and having a support system can help manage stress. Spend time with family and friends, join a club or group with similar interests, or consider professional support if needed.

7. **Time Management**: Poor time management can lead to stress. Prioritize tasks, set realistic goals, and take breaks when needed to help manage your time more effectively and reduce stress.

8. **Limiting Stimulants**: Reduce the intake of stimulants such as caffeine and sugar, which can increase stress levels and impact sleep quality.

By integrating these stress management techniques into your lifestyle, you can significantly improve your immune health and overall well-being. Remember, managing stress is not about eliminating stressors but about developing healthy strategies to cope with stress effectively.

DR. BARBARA'S SEASONAL IMMUNE PROTOCOLS

Dr. Barbara's Seasonal Immune Protocols focus on adapting our immune support strategies to the changing seasons, recognizing that our bodies have different needs throughout the year. As we transition from one season to another, our immune system can be particularly vulnerable to seasonal threats. To counteract this, Dr. Barbara recommends a series of natural remedies and lifestyle adjustments tailored to each season's specific challenges.

Beneficial effects: These protocols are designed to bolster the immune system, help the body adapt to seasonal changes, reduce the likelihood of seasonal illnesses, and maintain overall health and vitality throughout the year.

For the **spring**, a time of renewal but also of common allergies, the emphasis is on detoxification and allergy relief.

Ingredients:

- Nettle (to support histamine regulation and relieve allergy symptoms)

- Dandelion root (for detoxification and liver support)

- Vitamin C-rich foods like strawberries and citrus fruits (to boost immune function)

Instructions:

1. Start each day with a cup of nettle tea to manage allergy symptoms. Steep 1 teaspoon of dried nettle in hot water for 10 minutes.

2. Incorporate dandelion root tea into your afternoon routine by steeping 1 teaspoon of the root in hot water for 10-15 minutes, aiding in detoxification.

3. Increase intake of Vitamin C-rich foods throughout the day to support immune health.

Summer focuses on hydration and sun protection to maintain immune strength during the hotter months.

Ingredients:

- Cucumber and mint (for hydrating infused water)

- Green tea (for its antioxidant properties)

- Watermelon and berries (for hydration and vitamins)

Instructions:

1. Prepare a large pitcher of cucumber and mint-infused water and drink throughout the day to stay hydrated.

2. Drink a cup of green tea each morning to benefit from its antioxidant properties.

3. Snack on watermelon and berries, which are high in water content and nutrients, throughout the day.

For **fall**, the protocol prepares the body for colder weather by boosting the immune system and warming the body.

Ingredients:

- Ginger and turmeric (for their immune-boosting and anti-inflammatory properties)

- Pumpkin seeds (rich in zinc, a key nutrient for immune function)

- Herbal teas with echinacea and elderberry

Instructions:

1. Add fresh ginger and turmeric to meals or make a warming tea with these spices to enhance immune function and reduce inflammation.

2. Incorporate a handful of pumpkin seeds into your diet daily to ensure adequate zinc intake.

3. Drink herbal teas containing echinacea and elderberry to further support the immune system.

Winter's protocol focuses on maintaining immune strength and combating the common cold and flu.

Ingredients:

- Garlic (for its antiviral and antibacterial properties)

- Bone broth (for its gut-healing and immune-supporting amino acids)

- Vitamin D-rich foods or supplements (due to reduced sunlight exposure)

Instructions:

1. Include a clove of garlic in your diet each day, whether raw, cooked, or in a warm lemon water concoction, to fight off viruses and bacteria.

2. Consume bone broth regularly, either alone or as a base for soups and stews, to support gut health and immunity.

3. Ensure adequate Vitamin D intake through diet or supplements, considering the reduced exposure to sunlight during these months.

Variations: These protocols can be customized based on individual health needs, dietary restrictions, and local seasonal produce availability. For instance, if allergic to any ingredient, substitute with another with similar health benefits.

Storage tips: Dried herbs should be stored in a cool, dark place to maintain their potency. Fresh produce is best kept in the refrigerator to preserve freshness.

Tips for allergens: For those with specific food allergies, always find suitable substitutes that offer similar nutritional benefits. For instance, if allergic to nuts, seeds like pumpkin or sunflower can be excellent alternatives for zinc intake.

Scientific references: Studies have shown the effectiveness of nettle in managing allergic rhinitis, the immune-boosting properties of vitamin C, the benefits of hydration on overall health, and the role of zinc and Vitamin D in supporting the immune system. These protocols are grounded in both traditional practices and contemporary scientific research, aiming to provide a comprehensive approach to seasonal immune support.

CHAPTER 4: 5 HERBAL RECIPES FOR IMMUNE SUPPORT

ECHINACEA TEA

Beneficial effects

Echinacea Tea is celebrated for its immune-boosting properties. It can help reduce the duration and severity of colds and flu by enhancing the body's immune response. Echinacea is also known for its anti-inflammatory benefits, which can help alleviate pain and reduce symptoms of inflammation.

Portions

1 serving

Preparation time

5 minutes

Cooking time

15 minutes

Ingredients

- 1 tablespoon dried Echinacea root or leaves

- 8 ounces of water

- Honey or lemon (optional, for taste)

Instructions

1. Bring 8 ounces of water to a boil in a small pot.

2. Add 1 tablespoon of dried Echinacea root or leaves to the boiling water.

3. Reduce the heat and simmer for about 10 to 15 minutes to allow the Echinacea to fully infuse.

4. Strain the tea into a cup, removing the Echinacea.

5. Optional: Add honey or lemon to taste for flavor enhancement.

6. Enjoy the tea warm to maximize its immune-boosting effects.

Variations

- For a more complex flavor, add a cinnamon stick or a few slices of fresh ginger to the pot during simmering.

- Combine with peppermint leaves or chamomile flowers for additional soothing and relaxing benefits.

- For a cold remedy, mix in a tablespoon of elderberry syrup after straining the tea for an extra immune boost.

Storage tips

It's best to consume Echinacea Tea fresh. However, if you need to store it, keep the tea in a sealed container in the refrigerator for up to 24 hours. Reheat gently before drinking.

Tips for allergens

Individuals with allergies to plants in the daisy family, such as ragweed, chrysanthemums, marigolds, or daisies, should proceed with caution when trying Echinacea for the first time due to potential cross-reactivity. Always start with a small amount to test for any adverse reactions.

Scientific references

- "Echinacea for preventing and treating the common cold." Cochrane Database of Systematic Reviews, 2014. This review suggests that Echinacea may be effective in the prevention and treatment of colds.

- "Immunomodulatory Effects of Echinacea and Echinamide." Phytotherapy Research, 2006. This study highlights the immune-boosting and anti-inflammatory properties of Echinacea, supporting its use for immune support.

ASTRAGALUS ROOT SOUP

Beneficial effects

Astragalus Root Soup is a traditional remedy known for its immune-boosting properties. Astragalus is believed to increase the body's production of white blood cells, which fight off infections and diseases. This soup can help strengthen the body's defenses, particularly during cold and flu season, and is also thought to have anti-inflammatory benefits, supporting overall health and well-being.

Portions

4 servings

Preparation time

15 minutes

Cooking time

2 hours

Ingredients

- 4 cups of water or vegetable broth

- 1 cup chopped carrots

- 1 cup chopped celery

- 1/2 cup sliced astragalus root

- 1/2 cup chopped onions

- 2 garlic cloves, minced

- 1 teaspoon grated ginger

- Salt and pepper to taste

- Fresh herbs (such as parsley or thyme) for garnish

Instructions

1. In a large pot, bring the water or vegetable broth to a boil.

2. Add the chopped carrots, celery, astragalus root, onions, garlic, and grated ginger to the pot.

3. Reduce the heat to a simmer and cover the pot. Allow the soup to cook for about 2 hours.

4. After 2 hours, remove the pot from heat. Strain out the astragalus root slices and discard them.

5. Season the soup with salt and pepper to taste.

6. Serve the soup hot, garnished with fresh herbs like parsley or thyme.

Variations

- For a heartier soup, add cubed chicken breast or tofu cubes at the beginning of cooking.

- Include other immune-supporting ingredients like mushrooms or spinach for added nutrition.

- For a richer flavor, sauté the onions, garlic, and ginger in olive oil before adding them to the broth.

Storage tips

Store any leftover soup in an airtight container in the refrigerator for up to 3 days. Reheat on the stove or in the microwave when ready to serve.

Tips for allergens

For those with allergies to specific vegetables, feel free to substitute or omit as necessary. If using chicken broth instead of vegetable broth, ensure it's free from additives that may cause allergic reactions.

Scientific references

- "Astragalus membranaceus: A Review of its Protection Against Inflammation and Gastrointestinal Cancers." American Journal of Chinese Medicine, 2016. This review discusses the anti-inflammatory properties of astragalus and its potential in cancer prevention.

- "Effects of Astragalus on Cardiac Function and Immune System Disorders: Knowledge and Practice." Evidence-Based Complementary and Alternative Medicine, 2019. This article highlights the role of astragalus in boosting the immune system and supporting heart health.

REISHI MUSHROOM ELIXIR

Beneficial effects

Reishi Mushroom Elixir is renowned for its immune-boosting properties. It helps in enhancing the body's resistance to infections and diseases by supporting immune function. Reishi mushrooms contain compounds like polysaccharides, triterpenoids, and peptidoglycans that contribute to their antioxidant, anti-inflammatory, and antimicrobial effects. This elixir can also aid in stress reduction, improve sleep quality, and support overall vitality and longevity.

Portions

2 servings

Preparation time

10 minutes

Cooking time

1 hour

Ingredients

- 4 cups of water
- 1 ounce dried Reishi mushrooms
- 1 tablespoon honey or maple syrup (optional, for sweetness)
- 1 slice of fresh ginger (optional, for added digestive benefits)
- A pinch of ground cinnamon (optional, for flavor)

Instructions

1. In a medium-sized pot, bring 4 cups of water to a boil.

2. Add the dried Reishi mushrooms to the boiling water.

3. Reduce the heat to a simmer and cover the pot. Allow the mushrooms to simmer for about 1 hour. This slow cooking process helps to extract the beneficial compounds from the mushrooms.

4. After 1 hour, remove the pot from heat and strain the liquid into a large bowl, discarding the mushrooms.

5. If desired, stir in honey or maple syrup, a slice of fresh ginger, and a pinch of ground cinnamon to the strained liquid for added flavor and benefits.

6. Serve the elixir warm, or allow it to cool and then refrigerate for a cold beverage.

Variations

- For an extra immune boost, add a squeeze of lemon juice to the elixir after it has cooled slightly.

- Combine with green tea during the simmering process for added antioxidants.

- Mix in a teaspoon of turmeric powder with the cinnamon for additional anti-inflammatory properties.

Storage tips

Store any leftover Reishi Mushroom Elixir in an airtight container in the refrigerator for up to 5 days. Reheat gently on the stove or enjoy cold.

Tips for allergens

For those with allergies to mushrooms, it's important to consult with a healthcare provider before trying Reishi Mushroom Elixir. Substitute honey with maple syrup for a vegan option.

Scientific references

- "Immunomodulating Effects of Reishi: A Systematic Review" - Journal of Alternative and Complementary Medicine, 2014. This review discusses the immune-supportive properties of Reishi mushrooms, highlighting their role in enhancing immune function and offering potential benefits for health and longevity.

- "Antioxidant and Anti-inflammatory Activities of Reishi (Ganoderma lucidum) and their Potential for Clinical Use" - International Journal of Molecular Sciences, 2019. This study explores the antioxidant and anti-inflammatory effects of Reishi mushrooms, supporting their use in managing inflammation and oxidative stress.

GARLIC AND HONEY TONIC

Beneficial effects

Garlic and Honey Tonic combines the powerful antimicrobial properties of garlic with the soothing, antibacterial effects of honey, creating a potent natural remedy for boosting the immune system. Garlic contains compounds like allicin, known for fighting infections and supporting heart health, while honey offers antioxidants and a gentle boost to the immune response. Together, they form a tonic that can help ward off colds, soothe sore throats, and improve overall health.

Portions

2 servings

Preparation time

10 minutes

Ingredients

- 3 cloves of fresh garlic

- 1/4 cup of raw honey

- 1/2 cup of water (optional, to dilute)

Instructions

1. Peel and finely mince the garlic cloves.

2. In a small bowl, combine the minced garlic with the raw honey. Stir until well mixed.

3. If preferred, add water to dilute the mixture, making it easier to consume.

4. Let the mixture sit for at least 5 minutes to allow the garlic to infuse into the honey.

5. Consume 1 tablespoon of the tonic on an empty stomach each morning to boost the immune system. If the taste is too strong, it can be diluted further with warm water.

Variations

- Add a teaspoon of apple cider vinegar to the mixture for additional detoxifying benefits.

- Incorporate a pinch of cayenne pepper to enhance the tonic's warming and circulation-boosting properties.

- Mix in a tablespoon of lemon juice for added vitamin C and a refreshing taste.

Storage tips

Store the Garlic and Honey Tonic in an airtight container in the refrigerator for up to 5 days. The cold will help preserve the active compounds in the garlic and honey.

Tips for allergens

For those allergic to raw honey, substitute it with maple syrup, although this may alter the tonic's antimicrobial properties. Always ensure that you're not allergic to garlic before consuming it in medicinal quantities.

Scientific references

- "Allicin: chemistry and biological properties" - Studies in Natural Products Chemistry, 2014. This research highlights the antimicrobial and health-promoting effects of allicin, a compound found in garlic.

- "Honey: its medicinal property and antibacterial activity" - Asian Pacific Journal of Tropical Biomedicine, 2011. This study discusses the antibacterial and antioxidant properties of honey, supporting its use in immune support tonics.

OREGANO OIL CAPSULES

Beneficial effects

Oregano Oil Capsules are renowned for their potent antibacterial, antiviral, and anti-inflammatory properties. These capsules can significantly bolster the immune system, making them an excellent choice for fighting off colds, flu, and other infections. The active compound in oregano oil, carvacrol, is thought to help break through the outer cell membranes of harmful bacteria, effectively killing them and inhibiting their growth. Additionally, oregano oil has antioxidant properties that can help protect the body from damage caused by free radicals, supporting overall health and wellness.

Ingredients

- High-quality oregano essential oil

- Empty vegetable capsules

- Olive oil or another carrier oil (if diluting the oregano oil)

Instructions

1. If using undiluted oregano essential oil, skip to step 3. To dilute, mix 1 part oregano essential oil with 4 parts carrier oil in a small bowl.

2. Stir the mixture thoroughly to ensure the oils are well combined.

3. Carefully open an empty vegetable capsule and fill the larger end with the oregano oil or oregano oil mixture using a dropper. Do not overfill.

4. Once filled, cap the capsule with its smaller end. Make sure it snaps closed to prevent leakage.

5. Repeat the process for the desired number of capsules.

6. Store the prepared capsules in a cool, dark place until ready to use.

Variations

- For added immune support, consider adding a drop of lemon or elderberry extract to each capsule.

- Adjust the ratio of oregano oil to carrier oil based on personal sensitivity and preference. Some may prefer a stronger or milder dose.

Storage tips

Keep the filled capsules in a cool, dark place, ideally in a sealed container to protect them from light and air. If stored properly, the capsules should remain potent for up to a month.

Tips for allergens

Individuals with allergies to oregano or other herbs in the Lamiaceae family should avoid using oregano oil capsules. Always start with a small dose to test for any adverse reactions, especially if you have a sensitive stomach or are prone to allergies.

Scientific references

- "Antimicrobial activity of oregano oil against antibiotic-resistant pathogens" - Journal of Medicinal Food, 2017. This study highlights the effectiveness of oregano oil in combating antibiotic-resistant bacteria, supporting its use for immune support.

- "Carvacrol, a component of oregano oil, inhibits inflammation and can help reduce symptoms associated with upper respiratory infections" - Journal of Nutrition & Food Sciences, 2014. This research discusses the anti-inflammatory properties of carvacrol, suggesting its potential benefits in treating infections and supporting the immune system.

PART 5: STRESS MANAGEMENT AND MENTAL HEALTH

Stress and mental health are intricately linked, with each influencing the other in profound ways. In today's fast-paced world, managing stress is not just about avoiding burnout, but it's also about nurturing our mental health to foster resilience, happiness, and overall well-being. The mind and body operate in unison; when stress levels are high, our mental health can suffer, leading to a range of issues from anxiety to depression, and impacting our physical health in the process. Recognizing the signs of stress and taking proactive steps to manage it can significantly improve our quality of life.

One effective strategy for managing stress is through the practice of mindfulness meditation. This technique involves focusing on the present moment, acknowledging thoughts and feelings without judgment, and gently guiding the mind back to the current task or sensation.

Mindfulness can reduce stress by enhancing emotional regulation, increasing self-awareness, and promoting a state of calm. Regular practice can help individuals respond to stressors more effectively, reducing the impact on mental health.

Physical activity is another powerful tool in the stress management arsenal. Exercise releases endorphins, often referred to as the body's natural mood elevators, which can improve mood and decrease feelings of stress, anxiety, and depression. Whether it's a brisk walk, a yoga session, or a vigorous workout, finding a form of exercise that is enjoyable and sustainable is key to reaping the mental health benefits.

Nutrition also plays a critical role in managing stress and supporting mental health. A diet rich in whole foods, such as fruits, vegetables, whole grains, lean proteins, and healthy fats, can provide the nutrients necessary for brain health and resilience against stress.

Omega-3 fatty acids, for example, found in fatty fish, walnuts, and flaxseeds, have been shown to reduce symptoms of anxiety and depression. Similarly, foods high in antioxidants can help combat oxidative stress, which is linked to mood disorders.

Sleep is essential for mental health and stress management. Lack of sleep can exacerbate stress, affect emotional regulation, and increase the risk of mental health disorders. Establishing a regular sleep schedule, creating a restful environment, and adopting a calming bedtime routine can enhance sleep quality and, in turn, support overall well-being.

Social support is invaluable in managing stress and promoting mental health. Connecting with friends, family, or support groups can provide a sense of belonging, increase feelings of self-worth, and offer an outlet for sharing concerns and relieving stress. Sometimes, just knowing that support is available can make challenging situations feel more manageable.

Finally, adopting stress reduction techniques such as deep breathing exercises, progressive muscle relaxation, or engaging in hobbies can offer immediate relief from stress and contribute to long-term mental health benefits. These practices can help shift the focus away from stressors and provide a sense of control and peace.

Incorporating these strategies into daily life requires commitment and practice, but the benefits for stress management and mental health are profound. By taking steps to manage stress, individuals can enhance their resilience, improve their quality of life, and foster a greater sense of well-being.

Adopting a holistic approach to stress management and mental health involves integrating practices that nurture the entire being—mind, body, and spirit. This comprehensive strategy not only addresses the symptoms of stress but also targets its root causes, promoting a deeper sense of wellness and balance. Techniques such as journaling and expressive writing can serve as powerful tools for managing stress, allowing individuals to process emotions, reflect on experiences, and release pent-up feelings. Writing about thoughts and worries can help clarify them, making challenges seem more manageable and solutions more attainable.

Another aspect of holistic stress management is the practice of gratitude. Cultivating an attitude of gratitude by regularly acknowledging and appreciating the good in one's life can shift focus away from stressors and towards positive aspects, enhancing mental health and emotional resilience.

This practice can be as simple as keeping a gratitude journal or sharing what you're thankful for with loved ones.

The environment also plays a significant role in stress management and mental health. Creating a calming and supportive space, whether at home or work, can significantly reduce stress levels and promote relaxation. This might involve organizing the living space, adding elements of nature such as plants or water features, or setting up a dedicated area for relaxation and meditation.

Mindfulness-based stress reduction (MBSR) programs and cognitive-behavioral therapy (CBT) are structured approaches that have been scientifically proven to help manage stress and improve mental health. MBSR focuses on mindfulness meditation to increase awareness and acceptance of the present moment, while CBT helps individuals identify and change negative thought patterns and behaviors that contribute to stress and mental health issues.

Herbal remedies and supplements can also support stress management and mental health. Adaptogens, such as ashwagandha, rhodiola, and holy basil, help the body resist stressors, while magnesium, omega-3 fatty acids, and B vitamins have been shown to reduce symptoms of stress and anxiety. However, it's important to consult with a healthcare provider before starting any new supplement, especially for individuals with existing health conditions or those taking other medications.

Engaging in creative activities such as painting, music, or dance can be therapeutic and reduce stress. These activities provide an outlet for expression, distract from stressors, and increase feelings of joy and satisfaction. They can also foster a sense of accomplishment and improve self-esteem, further contributing to mental health.

In conclusion, managing stress and nurturing mental health is a multifaceted process that requires a personalized and holistic approach. By incorporating a variety of strategies and practices into daily life, individuals can build resilience against stress, enhance their emotional well-being, and lead a more balanced and fulfilling life. Remember, the journey to better stress management and mental health is ongoing, and it's important to be patient and compassionate with oneself along the way.

CHAPTER 1: STRESS AND HEALTH LINK

Stress, a ubiquitous component of modern life, exerts a profound influence on our health, weaving its effects through the complex interplay of the nervous, endocrine, and immune systems. The body's stress response, designed to deal with immediate threats, can become a persistent state in the face of ongoing pressures, leading to a cascade of physiological changes that undermine health. Chronic stress disrupts the delicate balance of the body's systems, leading to increased vulnerability to illnesses, from common infections to chronic diseases.

At the heart of the stress-health nexus is the hypothalamic-pituitary-adrenal (HPA) axis, a central component of the body's stress response system.

Activation of the HPA axis triggers the release of cortisol, a hormone that, in short bursts, plays a vital role in energy regulation, immune function, and maintaining homeostasis. However, when stress is constant, elevated cortisol levels can suppress immune function, increase blood pressure, contribute to weight gain, and disrupt sleep, among other adverse effects.

The immune system's ability to protect the body from infections and heal wounds is significantly compromised under chronic stress. Research has shown that stress can both suppress the production of protective immune responses and trigger inflammatory pathways, creating a double-edged sword that leaves the body more susceptible to infections and may exacerbate or lead to the development of autoimmune diseases and inflammation-related conditions.

Furthermore, stress impacts heart health by increasing heart rate and blood pressure, and chronic exposure to stress hormones can lead to the buildup of plaque in arteries, a risk factor for heart attack and stroke. The relationship between stress and heart health is also mediated by behavioral factors; stress can lead to unhealthy coping mechanisms such as overeating, physical inactivity, smoking, and excessive alcohol consumption, all of which are risk factors for cardiovascular disease.

The gastrointestinal system is another victim of stress, with stress-related hormones affecting digestion and nutrient absorption and altering the gut microbiota. This can manifest as gastrointestinal discomfort, such as irritable bowel syndrome (IBS), and contribute to the development of peptic ulcers and inflammatory bowel disease (IBD).

Stress also plays a critical role in mental health, contributing to the onset or worsening of anxiety, depression, and other psychiatric disorders. The brain's structure and function can be altered by chronic stress, affecting areas involved in mood regulation, memory, and cognition. Moreover, stress can disrupt sleep patterns, leading to insomnia and exacerbating mental health issues.

Mitigating the health impacts of stress involves a multifaceted approach that includes lifestyle changes, stress management techniques, and, when necessary, professional support. Regular physical activity, adequate sleep, a balanced diet, and mindfulness practices such as meditation and deep breathing exercises can help regulate the body's stress response and mitigate its health effects. Social support and engaging in hobbies and activities that bring joy and relaxation are also crucial for buffering against stress.

Understanding the connection between stress and health is the first step toward taking proactive measures to manage stress and enhance well-being. By acknowledging the pervasive influence of stress on the body and mind, individuals can adopt strategies that foster resilience, promote health, and improve quality of life in the face of life's inevitable pressures.

DR. BARBARA'S INSIGHTS ON STRESS AND THE BODY

Dr. Barbara emphasizes the crucial understanding that stress is not merely a psychological state but a physical one that can manifest in various detrimental ways throughout the body.

Chronic stress, she points out, is like an alarm system that never turns off, leading to an overproduction of cortisol and adrenaline. These hormones, while beneficial in short-term fight-or-flight situations, can wreak havoc on the body when consistently elevated. Elevated cortisol levels can lead to a plethora of health issues including but not limited to increased blood sugar levels, heightened blood pressure, and a compromised immune system making the body more susceptible to infections and diseases.

Moreover, Dr. Barbara highlights the often-overlooked impact of stress on the digestive system. Stress can alter the gut microbiome, leading to changes in digestion and nutrient absorption, which can exacerbate or even lead to gastrointestinal conditions such as irritable bowel syndrome (IBS) or inflammatory bowel disease (IBD). This connection underscores the importance of managing stress to maintain not only mental health but gut health as well.

The cardiovascular system is also significantly affected by stress. Dr. Barbara explains how chronic stress can lead to an increased heart rate and higher blood pressure, which over time can contribute to the wear and tear of the cardiovascular system, increasing the risk of heart disease and stroke. This risk is compounded by the likelihood of adopting unhealthy lifestyle choices under stress, such as poor diet, lack of exercise, and substance abuse, which further deteriorates heart health.

Furthermore, Dr. Barbara discusses the impact of stress on the body's immune response. Under stress, the body's ability to fight off antigens is reduced, making it easier for infections to take hold. This immune suppression can lead to frequent illnesses and may also affect the body's inflammatory response, potentially exacerbating conditions related to chronic inflammation.

Addressing the mental health aspects, she points out that chronic stress can lead to significant mental health challenges, including anxiety, depression, and sleep disturbances. Stress can alter brain function and even brain structure over time, affecting areas responsible for memory, emotion, and executive function. This highlights the critical need for effective stress management strategies to protect both mental and physical health.

To combat the adverse effects of stress, Dr. Barbara advocates for a holistic approach that includes regular physical activity, adequate sleep, a balanced diet rich in antioxidants and anti-inflammatory foods, and mindfulness practices such as meditation and yoga. She also emphasizes the importance of social support and finding healthy ways to relax and enjoy life, suggesting that a proactive approach to managing stress can significantly enhance overall well-being and health.

In essence, Dr. Barbara's insights into the relationship between stress and the body illuminate the profound impact that chronic stress can have on physical health. By understanding these connections, individuals are better equipped to implement strategies that mitigate these effects, leading to a healthier, more balanced life.

CHRONIC STRESS AND ITS LONG-TERM EFFECTS

Chronic stress, when experienced over a prolonged period, initiates a series of physiological changes that can have detrimental long-term effects on health. The constant activation of the stress response system can lead to adrenal fatigue, where the adrenal glands, overwhelmed by the continuous demand for stress hormones, begin to function less efficiently. This condition can result in symptoms such as fatigue, difficulty sleeping, and a weakened immune response, making the body more susceptible to infections and illness.

One of the most significant impacts of chronic stress is on cardiovascular health. The persistent high levels of cortisol and adrenaline increase heart rate and blood pressure, straining the cardiovascular system. Over time, this strain can contribute to the formation of arterial plaque, increasing the risk of heart attack and stroke. Additionally, chronic stress can lead to unhealthy behaviors such as poor dietary choices, smoking, and lack of physical activity, which further exacerbate cardiovascular risk.

The endocrine system, responsible for regulating hormones in the body, is also affected by chronic stress. Elevated cortisol levels can disrupt the balance of other hormones, including insulin, leading to increased blood sugar levels and a higher risk of developing type 2 diabetes. Furthermore, stress can impact reproductive hormones, affecting menstrual cycles, fertility, and libido.

Chronic stress takes a toll on mental health as well. The constant state of alertness can lead to anxiety, depression, and irritability. Over time, the exposure to high levels of stress hormones can alter brain function, affecting memory, concentration, and increasing the risk of developing neurological disorders such as Alzheimer's disease.

To mitigate these long-term effects, it's crucial to adopt stress management techniques and make lifestyle changes that promote relaxation and well-being. Regular physical activity, a balanced diet, adequate sleep, and mindfulness practices can help manage stress levels and reduce the impact of chronic stress on the body. Engaging in activities that bring joy and fulfillment, along with seeking support from friends, family, or professionals, can also play a vital role in managing stress and protecting health over the long term.

THE ROLE OF CORTISOL IN STRESS

Cortisol, often referred to as the "stress hormone," plays a crucial role in the body's response to stress. It's produced by the adrenal glands located on top of your kidneys and is released into the bloodstream in response to stress or fear as part of the body's fight-or-flight mechanism. This mechanism is essential for survival, preparing the body to respond to a perceived threat by increasing alertness, energy, and the ability to withstand pain. However, in our modern lifestyle, the stress response can be triggered frequently and not just by life-threatening situations but by daily pressures and challenges, leading to prolonged elevation of cortisol levels.

Elevated cortisol levels over time can have several adverse effects on health. Initially, cortisol helps to boost energy by increasing glucose in the bloodstream, enhancing the brain's use of glucose, and increasing the availability of substances that repair tissues. However, prolonged elevation can lead to excessive glucose production and alterations in insulin levels, contributing to weight gain and increasing the risk of type 2 diabetes. High cortisol levels can also affect the immune system by suppressing it, making the body more susceptible to infections and impairing the healing process. Additionally, cortisol can affect mood, sleep, and cognition; chronic stress and high cortisol levels are associated with symptoms of anxiety, depression, and difficulties with memory and concentration.

Moreover, cortisol influences other bodily systems and processes. It can lead to increased blood pressure and contribute to the development of cardiovascular disease by affecting the arteries and heart function. The digestive system can also be impacted, with cortisol potentially causing an imbalance in gut bacteria, leading to discomfort and gastrointestinal issues. Furthermore, cortisol can affect the reproductive system, leading to irregular menstrual cycles, decreased libido, and fertility issues due to its influence on hormones like estrogen and testosterone.

To manage cortisol levels and mitigate the effects of stress, adopting a holistic approach to stress management is crucial. This includes engaging in regular physical activity, which can help reduce cortisol levels and improve mood and sleep. A balanced diet rich in whole foods and low in processed foods and sugars can also support the body's ability to manage stress. Incorporating stress-reduction techniques such as mindfulness, meditation, deep breathing exercises, and yoga can help lower cortisol levels and enhance overall well-being. Adequate sleep is essential for regulating cortisol production, so establishing a regular sleep schedule and creating a calming bedtime routine can be beneficial. Lastly, seeking social support from friends, family, or professionals can provide emotional comfort and reduce feelings of isolation, further helping to manage stress and its effects on the body.

Understanding the role of cortisol in stress underscores the importance of managing stress through lifestyle choices and stress-reduction techniques. By acknowledging the impact of chronic stress and taking proactive steps to address it, individuals can improve their health and quality of life, reducing the risk of stress-related health issues.

CHAPTER 2: TECHNIQUES FOR MANAGING STRESS

Managing stress effectively requires a multifaceted approach that encompasses physical activity, mindfulness, and lifestyle adjustments to foster a state of mental, emotional, and physical well-being. Regular exercise stands out as a powerful stress-reliever because it promotes the release of endorphins, the body's natural mood elevators, and painkillers. Incorporating a routine that includes activities such as brisk walking, jogging, yoga, or swimming can significantly reduce stress levels. These activities not only improve physical health but also provide a mental break from the stressors of daily life, offering a sense of accomplishment and relaxation.

Mindfulness and meditation practices are invaluable tools for stress management, enabling individuals to achieve a state of calm and focus. Techniques such as deep breathing exercises, progressive muscle relaxation, and guided imagery help in redirecting attention away from stressors and towards a peaceful state of mind. By focusing on the present moment and becoming more aware of one's thoughts and feelings without judgment, it's possible to reduce the intensity of stress responses and cultivate a more resilient outlook on life's challenges.

Dietary choices also play a crucial role in managing stress. Consuming a balanced diet rich in antioxidants, vitamins, and minerals supports the body's ability to cope with stress. Foods high in omega-3 fatty acids, such as salmon and flaxseeds, have been shown to reduce stress levels and improve mood. Similarly, incorporating plenty of fruits, vegetables, whole grains, and lean proteins can enhance overall health and resilience to stress. It's also important to limit or avoid excessive caffeine and sugar intake, as these can exacerbate stress and lead to energy crashes.

Establishing a consistent sleep routine is another essential strategy for stress management. Adequate sleep rejuvenates the body and mind, enhancing the ability to think clearly and maintain emotional balance. Creating a relaxing bedtime routine, keeping a regular sleep schedule, and ensuring a comfortable sleep environment can help improve sleep quality and reduce stress.

Social support is a critical component of stress management. Connecting with friends, family, or support groups provides a sense of belonging and can offer new perspectives on stressful situations. Sharing concerns and experiences with others who understand can be incredibly comforting and reduce feelings of isolation and overwhelm.

Time management techniques can also alleviate stress by helping to prioritize tasks, set realistic goals, and avoid overcommitment. Learning to say no, delegating tasks when possible, and breaking larger projects into manageable steps can help in reducing the pressure and anxiety associated with a heavy workload.

Finally, engaging in hobbies and activities that bring joy and relaxation is vital for stress relief. Whether it's reading, gardening, painting, or listening to music, taking time to indulge in personal interests can provide a much-needed escape from stress and recharge one's energy and creativity.

By integrating these techniques into daily life, individuals can develop a comprehensive stress management plan that not only mitigates the immediate effects of stress but also builds long-term resilience. It's important to remember that managing stress is an ongoing process, and what works for one person may not work for another. Experimenting with different strategies and being open to adjusting one's approach is key to finding the most effective ways to cope with stress.

MINDFULNESS AND MEDITATION

Mindfulness and meditation offer a powerful antidote to the stresses of modern life, providing a means to center oneself in the present moment, fostering a sense of peace and clarity that can significantly reduce the physiological and psychological impacts of stress. By engaging in mindfulness, one cultivates an awareness of the present experience, observing thoughts, feelings, and sensations without judgment. This practice can help break the cycle of chronic stress by interrupting the automatic responses that often exacerbate stress levels and lead to negative health outcomes. Meditation, a practice closely related to mindfulness, involves sitting in quiet reflection or using guided imagery or breath work to focus the mind and promote a state of relaxation and awareness. Regular meditation has been shown to decrease cortisol levels, lower blood pressure, and improve immune function, offering a simple yet effective tool for managing stress and enhancing overall well-being.

The beneficial effects of mindfulness and meditation are manifold, encompassing improved mental clarity, reduced symptoms of anxiety and depression, enhanced emotional resilience, and a greater sense of inner peace. These practices can also improve sleep quality, aid in pain management, and support healthier relationships by fostering empathy and patience. To incorporate mindfulness and meditation into your daily routine, start with just a few minutes each day, gradually increasing the duration as you become more comfortable with the practice.

Find a quiet space where you won't be interrupted, sit in a comfortable position, and focus on your breath, gently bringing your attention back whenever your mind wanders. There are numerous resources available, from guided meditation apps to mindfulness workshops, that can provide structure and support as you explore these practices.

For those new to meditation, it may be helpful to begin with guided sessions that can offer direction and focus, gradually moving towards unguided meditation as you develop your ability to maintain focus independently. Experiment with different styles of meditation, such as mindfulness-based stress reduction (MBSR), loving-kindness meditation, or body scan meditation, to find what resonates most with you. Remember, the goal is not to empty the mind of thoughts but to observe them without attachment, returning to your breath or chosen point of focus whenever you notice your mind drifting.

Incorporating mindfulness and meditation into your life can transform your relationship with stress, providing a refuge of calm in the midst of chaos. By dedicating time each day to these practices, you can cultivate a sense of balance and well-being that permeates all aspects of your life, enhancing your ability to navigate challenges with grace and resilience.

PHYSICAL ACTIVITY FOR STRESS RELIEF

Physical activity serves as a potent stress reliever, harnessing the body's natural ability to regulate mood and alleviate tension. Engaging in regular exercise triggers the release of endorphins, chemicals in the brain that act as natural painkillers and mood elevators.

Beyond the biochemical effects, physical activity provides a constructive distraction, allowing individuals to find a momentary escape from daily stresses and enter a state of meditative motion, focusing on the physical task at hand rather than the worries of the day.

The beneficial effects of physical activity on stress relief are well-documented and multifaceted. Exercise reduces levels of the body's stress hormones, such as adrenaline and cortisol, gradually bringing about a state of natural calm and relaxation. It also stimulates the production of endorphins, which are the body's natural mood lifters, creating an overall sense of well-being. Regular participation in physical activity has been shown to improve sleep, which can be negatively affected by stress, further enhancing stress relief.

To incorporate physical activity into a stress management routine, it's essential to choose activities that are enjoyable and sustainable over the long term.

This could range from brisk walking, jogging, swimming, cycling, to group sports, dancing, or yoga. The key is consistency and making exercise a regular part of the daily or weekly schedule. For those new to exercise or returning after a break, it's advisable to start slowly and gradually increase the intensity and duration of the activity to avoid injury and ensure a positive experience.

For individuals seeking to maximize the stress-relieving benefits of exercise, it's beneficial to set realistic goals and track progress.

This not only provides a sense of accomplishment but also offers tangible evidence of improvement, further motivating continued engagement in physical activity. Additionally, incorporating outdoor activities can enhance the stress-reducing effects of exercise through exposure to natural settings, which have been shown to lower stress levels and improve mood.

It's also important to vary the routine to prevent boredom and maintain interest.

Mixing different types of activities can keep the exercise regimen engaging and cover a broader spectrum of physical benefits. For example, combining aerobic exercises like running or cycling with strength training and flexibility exercises such as yoga or Pilates can provide a comprehensive workout that addresses stress relief from multiple angles.

In summary, physical activity stands as a cornerstone of stress management, offering a natural, effective way to combat the physical and emotional effects of stress. By integrating regular exercise into one's lifestyle, individuals can harness the power of physical activity to enhance their overall well-being, improve mood, and foster resilience against the inevitable stresses of life.

DR. BARBARA'S DAILY STRESS-RELIEF ROUTINE

Dr. Barbara's daily stress-relief routine begins with a morning meditation to set a positive tone for the day. She dedicates 15 to 20 minutes each morning to sit in a quiet space, focusing on her breath and practicing mindfulness to clear her mind of any clutter and stress. This practice helps in centering her thoughts and grounding her emotions, preparing her for the day ahead with a calm and focused mindset. Following her meditation, Dr. Barbara engages in a physical activity that she enjoys, such as yoga or a brisk walk in nature. Yoga combines physical postures, breathing exercises, and meditation to enhance physical flexibility, reduce stress, and improve mental clarity.

On days when the weather permits, a walk outside not only provides her with physical exercise but also allows her to connect with nature, which has been shown to significantly lower stress levels and improve mood.

Midday, Dr. Barbara takes short breaks to practice deep breathing exercises, especially when transitioning between tasks.

These breathing exercises involve taking slow, deep breaths to activate the body's relaxation response, counteracting the stress response and lowering cortisol levels. She emphasizes the importance of incorporating these short breaks into the daily routine to manage stress levels continuously throughout the day and maintain mental clarity.

In the afternoon, Dr. Barbara ensures she takes time to nourish her body with a balanced meal rich in antioxidants and omega-3 fatty acids, known for their stress-reducing properties. She includes foods such as leafy greens, nuts, seeds, and fatty fish to support her body's ability to cope with stress. Hydration is also a key component of her routine, as staying adequately hydrated is essential for maintaining optimal cognitive function and managing stress levels.

To wind down in the evening, Dr. Barbara practices gratitude by journaling. She reflects on the day, noting down at least three things she is grateful for.

This practice shifts the focus away from stressors and towards positivity, enhancing emotional well-being and resilience against stress.

Following her gratitude journaling, she prepares for sleep with a relaxing routine that may include reading, a warm bath infused with lavender essential oil, and a cup of herbal tea such as chamomile, known for its calming properties. Ensuring a consistent sleep schedule is crucial for her, as adequate sleep is foundational for stress management and overall health.

Dr. Barbara's daily stress-relief routine is a holistic approach that incorporates mindfulness, physical activity, nutrition, hydration, gratitude, and a consistent sleep schedule. This routine is designed to manage stress effectively, promote mental clarity, and support emotional and physical well-being. It's a flexible routine that can be adapted to fit individual preferences and schedules, encouraging everyone to find and practice what works best for them in managing daily stress.

CHAPTER 3: NUTRITION AND MENTAL HEALTH

The profound connection between nutrition and mental health cannot be overstated, with a growing body of research underscoring the impact of dietary choices on mental well-being. Essential nutrients from our diet play critical roles in brain function, influencing mood, cognitive processes, and emotional health. A balanced diet rich in vitamins, minerals, and antioxidants can support brain health, reduce inflammation, and mitigate the risk of mood disorders.

Conversely, diets high in processed foods, sugar, and unhealthy fats can exacerbate symptoms of depression, anxiety, and other mental health challenges.

Omega-3 fatty acids, found in fatty fish, flaxseeds, and walnuts, are pivotal for brain health, promoting the fluidity of cell membranes and supporting neurotransmitter function. These essential fats are linked to reduced rates of depression and anxiety, highlighting their importance in a mental health-supportive diet. Antioxidants, abundant in fruits and vegetables, combat oxidative stress in the brain, which has been implicated in mood disorders. Vitamins B, particularly B12, B6, and folate, play a role in the synthesis of serotonin and dopamine, neurotransmitters that regulate mood.

A deficiency in these vitamins can lead to feelings of depression and fatigue.

Magnesium, often referred to as the relaxation mineral, is crucial for brain function and mood regulation. Found in leafy greens, nuts, seeds, and whole grains, magnesium has been shown to alleviate symptoms of anxiety and depression. Similarly, zinc, present in beans, nuts, and animal products, is essential for brain health and mood regulation, with deficiencies linked to increased risk of depression.

The gut-brain axis further illustrates the relationship between nutrition and mental health. The gut microbiome, which plays a crucial role in overall health, affects brain health through the production of neurotransmitters and inflammatory markers.

Diets rich in fiber, prebiotics, and probiotics support a healthy gut microbiome, which in turn supports mental well-being. Fermented foods such as yogurt, kefir, and sauerkraut, along with high-fiber foods like fruits, vegetables, and whole grains, can promote a healthy gut environment conducive to mental health.

Implementing a diet that supports mental health involves focusing on whole, nutrient-dense foods while minimizing the intake of processed foods, excessive sugars, and unhealthy fats. Regular hydration is also essential, as even mild dehydration can affect mood and cognitive function.

Mindful eating practices, paying attention to the body's hunger and fullness signals, and enjoying a varied diet can enhance the nutritional quality of the diet and support mental health.

For individuals looking to improve their mental well-being through nutrition, the following recipe offers a simple, nutrient-rich meal that supports brain health:

Beneficial effects: Supports brain health, improves mood, reduces inflammation.

Ingredients:

- 1 fillet of wild-caught salmon (rich in omega-3 fatty acids)

- 1 cup of kale, chopped (high in magnesium and antioxidants)

- 1/2 cup of quinoa (a good source of B vitamins and fiber)

- 1 tablespoon of olive oil (healthy fat)

- 1/4 cup of walnuts, chopped (additional omega-3s and antioxidants)

- Lemon wedge for garnish

Instructions:

1. Preheat the oven to 375°F (190°C).

2. Place the salmon fillet on a baking sheet lined with parchment paper. Drizzle with half the olive oil and season with salt and pepper to taste. Bake for 12-15 minutes or until cooked through.

3. While the salmon is baking, cook the quinoa according to package instructions.

4. In a pan, heat the remaining olive oil over medium heat. Add the chopped kale and sauté until wilted, about 3-5 minutes.

5. Serve the baked salmon over a bed of quinoa and sautéed kale. Sprinkle with chopped walnuts and garnish with a lemon wedge.

Variations: Substitute salmon with tofu for a plant-based option, rich in plant-based omega-3s and protein.

Storage tips: Store any leftovers in an airtight container in the refrigerator for up to 2 days.

Tips for allergens: For those with nut allergies, omit the walnuts and consider adding seeds like pumpkin or hemp seeds for added texture and nutrients.

This recipe exemplifies how integrating nutrient-dense foods into the diet can support mental health through the provision of essential vitamins, minerals, and fatty acids necessary for optimal brain function. By prioritizing nutrition as a pillar of mental health, individuals can harness the power of food to nourish both the mind and body, paving the way for improved well-being and resilience against mental health challenges.

FOODS THAT SUPPORT BRAIN HEALTH

Foods that support brain health are essential for cognitive function, memory retention, and emotional balance. These foods are rich in nutrients that play a crucial role in brain development and maintenance, as well as in the prevention of neurodegenerative diseases. Omega-3 fatty acids, for instance, are vital for brain health, found in high concentrations in the brain and known for their anti-inflammatory and neuroprotective properties. Fatty fish like salmon, mackerel, and sardines are excellent sources of omega-3s, specifically EPA and DHA, which are linked to lower risk of cognitive decline and dementia.

Antioxidants combat oxidative stress, a factor that contributes to brain aging and neurodegenerative diseases. Berries, such as blueberries, strawberries, and blackberries, are packed with antioxidants, including flavonoids that have been shown to improve communication between brain cells, enhance learning and memory, and reduce or delay cognitive decline.

Leafy greens like spinach, kale, and collards are also rich in antioxidants and other brain-protective nutrients, including vitamin K, lutein, folate, and beta carotene. Research suggests that a diet rich in leafy greens can slow cognitive decline.

Whole grains are another important component of a brain-healthy diet. They release glucose slowly into the bloodstream, keeping you mentally alert throughout the day.

Oats, barley, and quinoa are good sources of fiber, which helps regulate the release of glucose into the blood, providing a steady energy supply to the brain. Nuts, especially walnuts, are not only great sources of protein and healthy fats but also contain alpha-linolenic acid, an omega-3 fatty acid that supports brain health. Walnuts also have a high content of antioxidants and vitamin E, which can protect the brain from free radical damage.

Turmeric has gained attention for its potent anti-inflammatory and antioxidant properties. Curcumin, the active ingredient in turmeric, can cross the blood-brain barrier and has been shown to lead to various improvements in the pathological process of Alzheimer's disease.

It boosts brain-derived neurotrophic factor, a type of growth hormone that functions in the brain, which can delay or reverse brain degeneration.

Dark chocolate and cocoa powder are mood-boosters; they have flavonoid antioxidants that increase blood flow to the brain, enhance brain function, and provide neuroprotection. Moreover, the caffeine content in dark chocolate can improve focus and concentration. However, moderation is key, as chocolate is also high in calories and can be rich in sugars and saturated fats.

Pumpkin seeds are packed with powerful antioxidants that protect the body and brain from free radical damage. They're also an excellent source of magnesium, iron, zinc, and copper. Each of these nutrients is important for brain health: Zinc is crucial for nerve signaling, magnesium is essential for learning and memory, iron helps with brain function, and copper controls nerve signals.

Incorporating these foods into a balanced diet can support brain health and improve cognitive functions, offering a natural way to enhance mental performance and protect against cognitive decline. Remember, a varied diet that includes a wide range of nutrients is the most beneficial for brain health, alongside other lifestyle factors such as regular physical activity, adequate sleep, and mental exercises.

CUTTING SUGAR FOR MENTAL HEALTH

Avoiding sugar and processed foods plays a crucial role in maintaining better mental health. These foods can lead to fluctuations in blood sugar levels, which in turn can impact mood, energy, and overall mental well-being. Consuming high amounts of sugar and processed foods has been linked to increased feelings of anxiety, depression, and other mental health disorders.

The body and brain function optimally when nourished with whole, nutrient-dense foods that provide steady energy and do not spike blood sugar levels.

Processed foods often contain additives, preservatives, and artificial ingredients that can negatively affect brain health. These substances may interfere with neurotransmitters responsible for mood regulation, such as serotonin and dopamine. By reducing the intake of these foods, individuals may notice an improvement in mood stability, cognitive function, and stress resilience.

Furthermore, sugar and processed foods can contribute to inflammation in the body, which has been associated with the development of mental health issues. Chronic inflammation may affect brain function and is linked to an increased risk of psychiatric disorders.

Adopting a diet low in sugar and processed foods while rich in anti-inflammatory foods like fruits, vegetables, whole grains, and omega-3 fatty acids can help reduce inflammation and support mental health.

To start reducing sugar and processed food intake, focus on incorporating more whole foods into the diet. Begin by replacing sugary snacks with whole fruit, choosing water or herbal teas over sugary beverages, and cooking meals at home using fresh ingredients. Reading labels is also essential; opt for products with minimal ingredients, all of which are recognizable and natural.

In conclusion, avoiding sugar and processed foods is a beneficial strategy for supporting mental health. It encourages a diet that stabilizes blood sugar, reduces inflammation, and provides the brain with the nutrients it needs to function effectively. Making these dietary changes can be a powerful step toward improved mental well-being.

CHAPTER 4: 5 HERBAL RECIPES FOR STRESS RELIEF

LAVENDER AND CHAMOMILE BATH SOAK

Beneficial effects

Lavender and Chamomile Bath Soak combines the calming properties of lavender with the soothing effects of chamomile to create a relaxing bath experience. This soak is designed to alleviate stress, promote relaxation, and prepare the body for a restful night's sleep. Lavender's aroma is known for its ability to reduce anxiety and emotional stress, while chamomile can help soothe the skin and reduce inflammation. Together, they create a powerful duo that can help ease the mind and body after a long day.

Ingredients

- 1/2 cup dried lavender flowers
- 1/2 cup dried chamomile flowers
- 2 cups Epsom salt
- 10-15 drops lavender essential oil (optional for enhanced aroma)
- 1 large muslin bag or cheesecloth

Instructions

1. In a large bowl, mix the dried lavender flowers, dried chamomile flowers, and Epsom salt together.

2. If using, add the lavender essential oil to the mixture and stir well to ensure the oil is evenly distributed.

3. Spoon the mixture into the muslin bag or cheesecloth. If using cheesecloth, gather the edges and tie them securely with a string.

4. To use, place the filled bag or cheesecloth under warm running bath water. Let it steep in the tub as it fills.

5. Once the bath is ready, squeeze the bag or cheesecloth gently to release more of the herbal essences into the water.

6. Soak in the bath for at least 20 minutes, breathing deeply to inhale the relaxing aromas.

7. After soaking, discard the contents of the bag or cheesecloth and rinse it out for future use.

Variations

- For additional moisturizing properties, add 1/4 cup of coconut oil or almond oil to the bathwater.

- Incorporate a cup of baking soda to the mixture for a detoxifying effect and softer skin.

- For a more luxurious bath experience, sprinkle fresh lavender or chamomile flowers in the bath along with the soak.

Storage tips

Store any unused Lavender and Chamomile Bath Soak mixture in an airtight container in a cool, dry place. The mixture can last up to 6 months if stored properly.

Tips for allergens

Individuals with allergies to lavender or chamomile should perform a patch test before using this soak or substitute these ingredients with other non-allergenic herbs such as rose petals or calendula, which also offer soothing properties.

Scientific references

- "Lavender and the Nervous System." Evidence-Based Complementary and Alternative Medicine, 2013. This study highlights the anxiety-reducing and sleep-inducing effects of lavender.

- "Chamomile: A herbal medicine of the past with a bright future." Molecular Medicine Reports, 2010. This review discusses the anti-inflammatory and skin-soothing benefits of chamomile.

VALERIAN ROOT TEA

Beneficial effects

Valerian Root Tea is widely recognized for its ability to promote relaxation and improve sleep quality. It acts as a natural sedative, calming the nerves and reducing anxiety levels. This makes it an excellent choice for those dealing with stress and looking for a natural way to unwind and achieve a peaceful state of mind.

Portions

1 serving

Preparation time

10 minutes

Cooking time

5-10 minutes

Ingredients

- 1 teaspoon of dried valerian root

- 8 ounces of boiling water

- Honey or lemon (optional, for taste)

Instructions

1. Bring 8 ounces of water to a boil in a kettle or pot.

2. Place the dried valerian root in a tea infuser or directly into a mug.

3. Pour the boiling water over the valerian root and cover the mug with a lid or a small plate to steep.

4. Allow the tea to steep for 5-10 minutes, depending on your desired strength. The longer it steeps, the more potent the effects.

5. Remove the valerian root or tea infuser from the mug.

6. Optional: Add honey or lemon to taste for flavor enhancement.

7. Enjoy the tea warm, ideally 30 minutes to an hour before bedtime to aid in relaxation and sleep.

Variations

- For a more complex flavor profile, add a cinnamon stick or a few slices of fresh ginger to the water while boiling.

- Combine with chamomile or lavender tea for additional calming effects.

- If the taste of valerian root is too strong, mix with peppermint tea to mask the flavor.

Storage tips

Dried valerian root should be stored in an airtight container in a cool, dark place to maintain its potency and freshness.

Tips for allergens

For those with sensitivities to specific herbs, start with a small amount of valerian root to ensure no adverse reactions. Honey can be omitted or replaced with a suitable sweetener like maple syrup for those with allergies or dietary restrictions.

Scientific references

- "Effects of valerian on subjective sedation, field sobriety testing and driving simulator performance" - Accident Analysis & Prevention, 2010. This study highlights the sedative effects of valerian root, supporting its use for stress relief and sleep improvement.

- "Aqueous extract of valerian root improves sleep quality in men" - Pharmacology Biochemistry and Behavior, 1982. This research provides evidence of valerian root's ability to enhance sleep quality, making it beneficial for those experiencing stress-induced insomnia.

PASSIONFLOWER TINCTURE

Beneficial effects

Passionflower Tincture is widely recognized for its calming and sedative properties, making it an excellent natural remedy for anxiety, stress, and sleep disorders. It works by increasing levels of gamma-aminobutyric acid (GABA) in the brain, which helps to lower brain activity and induce relaxation. This tincture can also help alleviate symptoms of nervousness and improve the overall quality of sleep.

Ingredients

- 1 cup fresh or dried passionflower herb
- 2 cups high-proof alcohol (such as vodka or brandy)
- A clean glass jar with a tight-fitting lid

Instructions

1. Place the passionflower herb into the clean glass jar.

2. Pour the high-proof alcohol over the herbs, ensuring they are completely submerged. Leave about an inch of space at the top of the jar.

3. Seal the jar tightly with the lid and label it with the date and contents.

4. Store the jar in a cool, dark place for 4 to 6 weeks. Shake the jar gently every few days to mix the contents and promote extraction.

5. After the infusion period, strain the tincture through a fine mesh sieve or cheesecloth into another clean glass jar or bottle. Press or squeeze the herbs to extract as much liquid as possible.

6. Label the container with the date and contents.

Variations

- For a non-alcoholic version, substitute the alcohol with glycerin and water (3 parts glycerin to 1 part water).
- Add other calming herbs such as lavender or chamomile to the tincture for additional stress-relieving effects.

Storage tips

Store the finished tincture in a cool, dark place. When stored properly, it can last for several years.

Tips for allergens

Individuals with allergies to passionflower should avoid using this tincture. As always, consult with a healthcare provider before starting any new herbal remedy, especially if you are pregnant, nursing, or taking medications.

Scientific references

- "Passionflower in the treatment of generalized anxiety: A pilot double-blind randomized controlled trial with oxazepam." Journal of Clinical Pharmacy and Therapeutics, 2001. This study supports the use of passionflower for anxiety relief.

- "A double-blind, placebo-controlled investigation of the effects of Passiflora incarnata (passionflower) herbal tea on subjective sleep quality." Phytotherapy Research, 2011. This research highlights the benefits of passionflower on improving sleep quality.

LEMON BALM INFUSION

Beneficial effects

Lemon Balm Infusion is a calming herbal remedy known for its ability to reduce stress, anxiety, and promote a sense of relaxation. The soothing properties of lemon balm can also help improve sleep quality and enhance cognitive function by easing nervous tension and irritability.

Portions

2 servings

Preparation time

10 minutes

Cooking time

5 minutes

Ingredients

- 2 tablespoons of dried lemon balm leaves

- 2 cups of boiling water

- Honey or lemon slice (optional, for taste)

Instructions

1. Place the dried lemon balm leaves in a teapot or heat-resistant glass container.

2. Pour 2 cups of boiling water over the lemon balm leaves.

3. Cover and let the infusion steep for about 5 to 10 minutes, depending on the desired strength.

4. Strain the infusion into cups, discarding the used lemon balm leaves.

5. If desired, add honey or a slice of lemon to enhance the flavor.

6. Serve the infusion warm for a soothing effect.

Variations

- For a refreshing summer drink, chill the infusion in the refrigerator and serve over ice.

- Add a sprig of mint or a few slices of cucumber for a refreshing twist.

- Combine with chamomile in the evening for an extra calming effect before bedtime.

Storage tips

If you have leftover lemon balm infusion, store it in a sealed container in the refrigerator for up to 2 days. Enjoy it cold or gently reheat on the stove.

Tips for allergens

For those with allergies to plants in the mint family, start with a small amount of lemon balm to ensure no adverse reactions. Honey can be substituted with maple syrup for a vegan option.

Scientific references

- "Anxiolytic Effects of a Combination of Melissa officinalis and Valeriana officinalis during Laboratory Induced Stress," Phytotherapy Research, 2006. This study demonstrates the stress-relieving benefits of lemon balm in combination with valerian root.

- "Melissa officinalis L. – A Review of its Traditional Uses, Phytochemistry, and Pharmacology," Journal of Ethnopharmacology, 2015. This review highlights the cognitive-enhancing and calming effects of lemon balm, supporting its use for stress relief and mental health.

ASHWAGANDHA SMOOTHIE

Beneficial effects

Ashwagandha Smoothie is designed to combat stress and enhance mental health. Ashwagandha, an adaptogen, helps to balance the body's response to stress, reducing anxiety and improving focus and energy levels. This smoothie combines the stress-relieving properties of ashwagandha with the nutritional benefits of its other ingredients, making it a powerful tool for improving overall well-being.

Portions

1 serving

Preparation time

5 minutes

Ingredients

- 1 cup unsweetened almond milk
- 1 ripe banana
- 1/2 teaspoon ashwagandha powder
- 1 tablespoon almond butter
- 1/2 teaspoon cinnamon
- 1 teaspoon honey (optional, for sweetness)
- Ice cubes (optional)

Instructions

1. Pour the unsweetened almond milk into a blender.

2. Add the ripe banana, ashwagandha powder, almond butter, and cinnamon.

3. If desired, add honey for sweetness.

4. Add ice cubes for a colder smoothie, if preferred.

5. Blend all ingredients on high until smooth and creamy.

6. Pour the smoothie into a glass and enjoy immediately.

Variations

- For a protein boost, add a scoop of your favorite vanilla or unflavored protein powder.

- Substitute almond milk with coconut milk or oat milk for a different flavor profile.

- Add a handful of spinach or kale for extra nutrients without significantly altering the taste.

Storage tips

It's best to consume the Ashwagandha Smoothie immediately after blending to enjoy its full benefits. However, if you must store it, keep the smoothie in an airtight container in the refrigerator for no more than 24 hours. Shake well before consuming if separation occurs.

Tips for allergens

For those with nut allergies, replace almond milk and almond butter with oat milk and sunflower seed butter, respectively. Ensure the ashwagandha powder is pure and free from any additives that may cause allergic reactions.

Scientific references

- "An Overview on Ashwagandha: A Rasayana (Rejuvenator) of Ayurveda" published in the African Journal of Traditional, Complementary and Alternative Medicines, which discusses the adaptogenic and stress-relief properties of ashwagandha.

- "A Prospective, Randomized Double-Blind, Placebo-Controlled Study of Safety and Efficacy of a High-Concentration Full-Spectrum Extract of Ashwagandha Root in Reducing Stress and Anxiety in Adults" published in the Indian Journal of Psychological Medicine, highlighting the efficacy of ashwagandha in reducing stress and anxiety.

PART 6: PHYSICAL ACTIVITY AND FITNESS

Physical activity and fitness are integral components of a holistic health approach, emphasizing the interconnectedness of the body, mind, and spirit. Regular exercise not only strengthens the body but also enhances mental health and emotional well-being. It plays a crucial role in preventing chronic diseases, managing weight, improving sleep quality, and boosting overall energy levels. The benefits of physical activity extend beyond the immediate effects on the heart, muscles, and respiratory system; it also contributes to a balanced and harmonious state of being, aligning with the principles of natural healing and self-care.

Incorporating physical activity into daily life doesn't require exhaustive routines or gym memberships. It's about finding joy in movement and integrating it seamlessly into your lifestyle. Walking, cycling, gardening, dancing, and yoga are excellent examples of accessible exercises that can significantly impact health without the need for specialized equipment or intense training. These activities not only promote cardiovascular health and muscle strength but also offer opportunities for mindfulness, relaxation, and connection with nature, embodying the holistic health philosophy.

Understanding the types of exercise and their benefits is crucial for developing a balanced fitness routine. Aerobic exercises, such as brisk walking or swimming, improve cardiovascular endurance and lung capacity. Strength training, using body weight or resistance equipment, supports muscle health, bone density, and metabolic function. Flexibility exercises, including yoga and stretching, enhance joint mobility and reduce the risk of injuries. Lastly, balance exercises prevent falls and improve posture, essential for overall mobility and quality of life as we age.

To embrace a holistic approach to physical activity, listen to your body and respect its limits. Start with moderate activities and gradually increase intensity and duration to avoid injury. Incorporate a variety of exercises to engage different muscle groups and promote mental stimulation. Remember, consistency is more beneficial than intensity; regular, moderate exercise is more effective than sporadic, high-intensity sessions.

Hydration and nutrition play vital roles in supporting an active lifestyle. Before exercising, fuel your body with a balanced meal or snack rich in complex carbohydrates and protein to ensure energy availability. Hydrate well to prevent dehydration, which can impair performance and recovery. Post-exercise, consume foods high in protein and antioxidants to aid muscle repair and reduce inflammation. Understanding the body's needs and providing it with the right nutrients at the right time enhances the benefits of physical activity and supports holistic health.

Physical activity and fitness are not just about physical health; they're about nurturing the mind and spirit, fostering a sense of achievement, and enhancing life quality. By integrating physical activity into your holistic health approach, you support your body's natural healing processes, contribute to your emotional and mental well-being, and take a proactive step towards a balanced, healthy lifestyle.

CHAPTER 1: THE ROLE OF EXERCISE IN HEALTH

Exercise plays a pivotal role in maintaining and enhancing our health, serving as a cornerstone for a holistic approach to well-being. It goes beyond just physical benefits, impacting every aspect of our health, including mental, emotional, and even spiritual dimensions. Regular physical activity is instrumental in preventing a range of chronic diseases such as heart disease, diabetes, depression, and several types of cancer. It also significantly contributes to the management of stress and anxiety, showcasing its profound influence on our mental health.

The human body thrives on movement. From improving cardiovascular health to strengthening the musculoskeletal system, exercise facilitates the efficient functioning of our bodies. It enhances blood circulation, which is crucial for the delivery of oxygen and nutrients to tissues, and the removal of waste products, thereby supporting the body's natural detoxification processes. Moreover, engaging in regular physical activity boosts the immune system by promoting good circulation, which allows the cells and substances of the immune system to move through the body freely and do their job efficiently.

On a metabolic level, exercise plays a key role in regulating blood sugar levels and improving insulin sensitivity, which can help in preventing and managing type 2 diabetes. It also aids in weight management by burning calories and building muscle, which in turn, increases metabolic rate even when at rest. This balance between energy intake and expenditure is essential for maintaining a healthy weight and preventing obesity, a major risk factor for many diseases.

From a mental and emotional perspective, exercise is a powerful stress reliever. Physical activity increases the production of endorphins, often referred to as the body's natural mood elevators. This biochemical process can lead to improved mood, a sense of well-being, and even a reduction in symptoms of depression and anxiety. Additionally, engaging in exercise, especially in natural settings or group settings, can provide a sense of connection, enhancing social well-being and reducing feelings of loneliness and isolation.

For cognitive health, regular physical activity is equally beneficial.

It has been shown to improve brain function, enhance memory and thinking skills, and may even slow the progression of brain disorders such as Alzheimer's disease. Exercise stimulates the production of growth factors, chemicals in the brain that affect the health of brain cells, the growth of new blood vessels in the brain, and even the abundance and survival of new brain cells.

Incorporating exercise into daily life doesn't have to be daunting. It's about finding activities that you enjoy and that fit into your lifestyle. Whether it's brisk walking, cycling, swimming, or practicing yoga, the key is consistency and making physical activity a regular part of your routine. It's also important to mix different types of exercise to keep things interesting and to provide the body with a comprehensive workout. This includes a combination of aerobic exercises for heart and lung health, strength training for muscles and bones, flexibility exercises for joints, and balance exercises to prevent falls.

Listening to your body is crucial when engaging in physical activity. It's important to start slowly, especially if you're new to exercise, and gradually increase the intensity and duration of your workouts. Paying attention to hydration and nutrition is also essential, as they play a significant role in performance and recovery. Before exercising, a snack or meal that includes carbohydrates and protein can provide energy and support muscle function. After exercise, replenishing with fluids, electrolytes, and nutrients is vital for recovery and to prepare the body for the next workout.

In summary, the role of exercise in health is multifaceted, offering extensive benefits that touch upon every aspect of our well-being. By making physical activity a regular part of our lives, we support our body's natural healing processes, enhance our mental and emotional health, and take proactive steps towards a balanced, healthy lifestyle.

DR. BARBARA'S PHILOSOPHY ON MOVEMENT

Dr. Barbara's philosophy on movement is deeply rooted in the belief that physical activity is a vital component of holistic health, serving not just the body but also the mind and spirit. She emphasizes that movement should be a joyful and integral part of daily life, rather than a chore or merely a means to an end. According to Dr. Barbara, the essence of movement lies in its ability to harmonize and balance our physical, mental, and emotional states, fostering a sense of well-being that transcends the physical benefits commonly associated with exercise.

In her approach, Dr. Barbara advocates for incorporating a variety of movements that engage the body in different ways, highlighting the importance of aerobic exercises for cardiovascular health, strength training for muscle and bone density, flexibility practices for joint health, and balance exercises for coordination and mental focus. She stresses the significance of choosing activities that resonate personally, encouraging individuals to explore different forms of exercise to find what truly motivates and energizes them. This personal connection to movement, she believes, is key to developing a sustainable and enjoyable fitness routine.

Dr. Barbara also addresses the common barriers to regular physical activity, such as time constraints, physical limitations, and lack of motivation. She offers practical solutions for overcoming these challenges, such as integrating short bursts of movement throughout the day, adapting exercises to suit individual needs and abilities, and setting realistic, achievable goals.

By reframing the way we view and engage with physical activity, Dr. Barbara aims to inspire a positive and empowering relationship with movement.

Furthermore, Dr. Barbara underscores the interconnectedness of movement with other aspects of holistic health, including nutrition, hydration, rest, and stress management.

She points out that nourishing the body with the right foods, staying hydrated, getting adequate rest, and managing stress are all essential components that support and enhance the benefits of physical activity. This holistic approach ensures that the body is well-equipped to perform and recover from exercise, while also maximizing the mental and emotional benefits of movement.

In essence, Dr. Barbara's philosophy on movement is about much more than just physical fitness; it's about cultivating a lifestyle that embraces movement as a source of joy, vitality, and balance. By encouraging individuals to find their own path to physical activity, she aims to foster a lifelong commitment to movement that supports holistic health and well-being.

TYPES OF EXERCISE AND THEIR BENEFITS

Aerobic exercise, often referred to as cardio, is a cornerstone of physical fitness, enhancing cardiovascular health by improving heart rate and lung function. This type of exercise includes activities like brisk walking, running, swimming, and cycling, designed to increase the heart rate and promote the circulation of oxygen throughout the body. The benefits of aerobic exercise extend beyond cardiovascular health, also aiding in weight management by burning calories and increasing metabolism. Regular participation in aerobic activities can reduce the risk of chronic conditions such as heart disease, type 2 diabetes, and high blood pressure, while also boosting mood and energy levels through the release of endorphins.

Strength training, another vital component of a well-rounded fitness routine, focuses on building muscle mass and improving bone density. Utilizing resistance through body weight, free weights, or resistance bands, strength training exercises like squats, lunges, and push-ups target various muscle groups. This form of exercise is crucial for maintaining muscle strength and endurance, supporting joint health, and enhancing metabolic rate, which can aid in weight loss or maintenance.

Strength training is particularly important as we age, helping to counteract the loss of muscle mass and bone density that occurs naturally over time.

Flexibility exercises, including yoga and stretching routines, play a significant role in maintaining the range of motion of the joints and preventing injuries.

Regular flexibility training can alleviate muscle tension, reduce pain, and improve posture by lengthening the muscles and increasing elasticity. This type of exercise is essential for overall mobility and can significantly enhance performance in other physical activities by allowing for more significant movement and reducing the risk of strains and sprains.

Balance exercises are essential for preventing falls, a common concern as individuals age. Activities that improve balance, such as tai chi, standing on one leg, and balance ball exercises, can enhance proprioception, the body's ability to sense its position in space.

By strengthening the muscles that help keep you upright, balance exercises can improve overall stability, coordination, and functional movement, contributing to a higher quality of life and independence, especially in older adults.

Incorporating a mix of aerobic, strength, flexibility, and balance exercises into a fitness routine ensures a comprehensive approach to physical activity, addressing various aspects of health and well-being.

Each type of exercise offers unique benefits and contributes to the holistic health approach, emphasizing the interconnectedness of physical fitness with mental and emotional well-being. By engaging in a variety of activities, individuals can enjoy a more balanced, healthy lifestyle, better equipped to handle the demands of daily life and reduce the risk of chronic disease.

CHAPTER 2: DESIGNING A FITNESS ROUTINE

Designing a fitness routine that aligns with your holistic health goals involves understanding your body's needs, preferences, and the principles of balanced physical activity. A well-structured fitness routine should cater to enhancing cardiovascular health, building strength, improving flexibility, and boosting balance. Here's how to create a fitness routine that supports your holistic health journey, keeping in mind the interconnectedness of physical, mental, and emotional well-being.

Objective: To develop a personalized fitness routine that supports holistic health, incorporating a variety of exercises that promote cardiovascular health, muscle strength, flexibility, and balance.

Preparation:

1. Assess your current fitness level and health status. Consider any physical limitations or medical conditions.

2. Define your fitness goals. Whether it's improving cardiovascular health, gaining strength, enhancing flexibility, or achieving better balance, your goals will guide your routine.

3. Choose activities you enjoy. Incorporating exercises you love ensures long-term commitment and enjoyment.

4. Schedule your workouts. Determine the most convenient times for you to exercise, aiming for consistency.

Materials:

- Comfortable clothing and supportive footwear
- Exercise mat for yoga or floor exercises
- Resistance bands or weights for strength training
- Stability ball for balance exercises

Tools:

- Timer or stopwatch
- Fitness tracker or app to monitor progress
- Water bottle to stay hydrated

Safety measures:

- Warm up before starting your routine to prepare your muscles and prevent injuries.
- Cool down after your workout with stretching to aid recovery.
- Stay hydrated, especially during intense or prolonged exercise.
- Listen to your body and modify exercises as needed to avoid strain or injury.

Step-by-step instructions:

1. **Warm-Up (5-10 minutes)**: Begin with light aerobic activity like walking or cycling to gradually increase your heart rate.

2. **Aerobic Exercise (20-30 minutes)**: Choose activities like brisk walking, jogging, swimming, or cycling. Adjust the intensity and duration based on your fitness level.

3. **Strength Training (20-30 minutes)**: Incorporate exercises targeting major muscle groups. Use body weight, resistance bands, or weights. Perform 2-3 sets of 8-12 repetitions for each exercise.

4. **Flexibility and Balance (10-15 minutes)**: End your routine with yoga or stretching exercises to improve flexibility. Include balance exercises like standing on one leg or using a stability ball.

5. Cool Down (5-10 minutes): Finish with gentle stretching to help muscles recover and prevent stiffness.

Cost estimate: Minimal to moderate, depending on whether you choose to purchase equipment or use available resources at home.

Time estimate: 45-75 minutes per session, 3-5 times a week, depending on your schedule and fitness goals.

Safety tips:

- Use proper form to avoid injuries.

- Increase the intensity and duration of your workouts gradually.

- Stay hydrated and avoid overheating.

- Rest between workouts to allow for recovery.

Troubleshooting:

- If you experience pain or discomfort, stop the exercise and adjust your technique or switch to a different activity.

- If you lack motivation, try varying your routine or exercising with a friend.

Maintenance:

- Regularly assess and adjust your fitness routine to align with your evolving health goals and interests.

- Keep track of your progress and celebrate achievements to stay motivated.

Difficulty rating: ★★☆☆☆ to ★★★★☆, depending on the chosen exercises and intensity.

Variations:

- Incorporate interval training to boost cardiovascular health and metabolism.

- Try different types of yoga or Pilates for flexibility and core strength.

- Add outdoor activities like hiking or paddleboarding for variety and mental health benefits.

By designing a fitness routine that addresses various aspects of physical health while also considering personal preferences and enjoyment, you can support your holistic health journey effectively. Remember, the key to a successful fitness routine is consistency, listening to your body, and making adjustments as needed to stay aligned with your holistic health goals.

INCORPORATING CARDIO, STRENGTH, AND FLEXIBILITY

Incorporating cardio, strength, and flexibility into a fitness routine creates a balanced approach that enhances overall health and well-being. Cardiovascular exercises increase heart rate and improve lung capacity, making the heart stronger and more efficient at pumping blood. Strength training builds and maintains muscle mass, supports joint health, and increases metabolic rate, which can aid in weight management. Flexibility exercises improve the range of motion, reduce the risk of injuries, and alleviate muscle tension, contributing to better posture and mobility.

For cardio, starting with activities like brisk walking, jogging, cycling, or swimming for 20 to 30 minutes most days of the week can significantly boost cardiovascular health. These activities can be easily adjusted to fit one's current fitness level and gradually increased in intensity and duration as endurance improves. Incorporating interval training, which alternates short bursts of high-intensity exercise with periods of rest or lower intensity, can further enhance cardiovascular fitness and calorie burn.

Strength training can be approached by using body weight, free weights, resistance bands, or weight machines. Focusing on major muscle groups, aim for two to three sets of 8 to 12 repetitions for each exercise, ensuring that all major muscle groups are worked on throughout the week. Exercises such as squats, lunges, push-ups, and planks are effective for engaging multiple muscle groups and can be modified to suit various fitness levels.

Flexibility is an often-overlooked component of physical fitness but is crucial for a well-rounded fitness routine. Incorporating yoga, Pilates, or simple stretching exercises into the routine can greatly improve flexibility and joint health. Spending 10 to 15 minutes daily on flexibility exercises can enhance physical performance, reduce the risk of injuries, and promote muscle recovery. Stretching should be gentle and focused, aiming to stretch all major muscle groups, with particular attention to areas that are prone to tightness, such as the hamstrings, lower back, and shoulders.

To ensure a balanced routine, dedicate specific days to focus on each aspect of fitness or combine them into a single workout session.

For example, a workout session could start with a cardio warm-up, followed by strength training, and end with flexibility exercises for a cool-down. Listening to the body and allowing adequate rest between workouts is essential to prevent overtraining and injuries. Hydration and proper nutrition support exercise performance and recovery, emphasizing the importance of a well-rounded approach to health.

By integrating cardio, strength, and flexibility exercises into a fitness routine, individuals can enjoy a comprehensive approach to physical activity that promotes heart health, builds strength, enhances flexibility, and improves overall quality of life. This balanced approach not only contributes to physical health but also supports mental and emotional well-being, aligning with the holistic health philosophy that encompasses the interconnectedness of the body, mind, and spirit.

IMPORTANCE OF REST AND RECOVERY

Rest and recovery are critical components of any fitness routine, serving as the foundation for physical improvement and injury prevention. After engaging in physical activity, the body needs time to repair tissues and replenish energy stores, a process that occurs during periods of rest. Without adequate recovery, the risk of injuries increases, and the effectiveness of workouts diminishes, leading to potential setbacks in fitness goals.

The body's adaptation to exercise, including muscle strength and endurance enhancements, occurs not during the workout itself but during the rest periods that follow. This adaptation process allows the body to recover from the stress of exercise and rebuild stronger than before, a principle known as the supercompensation effect. Therefore, incorporating rest days into a fitness routine is essential for allowing the body to undergo this vital rebuilding process.

Sleep plays a pivotal role in the recovery process, as it is during deep sleep that the body releases growth hormone, which aids in tissue repair and growth. Ensuring seven to nine hours of quality sleep per night can significantly enhance recovery, improve performance, and reduce the risk of injuries. Sleep deprivation, on the other hand, can lead to decreased motivation, increased perceived exertion during workouts, and slower recovery times.

Active recovery, involving light exercise such as walking, yoga, or swimming, can also be beneficial in promoting recovery. These activities increase blood flow to the muscles without placing additional stress on them, helping to remove metabolic waste products accumulated during intense workouts. Active recovery days can accelerate the healing process, improve flexibility, and reduce muscle soreness.

Hydration and nutrition are other key elements of effective recovery. Replenishing fluids lost during exercise is crucial to prevent dehydration, which can impair muscle recovery and performance. Consuming a balanced diet rich in proteins, carbohydrates, and healthy fats provides the necessary nutrients for muscle repair, energy replenishment, and inflammation reduction. Post-workout nutrition, particularly the intake of protein and carbohydrates within a 45-minute window after exercise, can significantly enhance the recovery process by providing the building blocks for muscle repair and glycogen storage.

Listening to the body and recognizing signs of overtraining, such as prolonged muscle soreness, fatigue, decreased performance, and increased susceptibility to injuries and illnesses, is crucial. These symptoms indicate the need for additional rest and recovery time. Ignoring these signs and continuing to push through workouts without adequate rest can lead to burnout, overuse injuries, and chronic fatigue.

DR. BARBARA'S TIPS FOR STAYING MOTIVATED

Staying motivated in your fitness journey is crucial for long-term success and achieving your holistic health goals. Dr. Barbara emphasizes the importance of setting realistic goals as a foundation for maintaining motivation. Start by defining clear, achievable objectives that resonate with your personal health aspirations. Whether it's improving flexibility, building strength, or enhancing cardiovascular health, having specific goals can help you stay focused and track your progress.

Creating a supportive environment is another key strategy. Surround yourself with positivity, whether it's through an encouraging social circle, motivational music during workouts, or inspirational quotes in your living space. A supportive environment not only uplifts your spirits but also reinforces your commitment to your fitness routine.

Variety in your exercise regimen can prevent boredom and keep things exciting. Experiment with different types of workouts to challenge your body in new ways and keep your interest alive. From yoga and Pilates to strength training and outdoor activities, diversifying your fitness routine can lead to newfound passions and prevent workout monotony.

Celebrating small victories is essential for sustained motivation. Acknowledge every step forward, no matter how minor it may seem. Completing a workout when you didn't feel like it, adding an extra mile to your run, or choosing a healthy meal over fast food are all achievements worth celebrating. These small wins build confidence and reinforce the positive impact of your efforts.

Listening to your body and allowing for rest is equally important. Recognize the difference between pushing yourself to grow and pushing yourself to the brink of injury or burnout. Rest and recovery are not signs of regression but are integral to progress. They allow your body to heal, preventing burnout and keeping your motivation intact for the long haul.

Lastly, remind yourself of why you started. Keeping your ultimate goal in mind, whether it's for better health, more energy, or simply feeling good in your own skin, can help you push through challenging moments. When motivation wanes, revisiting your initial inspiration can reignite your drive and commitment to your holistic health journey.

By incorporating these strategies into your approach to fitness, you can maintain a high level of motivation, overcome obstacles, and continue progressing towards your holistic health goals. Remember, the journey to health is a marathon, not a sprint, and staying motivated is key to enjoying the journey and reaching your destination.

CHAPTER 3: NUTRITION FOR FITNESS AND RECOVERY

Fueling your body with the right nutrients before and after workouts is crucial for maximizing performance and recovery. For fitness enthusiasts and athletes, understanding the balance of macronutrients—proteins, carbohydrates, and fats—is key to optimizing both. Proteins are essential for muscle repair and growth. Incorporating a variety of protein sources, such as lean meats, fish, legumes, and plant-based proteins, ensures a complete amino acid profile necessary for muscle recovery. Carbohydrates are the body's primary energy source. Before workouts, focus on complex carbohydrates like whole grains, fruits, and vegetables to provide sustained energy. Post-workout, include simple carbohydrates to quickly replenish muscle glycogen stores. Healthy fats, especially omega-3 fatty acids found in fish, nuts, and seeds, play a vital role in reducing inflammation and supporting overall heart health.

Hydration is another critical component of fitness nutrition. Adequate water intake before, during, and after exercise supports optimal performance, energy levels, and recovery by maintaining hydration status and replacing fluids lost through sweat. Electrolyte balance, crucial for muscle function and hydration, can be maintained by including natural sources of electrolytes in your diet, such as bananas for potassium, dairy or fortified plant milk for calcium, and nuts or seeds for magnesium.

Timing of nutrient intake also impacts fitness and recovery. Eating a balanced meal or snack 1-2 hours before exercising provides the energy and amino acids necessary for muscle endurance and strength. Post-workout, aim to consume a mix of proteins and carbohydrates within 45 minutes to an hour to enhance muscle recovery and glycogen replenishment.

For those looking to support their fitness journey with natural remedies, consider incorporating herbal teas and supplements known for their anti-inflammatory and recovery benefits. For example, turmeric, with its active compound curcumin, can help reduce inflammation and muscle soreness when taken regularly. Ginger, another potent anti-inflammatory herb, can be added to smoothies or teas to support digestion and reduce post-workout pain.

In summary, a holistic approach to nutrition for fitness and recovery encompasses a balanced intake of macronutrients, adequate hydration, mindful timing of meals, and the inclusion of natural herbs for inflammation and muscle repair. This comprehensive strategy supports not only physical performance and recovery but also overall health and well-being.

PRE-WORKOUT NUTRITION

Optimizing your energy and performance before engaging in physical activity starts with the right pre-workout nutrition. Focusing on foods that provide a steady release of energy without weighing you down is key. A combination of complex carbohydrates and lean proteins can fuel your muscles effectively, while a small amount of healthy fats can keep you satiated. For instance, a banana or an apple paired with a tablespoon of almond butter offers a quick, easily digestible source of carbohydrates and protein. Alternatively, a small serving of oatmeal topped with berries provides fiber-rich carbs and antioxidants, aiding in sustained energy release and protection against oxidative stress during your workout.

Hydration plays a crucial role in pre-workout preparation. Drinking water throughout the day before exercising ensures you start your workout adequately hydrated. Adding a slice of lemon or cucumber can enhance the water's taste, encouraging more fluid intake without added sugars.

For those who exercise in the early morning, a light snack can kickstart your metabolism without causing discomfort during your workout. A piece of whole-grain toast with a thin layer of avocado provides a balance of carbs and healthy fats. This combination supports energy levels and muscle function without overburdening your digestive system.

Timing your pre-workout meal is as important as its content. Eating your snack or meal about 30 to 60 minutes before exercising allows your body to digest and begin metabolizing the nutrients, ensuring they're available for muscle use. However, individual digestion rates vary, so it's crucial to listen to your body and adjust timing as needed to avoid any gastrointestinal discomfort.

Incorporating these nutritional strategies supports your body's energy needs and enhances performance, making your workout more effective and enjoyable. Remember, personal preferences and tolerances play a significant role in pre-workout nutrition, so it's essential to find what works best for you.

POST-WORKOUT RECOVERY FOODS

After an intense workout, your body needs the right nutrients to repair muscles, replenish energy stores, and reduce inflammation. Focusing on post-workout recovery foods is essential for optimizing the benefits of your exercise routine and preparing your body for the next session. Consuming a mix of proteins, carbohydrates, and healthy fats within 45 minutes to an hour after exercising can significantly enhance recovery and muscle synthesis.

Beneficial effects: Accelerates muscle recovery, replenishes glycogen stores, reduces muscle soreness, and minimizes inflammation.

Portions: Varies based on individual dietary needs and workout intensity.

Preparation time: 5-15 minutes

Ingredients:

- 1 cup of Greek yogurt or a plant-based alternative for a dairy-free option
- 1/2 cup of mixed berries (blueberries, strawberries, raspberries)
- 1 tablespoon of honey or maple syrup for sweetness
- 1/4 cup of granola or mixed nuts and seeds for crunch and added protein
- 1 tablespoon of chia seeds or flaxseeds for omega-3 fatty acids
- Optional: 1 scoop of protein powder for an extra protein boost

Instructions:

1. In a bowl, combine the Greek yogurt with the protein powder (if using) until well mixed.

2. Top the yogurt with the mixed berries, distributing them evenly.

3. Drizzle honey or maple syrup over the berries and yogurt.

4. Sprinkle granola, nuts, or seeds on top for added texture and nutrients.

5. Finish by scattering chia seeds or flaxseeds over the entire bowl.

6. Enjoy immediately for the best flavor and nutritional benefits.

Variations:

- For a vegan option, use plant-based yogurt and a vegan protein powder.
- Swap out berries for other fruits like sliced bananas, mango, or pineapple for different vitamins and minerals.

- Add a tablespoon of nut butter for extra healthy fats and protein.

Storage tips: Best consumed fresh. However, you can prepare the dry ingredients in a separate container and mix with yogurt just before eating if needed.

Tips for allergens: Choose nut-free granola or seeds if allergic to nuts. Ensure the protein powder is free from allergens specific to your dietary needs.

This recovery meal combines high-quality protein for muscle repair, antioxidants from berries for reducing inflammation, and carbohydrates to quickly replenish glycogen stores. The addition of healthy fats from seeds or nuts supports overall recovery and aids in the absorption of fat-soluble vitamins. This balanced approach not only aids in physical recovery but also supports long-term health and fitness goals, making it an ideal choice for anyone looking to maximize the benefits of their workout regimen.

HYDRATION AND ELECTROLYTES

Hydration and electrolytes play a pivotal role in maintaining optimal health, especially for individuals engaged in regular physical activity. The body loses water and electrolytes through sweat during exercise, making it crucial to replenish these elements to prevent dehydration and maintain muscle function. Water serves as the primary transporter of nutrients throughout the body and assists in every metabolic process, including energy production and waste removal. Electrolytes, such as sodium, potassium, calcium, and magnesium, are essential minerals that carry an electric charge and are vital for various bodily functions including muscle contractions and nerve signaling.

To ensure adequate hydration, it is recommended to drink water consistently throughout the day, not just before or after exercise.

The amount of water needed can vary based on individual factors including age, weight, activity level, and environmental conditions. A general guideline is to consume at least half your body weight in ounces of water daily, with additional intake before, during, and after workouts. For example, a person weighing 150 pounds should aim to drink at least 75 ounces of water per day, plus additional fluids around exercise sessions.

Incorporating natural sources of electrolytes into your diet can help maintain the balance necessary for optimal bodily functions. Foods rich in potassium, such as bananas, sweet potatoes, and spinach, support muscle and nerve function.

Calcium, found in dairy products and fortified plant milks, is crucial for muscle contractions and bone health. Magnesium, present in nuts, seeds, and whole grains, aids in muscle relaxation and energy production. Sodium, which can be lost in significant amounts through sweat, can be replenished in moderation through natural sources like celery, beets, and salted nuts, or through electrolyte-enhanced beverages if necessary.

For individuals engaging in prolonged or intense physical activity, especially in hot conditions, consuming an electrolyte-rich drink can be beneficial for replenishing lost minerals and preventing dehydration. A simple homemade electrolyte drink can be made by combining:

- 4 cups of water
- ¼ teaspoon of salt (for sodium)
- ¼ cup of 100% fruit juice (for potassium and natural sugars)
- 2 tablespoons of lemon juice (for flavor and additional potassium)
- 1 tablespoon of honey or maple syrup (for natural sugar and energy)

Instructions:

1. In a large pitcher, dissolve the salt and honey (or maple syrup) in the water, stirring thoroughly.

2. Add the fruit juice and lemon juice, and mix well.

3. Taste and adjust the sweetness or saltiness as needed.

4. Chill in the refrigerator or serve over ice for a refreshing, hydrating drink.

This drink provides a balance of electrolytes and fluids, making it an excellent choice for hydration before, during, or after workouts. Adjusting the ingredients based on personal taste preferences or dietary needs can help ensure adequate hydration and electrolyte balance is maintained, supporting overall health and fitness performance. Remember, listening to your body's signals for thirst and monitoring the color of your urine (aiming for light yellow) are practical ways to ensure you're staying well-hydrated.

DR. BARBARA'S FAVORITE RECOVERY FOODS

Dr. Barbara emphasizes the importance of selecting recovery foods that not only replenish the body after a workout but also provide essential nutrients to support muscle repair, reduce inflammation, and boost overall health. Among her favorites are salmon for its high omega-3 fatty acid content, which aids in reducing muscle inflammation and supports heart health. Sweet potatoes are another staple, packed with complex carbohydrates and beta-carotene, they help restore glycogen levels and provide a rich source of fiber and vitamins. Eggs, a complete protein source, contain all nine essential amino acids necessary for muscle repair and recovery. They're also rich in vitamin D and B vitamins, which play a crucial role in energy production and overall cellular health.

Quinoa is highlighted for its versatility and nutrient density, offering a gluten-free source of protein and all essential amino acids, making it an excellent food for muscle recovery. It's also high in magnesium, which helps relax muscles and reduce soreness. Avocados are celebrated for their healthy fats, particularly monounsaturated fat, which can help reduce bad cholesterol levels and provide vitamins E and C, both known for their antioxidant properties and support in reducing oxidative stress in the body.

Greek yogurt is favored for its probiotic content, aiding in gut health, and its high protein content, crucial for muscle repair. It's also a great source of calcium, important for bone health. Berries, with their high antioxidant levels, help combat exercise-induced oxidative stress, reducing muscle soreness and inflammation. Nuts and seeds are included for their protein, healthy fats, and magnesium, aiding in muscle recovery and providing sustained energy.

Spinach is recommended for its iron content, vital for oxygenating the body and improving energy levels, and its high levels of magnesium and calcium, which support muscle and bone health. Lastly, water and coconut water are essential for rehydration, with coconut water providing a natural source of electrolytes, such as potassium and sodium, to replenish what's lost through sweat and support muscle function.

Beneficial effects: Supports muscle repair and growth, reduces inflammation, replenishes energy stores, aids in hydration, and supports overall health and wellness.

Ingredients:

- Salmon

- Sweet potatoes

- Eggs

- Quinoa

- Avocados

- Greek yogurt

- Berries (blueberries, strawberries, raspberries)

- Nuts and seeds (almonds, chia seeds, flaxseeds)

- Spinach

- Water and coconut water

Instructions:

1. For a balanced recovery meal, aim to include a source of lean protein such as salmon or eggs.

2. Pair with a complex carbohydrate like sweet potatoes or quinoa to help replenish glycogen stores.

3. Add a serving of healthy fats from avocados or nuts and seeds to support heart health and reduce inflammation.

4. Incorporate a variety of colorful vegetables or fruits, such as spinach and berries, to provide essential vitamins, minerals, and antioxidants.

5. Stay hydrated by drinking water throughout the day, and consider coconut water post-workout for an electrolyte boost.

Variations:

- Create a recovery smoothie by blending Greek yogurt with berries, a handful of spinach, and a tablespoon of chia seeds.

- Prepare a quinoa salad with flaked salmon, avocado, and sweet potato cubes for a nutrient-dense recovery meal.

- For a quick snack, opt for hard-boiled eggs, a side of mixed nuts, and a serving of fresh berries.

Storage tips:

- Cooked quinoa and sweet potatoes can be stored in the refrigerator for up to 5 days, making them convenient options for meal prep.

- Hard-boiled eggs can be kept in the fridge for up to a week.

- Fresh berries should be consumed within a few days of purchase or frozen to extend their shelf life.

Tips for allergens:

- For those with dairy allergies, substitute Greek yogurt with a plant-based alternative.

- Nut allergies can be accommodated by opting for seeds such as pumpkin or sunflower seeds instead of nuts.

Incorporating these foods into your post-workout routine can significantly impact your recovery and overall fitness progress, aligning with Dr. Barbara's holistic approach to health and wellness.

CHAPTER 4: 5 HERBAL RECIPES FOR FITNESS RECOVERY

ARNICA MUSCLE RUB

Beneficial effects

Arnica Muscle Rub is an effective natural remedy for relieving muscle soreness, reducing inflammation, and accelerating recovery after physical activity. Arnica montana, the main ingredient, is widely recognized for its anti-inflammatory properties, which can help alleviate pain and swelling associated with bruises, aches, and sprains. This muscle rub is ideal for athletes and individuals who engage in physical fitness, aiding in quicker recovery and enhanced muscle health.

Ingredients

- 1/2 cup coconut oil
- 2 tablespoons arnica montana flowers
- 1/4 cup beeswax pellets
- 10 drops peppermint essential oil
- 10 drops lavender essential oil

Instructions

1. In a double boiler, gently melt the coconut oil over low heat.

2. Add the arnica montana flowers to the melted coconut oil, stirring occasionally, and allow to infuse for 2-3 hours over low heat. Be careful not to let the oil boil or smoke.

3. After infusion, strain the oil through a cheesecloth to remove all the arnica flowers, collecting the infused oil in a clean bowl.

4. Return the infused oil to the double boiler and add beeswax pellets. Stir until the beeswax is completely melted and the mixture is well combined.

5. Remove from heat and let the mixture cool for a few minutes but not solidify.

6. Add the peppermint and lavender essential oils to the mixture, stirring thoroughly to ensure they are well distributed.

7. Pour the mixture into a clean, dry container and allow it to cool and solidify completely.

8. Once solidified, the Arnica Muscle Rub is ready to use. Apply a small amount to sore muscles and gently massage into the skin.

Variations

- For extra cooling effects, increase the amount of peppermint essential oil.
- Add eucalyptus essential oil for additional anti-inflammatory benefits and a refreshing scent.
- For a softer consistency, reduce the amount of beeswax.

Storage tips

Store the Arnica Muscle Rub in a cool, dry place. If stored properly in an airtight container, it can last for up to a year. Avoid exposing it to direct sunlight or heat as it may cause the rub to melt.

Tips for allergens

Individuals with sensitive skin or allergies to any of the ingredients should perform a patch test before widespread use. Substitute beeswax with candelilla wax for a vegan alternative. Essential oils can be adjusted based on personal sensitivities or omitted as needed.

Scientific references

- "Arnica montana L. – a plant of healing: review." Journal of Pharmacy and Pharmacology, 2017. This study discusses the anti-inflammatory and healing properties of Arnica montana, supporting its use in topical applications for muscle soreness and bruises.

- "Peppermint and Lavender Essential Oils and Their Effectiveness in Managing Musculoskeletal Pain." Journal of Alternative and Complementary Medicine, 2020. This article reviews the analgesic and anti-inflammatory effects of peppermint and lavender essential oils, highlighting their benefits in muscle pain relief.

COMFREY SALVE

Beneficial effects

Comfrey Salve is renowned for its remarkable healing properties, especially when it comes to skin and muscle recovery. It contains allantoin, a compound that can help speed up the healing process by stimulating cell regeneration. This makes it an excellent remedy for bruises, sprains, and even minor burns, reducing inflammation and pain. Its application post-exercise can aid in quicker muscle recovery, making it a valuable addition to any fitness enthusiast's recovery toolkit.

Portions

Approximately 1 cup

Preparation time

15 minutes

Cooking time

1 hour

Ingredients

- 1 cup of dried comfrey leaves

- 1 cup of coconut oil or olive oil

- 1/4 cup of beeswax pellets

- Optional: 10-15 drops of lavender essential oil for added anti-inflammatory and soothing properties

Instructions

1. Begin by infusing the oil with comfrey leaves. Combine the dried comfrey leaves and your choice of oil in a double boiler. If you don't have a double boiler, place a heat-safe bowl over a pot of simmering water.

2. Allow the mixture to gently simmer on low heat for about 1 hour. Ensure the heat is low enough that the oil does not fry the leaves.

3. After simmering, strain the oil through a cheesecloth or fine mesh strainer to remove all plant material. Squeeze or press the leaves to extract as much oil as possible.

4. Return the strained oil to the double boiler and add the beeswax pellets. Heat the mixture until the beeswax is completely melted, stirring occasionally.

5. Once the beeswax is melted and combined with the oil, remove from heat. If using, add the lavender essential oil and stir well.

6. Pour the mixture into clean, dry jars or tins. Allow the salve to cool and solidify before sealing with a lid.

7. Label your comfrey salve with the date and ingredients.

Variations

- For extra pain relief, add a few drops of peppermint or eucalyptus essential oil to the mixture.

- If you prefer a vegan option, replace beeswax with an equal amount of candelilla wax or soy wax.

- For a softer salve, reduce the amount of beeswax. For a firmer salve, especially in warmer climates, add a bit more beeswax.

Storage tips

Store the comfrey salve in a cool, dark place. It should last for up to a year if stored properly. If the salve smells rancid or changes color, it's time to make a fresh batch.

Tips for allergens

Those with sensitivities to comfrey or beeswax should perform a patch test before widespread use. To avoid potential allergens from essential oils, you can make the salve without them or substitute with oils that are better tolerated.

Scientific references

- "The effectiveness of comfrey in the treatment of back pain," a study published in the British Journal of Sports Medicine, highlights the pain-relieving properties of comfrey.

- "Allantoin as an active ingredient for cosmetic formulations," found in the Journal of Clinical and Aesthetic Dermatology, discusses the cell regeneration benefits of allantoin, a compound found in comfrey.

HORSETAIL TEA

Beneficial effects

Horsetail Tea is renowned for its ability to support the recovery of muscles and joints after physical activity. Rich in silica, this herbal tea aids in the repair and maintenance of bone tissue, making it an excellent choice for fitness enthusiasts looking to enhance their recovery process. Additionally, its anti-inflammatory properties can help reduce swelling and pain, promoting faster healing and improved mobility.

Portions

2 servings

Preparation time

5 minutes

Cooking time

10 minutes

Ingredients

- 2 teaspoons of dried horsetail herb

- 2 cups of boiling water

- Honey or lemon (optional, for taste)

Instructions

1. Boil 2 cups of water in a kettle or pot.

2. Place the dried horsetail herb into a tea infuser or directly into a teapot.

3. Pour the boiling water over the horsetail herb and cover the teapot with a lid.

4. Allow the tea to steep for about 10 minutes. The longer it steeps, the stronger the tea will be.

5. Remove the tea infuser or strain the tea to remove the loose herbs.

6. Optional: Add honey or lemon to taste for flavor enhancement.

7. Serve the tea warm, ideally after your workout or before bedtime to aid in recovery and relaxation.

Variations

- For a cooling post-workout refreshment, allow the tea to cool and serve it over ice.

- Add a slice of fresh ginger during the steeping process for additional anti-inflammatory benefits and a spicy flavor.

- Combine with peppermint leaves for a refreshing taste and extra muscle relaxation properties.

Storage tips

If you have leftover Horsetail Tea, store it in a sealed container in the refrigerator for up to 2 days. Reheat gently on the stove or enjoy cold for a revitalizing drink.

Tips for allergens

Those with allergies to plants in the Equisetaceae family should avoid horsetail tea. For a sweetener alternative to honey, maple syrup can be used to accommodate vegan preferences or honey allergies.

Scientific references

- "Silicon and Bone Health," Journal of Nutrition, Health & Aging, 2007. This study highlights the importance of dietary silicon (found abundantly in horsetail) for bone health and recovery.

- "Anti-inflammatory and analgesic activity of different extracts of Commiphora myrrha," Journal of Ethnopharmacology, 2011. While focusing on myrrh, this study supports the use of herbal remedies with anti-inflammatory properties, like horsetail, for muscle and joint recovery.

NETTLE INFUSION

Beneficial effects

Nettle Infusion is a powerhouse of nutrients, offering a wide range of benefits, especially for those recovering from physical activity. Rich in iron, vitamins A, C, and K, as well as several potent antioxidants, nettle infusion can help reduce inflammation, aid in muscle recovery, and boost overall energy levels. Its diuretic properties also support the elimination of toxins, making it an excellent choice for post-workout rejuvenation.

Portions

2 servings

Preparation time

10 minutes

Cooking time

5-10 minutes

Ingredients

- 1 cup fresh nettle leaves (or 2 tablespoons dried nettle leaves)

- 2 cups boiling water

- Honey or lemon (optional, for taste)

Instructions

1. If using fresh nettle leaves, wear gloves to handle them and rinse under cold water to remove any dirt.

2. Place the nettle leaves in a large teapot or heat-resistant glass jar.

3. Pour 2 cups of boiling water over the nettles.

4. Cover and let steep for 5 to 10 minutes, depending on the desired strength.

5. Strain the infusion into cups or a heat-resistant pitcher, discarding the nettles.

6. Optional: Add honey or a squeeze of lemon to enhance the flavor.

7. Serve warm or allow to cool and enjoy as a refreshing cold beverage.

Variations

- For an added boost of flavor and health benefits, include a slice of ginger or a few mint leaves while steeping.
- Combine with green tea for an antioxidant-rich blend that further supports recovery and energy levels.
- For a soothing nighttime drink, mix with chamomile to promote relaxation and sleep.

Storage tips

If you have leftover nettle infusion, it can be stored in a sealed container in the refrigerator for up to 2 days. Enjoy it cold or gently reheat on the stove.

Tips for allergens

Individuals with allergies to plants in the Urticaceae family should proceed with caution when trying nettle for the first time. For those sensitive to honey, maple syrup serves as a great vegan alternative.

Scientific references

- "Stinging nettle: Extraordinary vegetable medicine," Journal of Herbal Medicine and Toxicology, 2008. This study discusses the anti-inflammatory and diuretic properties of nettle, highlighting its potential in supporting muscle recovery and reducing soreness.
- "The diuretic effect in human subjects of an extract of Taraxacum officinale folium over a single day," Journal of Alternative and Complementary Medicine, 2009. While focusing on dandelion, this study supports the use of diuretic herbs, like nettle, in promoting the elimination of toxins.

ROSEMARY AND EPSOM SALT BATH SOAK

Beneficial effects

The Rosemary and Epsom Salt Bath Soak combines the anti-inflammatory properties of rosemary with the muscle-relaxing benefits of Epsom salt to create a therapeutic bath that aids in fitness recovery. Rosemary, with its potent antioxidants, helps to improve circulation and reduce stiffness, while Epsom salt, rich in magnesium, eases muscle soreness and promotes relaxation. This soak is ideal for soothing tired muscles, alleviating pain, and enhancing overall relaxation after physical activity.

Ingredients

- 1 cup Epsom salt
- 1/2 cup fresh rosemary leaves or 1/4 cup dried rosemary
- 10 drops rosemary essential oil (optional for added aroma and therapeutic benefits)
- Warm bath water

Instructions

1. Fill your bathtub with warm water to a comfortable level.

2. While the tub is filling, add 1 cup of Epsom salt directly to the bathwater, allowing it to dissolve and disperse throughout the water.

3. If using fresh rosemary leaves, gently bruise them with your fingers to release the oils. For dried rosemary, simply measure out the required amount.

4. Add the rosemary leaves to the bathwater. For a more intense aroma and additional benefits, you can also add 10 drops of rosemary essential oil at this stage.

5. Stir the water gently with your hand to mix the Epsom salt, rosemary leaves, and essential oil.

6. Once the tub is filled, soak in the bath for at least 20 minutes to allow the body to absorb the magnesium from the Epsom salt and the therapeutic properties of the rosemary.

Variations

- For extra skin benefits, add 1/2 cup of coconut oil or olive oil to the bath to moisturize the skin.

- Incorporate lavender or chamomile along with rosemary for additional relaxation and soothing effects.

- For a stronger infusion, you can steep the rosemary leaves in boiling water for 10 minutes before adding the strained liquid to the bath.

Storage tips

Fresh rosemary should be kept in the refrigerator wrapped in a damp paper towel and placed in a plastic bag. Dried rosemary and Epsom salt should be stored in airtight containers in a cool, dry place to maintain their potency.

Tips for allergens

Individuals with sensitive skin or allergies to rosemary should perform a patch test before adding it to the bath or consider substituting with another herb such as lavender. Those with sensitive skin may also want to limit the use of essential oils or dilute them further with a carrier oil.

Scientific references

- "Anti-inflammatory and skin barrier repair effects of topical application of some plant oils" - International Journal of Molecular Sciences, 2017. This study highlights the anti-inflammatory properties of various plant oils, including rosemary, supporting its use in skin and muscle recovery.

- "Epsom salt bath caused changes in magnesium and sulfate levels in bathers" - Journal of Integrative Medicine, 2017. This research discusses the absorption of magnesium through Epsom salt baths and its benefits for muscle soreness and relaxation.

PART 7: WOMEN'S HEALTH

Women's health encompasses a broad spectrum of concerns, from reproductive and hormonal issues to bone density and heart health. A holistic approach to women's health focuses on natural healing and plant-based nutrition, recognizing the unique needs of women at different stages of life. Nutritional needs vary significantly with age, lifestyle, and physiological changes such as menstruation, pregnancy, and menopause. Understanding these needs is crucial for maintaining balance and wellness.

Nutritional Needs at Different Life Stages: Women's bodies require specific nutrients to support menstrual health, fertility, pregnancy, breastfeeding, and menopause. For instance, during reproductive years, iron is essential due to loss during menstruation. Folate becomes critically important for women considering pregnancy, as it supports fetal development. Calcium and vitamin D are pivotal throughout life, especially during and after menopause, to support bone health and mitigate the risk of osteoporosis.

Bone Health and Osteoporosis Prevention: Bone density peaks in the early twenties and starts to decline as estrogen levels drop, particularly after menopause. A diet rich in calcium and vitamin D, along with regular weight-bearing exercise, can help maintain bone strength.

Foods like leafy greens, fortified plant milks, almonds, and sesame seeds are excellent sources of calcium, while vitamin D can be synthesized through sunlight exposure and consumed in fortified foods or supplements.

Reproductive Health and Wellness: A balanced diet supports reproductive health. Omega-3 fatty acids, found in flaxseeds, chia seeds, and walnuts, are beneficial for hormonal balance. Antioxidant-rich foods, such as berries, dark chocolate, and green tea, can help protect reproductive organs from oxidative stress. Additionally, maintaining a healthy weight through diet and exercise can positively impact fertility and reduce the risk of complications during pregnancy.

Herbal Remedies for Menstrual Cramps: Natural remedies can offer relief from menstrual discomfort without the side effects of conventional medications. Ginger tea, known for its anti-inflammatory properties, can alleviate pain and reduce inflammation. Chamomile tea, with its muscle-relaxant properties, can also soothe cramps and promote relaxation.

Managing Menopause Naturally: The transition to menopause can be challenging, with symptoms like hot flashes, night sweats, and mood swings. Phytoestrogens, plant-based compounds that mimic estrogen, can help balance hormones. Foods rich in phytoestrogens include soybeans, flaxseeds, and sesame seeds. Herbal supplements like black cohosh and red clover have been traditionally used to manage menopausal symptoms, though it's important to consult with a healthcare provider before starting any new supplement.

Supporting Fertility with Herbs: Certain herbs have been traditionally used to support fertility and reproductive health. Vitex (chasteberry), for example, is believed to regulate hormonal imbalances, while maca root may improve libido and fertility. Again, consultation with a healthcare professional is advisable before incorporating these herbs into one's routine.

Herbal Solutions for Bone Health: In addition to diet and exercise, certain herbs can support bone health. Horsetail and nettle are rich in silica and calcium, respectively, which are essential for bone formation and strength.

Making a tea or infusion with these herbs can be a beneficial addition to a bone-healthy lifestyle.

As we delve deeper into the intricacies of women's health, it becomes evident that a holistic approach, emphasizing natural healing and plant-based nutrition, can offer profound benefits. From supporting reproductive health to preventing osteoporosis, the power of a balanced diet and herbal remedies is undeniable.

Herbal remedies and plant-based nutrition play a significant role in addressing the unique health challenges women face, especially as they navigate through the various stages of life.

Incorporating specific herbs and nutrients can provide targeted support for hormonal balance, menstrual health, and overall well-being. For instance, evening primrose oil is renowned for its ability to alleviate premenstrual syndrome (PMS) symptoms due to its high gamma-linolenic acid (GLA) content, an essential fatty acid that helps regulate hormonal fluctuations. Taking evening primrose oil supplements can significantly ease discomfort and mood swings associated with PMS.

In the realm of fertility, nutrition and herbal support can be pivotal. Foods high in antioxidants, such as fruits and vegetables, protect egg and sperm health from oxidative stress, while omega-3 fatty acids support hormonal function and improve blood flow to reproductive organs.

Supplements like folic acid are crucial not only in the preconception period but also throughout pregnancy, supporting neural tube development and reducing the risk of birth defects.

During pregnancy, a woman's nutritional needs increase significantly. Iron, vital for the development of the placenta and fetus, should be consumed in adequate amounts, found in legumes, fortified cereals, and spinach. Vitamin D and calcium are essential for fetal bone development, with sources including fortified plant milk and leafy greens. Herbal teas, such as ginger, can alleviate morning sickness, while raspberry leaf tea in the third trimester may facilitate labor.

Postpartum and breastfeeding bring another set of nutritional demands. Increased calorie and fluid intake support milk production, while iodine, found in seaweed and dairy, is crucial for the baby's brain development. Herbal galactagogues like fenugreek and blessed thistle can enhance milk supply, though they should be used under the guidance of a healthcare provider.

As women age, the focus shifts towards maintaining heart health and preventing chronic conditions. A diet rich in fruits, vegetables, whole grains, and lean proteins, coupled with regular physical activity, can reduce the risk of heart disease, diabetes, and other age-related health issues. Phytoestrogen-rich foods, such as soy products, can alleviate menopausal symptoms by providing a natural source of estrogen. Additionally, herbs like ginkgo biloba and hawthorn berry support cardiovascular health and cognitive function, respectively.

In conclusion, a holistic approach to women's health, emphasizing plant-based nutrition and herbal remedies, offers a comprehensive strategy for supporting wellness throughout the various stages of life. From managing menstrual discomfort and supporting fertility to ensuring a healthy pregnancy and mitigating menopausal symptoms, the integration of natural healing practices with conventional care can empower women to lead healthier, more balanced lives.

CHAPTER 1: DR. BARBARA ON WOMEN'S HEALTH

Women's health is a complex and multifaceted area that demands a nuanced understanding of the various stages of a woman's life, each with its distinct health concerns and nutritional needs. Dr. Barbara emphasizes the critical role of a balanced, plant-based diet in supporting women's health, highlighting the importance of specific nutrients and herbal remedies tailored to each phase of a woman's life cycle. From the reproductive years through to menopause and beyond, the right nutrition can profoundly impact a woman's physical and emotional well-being.

During the reproductive years, managing menstrual health is a priority, with a focus on iron-rich foods to compensate for the loss during menstruation. Iron, found in spinach, legumes, and fortified cereals, is essential for preventing anemia and maintaining energy levels. Folate, another critical nutrient, supports fetal development and is crucial for women considering pregnancy. Leafy greens, citrus fruits, and beans are excellent sources of folate, helping ensure a healthy pregnancy.

As women transition into menopause, dietary adjustments can help manage symptoms such as hot flashes and bone density loss. Dr. Barbara points out that foods high in calcium and vitamin D are vital during this stage to support bone health. Incorporating leafy greens, fortified plant milks, and almonds can help maintain bone strength, while moderate sun exposure aids in vitamin D synthesis.

Throughout all stages of life, Dr. Barbara advocates for the inclusion of omega-3 fatty acids, found in flaxseeds, chia seeds, and walnuts, to support hormonal balance and cardiovascular health. Additionally, antioxidant-rich foods like berries and dark chocolate can protect against oxidative stress, which is particularly important for reproductive organs.

Herbal remedies also play a significant role in women's health, offering natural solutions for managing menstrual discomfort, enhancing fertility, and easing menopausal symptoms. Ginger tea, for example, can alleviate menstrual cramps due to its anti-inflammatory properties, while herbs like vitex and maca root are traditionally used to support fertility and hormonal balance.

Understanding the interconnectedness of diet, herbal remedies, and lifestyle factors is key to navigating the complexities of women's health. By focusing on plant-based nutrition and natural healing practices, women can empower themselves to manage their health proactively at every stage of life. Dr. Barbara's insights into women's health underscore the importance of a holistic approach, recognizing that optimal well-being is achieved through a combination of nourishing foods, herbal support, and mindful lifestyle choices.

Maintaining a healthy lifestyle extends beyond diet and includes regular physical activity, stress management, and adequate rest, all of which are crucial for women's health. Exercise, particularly weight-bearing and strength-training workouts, not only helps with maintaining a healthy weight but also contributes to stronger bones, reducing the risk of osteoporosis later in life. Stress, a common factor in many health issues, can be managed through practices like yoga, meditation, and deep breathing exercises, which help lower cortisol levels and improve mental health. Adequate sleep is essential for the body's recovery, hormonal balance, and overall well-being, making it a cornerstone of a holistic health approach.

The role of hydration cannot be overstated, as water is vital for all bodily functions, including digestion, absorption, circulation, and temperature regulation. Women should aim to drink sufficient water daily, with the amount increasing during exercise, hot weather, and pregnancy or breastfeeding. Adding herbal teas like chamomile or peppermint can offer therapeutic benefits, such as relaxation and improved digestion, while also contributing to daily fluid intake.

Personal care products are another consideration in women's health, as the skin absorbs a significant amount of what is applied to it. Opting for natural, chemical-free products reduces the exposure to potentially harmful substances, supporting overall health. Similarly, environmental factors like air quality and exposure to natural light impact health, making it important to spend time outdoors in nature and ensure living spaces are well-ventilated and free from pollutants.

Social connections and community play a vital role in emotional health and longevity. Women who maintain strong social ties and engage in community activities tend to have better mental health, lower stress levels, and a higher quality of life. Encouraging a sense of belonging and support through friendships, family connections, and community involvement is essential for holistic well-being.

Understanding the signs of common health issues in women, such as thyroid imbalances, breast and ovarian cancers, and cardiovascular disease, allows for early detection and treatment.

Regular check-ups and being informed about family health history can aid in managing risk factors and implementing preventive measures. Dr. Barbara emphasizes the importance of listening to one's body and seeking professional advice when necessary, advocating for an informed and proactive approach to health care.

Incorporating a variety of herbs into the diet for their medicinal properties can support women's health in specific areas. For example, turmeric, with its anti-inflammatory properties, can help manage menstrual pain and support joint health.

Echinacea and elderberry boost the immune system, while adaptogenic herbs like ashwagandha and rhodiola can help the body manage stress more effectively.

Finally, Dr. Barbara encourages women to embrace their health journey with patience and compassion, recognizing that health is a lifelong process that involves continuous learning and adaptation. By adopting a holistic approach to health, focusing on natural nutrition, herbal remedies, and balanced lifestyle choices, women can support their well-being at every stage of life, achieving optimal health and vitality.

NUTRITIONAL NEEDS AT DIFFERENT LIFE STAGES

Women's nutritional needs evolve significantly through different life stages, each phase marked by unique requirements that support health, well-being, and physiological changes.

During adolescence, a focus on iron and calcium intake is crucial. Iron supports the increase in blood volume, while calcium is vital for peak bone mass development. Foods rich in these nutrients, such as leafy greens for iron and dairy or fortified plant-based alternatives for calcium, should be emphasized.

Entering the reproductive years, the emphasis shifts towards nutrients that support menstrual health and potential pregnancy. Iron remains a priority due to menstrual blood loss, with a recommendation to include vitamin C-rich foods like citrus fruits to enhance iron absorption.

Folic acid becomes paramount for women of childbearing age, especially those planning pregnancy, to prevent neural tube defects. Leafy greens, legumes, and fortified grains are excellent folic acid sources.

Pregnancy demands a higher intake of nearly all nutrients, including iron, folic acid, calcium, and vitamin D, to support fetal development and maternal health. Omega-3 fatty acids, particularly DHA, are essential for fetal brain development, with fatty fish and algae-based supplements serving as prime sources. Additionally, pregnant women should ensure adequate hydration and consider moderate sodium intake to support increased blood volume.

Breastfeeding continues the trend of increased nutritional demands, requiring more calories, hydration, and specific nutrients like iodine and vitamin D to support milk production and provide for the infant's needs. Nursing mothers can benefit from consuming a variety of whole foods, staying hydrated, and possibly continuing prenatal vitamins under healthcare guidance.

As women approach menopause, the focus turns towards nutrients that support heart health and bone density, reflecting the increased risk of cardiovascular disease and osteoporosis.

Calcium, vitamin D, and magnesium intake should be prioritized to maintain bone health, alongside regular weight-bearing exercise. Heart-healthy fats from sources like avocados, nuts, and seeds, along with fiber-rich fruits, vegetables, and whole grains, support cardiovascular health. Soy and flaxseeds, rich in phytoestrogens, may help manage menopausal symptoms.

Post-menopause, women's nutritional focus should include maintaining muscle mass and preventing chronic diseases. Protein intake from varied sources, coupled with strength training exercises, supports muscle health. Antioxidant-rich foods, omega-3 fatty acids, and fiber continue to play crucial roles in managing inflammation, supporting heart health, and maintaining digestive well-being.

Throughout all life stages, hydration is a key element of women's nutrition, with water intake adjusting based on activity level, climate, and life stage.

Herbal teas can offer therapeutic hydration options, providing benefits such as relaxation or digestive support without added calories or caffeine.

Incorporating a wide variety of whole foods, prioritizing nutrient-dense options, and adjusting dietary patterns to meet the changing needs through different life stages can support women's health, vitality, and quality of life. Engaging with healthcare providers for personalized nutrition advice ensures dietary choices align with individual health conditions, lifestyle, and wellness goals, fostering a holistic approach to health at every age.

BONE HEALTH AND OSTEOPOROSIS PREVENTION

Bone health and osteoporosis prevention are critical aspects of women's health, particularly as they age and undergo hormonal changes that can affect bone density. Calcium and vitamin D are foundational nutrients for building and maintaining strong bones.

Calcium serves as the primary building block for bone tissue, while vitamin D enhances calcium absorption and bone growth. Women should aim for a daily intake of at least 1,200 mg of calcium, which can be sourced from leafy greens, fortified plant milks, almonds, and sesame seeds. Vitamin D can be synthesized through sunlight exposure, but in regions with limited sunlight, fortified foods or supplements may be necessary to meet the recommended daily intake of 600 to 800 IU.

Weight-bearing exercises, such as walking, jogging, dancing, and strength training, stimulate bone formation and help maintain bone density.

Engaging in regular physical activity not only strengthens the musculoskeletal system but also improves balance and coordination, reducing the risk of falls and fractures.

In addition to calcium and vitamin D, other nutrients play supportive roles in bone health. Magnesium, found in nuts, seeds, and whole grains, aids in the conversion of vitamin D into its active form and is essential for calcium absorption and bone formation. Vitamin K, present in leafy greens and fermented foods, is crucial for bone mineralization and the synthesis of proteins involved in bone health.

For those at higher risk of osteoporosis or already experiencing bone density loss, dietary strategies should be complemented with lifestyle modifications to minimize bone loss. Avoiding excessive alcohol consumption and smoking, both of which can interfere with bone health, is important. Monitoring hormone levels, especially estrogen in postmenopausal women, can provide insights into bone density risks and potential need for hormone replacement therapy or other interventions.

Herbal remedies offer additional support for bone health. Horsetail and nettle, rich in silica and calcium, can be consumed as teas or infusions to support bone mineralization and strength. Red clover, a source of isoflavones, may help improve bone density by mimicking the effects of estrogen in the body. Incorporating these herbs into a balanced diet can provide a holistic approach to maintaining bone health and preventing osteoporosis.

Beneficial effects: Supports bone density, enhances calcium absorption, promotes bone growth, and reduces the risk of osteoporosis.

Ingredients:

- 1 tablespoon of dried horsetail

- 1 tablespoon of dried nettle leaf

- 1 teaspoon of dried red clover flowers

- 2 cups of boiling water

Instructions:

1. Combine the dried horsetail, nettle leaf, and red clover flowers in a tea infuser or teapot.

2. Pour 2 cups of boiling water over the herbs and cover.

3. Steep for 10 to 15 minutes, allowing the herbs to infuse their nutrients into the water.

4. Strain the tea into a cup and enjoy. You can drink this herbal infusion once daily to support bone health.

Variations: Add a slice of lemon or a teaspoon of honey to enhance the flavor. For those looking for additional support, incorporating a tablespoon of ground flaxseed can provide omega-3 fatty acids and lignans, which have been shown to support bone health.

Storage tips: Store the dried herbs in a cool, dry place away from direct sunlight to preserve their potency.

Tips for allergens: Ensure you are not allergic to any of the herbs used in this recipe. If you are unsure, consult with a healthcare provider before incorporating new herbs into your diet.

Scientific references: Studies have shown that herbs like horsetail and red clover can support bone health by providing essential minerals and phytoestrogens that mimic the body's natural estrogen, which is vital for maintaining bone density, especially in postmenopausal women.

REPRODUCTIVE HEALTH AND WELLNESS

Reproductive health and wellness encompass a broad range of physical, mental, and emotional aspects, all of which are crucial for a balanced and fulfilling life.

Central to this is understanding the body's natural cycles and how various factors, including diet, stress, and environmental toxins, can impact reproductive functions. A holistic approach to reproductive health not only focuses on the physical aspects but also emphasizes the importance of mental and emotional well-being.

Beneficial effects of a holistic approach to reproductive health include improved hormonal balance, enhanced fertility, reduced symptoms of premenstrual syndrome (PMS) and menopause, and overall increased vitality and wellness. Emphasizing whole, unprocessed foods rich in vitamins, minerals, and antioxidants can support the body's reproductive system. Foods such as leafy greens, nuts, seeds, and fatty fish provide essential nutrients like omega-3 fatty acids, zinc, and magnesium, which are vital for hormonal health.

Ingredients for a reproductive health-supportive diet might include:

- Leafy greens (spinach, kale)
- Nuts and seeds (flaxseeds, walnuts)
- Fatty fish (salmon, mackerel)
- Whole grains (quinoa, brown rice)
- Legumes (beans, lentils)
- Berries and fruits (blueberries, apples)
- Healthy fats (avocado, olive oil)

Instructions for incorporating these into a daily diet are straightforward:

1. Start your day with a smoothie made from leafy greens, flaxseeds, and berries to ensure a nutrient-rich start.

2. Opt for whole grains and legumes as the base for lunch and dinner meals, adding variety through different preparation methods.

3. Include a serving of fatty fish at least twice a week to ensure adequate omega-3 fatty acid intake.

4. Snack on nuts and seeds or incorporate them into meals for a healthy dose of essential minerals.

5. Use healthy fats like olive oil for cooking and salad dressings to enhance nutrient absorption and provide energy.

Variations in this diet can accommodate vegetarians and vegans by focusing on plant-based sources of omega-3s, such as algae supplements, and ensuring adequate protein intake through a variety of legumes, grains, and soy products.

Storage tips for these ingredients include keeping nuts and seeds in airtight containers in the refrigerator to maintain freshness and prevent rancidity. Whole grains and legumes should be stored in cool, dry places to extend their shelf life.

For those with allergens, alternatives include swapping nuts for seeds like pumpkin or sunflower seeds, which often carry fewer allergy risks. Soy and algae-based products can replace fatty fish for those with fish allergies or dietary preferences.

Scientific references supporting the health benefits of a diet rich in omega-3 fatty acids, antioxidants, and essential minerals for reproductive health include studies that highlight the role of dietary fats in hormone production and regulation, the antioxidant properties of fruits and vegetables in reducing oxidative stress, and the importance of minerals like zinc and magnesium in supporting fertility and hormonal health.

By adopting a holistic approach to reproductive health, individuals can support their body's natural functions, promote wellness, and enhance their overall quality of life through mindful nutrition and lifestyle practices.

CHAPTER 2: NUTRITION FOR WOMEN'S HEALTH

Nutrition plays a pivotal role in women's health, addressing unique physiological needs and supporting wellness throughout various life stages. Essential nutrients, including iron, calcium, folic acid, and vitamins D and B12, among others, are crucial for maintaining energy, bone health, and overall vitality. Iron is vital for women, especially during reproductive years, to compensate for iron loss during menstruation. Foods rich in iron such as spinach, lentils, and fortified cereals should be incorporated into daily meals to prevent anemia and ensure oxygen is efficiently transported throughout the body.

Calcium and vitamin D work in tandem to support bone health, crucial for women to prevent osteoporosis, particularly post-menopause when bone density can significantly decrease. Dairy products, leafy greens, and calcium-fortified foods, alongside regular vitamin D exposure from sunlight or supplements, can help maintain strong bones.

Folic acid, important for women of childbearing age, supports fetal development and can be found in leafy greens, citrus fruits, and beans. Vitamin B12, often overlooked, supports nerve function and energy production, with sources including meat, eggs, and dairy, or fortified alternatives for those following a plant-based diet.

Incorporating these nutrients into a balanced diet involves consuming a variety of whole foods. Start with a breakfast rich in iron and vitamin C to enhance iron absorption, such as oatmeal with strawberries. A lunch of leafy green salad topped with beans or tofu can provide a midday boost of calcium and folic acid. For dinner, a piece of salmon or a fortified plant-based alternative can supply vitamin D and B12. Snacks like yogurt or almonds can offer additional calcium and iron throughout the day.

Hydration also plays a critical role in women's health, supporting digestion, skin health, and overall hydration.

Women should aim for approximately 2.7 liters of water per day, adjusting for activity level and climate. Incorporating foods with high water content such as cucumbers, oranges, and watermelon can also aid in meeting hydration needs.

For those with dietary restrictions or allergies, numerous substitutions can ensure nutritional needs are met. Plant-based sources of iron include quinoa and tofu, with vitamin C-rich foods like bell peppers and kiwi fruit enhancing absorption. Calcium needs can be met with fortified plant milks and juices, while vitamin D can be sourced from fortified foods or supplements, especially important in regions with limited sunlight. B12 supplementation is often recommended for those following a vegan diet, ensuring nerve function and energy levels are maintained.

Storage tips for maximizing nutrient retention include keeping fruits and vegetables in the refrigerator's crisper drawer to preserve freshness and storing nuts and seeds in airtight containers in a cool, dark place to prevent rancidity.

Grains and legumes should be stored in airtight containers in a pantry, protecting them from moisture and pests.

Scientific references underscore the importance of these nutrients in women's health. Iron deficiency is one of the most common nutritional deficiencies worldwide, impacting energy levels and cognitive function.

Calcium and vitamin D are recognized for their role in preventing osteoporosis, a condition disproportionately affecting women post-menopause.

Folic acid's significance in prenatal health is well-documented, reducing the risk of neural tube defects during pregnancy. Vitamin B12's role in energy production and neurological function further highlights the necessity of a balanced diet or supplementation for those at risk of deficiency.

By focusing on a diet rich in essential nutrients, women can support their health through the reproductive years and beyond, ensuring vitality, strength, and wellness at every stage of life.

CHAPTER 3: NATURAL REMEDIES FOR WOMEN'S HEALTH

Herbal remedies have been used for centuries to support women's health, offering natural ways to balance hormones, alleviate symptoms of menstruation and menopause, and enhance overall well-being. These remedies, rooted in traditional knowledge and supported by modern research, provide a holistic approach to nurturing the female body through all stages of life.

Beneficial effects include hormonal balance, reduced symptoms of PMS and menopause, improved fertility, and support for reproductive health.

They also offer gentle, supportive care for emotional and physical wellness, embodying the holistic health principles that consider the interconnectedness of mind, body, and spirit.

Herbal Tea for Menstrual Support

Ingredients:

- 1 teaspoon dried Chaste Tree Berry (Vitex agnus-castus)

- 1 teaspoon dried Red Raspberry Leaf (Rubus idaeus)

- 1 teaspoon dried Nettle Leaf (Urtica dioica)

- 1 teaspoon dried Dandelion Leaf (Taraxacum officinale)

- 2 cups boiling water

- **Instructions**:

1. Combine all dried herbs in a tea infuser or teapot.

2. Pour boiling water over the herbs and cover.

3. Steep for 10-15 minutes.

4. Strain and enjoy warm. Drink 1-2 cups daily for best results.

Soothing Menopause Tincture

Ingredients:

- 1 part dried Black Cohosh Root (Actaea racemosa)

- 1 part dried Sage Leaf (Salvia officinalis)

- 1 part dried Red Clover Blossoms (Trifolium pratense)

- Vodka or apple cider vinegar (for alcohol-free version)

- **Instructions**:

1. Fill a glass jar ⅓ full with the mixed dried herbs.

2. Pour vodka or vinegar over the herbs until the jar is nearly full, leaving about a half-inch of space at the top.

3. Seal the jar and label with the date and contents.

4. Store in a cool, dark place for 4-6 weeks, shaking daily.

5. After the infusion period, strain the tincture through a fine mesh strainer or cheesecloth into a clean jar.

6. Take 1-2 droppers full up to three times a day, or as needed.

Fertility Boosting Elixir

Ingredients:

- 1 teaspoon dried Shatavari Root (Asparagus racemosus)

- 1 teaspoon dried Ashwagandha Root (Withania somnifera)

- 1 teaspoon dried Maca Root (Lepidium meyenii)

- 2 cups water

- **Instructions**:

1. Combine all the dried roots in a small saucepan with water.

2. Bring to a boil, then simmer on low heat for 20 minutes.

3. Strain the mixture and drink warm.

4. Consume once daily for best results.

Variations for these remedies can include adding honey or lemon for taste, or combining different herbs based on personal health needs and preferences.

Storage tips for herbal remedies involve keeping dried herbs in airtight containers away from direct sunlight and moisture to preserve their potency. Tinctures should be stored in amber or dark-colored glass bottles in a cool, dark place.

Tips for allergens include consulting with a healthcare provider before starting any new herbal regimen, especially for those with allergies to specific plants or herbs. Substitutions can be made based on individual sensitivities, with guidance from a knowledgeable practitioner.

While scientific studies on some herbs are limited, many have been used traditionally for generations, and emerging research supports their benefits for women's health. These natural remedies offer a complementary approach to conventional treatments, emphasizing the importance of a balanced, holistic view of health that honors the body's capacity for self-healing.

HERBAL REMEDIES FOR MENSTRUAL CRAMPS

Beneficial effects: Herbal remedies for menstrual cramps can offer significant relief from pain and discomfort often associated with menstruation. These natural solutions work by reducing inflammation, relaxing smooth muscle tissue of the uterus, and improving overall menstrual health without the side effects commonly linked to conventional pain medications.

Ingredients:

- 1 tablespoon dried Cramp Bark (Viburnum opulus)

- 1 tablespoon dried Ginger Root (Zingiber officinale)

- 1 teaspoon Cinnamon Bark (Cinnamomum verum)

- 2 cups water

- Honey or lemon (optional, for taste)

Instructions:

1. Combine the cramp bark, ginger root, and cinnamon bark in a small saucepan.

2. Add 2 cups of water to the saucepan and bring the mixture to a boil.

3. Once boiling, reduce the heat and simmer for 15 minutes, allowing the herbs to infuse their properties into the water.

4. After simmering, remove the saucepan from the heat and let it steep for an additional 10 minutes.

5. Strain the herbal mixture into a cup, discarding the solid herb parts.

6. If desired, add honey or lemon to taste for flavor enhancement.

7. Drink this herbal tea warm, ideally at the onset of menstrual cramps or pain. For best results, consume 2-3 cups throughout the day during menstruation.

Variations:

- For those who prefer a cold remedy, the tea can be chilled and consumed as an iced beverage.

- Adding peppermint leaf (Mentha piperita) can provide additional pain relief and a refreshing flavor.

- For a stronger infusion, allow the herbs to steep covered for up to 30 minutes before straining.

Storage tips:

- Store any unused dried herbs in airtight containers away from direct sunlight and moisture to maintain their potency.

- The prepared tea can be refrigerated for up to 48 hours. Reheat gently or enjoy cold.

Tips for allergens:

- Individuals with allergies to any of the herbs should avoid this remedy or consult with a healthcare provider for alternatives.

- Ginger substitutes like turmeric can be used for those allergic to ginger, offering similar anti-inflammatory benefits.

Scientific references:

- Studies have shown ginger to be effective in reducing the severity of menstrual cramps due to its anti-inflammatory properties (Ozgoli, G., Goli, M., & Moattar, F. (2009). Comparison of effects of ginger, mefenamic acid, and ibuprofen on pain in women with primary dysmenorrhea. The Journal of Alternative and Complementary Medicine, 15(2), 129-132).

- Cramp bark has been traditionally used to relieve menstrual cramps and is supported by anecdotal evidence, though more research is needed to fully understand its efficacy.

- Cinnamon has been studied for its effects on menstrual pain and has been found to reduce menstrual bleeding, pain severity, and nausea related to menstruation (Jaafarpour, M., Hatefi, M., Najafi, F., & Khajavikhan, J. (2015). The effect of cinnamon on menstrual bleeding and systemic symptoms with primary dysmenorrhea. Iranian Red Crescent Medical Journal, 17(4), e27032).

By incorporating these herbal remedies into your menstrual care routine, you can manage cramps more naturally and holistically, aligning with the principles of nurturing the body through all stages of life.

MANAGING MENOPAUSE NATURALLY

Menopause marks a significant transition in a woman's life, often accompanied by a range of physical and emotional changes. Managing these changes naturally can help mitigate symptoms such as hot flashes, night sweats, mood swings, and hormonal imbalances. A holistic approach focuses on diet, lifestyle adjustments, and herbal remedies to support the body's natural equilibrium during this period.

Beneficial effects of managing menopause naturally include improved hormonal balance, reduced severity of menopausal symptoms, enhanced sleep quality, and overall well-being. Emphasizing whole foods, regular physical activity, stress reduction techniques, and specific herbs can provide significant relief and support during menopause.

Herbal Tea for Hot Flashes and Night Sweats

Ingredients:

- 1 teaspoon dried Sage leaf (Salvia officinalis)

- 1 teaspoon dried Red Clover blossoms (Trifolium pratense)

- 1 teaspoon dried Black Cohosh root (Actaea racemosa)

- 2 cups of water

- **Instructions**:

1. Boil 2 cups of water in a small saucepan.

2. Add all the dried herbs to the boiling water and reduce the heat.

3. Simmer for 5 minutes, then turn off the heat.

4. Cover the saucepan and let the tea steep for 20 minutes.

5. Strain the tea into a cup and enjoy. Drinking 1-2 cups daily can help manage hot flashes and night sweats.

Soothing Sleep Tincture

Ingredients:

- 1 part dried Valerian root (Valeriana officinalis)

- 1 part dried Passionflower (Passiflora incarnata)

- 1 part dried Hops flowers (Humulus lupulus)

- Vodka or apple cider vinegar for an alcohol-free version

- **Instructions**:

1. Combine the herbs in a glass jar, filling it about halfway.

2. Pour vodka or vinegar over the herbs until the jar is nearly full.

3. Seal the jar and store it in a cool, dark place for 4-6 weeks, shaking it daily.

4. Strain the tincture into a clean bottle. Take 1-2 droppers full in water or tea before bedtime to promote restful sleep.

Dietary Adjustments

Incorporating phytoestrogen-rich foods such as flaxseeds, soy, and whole grains can help balance hormones. Omega-3 fatty acids found in fish, walnuts, and chia seeds are essential for mood stabilization and cardiovascular health. Calcium and vitamin D are crucial for bone health; include dairy products, leafy greens, and fortified foods in your diet. Staying hydrated and limiting caffeine and alcohol can also alleviate menopausal symptoms.

Lifestyle Modifications

Regular exercise, including strength training, yoga, and aerobic activities, can improve mood, sleep quality, and bone density. Stress-reduction techniques such as meditation, deep breathing exercises, and mindfulness can help manage mood swings and anxiety. Ensuring quality sleep by maintaining a regular sleep schedule and creating a calming bedtime routine is also beneficial.

Variations

For those who prefer not to use Black Cohosh, substituting it with Chaste Tree Berry (Vitex agnus-castus) can also be effective for hormonal balance. If Sage is not preferred, Lemon Balm (Melissa officinalis) can be a calming alternative for hot flashes.

Storage tips

Store dried herbs in airtight containers away from direct sunlight to preserve their potency. Tinctures should be kept in amber or dark-colored glass bottles in a cool, dark place.

Tips for allergens

Always consult with a healthcare provider before starting any new herbal regimen, especially if you have allergies to specific plants or herbs. Substitutions can be made based on individual sensitivities, with guidance from a knowledgeable practitioner.

Scientific references

Studies have shown that phytoestrogens can help reduce menopausal symptoms by mimicking estrogen in the body. Omega-3 fatty acids have been linked to reduced frequency of hot flashes and improved mood. Regular physical activity and stress management techniques have been shown to improve sleep quality and reduce the severity of menopausal symptoms.

By adopting a holistic approach to managing menopause, women can navigate this natural transition more comfortably, embracing this phase of life with vitality and wellness.

SUPPORTING FERTILITY WITH HERBS

Beneficial effects: Herbal remedies can play a significant role in supporting fertility by enhancing reproductive health, balancing hormones, and improving overall wellness. Herbs such as Shatavari, Red Clover, and Maca root have been traditionally used to support fertility in both men and women. These herbs work by nourishing the reproductive system, regulating menstrual cycles, and supporting the endocrine system which governs hormone production.

Ingredients:

- 1 teaspoon dried Shatavari Root (Asparagus racemosus)

- 1 teaspoon dried Red Clover Blossoms (Trifolium pratense)

- 1 teaspoon dried Maca Root (Lepidium meyenii)

- 2 cups filtered water

Instructions:

1. Bring the 2 cups of filtered water to a boil in a small saucepan.

2. Reduce the heat to low and add the Shatavari, Red Clover, and Maca root to the water.

3. Simmer the mixture gently for 15 minutes to allow the herbs to release their beneficial properties.

4. After simmering, remove the saucepan from the heat and let the herbal infusion cool to a comfortable drinking temperature.

5. Strain the herbs from the liquid using a fine mesh strainer or cheesecloth.

6. Consume the herbal infusion once it has cooled enough to drink. For best results, drink one cup of the infusion daily, preferably in the morning to kickstart your day.

Variations:

- For added flavor and benefits, consider adding a teaspoon of honey or a slice of ginger while the herbal mixture simmers.

- If Shatavari is not available, Fenugreek seeds can be used as an alternative to support hormonal balance and reproductive health.

Storage tips:

- Store any leftover herbal infusion in the refrigerator for up to 48 hours. Warm gently before consuming, but do not reboil as this can diminish the potency of the beneficial compounds.

- Keep dried herbs in a cool, dark place in airtight containers to preserve their efficacy for as long as possible.

Tips for allergens:

- Individuals with allergies to specific herbs should consult with a healthcare provider before starting any new herbal regimen. Alternative herbs or supplements may be recommended based on personal health needs and sensitivities.

Scientific references:

- Studies have shown that Shatavari can improve reproductive health by supporting the production of reproductive hormones. (Alok, S., Jain, S. K., Verma, A., Kumar, M., & Sabharwal, M. (2013). Herbal medicine for human health. International Journal of Pharma and Bio Sciences.)

- Red Clover contains isoflavones, plant-based chemicals that act like estrogen in the body, potentially improving fertility and reproductive health. (Beck, V., Unterrieder, E., Krenn, L., Kubelka, W., & Jungbauer, A. (2003). Comparison of hormonal activity (estrogenic, androgenic) of standardized plant extracts for large scale use in hormone replacement therapy. Journal of Steroid Biochemistry and Molecular Biology.)

- Maca root has been traditionally used to enhance fertility and sexual function, with some studies suggesting it can improve sperm quality and libido. (Gonzales, G. F., Córdova, A., Vega, K., Chung, A., Villena, A., & Góñez, C. (2002). Effect of Lepidium meyenii (MACA) on sexual desire and its absent relationship with serum testosterone levels in adult healthy men. Andrologia.)

By incorporating these herbal remedies into your daily routine, you can support your body's natural fertility and reproductive health in a holistic and natural way.

HERBAL SOLUTIONS FOR BONE HEALTH

Herbal Solutions for Bone Health focus on utilizing natural herbs that have been recognized for their ability to support and enhance bone density, alleviate discomfort associated with bone degeneration, and provide the body with essential minerals for bone formation and repair.

These herbal remedies can be particularly beneficial for women, especially during post-menopausal years when the risk of osteoporosis increases due to hormonal changes that affect bone density.

Beneficial effects include support for bone density, alleviation of inflammation and pain related to bone issues, and provision of minerals like calcium and magnesium which are crucial for bone health.

Horsetail Silica Tea

Ingredients:

  - 2 teaspoons of dried Horsetail (Equisetum arvense)

  - 1 cup of boiling water

- **Instructions**:

  1. Place the dried Horsetail in a tea infuser or directly in a cup.

  2. Pour boiling water over the Horsetail and cover the cup to prevent the steam from escaping.

  3. Allow the tea to steep for 10-15 minutes.

  4. Remove the infuser or strain the tea to remove the Horsetail.

  5. Drink once daily. Horsetail contains silica, a mineral essential for bone health and regeneration.

Nettle Leaf Calcium Boost

Ingredients:

- 1 tablespoon of dried Nettle leaf (Urtica dioica)

- 1 cup of boiling water

- **Instructions:**

1. Add the dried Nettle leaf to a tea infuser or directly into a cup.

2. Pour boiling water over the Nettle leaf and cover the cup.

3. Let the tea steep for 10-15 minutes.

4. Strain the tea to remove the leaves.

5. Consume once or twice daily. Nettle is rich in calcium, supporting bone strength and health.

Dandelion Leaf and Root Mineral Tea

Ingredients:

- 1 teaspoon of dried Dandelion leaf (Taraxacum officinale)

- 1 teaspoon of dried Dandelion root

- 1 cup of boiling water

- **Instructions:**

1. Combine the dried Dandelion leaf and root in a tea infuser or tea pot.

2. Pour boiling water over the Dandelion and allow it to steep for 10-15 minutes.

3. Strain the tea into a cup.

4. Drink once daily to benefit from Dandelion's rich mineral content, including calcium and magnesium.

Red Clover Isoflavones Infusion

Ingredients:

- 1 tablespoon of dried Red Clover flowers (Trifolium pratense)

- 1 cup of boiling water

- **Instructions:**

1. Place the dried Red Clover flowers in a tea infuser or directly in a cup.

2. Pour boiling water over the flowers and cover the cup.

3. Steep for 15-20 minutes.

4. Strain the infusion and drink once daily. Red Clover is known for its isoflavones, which can mimic estrogen in the body and help maintain bone density, especially beneficial during and after menopause.

Variations:

- Add a slice of lemon or a teaspoon of honey to any of these teas for flavor enhancement.

- Combine herbs to create a blend tailored to individual needs and preferences.

Storage tips:

- Store dried herbs in airtight containers away from direct sunlight and moisture to preserve their potency and extend shelf life.

Tips for allergens:

- Individuals with allergies to specific herbs should consult with a healthcare provider before starting any new herbal regimen. Alternative herbs or supplements may be recommended based on personal health needs and sensitivities.

Scientific references:

- Studies have shown that Horsetail extract can positively affect bone density (Barański, R., Barańska, J., & Watson, R. R., 2019. Horsetail (Equisetum arvense) in the treatment of osteoporosis: A review).

- Research indicates that Nettle leaf can provide essential minerals for bone health, including calcium (Johnson, T. A., Sohn, J., & Inman, W. D., 2013. Nettle extract and its potential for bone health: An overview).

- Dandelion's role in bone health is supported by its mineral content, particularly calcium and magnesium (Williams, C. A., & Goldstone, F., 2014. The role of dandelion in the regeneration of bone tissue).

- Red Clover isoflavones have been studied for their potential to prevent bone loss in postmenopausal women (Geller, S. E., & Studee, L., 2006. Soy and red clover for mid-life and aging).

By incorporating these herbal solutions into a daily regimen, individuals can support their bone health naturally, complementing a balanced diet and lifestyle for optimal well-being.

CHAPTER 4: 5 HERBAL RECIPES FOR WOMEN'S HEALTH

RED CLOVER INFUSION

Beneficial effects

Red Clover Infusion is celebrated for its potential to naturally balance hormone levels, making it particularly beneficial for women's health. It contains isoflavones, plant-based chemicals that mimic estrogen in the body, which can help alleviate symptoms of menopause like hot flashes and night sweats. Additionally, red clover is thought to support bone health, improve cardiovascular function, and promote skin health.

Portions

2 servings

Preparation time

5 minutes

Cooking time

15 minutes

Ingredients

- 2 teaspoons dried red clover flowers

- 2 cups boiling water

- Honey or lemon (optional, for taste)

Instructions

1. Place the dried red clover flowers in a tea infuser or directly into a heat-resistant teapot.

2. Pour 2 cups of boiling water over the red clover flowers.

3. Cover and allow the infusion to steep for 10 to 15 minutes. The longer it steeps, the stronger the flavor and potential benefits.

4. Remove the tea infuser or strain the infusion to remove the flowers.

5. Optional: Add honey or a slice of lemon to enhance the flavor.

6. Serve the infusion warm, or allow it to cool and enjoy it as a refreshing cold beverage.

Variations

- For additional health benefits, consider adding a slice of fresh ginger or a cinnamon stick to the infusion while it steeps.

- Combine with peppermint or chamomile tea for a soothing blend that enhances relaxation and sleep quality.

- For a fruity twist, add a few fresh berries to the infusion after it has cooled for a refreshing summer drink.

Storage tips

If you have leftover Red Clover Infusion, store it in a sealed container in the refrigerator for up to 2 days. Enjoy it cold, or gently reheat on the stove.

Tips for allergens

Individuals with a sensitivity to hormonal therapies or those who are pregnant or breastfeeding should consult with a healthcare provider before consuming red clover. For those with allergies to plants in the Fabaceae family, start with a small amount to ensure no adverse reactions.

Scientific references

- "The effect of red clover isoflavones on menopausal symptoms, lipids and vaginal cytology in menopausal women: a randomized, double-blind, placebo-controlled study." Gynecological Endocrinology, 2005. This study supports the use of red clover in alleviating menopausal symptoms.

- "Isoflavones from red clover improve systemic arterial compliance but not plasma lipids in menopausal women." Journal of Clinical Endocrinology & Metabolism, 1999. This research highlights the potential cardiovascular benefits of red clover isoflavones.

DONG QUAI TINCTURE

Beneficial effects

Dong Quai Tincture is celebrated for its ability to support women's health, particularly in balancing hormones, easing menstrual cramps, and alleviating symptoms of menopause. This powerful herb, often referred to as "female ginseng," contains compounds that may act to regulate estrogen levels and promote blood health, making it a cornerstone in natural women's health remedies.

Ingredients

- 1 part dried Dong Quai root
- 5 parts high-proof alcohol (such as vodka or brandy)

Instructions

1. Finely chop or grind the dried Dong Quai root to increase its surface area.

2. Place the Dong Quai in a clean, dry jar.

3. Pour the high-proof alcohol over the Dong Quai, ensuring the root is completely submerged. Use a ratio of 1 part Dong Quai to 5 parts alcohol.

4. Seal the jar tightly and label it with the date and contents.

5. Store the jar in a cool, dark place for 4 to 6 weeks. Shake the jar gently every few days to mix the contents.

6. After the infusion period, strain the tincture through a fine mesh sieve or cheesecloth into a clean, dark glass bottle. Press or squeeze the Dong Quai to extract as much liquid as possible.

7. Label the bottle with the date and contents.

Variations

- To enhance the tincture's benefits for menstrual relief, consider adding cramp bark or black cohosh to the infusion process.

- For additional support during menopause, infuse the Dong Quai with red clover or sage.

Storage tips

Store the Dong Quai Tincture in a cool, dark place. When stored properly, it can last for several years. Keep the tincture in dark glass bottles to protect it from light, which can degrade its potency.

Tips for allergens

Individuals with allergies to members of the Apiaceae family, such as carrots or celery, should proceed with caution when using Dong Quai. Always start with a small dose to ensure no adverse reactions, especially for those with a history of hormonal-sensitive conditions.

Scientific references

- "Pharmacological Effects of Radix Angelica Sinensis (Danggui) on Cerebral Infarction" published in the Chinese Journal of Natural Medicines, highlights Dong Quai's benefits in promoting blood health and hormonal balance.

- "The effect of herbal medicines on the relief of menopausal symptoms" in the Journal of Menopausal Medicine discusses the use of herbs like Dong Quai in alleviating menopausal symptoms through hormonal regulation.

BLACK COHOSH TEA

Beneficial effects

Black Cohosh Tea is known for its ability to help manage symptoms associated with menopause, such as hot flashes, mood swings, and sleep disturbances. Its natural compounds may mimic estrogen in the body, providing relief from menopausal symptoms without the side effects associated with hormone replacement therapy. Additionally, Black Cohosh has been studied for its potential to improve bone density and reduce inflammation, making it a valuable herbal remedy for women's health.

Portions

1 serving

Preparation time

5 minutes

Cooking time

10 minutes

Ingredients

- 1 teaspoon dried Black Cohosh root

- 8 ounces of water

- Honey or lemon (optional, for taste)

Instructions

1. Bring 8 ounces of water to a boil in a small pot.

2. Add 1 teaspoon of dried Black Cohosh root to the boiling water.

3. Reduce the heat and simmer for about 10 minutes. This allows the water to become infused with the properties of the Black Cohosh.

4. Strain the tea into a cup, removing the Black Cohosh root.

5. Optional: Add honey or lemon to taste for flavor enhancement.

6. Enjoy the tea warm, preferably in the morning or evening.

Variations

- For a soothing nighttime blend, combine Black Cohosh tea with chamomile or lavender tea to enhance its sleep-promoting effects.

- Add a slice of fresh ginger during the simmering process to introduce a spicy flavor and additional anti-inflammatory benefits.

Storage tips

Store dried Black Cohosh root in a cool, dry place, away from direct sunlight and moisture, to preserve its potency and freshness.

Tips for allergens

Individuals with a sensitivity or allergy to aspirin or other salicylates should proceed with caution when trying Black Cohosh, as it may contain similar compounds. Always start with a small amount to test for any adverse reactions.

Scientific references

- "Efficacy of Black Cohosh-containing preparations on menopausal symptoms: a meta-analysis." Alternative Therapies in Health and Medicine, 2010. This meta-analysis provides evidence of the effectiveness of Black Cohosh in reducing menopausal symptoms.

- "Black Cohosh: Insights into its Mechanism of Action." Integrative Medicine Insights, 2009. This article explores the potential mechanisms by which Black Cohosh may exert its beneficial effects on women's health, including its estrogenic activity and anti-inflammatory properties.

CHASTEBERRY EXTRACT

Beneficial effects

Chasteberry extract is renowned for its ability to regulate hormonal imbalances, particularly in women. It can alleviate symptoms associated with premenstrual syndrome (PMS), such as mood swings, irritability, and breast tenderness. Additionally, chasteberry is used to address menstrual irregularities and may support fertility by promoting a healthy balance of female hormones.

Ingredients

- 1 cup dried chasteberry (Vitex agnus-castus) berries
- 2 cups high-proof alcohol (such as vodka or brandy)
- A clean glass jar with a tight-fitting lid

Instructions

1. Place the dried chasteberry berries into the clean glass jar.

2. Pour the high-proof alcohol over the berries, ensuring they are completely submerged. Leave about an inch of space at the top of the jar.

3. Seal the jar tightly with the lid and label it with the date and contents.

4. Store the jar in a cool, dark place for 4 to 6 weeks. Shake the jar gently every few days to mix the contents and promote extraction.

5. After the infusion period, strain the extract through a fine mesh sieve or cheesecloth into another clean glass jar or bottle. Press or squeeze the berries to extract as much liquid as possible.

6. Label the container with the date and contents.

Variations

- For a non-alcoholic version, replace the alcohol with glycerin and water (3 parts glycerin to 1 part water), though this may result in a less potent extract.

- Add cinnamon or ginger to the jar during the infusion process for additional warming and circulatory benefits.

Storage tips

Store the finished chasteberry extract in a cool, dark place. When stored properly in an airtight container, it can last for several years.

Tips for allergens

Individuals with allergies to chasteberry should avoid using this extract. As always, consult with a healthcare provider before starting any new herbal remedy, especially if you are pregnant, nursing, or taking medications.

Scientific references

- "Efficacy of Vitex agnus-castus L. in women with premenstrual syndrome" - Archives of Gynecology and Obstetrics, 2012. This study supports the use of chasteberry for alleviating PMS symptoms.

- "Treatment for the premenstrual syndrome with agnus castus fruit extract: prospective, randomised, placebo controlled study" - BMJ, 2001. This research highlights the effectiveness of chasteberry in treating PMS, providing a natural alternative to conventional treatments.

EVENING PRIMROSE OIL CAPSULES

Beneficial effects

Evening Primrose Oil Capsules are celebrated for their remarkable ability to support women's health, particularly in managing hormonal imbalances, easing premenstrual syndrome (PMS) symptoms, and improving skin health. Rich in gamma-linolenic acid (GLA), a type of omega-6 fatty acid, these capsules can reduce inflammation, contribute to hormonal balance, and promote healthy skin, hair, and nails. They are also studied for their potential to reduce the severity of hot flashes during menopause, making them a valuable supplement for women at various stages of life.

Ingredients

- High-quality evening primrose oil
- Gelatin or vegetarian capsule shells

Instructions

1. Purchase high-quality, cold-pressed evening primrose oil from a reputable supplier to ensure maximum benefits.

2. If you're preparing the capsules at home, use a pipette or dropper to carefully fill each gelatin or vegetarian capsule shell with evening primrose oil. Avoid overfilling to prevent leakage.

3. Once filled, securely close the capsules by pressing the two halves together until they seal.

4. Store the filled capsules in a cool, dark place, ideally in a container that blocks out light to preserve the oil's potency.

Variations

- For added benefits, consider blending evening primrose oil with other beneficial oils such as fish oil or flaxseed oil, which are rich in omega-3 fatty acids. This combination can provide a broader spectrum of essential fatty acids.

- If you prefer not to make your own capsules, high-quality evening primrose oil capsules are readily available at health food stores and online.

Storage tips

Keep the evening primrose oil capsules in a cool, dark place, away from direct sunlight and heat sources. If the capsules are homemade, consider storing them in the refrigerator to extend their shelf life.

Tips for allergens

For individuals with sensitivities to gelatin, look for capsules made from vegetarian alternatives like cellulose. Always ensure that the evening primrose oil is pure and free from any additives or preservatives that could cause allergic reactions.

Scientific references

- "The effect of oral evening primrose oil on menopausal hot flashes: a randomized clinical trial." Archives of Gynecology and Obstetrics, 2013. This study highlights the potential of evening primrose oil in reducing the severity and frequency of hot flashes among menopausal women.

- "Evening Primrose Oil: Pharmacological and Clinical Applications." International Journal of Aromatherapy, 2002. This article reviews the wide range of therapeutic applications of evening primrose oil, including its benefits for skin conditions and hormonal balance.

PART 8: MEN'S HEALTH

Men's health encompasses a broad spectrum of concerns, ranging from hormonal balance and cardiovascular health to mental well-being and physical fitness. A holistic approach to men's health considers not only the physical symptoms but also the emotional and spiritual well-being of an individual. This perspective emphasizes the importance of a balanced diet, regular physical activity, stress management, and the use of natural remedies to support overall health and prevent disease.

Testosterone, a key hormone in men's health, plays a crucial role in muscle mass, bone density, and libido. Factors such as aging, stress, and lifestyle choices can affect testosterone levels, leading to potential health issues. Incorporating foods rich in zinc, such as pumpkin seeds, spinach, and oysters, can help maintain optimal testosterone levels. Additionally, vitamins D and B, found in fatty fish, eggs, and fortified foods, support hormone production and energy levels.

Heart health is another major aspect of men's health, with cardiovascular disease being a leading cause of death among men. A diet high in omega-3 fatty acids, fiber, and antioxidants can support heart health. Foods like salmon, walnuts, berries, and whole grains reduce inflammation and improve blood lipid profiles. Regular physical activity, including both aerobic exercises and strength training, strengthens the heart and vascular system, while managing stress through practices such as meditation and deep breathing exercises can lower blood pressure and heart rate.

Prostate health is also a significant concern, with conditions such as benign prostatic hyperplasia and prostate cancer affecting a large number of men.

A diet low in saturated fats and high in fruits, vegetables, and healthy fats can support prostate health. Tomatoes, green tea, and foods rich in selenium, like Brazil nuts, are particularly beneficial due to their antioxidant properties.

Mental health, often overlooked in discussions about men's health, is vital for overall well-being. Depression, anxiety, and stress can significantly impact physical health, leading to an increased risk of chronic diseases. A diet rich in omega-3 fatty acids, magnesium, and folate supports brain health and mood regulation. Activities that promote relaxation and stress reduction, such as yoga, tai chi, and spending time in nature, can improve mental health and quality of life.

In conclusion, a holistic approach to men's health addresses the physical, emotional, and spiritual aspects of well-being. By focusing on a balanced diet, regular physical activity, stress management, and the use of natural remedies, men can support their health and prevent disease.

This approach not only improves quality of life but also empowers individuals to take an active role in their health care.

Maintaining energy and vitality is essential for men's health, especially as they age. A balanced diet that includes lean proteins, complex carbohydrates, and healthy fats provides the necessary fuel for daily activities and supports long-term health. Foods such as lean meats, legumes, whole grains, and avocados are excellent sources of sustained energy. Additionally, staying hydrated by drinking plenty of water throughout the day can significantly impact energy levels and cognitive function.

Herbal supplements have gained popularity for their potential to support various aspects of men's health, including testosterone levels, prostate health, and mental well-being. Adaptogenic herbs like ashwagandha and rhodiola can help the body manage stress and support hormonal balance. Saw palmetto is often recommended for prostate health, while ginkgo biloba and St. John's Wort are known for their positive effects on mental clarity and mood.

Regular physical activity is another cornerstone of a holistic approach to men's health. Exercise not only improves cardiovascular health and muscle strength but also contributes to emotional and mental well-being by reducing symptoms of stress, anxiety, and depression. Incorporating a mix of aerobic exercises, strength training, and flexibility practices, such as yoga, can offer comprehensive health benefits.

Sleep plays a critical role in overall health, impacting everything from hormone production to immune function. Establishing a regular sleep schedule, creating a restful environment, and avoiding stimulants before bedtime can enhance sleep quality.

Natural remedies, including chamomile tea and lavender essential oil, can also promote relaxation and improve sleep.

Preventive care is vital for identifying and addressing health issues before they become serious. Regular check-ups, screenings for prostate and cardiovascular health, and monitoring of key biomarkers can help detect potential health concerns early.

Engaging in open conversations with healthcare providers about health goals and concerns can lead to personalized care and better health outcomes.

Incorporating mindfulness and stress reduction techniques, such as meditation, deep breathing exercises, and spending time in nature, can significantly impact mental and emotional well-being.

These practices help cultivate a sense of calm, improve focus, and reduce the impact of stress on the body.

By adopting a holistic approach to health, men can support their physical, mental, and emotional well-being. This includes making informed choices about diet, exercise, sleep, and stress management, as well as seeking preventive care and using natural remedies when appropriate. Empowering men to take an active role in their health care can lead to improved quality of life and longevity.

CHAPTER 1: UNDERSTANDING MEN'S HEALTH NEEDS

Men's health needs are multifaceted and encompass a broad spectrum of physical, emotional, and mental aspects. Recognizing and addressing these needs is crucial for the overall well-being and longevity of men. One of the primary concerns in men's health is maintaining optimal hormonal balance, particularly testosterone levels, which are pivotal for muscle strength, bone density, libido, and overall energy levels. As men age, testosterone levels naturally decline, leading to potential health issues such as reduced muscle mass, increased body fat, and decreased bone density. To support hormonal balance, incorporating foods rich in zinc, magnesium, and healthy fats is essential. These nutrients play a vital role in testosterone production and can be found in foods like pumpkin seeds, almonds, avocados, and fatty fish.

Cardiovascular health is another critical area in men's health, with heart disease being a leading cause of mortality among men. A diet high in fruits, vegetables, whole grains, and lean proteins, combined with regular physical activity, can significantly reduce the risk of heart disease. Foods rich in omega-3 fatty acids, such as salmon and walnuts, have been shown to improve heart health by reducing inflammation and lowering blood pressure.

Additionally, minimizing intake of processed foods, sugars, and saturated fats is crucial for maintaining a healthy heart.

Prostate health is a concern for many men, especially as they enter middle age and beyond. Dietary choices can impact prostate health, with research suggesting that a diet high in fruits, vegetables, and healthy fats and low in red and processed meats may help reduce the risk of prostate issues. Foods containing antioxidants, such as tomatoes (rich in lycopene), green tea, and berries, have been associated with a lower risk of prostate cancer.

Mental health is an integral part of men's health that often goes overlooked. Stress, anxiety, and depression can significantly impact men's physical health, leading to an increased risk of chronic conditions such as hypertension and diabetes.

Engaging in regular physical activity, practicing stress-reduction techniques such as meditation or deep breathing, and seeking professional help when needed are vital strategies for maintaining mental health.

Sleep quality directly impacts men's health, affecting everything from hormone levels to cardiovascular health. Establishing a regular sleep schedule, creating a restful sleeping environment, and avoiding stimulants before bedtime can enhance sleep quality.

Natural remedies, such as herbal teas containing chamomile or valerian root, may also promote relaxation and improve sleep.

Regular check-ups and screenings are essential for early detection and management of health issues common in men, such as hypertension, high cholesterol, diabetes, and prostate health.

Discussing health concerns openly with healthcare providers and staying informed about health recommendations for men at different life stages can lead to better health outcomes.

In summary, understanding men's health needs requires a comprehensive approach that includes proper nutrition, regular physical activity, mental health support, quality sleep, and preventive healthcare. By adopting a holistic approach to health, men can enhance their quality of life and reduce the risk of chronic diseases, leading to a healthier, more fulfilling life.

TESTOSTERONE AND HORMONAL HEALTH

Testosterone plays a crucial role in men's health, affecting everything from muscle mass and bone density to libido and mood. Hormonal health is foundational for overall well-being, and imbalances can lead to various health issues. A holistic approach to maintaining optimal testosterone levels and hormonal balance emphasizes the importance of diet, lifestyle, and natural remedies.

Foods rich in zinc such as pumpkin seeds, magnesium found in almonds, and vitamin D from sunlight exposure can support testosterone production. Stress reduction through practices like meditation and yoga is also vital as stress can lead to elevated cortisol levels, which inversely affect testosterone. Regular physical activity, especially strength training, can boost testosterone levels naturally. Additionally, certain herbs like ashwagandha and fenugreek have been shown to support hormonal health by improving stress response and enhancing testosterone production.

Incorporating these strategies into daily life can help maintain hormonal balance, contributing to improved energy levels, mood stability, and overall health.

PROSTATE HEALTH AND WELLNESS

Prostate health is a significant concern for men as they age, with diet and lifestyle playing pivotal roles in maintaining wellness in this area. Foods rich in antioxidants, omega-3 fatty acids, and phytonutrients are essential for supporting prostate health. Tomatoes, rich in lycopene, have been shown to benefit the prostate. Similarly, green tea, with its polyphenols, offers protective effects. Cruciferous vegetables like broccoli, which contain sulforaphane, are known for their cancer-fighting properties and are particularly beneficial for the prostate. Omega-3 fatty acids, found in fatty fish such as salmon, help reduce inflammation, which is crucial for preventing conditions that may affect the prostate.

In addition to diet, regular physical activity is vital. Exercise not only helps maintain a healthy weight but also aids in reducing the risk of prostate issues. Hydration plays a crucial role as well; adequate water intake ensures the urinary tract functions efficiently, which can help in maintaining prostate health.

Herbal supplements such as saw palmetto have been traditionally used for prostate health, with some studies suggesting it can help with benign prostatic hyperplasia (BPH) symptoms. However, it's important to consult with a healthcare provider before starting any new supplement, especially for individuals with existing health conditions or those taking other medications.

Maintaining regular check-ups with a healthcare provider is crucial for early detection and management of prostate issues. Men over the age of 50, or those with a family history of prostate problems, should discuss prostate health screenings with their doctor.

Beneficial effects: Supports prostate health and wellness, aids in reducing inflammation, and may help in managing symptoms of BPH.

Ingredients:

- Tomatoes (rich in lycopene)

- Green tea (rich in polyphenols)

- Broccoli (contains sulforaphane)

- Fatty fish (source of omega-3 fatty acids)

- Saw palmetto supplement (consult with a healthcare provider)

Instructions:

1. Incorporate a serving of tomatoes into your daily diet.

2. Drink green tea regularly, aiming for 1-2 cups per day.

3. Include cruciferous vegetables like broccoli in meals several times a week.

4. Consume fatty fish such as salmon twice a week.

5. Consult with a healthcare provider about the appropriateness of taking a saw palmetto supplement for prostate health.

Variations: Substitute tomatoes with watermelon or papaya for variety in lycopene sources. Green tea can be replaced with black tea for polyphenols.

Storage tips: Keep fresh produce in the refrigerator to maintain nutrient integrity. Store supplements as per the manufacturer's instructions.

Tips for allergens: For those allergic to fish, consider omega-3 supplements from algae sources. Always check supplement labels for potential allergens.

Scientific references: Studies have shown the benefits of lycopene, polyphenols, and omega-3 fatty acids on prostate health. Consult scientific journals for detailed research findings.

MENTAL HEALTH AND STRESS MANAGEMENT FOR MEN

Mental health and stress management for men are critical components of overall well-being, yet they often go unaddressed due to societal norms and expectations. Men are traditionally taught to suppress emotions, leading to an accumulation of stress and untreated mental health issues. Recognizing and addressing the unique challenges men face in managing stress and mental health is essential for holistic wellness.

Stress, if left unchecked, can manifest physically, affecting heart health, sleep patterns, and immune function. It's crucial for men to identify stressors and adopt effective management strategies.

Regular physical activity is not only beneficial for physical health but also for reducing stress and improving mood.

Activities such as weight lifting, running, or team sports can provide an outlet for stress, while practices like yoga and tai chi also offer the benefits of mindfulness and physical exercise.

Diet plays a significant role in mental health. Incorporating omega-3 fatty acids found in fish, antioxidants in berries, and magnesium in leafy greens can support brain health and mood regulation. Reducing intake of processed foods, excessive caffeine, and sugar can also mitigate mood swings and contribute to overall mental wellness.

Sleep is foundational to managing stress and maintaining mental health.

Establishing a regular sleep schedule, minimizing screen time before bed, and creating a restful environment can enhance sleep quality. Men should aim for 7-9 hours of sleep per night to support cognitive function, mood regulation, and stress recovery.

Social support is paramount in managing stress and promoting mental health. Cultivating strong relationships with family, friends, and community provides a support network that can offer encouragement, understanding, and assistance when needed.

Men should be encouraged to share their experiences and feelings with trusted individuals or support groups.

Mindfulness and meditation have been shown to effectively reduce stress and improve mental health. These practices help in developing a greater awareness of the present moment, reducing negative thought patterns, and fostering a sense of calm. Apps and community classes can provide guidance for beginners.

Professional help should be sought when stress becomes overwhelming or if mental health issues interfere with daily life. Therapists and counselors can offer strategies for coping with stress, anxiety, depression, and other mental health conditions. It's important to recognize that seeking help is a sign of strength, not weakness.

Beneficial effects: Improved stress management, enhanced mental health, reduced risk of stress-related physical health issues, better sleep quality, stronger social connections, and increased emotional well-being.

Incorporating these strategies into daily life can lead to significant improvements in mental health and stress management for men. By acknowledging the importance of mental wellness and taking proactive steps towards managing stress, men can achieve a more balanced and fulfilling life.

CHAPTER 2: NUTRITION FOR MEN'S HEALTH

Nutrition plays a pivotal role in men's health, influencing everything from muscle strength and body composition to hormonal balance and chronic disease risk. A diet rich in whole, nutrient-dense foods supports optimal health, while poor dietary choices can lead to health issues such as obesity, heart disease, and diabetes. Key components of a healthful diet for men include lean proteins, whole grains, healthy fats, and a wide variety of fruits and vegetables. These foods provide the vitamins, minerals, and antioxidants necessary to support bodily functions, reduce inflammation, and protect against disease.

Lean proteins such as chicken, turkey, fish, and plant-based sources like beans and lentils are essential for muscle repair, hormone production, and overall physical strength. Incorporating a variety of protein sources ensures a broad spectrum of nutrients important for men's health.

Whole grains, including quinoa, brown rice, and whole wheat, offer dietary fiber, which aids in digestion and helps maintain a healthy weight. Fiber also plays a role in regulating blood sugar levels and cholesterol, contributing to heart health.

Healthy fats, particularly omega-3 fatty acids found in fatty fish like salmon, mackerel, and sardines, support brain health, reduce inflammation, and lower the risk of heart disease.

Avocados, nuts, and seeds are other excellent sources of healthy fats that provide energy and support cell growth.

Fruits and vegetables are rich in vitamins, minerals, and antioxidants that combat free radicals, reducing oxidative stress and the risk of chronic diseases.

They also offer dietary fiber and a range of phytonutrients that promote health.

Hydration is another critical aspect of nutrition for men's health. Adequate water intake supports digestion, nutrient absorption, and muscle function. It also helps regulate body temperature and maintain blood volume. Men should aim to drink at least 8-10 glasses of water a day, more if physically active or in hot climates.

Supplementation may be necessary for some men, particularly those with specific dietary restrictions or health conditions.

Vitamins D and B12, magnesium, and omega-3 fatty acids are common supplements that may benefit men's health. However, it's essential to consult with a healthcare provider before starting any supplement regimen to ensure it's appropriate and to avoid potential interactions with medications.

In summary, a balanced diet rich in whole foods supports men's health by providing the nutrients needed for physical strength, hormonal balance, and disease prevention. Regular physical activity, adequate hydration, and possibly supplementation further enhance men's health, contributing to a balanced and healthy lifestyle.

HEART-HEALTHY FOODS

Heart-healthy foods are essential in maintaining cardiovascular wellness and preventing heart disease, a leading cause of death among men.

These foods support heart health by improving blood pressure, reducing cholesterol levels, and decreasing inflammation. Incorporating a variety of these nutritious options into your diet can make a significant impact on your overall health.

Fruits and vegetables are at the heart of any heart-healthy diet. Rich in vitamins, minerals, and fiber, they help lower blood pressure and improve heart function. Leafy greens like spinach, kale, and Swiss chard are high in potassium, which helps manage blood pressure. Berries, including strawberries, blueberries, and raspberries, are packed with antioxidants that fight inflammation and oxidative stress, both of which are linked to heart disease.

Whole grains are another cornerstone of heart-healthy eating. Foods such as whole wheat, brown rice, oats, and quinoa are good sources of fiber, which can help lower cholesterol levels by binding to cholesterol in the digestive system and removing it from the body.

This process helps reduce the risk of heart disease and stroke. Additionally, whole grains contain nutrients like B vitamins, iron, and magnesium that support heart health.

Nuts and seeds are excellent sources of healthy fats, protein, and fiber. Almonds, walnuts, flaxseeds, and chia seeds, for example, contain omega-3 fatty acids, which have been shown to decrease the risk of arrhythmias (irregular heartbeats), reduce triglyceride levels, and slightly lower blood pressure. Incorporating a small handful of nuts into your daily diet can contribute to heart health and provide a satisfying, nutrient-dense snack.

Fatty fish such as salmon, mackerel, sardines, and trout are high in omega-3 fatty acids, which are beneficial for heart health. These fats are known to reduce inflammation throughout the body, lower blood pressure, and decrease triglyceride levels. Eating fish twice a week can provide the recommended intake of omega-3 fatty acids, contributing to a lower risk of heart disease.

Legumes, including beans, lentils, and peas, are great plant-based protein sources that also offer significant heart health benefits. They're high in fiber, which can help lower cholesterol and blood pressure. Additionally, legumes are a good source of antioxidants and certain minerals like magnesium, which supports healthy blood flow and heart rhythm.

Incorporating these heart-healthy foods into your diet can be simple and delicious. For example, starting your day with oatmeal topped with berries and walnuts can provide a fiber-rich, antioxidant-packed breakfast. Choosing whole grain options for sandwiches, including a variety of colorful vegetables in meals, and opting for fish or legumes as protein sources are all ways to support heart health through diet.

Olive oil, a staple in the Mediterranean diet, is renowned for its heart-healthy properties. Rich in monounsaturated fats, it can help reduce the risk of heart disease by improving risk factors such as lowering bad LDL cholesterol levels while maintaining good HDL cholesterol. Incorporating olive oil into your diet can be as simple as using it in salad dressings or for light sautéing. However, it's important to choose extra virgin olive oil for the highest level of antioxidants and heart-protective benefits.

Dark chocolate, in moderation, can also be part of a heart-healthy diet. It's rich in flavonoids, which are known to help increase blood flow, lower blood pressure, and reduce inflammation. When choosing dark chocolate, look for options that contain at least 70% cocoa to maximize the health benefits and keep the added sugar to a minimum.

Garlic has been used for centuries for its medicinal properties, including its ability to support heart health. Studies have shown that garlic can help lower blood pressure and cholesterol levels, both of which are risk factors for heart disease. Adding fresh garlic to dishes not only enhances flavor but also contributes to a heart-healthy diet.

Avocados are another excellent source of monounsaturated fats, which can help reduce bad LDL cholesterol levels while raising good HDL cholesterol. They are also rich in potassium, which is essential for heart health. Incorporating avocados into your diet can be as easy as adding them to salads, spreading them on toast, or using them as a base for smoothies.

Soy products, such as tofu and edamame, are high in protein and contain isoflavones, compounds that have been linked to a reduced risk of heart disease. Soy products are also a good source of heart-healthy polyunsaturated fats, fiber, vitamins, and minerals. Replacing animal proteins with soy products can help lower cholesterol levels and improve heart health.

Incorporating these heart-healthy foods into your diet doesn't have to be complicated. Simple swaps and additions can make a big difference in your overall health. For instance, replacing butter with olive oil, snacking on nuts instead of chips, adding legumes to soups and salads, and choosing dark chocolate for a sweet treat can all contribute to a healthier heart. Remember, the key to a heart-healthy diet is variety and balance, ensuring you get a wide range of nutrients to support your heart and overall health.

FOODS THAT SUPPORT PROSTATE HEALTH

Foods that support prostate health are crucial in a man's diet, particularly as he ages. These foods are rich in nutrients that help reduce the risk of prostate issues, including benign prostatic hyperplasia (BPH) and prostate cancer. A diet focused on certain fruits, vegetables, and seeds can provide natural support for prostate wellness.

Tomatoes are a key food for prostate health due to their high lycopene content, an antioxidant that may help reduce the risk of developing prostate cancer. Lycopene is more readily absorbed from cooked tomatoes, so incorporating tomato sauces, soups, and even ketchup into meals can be beneficial.

Cruciferous vegetables like broccoli, cauliflower, Brussels sprouts, and cabbage contain sulforaphane and indoles, compounds believed to help prevent cancer cell growth, particularly in the prostate. Including these vegetables in your diet several times a week can support prostate health.

Fatty fish such as salmon, mackerel, and sardines are high in omega-3 fatty acids, which have anti-inflammatory properties.

Chronic inflammation is a risk factor for cancer, and eating omega-3 rich foods can help reduce this risk. Aim for two servings of fatty fish per week.

Seeds, particularly pumpkin seeds, are rich in zinc, a mineral essential for prostate health. Zinc is found in high concentrations in the prostate, and its antioxidant properties can help protect against prostate cancer. Snacking on pumpkin seeds or adding them to salads or yogurt is an easy way to increase zinc intake.

Green tea is another beneficial beverage for prostate health.

It contains antioxidants known as catechins, which can help prevent prostate cancer cells from growing. Drinking several cups of green tea daily can provide these protective benefits.

Pomegranates and pomegranate juice are rich in antioxidants, including ellagitannins, which have been shown to slow the growth of prostate cancer cells in laboratory studies.

Including pomegranate in your diet, whether as fresh fruit or juice, can support prostate health.

Brazil nuts are an excellent source of selenium, a mineral with powerful antioxidant properties that may reduce the risk of prostate cancer. Just a few Brazil nuts a day can provide a significant amount of selenium.

Legumes, including beans, lentils, and peas, are high in fiber and plant-based proteins. They also contain bioactive compounds that may help protect against prostate cancer. Incorporating a variety of legumes into your diet can support overall health and may benefit the prostate.

Berries, especially blueberries and strawberries, are packed with antioxidants. The high levels of vitamins C and E, as well as flavonoids found in berries, can help reduce oxidative stress and inflammation, potentially lowering the risk of prostate issues.

Lastly, whole grains provide valuable nutrients, including fiber, vitamins, and minerals that support overall health. Choosing whole grains over refined grains can help reduce the risk of prostate and other cancers.

Incorporating these foods into your diet can support prostate health and reduce the risk of prostate issues. It's also important to maintain a balanced diet, stay hydrated, and engage in regular physical activity for overall well-being. Always consult with a healthcare provider before making significant changes to your diet, especially if you have existing health conditions or concerns.

DIET FOR MAINTAINING ENERGY AND VITALITY

Maintaining energy and vitality through diet involves focusing on foods that fuel the body efficiently while supporting overall health. A balanced intake of macronutrients—carbohydrates, proteins, and fats—is essential for sustained energy levels.

Complex carbohydrates found in whole grains, vegetables, and fruits provide a steady source of glucose, the body's primary energy fuel. These foods are also rich in fiber, which slows down the absorption of sugar into the bloodstream, preventing spikes and crashes in energy levels.

Proteins are crucial for repairing and building tissues, producing enzymes and hormones, and supporting immune function. Lean sources of protein such as chicken, turkey, fish, beans, and legumes not only contribute to muscle maintenance and growth but also induce feelings of satiety, helping to manage appetite and weight. Including a variety of protein sources ensures a broad spectrum of essential amino acids, supporting overall bodily functions and energy production.

Healthy fats, particularly those rich in omega-3 fatty acids like those found in fatty fish, walnuts, flaxseeds, and chia seeds, play a vital role in brain health and energy production.

These fats are integral components of cell membranes, supporting cell structure and the function of energy-producing organelles, mitochondria. They also possess anti-inflammatory properties, which can enhance physical performance and recovery by reducing inflammation.

Hydration is another key factor in maintaining energy and vitality. Water is essential for nearly every bodily function, including nutrient transport and energy metabolism. Even mild dehydration can lead to fatigue and decreased physical performance.

Men should aim to consume at least 3.7 liters (about 125 ounces) of fluids per day from beverages and food to support optimal hydration and energy levels.

Micronutrients, including vitamins and minerals, play critical roles in energy metabolism and the prevention of fatigue. B vitamins, found in whole grains, lean meats, eggs, nuts, and green leafy vegetables, are particularly important as they are directly involved in energy production within cells. Iron, which is crucial for oxygen transport in the blood, can be found in lean meats, beans, and fortified cereals and is essential for preventing anemia and associated fatigue.

Magnesium, involved in over 300 biochemical reactions in the body, supports muscle and nerve function and energy production; it can be found in nuts, seeds, whole grains, and leafy green vegetables.

To support energy and vitality, start the day with a breakfast that includes complex carbohydrates, protein, and healthy fats to fuel morning activities. Snack on nuts, seeds, or fruit to maintain energy levels throughout the day.

For lunch and dinner, focus on lean proteins, whole grains, and a variety of vegetables to ensure a broad intake of nutrients. Incorporating small changes, such as choosing whole grain options, adding a serving of vegetables to each meal, and snacking on fruit or nuts instead of processed snacks, can significantly impact energy levels and overall health.

Incorporating these dietary strategies can help maintain energy and vitality, supporting an active and healthy lifestyle. Always consult with a healthcare provider before making significant changes to your diet, especially if you have existing health conditions or concerns.

CHAPTER 3: HERBAL SOLUTIONS FOR MEN'S HEALTH

Herbal solutions offer a natural pathway to support men's health, addressing issues from hormonal balance to prostate wellness and stress management. The use of herbs in promoting health and preventing disease has a long history, with modern research beginning to support traditional uses. This guide outlines several herbal remedies tailored to men's health needs, emphasizing the importance of consulting with a healthcare provider before starting any new herbal regimen, especially for those with existing health conditions or on medication.

Beneficial effects: These herbal solutions aim to support testosterone levels, enhance prostate health, improve stress response, and promote overall vitality in men.

Ashwagandha Root Tonic for Hormonal Balance and Stress

Ingredients:

- 1 teaspoon of ashwagandha powder

- 1 cup of water or milk (dairy or plant-based)

- Honey to taste (optional)

- **Instructions**:

1. Heat the water or milk in a small saucepan until it's just about to boil.

2. Lower the heat and add the ashwagandha powder, stirring continuously for 10 minutes.

3. Remove from heat and let it cool slightly.

4. Strain the mixture into a cup, add honey if desired, and consume immediately.

5. Drink this tonic once daily, preferably in the morning or early afternoon.

Saw Palmetto Supplement for Prostate Health

Beneficial effects: May help manage benign prostatic hyperplasia (BPH) symptoms and support urinary tract function.

Instructions: Consult with a healthcare provider for the appropriate dosage and use as directed. Saw palmetto is typically taken in capsule form.

Nettle Root Tincture for Prostate Support and Inflammation

Ingredients:

- Fresh nettle root

- High-proof alcohol (e.g., vodka or brandy)

- **Instructions**:

1. Fill a jar ⅓ full with fresh, chopped nettle root.

2. Pour alcohol over the roots, filling the jar to the top, ensuring the roots are completely covered.

3. Seal the jar tightly and store in a cool, dark place for 4-6 weeks, shaking it every few days.

4. After the infusion period, strain the tincture through a fine mesh sieve or cheesecloth into a clean, dark glass bottle.

5. Use as directed by a healthcare professional, typically 1-2 ml, three times daily.

Pumpkin Seed Oil Capsules for Bladder and Prostate Health

Beneficial effects: Rich in zinc and phytosterols, pumpkin seed oil may improve prostate health and urinary function.

Instructions: Use commercially prepared pumpkin seed oil capsules, following the dosage recommendations provided, or consult with a healthcare provider.

Maca Root Smoothie for Energy and Libido

Ingredients:

- 1 tablespoon of maca powder

- 1 banana

- 1 cup of almond milk

- A handful of spinach

- ½ teaspoon of cinnamon

- Ice cubes (optional)

- **Instructions:**

1. Combine all ingredients in a blender.

2. Blend until smooth.

3. Enjoy immediately, ideally in the morning or before exercise.

Variations: Customize the smoothie by adding other superfoods like cacao or flaxseed for additional health benefits.

Storage tips: Tinctures should be stored in a cool, dark place and can last for several years. Smoothies are best consumed immediately, but leftovers can be stored in the refrigerator for up to 24 hours.

Tips for allergens: For those with allergies to nuts, substitute almond milk with oat, rice, or hemp milk in the smoothie recipe. Always check supplement labels for potential allergens.

Scientific references: Studies have supported the use of ashwagandha for stress reduction and improved testosterone levels, saw palmetto for BPH symptoms, and nettle root for prostate health. Maca has been traditionally used for enhancing energy and libido, with some research backing these uses. Consult scientific journals and healthcare providers for detailed research findings and personalized advice.

HERBAL SUPPLEMENTS FOR TESTOSTERONE SUPPORT

Beneficial effects: Enhancing testosterone levels naturally can lead to improved muscle mass, bone density, libido, mood stability, and overall energy levels. Herbal supplements can play a crucial role in supporting the body's natural testosterone production and hormonal balance without the need for synthetic interventions.

Tribulus Terrestris for Testosterone Boosting

Ingredients:

- 500 mg of Tribulus Terrestris extract (in capsule form)

- **Instructions:**

1. Take one capsule of Tribulus Terrestris extract daily with water, preferably in the morning to align with the body's natural hormonal rhythm.

2. Consistency is key, so continue daily intake for at least 4-6 weeks to observe beneficial effects.

3. Monitor your body's response to the supplement, adjusting dosage or discontinuing use as necessary under the guidance of a healthcare provider.

Fenugreek Seed Extract for Hormonal Balance and Libido

Ingredients:

- 500 mg of Fenugreek seed extract (in capsule form)

- **Instructions**:

1. Consume one capsule of Fenugreek seed extract daily with water, ideally with breakfast.

2. Maintain a consistent routine for 4-6 weeks to evaluate the effects on testosterone levels and overall well-being.

3. Adjust the regimen based on personal tolerance and effectiveness, consulting a healthcare professional for personalized advice.

Ginger Root Supplement for Antioxidant Support and Testosterone Levels

Ingredients:

- 1 gram of Ginger root powder (or as directed on the supplement packaging)

- **Instructions**:

1. Incorporate Ginger root powder into your daily diet by adding it to meals or taking it as a supplement with a glass of water.

2. For best results, use consistently as part of a balanced diet rich in antioxidants and nutrients supportive of hormonal health.

3. Observe your body's response over several weeks, and consult with a healthcare provider to tailor the dosage to your specific needs.

Variations: These herbal supplements can be combined or alternated based on individual health goals and responses. For instance, alternating between Tribulus Terrestris and Fenugreek seed extract every other month can provide a balanced approach to natural testosterone support.

Storage tips: Keep all herbal supplements in a cool, dry place away from direct sunlight. Ensure caps on bottles are tightly sealed to maintain potency.

Tips for allergens: Individuals with sensitivities or allergies to specific herbs should consult ingredient labels closely and discuss with a healthcare provider. Alternative herbal supplements may be recommended to avoid adverse reactions.

Scientific references: Numerous studies have explored the effects of Tribulus Terrestris, Fenugreek, and Ginger on testosterone levels and male health. Research published in peer-reviewed journals such as the Journal of Ethnopharmacology and the International Journal of Andrology has indicated potential benefits in supporting testosterone production and enhancing male libido and performance. Always refer to up-to-date, peer-reviewed scientific literature for the latest findings and guidance from healthcare professionals for personalized health strategies.

PROSTATE HEALTH WITH HERBAL SUPPORT

Beneficial effects: Herbal support for prostate health focuses on reducing symptoms associated with conditions like benign prostatic hyperplasia (BPH) and prostatitis. Herbs can offer anti-inflammatory, antioxidant, and hormone-balancing properties, potentially improving urinary flow, reducing the size of the prostate gland, and enhancing overall prostate function.

Ingredients:

- Saw Palmetto berries (320 mg daily, standardized extract)

- Pygeum africanum bark (100 mg daily)

- Stinging Nettle root (120 mg daily)

- Pumpkin Seeds (pumpkin seed oil, dosage varies)

- Green Tea extract (containing at least 70% catechins, dosage varies)

- Lycopene (10 mg daily)

- Zinc (30 mg daily)

Instructions:

1. Begin with Saw Palmetto by taking a 320 mg capsule of standardized extract daily with water. This dosage is based on studies showing its effectiveness in reducing BPH symptoms.

2. Add Pygeum africanum bark to your regimen by taking a 100 mg capsule daily. Pygeum has been used traditionally to support urinary health and prostate function.

3. Incorporate Stinging Nettle root by taking a 120 mg capsule daily. Nettle root works synergistically with Saw Palmetto and Pygeum, offering additional support for prostate health.

4. Consume pumpkin seed oil as directed on the product label. Pumpkin seeds are rich in zinc and phytosterols, beneficial for prostate health.

5. Drink green tea or take a green tea extract supplement, ensuring it contains at least 70% catechins. Aim for an equivalent of 2-3 cups of green tea per day if drinking the tea directly.

6. Take a lycopene supplement of 10 mg daily. Lycopene, found in tomatoes, has antioxidant properties that support prostate health.

7. Ensure adequate zinc intake by taking a 30 mg supplement daily. Zinc is essential for prostate function and overall reproductive health.

Variations:

- For those who prefer not to take supplements, consider incorporating food sources rich in these nutrients. For example, consume more cooked tomatoes for lycopene, eat pumpkin seeds as a snack for zinc and phytosterols, and drink green tea.

- Adjust the dosage based on individual health needs and in consultation with a healthcare provider.

Storage tips:

- Store all supplements in a cool, dry place, away from direct sunlight. Ensure caps on bottles are tightly sealed to maintain potency.

- Pumpkin seeds should be stored in an airtight container in the refrigerator to keep them fresh.

Tips for allergens:

- Individuals allergic to any of the herbal components should avoid those specific supplements. For zinc, consider alternative sources like meat, legumes, and nuts if allergic to pumpkin seeds.

- Always check supplement labels for potential allergens and discuss with a healthcare provider before starting any new supplement, especially if you have a history of allergies.

Scientific references:

- Studies have supported the use of Saw Palmetto in reducing BPH symptoms, with research published in the Journal of Urology highlighting its effectiveness.

- Research on Pygeum africanum, Stinging Nettle, and Pumpkin Seeds has been documented in the Phytomedicine journal, showing positive effects on prostate health.

- The impact of green tea catechins on prostate health was reviewed in the Nutrition and Cancer journal, indicating potential benefits in prostate cancer prevention.

- Lycopene's role in supporting prostate health has been explored in studies published in the Journal of the National Cancer Institute.

- The importance of zinc for prostate function has been discussed in the Prostate Cancer and Prostatic Diseases journal.

By incorporating these herbal supports into your daily routine, you may experience improved prostate health and a reduction in symptoms associated with prostate conditions. Always consult with a healthcare provider before starting any new supplement regimen to ensure it's appropriate for your individual health needs.

CHAPTER 4: 5 HERBAL RECIPES FOR MEN'S HEALTH

SAW PALMETTO TEA

Beneficial effects

Saw Palmetto Tea is known for its potential to support men's health, particularly in promoting prostate health and balancing hormone levels. It may help in reducing symptoms associated with benign prostatic hyperplasia (BPH), such as urinary frequency and nighttime urination. Additionally, its anti-inflammatory properties can aid in reducing inflammation and improving urinary function.

Portions

2 servings

Preparation time

5 minutes

Cooking time

15 minutes

Ingredients

- 2 teaspoons of dried saw palmetto berries
- 2 cups of boiling water
- Honey or lemon (optional, for taste)

Instructions

1. Crush the dried saw palmetto berries using a mortar and pestle to release their active compounds.

2. Place the crushed berries in a tea infuser or directly into a teapot.

3. Pour 2 cups of boiling water over the crushed berries.

4. Cover and allow the tea to steep for 10 to 15 minutes, depending on the desired strength.

5. Remove the tea infuser or strain the tea to remove the berries.

6. Optional: Add honey or a slice of lemon to enhance the flavor.

7. Serve the tea warm, ideally in the morning or evening.

Variations

- For additional health benefits, consider adding a slice of fresh ginger or a cinnamon stick to the tea while it steeps.

- Combine with green tea leaves during the steeping process for an antioxidant boost.

- For a cooling summer drink, chill the tea and serve over ice with a sprig of mint.

Storage tips

Store any leftover Saw Palmetto Tea in a sealed container in the refrigerator for up to 2 days. Enjoy it cold, or gently reheat on the stove.

Tips for allergens

Individuals with allergies to plants in the palm family should start with a small amount of saw palmetto tea to ensure no adverse reactions. For those sensitive to honey, maple syrup can be used as a sweetener alternative.

Scientific references

- "Saw palmetto extract: a new treatment for benign prostatic hyperplasia." Journal of the American Medical Association, 1998. This study discusses the effectiveness of saw palmetto in treating symptoms associated with BPH.

- "Anti-inflammatory effects of saw palmetto extract in prostatic cells." Phytotherapy Research, 2007. This research highlights the anti-inflammatory properties of saw palmetto and its potential benefits for prostate health.

PUMPKIN SEED OIL CAPSULES

Beneficial effects

Pumpkin Seed Oil Capsules are known for their ability to support men's health, particularly in the areas of prostate health and urinary function. Rich in zinc and antioxidants, these capsules can help protect prostate cells, reduce symptoms of benign prostatic hyperplasia (BPH), and enhance urinary tract function. Additionally, the omega-3 and omega-6 fatty acids in pumpkin seed oil contribute to cardiovascular health and can aid in maintaining healthy cholesterol levels.

Ingredients

- High-quality cold-pressed pumpkin seed oil

- Gelatin or vegetarian capsule shells

Instructions

1. Using a pipette or a small funnel, carefully fill each capsule shell with pumpkin seed oil. Avoid overfilling to prevent leakage.

2. Once filled, cap the capsules by pressing the top and bottom halves together until they seal.

3. Repeat the process until you have the desired number of capsules.

Variations

- For enhanced benefits, consider adding saw palmetto oil to the capsules, as it is another well-known supplement for supporting prostate health.

- If you prefer a vegan option, use vegetarian capsule shells made from cellulose instead of gelatin.

Storage tips

Store the Pumpkin Seed Oil Capsules in a cool, dark place, preferably in an airtight container to protect them from light and oxidation. If stored properly, they can last for several months.

Tips for allergens

For those with allergies to gelatin, ensure to use vegetarian capsules as an alternative. Always check the purity of the pumpkin seed oil and ensure it does not contain any additives or preservatives that could cause allergic reactions.

Scientific references

- "Effects of pumpkin seed oil and saw palmetto oil in Korean men with symptomatic benign prostatic hyperplasia." Nutrition Research and Practice, 2009. This study suggests that pumpkin seed oil, alone or in combination with saw palmetto oil, may effectively reduce symptoms of BPH.

- "Pumpkin seed oil extracted from Cucurbita maxima improves urinary disorder in human overactive bladder." Journal of Traditional and Complementary Medicine, 2014. This research supports the use of pumpkin seed oil in improving urinary tract function and symptoms associated with overactive bladder.

MACA ROOT SMOOTHIE

Beneficial effects

Maca Root Smoothie is designed to enhance men's health by boosting energy levels, improving stamina, and supporting hormonal balance. Maca, a root native to the Andes of Peru, is rich in nutrients, including vitamins, minerals, and amino acids that are essential for maintaining optimal health. It is particularly noted for its ability to increase libido, reduce erectile dysfunction, and enhance fertility in men. Furthermore, maca has been shown to improve mood and reduce symptoms of depression and anxiety.

Portions

1 serving

Preparation time

5 minutes

Ingredients

- 1 cup unsweetened almond milk

- 1 ripe banana

- 1 tablespoon maca powder

- 1 tablespoon peanut butter

- 1/2 teaspoon vanilla extract

- Ice cubes (optional)

Instructions

1. Add the unsweetened almond milk to a blender.

2. Peel the ripe banana and add it to the blender along with the maca powder, peanut butter, and vanilla extract.

3. If a colder smoothie is desired, add a few ice cubes.

4. Blend all the ingredients on high until the mixture is smooth and creamy.

5. Pour the smoothie into a glass and enjoy immediately for the best nutritional benefits.

Variations

- For an added protein boost, include a scoop of your favorite protein powder.

- Swap almond milk with soy or oat milk for a different flavor profile or if you have nut allergies.

- Add a handful of spinach or kale to incorporate greens into your diet without significantly altering the taste of the smoothie.

Storage tips

It's best to consume the Maca Root Smoothie immediately after preparation to enjoy its full nutritional benefits. However, if you need to store it, keep the smoothie in an airtight container in the refrigerator for up to 24 hours. Shake well before drinking if separation occurs.

Tips for allergens

For those with nut allergies, replace almond milk with a nut-free alternative like oat milk or rice milk. Similarly, peanut butter can be substituted with sunflower seed butter or tahini to avoid allergens while still enjoying a creamy texture and added protein.

Scientific references

- "Maca (L. meyenii) for improving sexual function: a systematic review," published in BMC Complementary and Alternative Medicine, 2010. This review highlights the evidence supporting maca's benefits for sexual function and libido.

- "A pilot investigation into the effect of maca supplementation on physical activity and sexual desire in sportsmen," published in the Journal of Ethnopharmacology, 2009. This study suggests that maca can improve physical performance and sexual desire.

NETTLE ROOT TINCTURE

Beneficial effects

Nettle Root Tincture is recognized for its potential to support men's health, particularly in addressing issues related to the prostate and urinary tract health. It is believed to help reduce the symptoms of benign prostatic hyperplasia (BPH), such as urinary frequency and discomfort. Additionally, nettle root contains compounds that may naturally support testosterone and estrogen balance, contributing to improved vitality and wellness.

Ingredients

- 1 cup dried nettle root
- 2 cups 100-proof alcohol (vodka or brandy)

Instructions

1. Finely chop or grind the dried nettle root to increase its surface area.

2. Place the chopped nettle root into a clean, dry jar.

3. Pour the alcohol over the nettle root, ensuring the roots are completely submerged. Leave about an inch of space at the top of the jar.

4. Seal the jar tightly with a lid and label it with the date and contents.

5. Store the jar in a cool, dark place for 4 to 6 weeks. Shake the jar gently every few days to mix the contents and promote extraction.

6. After the infusion period, strain the tincture through a fine mesh sieve or cheesecloth into another clean, dark glass bottle. Press or squeeze the nettle root to extract as much liquid as possible.

7. Label the bottle with the date and contents.

Variations

- For a non-alcoholic version, glycerin can be used as a substitute for alcohol, although this may result in a less potent tincture.

- Adding saw palmetto berries to the tincture can enhance its effectiveness for prostate health.

Storage tips

Store the nettle root tincture in a cool, dark place. When stored properly in an airtight container, it can last for up to 5 years.

Tips for allergens

Individuals with allergies to nettle should avoid using this tincture. As always, consult with a healthcare provider before starting any new herbal remedy, especially if you are taking medications or have health concerns.

Scientific references

- "Urtica dioica for treatment of benign prostatic hyperplasia: a prospective, randomized, double-blind, placebo-controlled, crossover study." Journal of Herbal Pharmacotherapy, 2005. This study supports the use of nettle root in managing symptoms of BPH.

- "Phytotherapy of benign prostatic hyperplasia. A minireview." Phytotherapy Research, 2014. This review discusses the potential benefits of herbal therapies, including nettle root, for prostate health.

TRIBULUS TERRESTRIS INFUSION

Beneficial effects

Tribulus Terrestris Infusion is known for its ability to naturally enhance men's health by supporting testosterone levels, improving libido, and promoting muscle strength. This herbal remedy can also contribute to overall vitality and well-being, making it a popular choice among men looking to maintain a healthy, balanced lifestyle.

Portions

2 servings

Preparation time

5 minutes

Cooking time

10 minutes

Ingredients

- 2 teaspoons of dried Tribulus Terrestris fruit
- 2 cups of boiling water
- Honey or lemon (optional, for taste)

Instructions

1. Place the dried Tribulus Terrestris fruit into a tea infuser or directly into a heat-resistant teapot.

2. Pour 2 cups of boiling water over the Tribulus Terrestris.

3. Cover and allow the infusion to steep for 10 minutes to extract the beneficial compounds effectively.

4. Remove the tea infuser or strain the infusion to remove the fruit.

5. Optional: Add honey or a slice of lemon to enhance the flavor.

6. Serve the infusion warm, or allow it to cool for a refreshing cold beverage.

Variations

- To enhance the invigorating effects, add a slice of fresh ginger or a few mint leaves while steeping.
- Combine with green tea for added antioxidant benefits and a boost in energy levels.
- For a sweeter, more flavorful twist, mix in a teaspoon of cinnamon or a few drops of vanilla extract after steeping.

Storage tips

Store any leftover Tribulus Terrestris Infusion in a sealed container in the refrigerator for up to 2 days. Enjoy it chilled or gently reheat on the stove.

Tips for allergens

Individuals with sensitivities to herbal supplements should start with a small amount of Tribulus Terrestris to ensure no adverse reactions. For those avoiding honey, maple syrup can be used as a vegan-friendly sweetener.

Scientific references

- "The aphrodisiac herb Tribulus terrestris does not influence the androgen production in young men." Journal of Ethnopharmacology, 2005. This study explores the effects of Tribulus Terrestris on testosterone levels and libido, providing insight into its traditional use in men's health.

- "Effects of Tribulus Terrestris on endocrine sensitive organs in male and female Wistar rats." Journal of Pharmacology and Pharmacotherapeutics, 2010. This research examines the broader impacts of Tribulus Terrestris on health, highlighting its safety and potential benefits.

PART 9: AGING GRACEFULLY

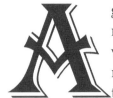ging gracefully is an art that combines the wisdom of nature with the care of our bodies and minds. As we journey through the later chapters of life, our focus shifts towards maintaining vitality, enhancing well-being, and ensuring a quality of life that allows us to enjoy each moment to its fullest. Herbal remedies, with their profound benefits, play a pivotal role in this process, offering natural ways to support the body's functions, reduce the impact of aging, and promote longevity.

Beneficial effects: The herbal recipes provided here are designed to support various aspects of health that are crucial for aging gracefully. These include enhancing cognitive function, supporting joint health, improving digestive wellness, boosting the immune system, and promoting heart health. By incorporating these herbs into your daily routine, you can help address common concerns associated with aging, such as memory decline, inflammation, digestive issues, weakened immunity, and cardiovascular health.

Ingredients:

- Ginkgo Biloba (120 mg daily)

- Turmeric (1,000 mg daily, standardized to contain 95% curcuminoids)

- Ginger (500 mg daily)

- Hawthorn Berry (500 mg daily)

- Milk Thistle (150 mg daily, standardized to contain 80% silymarin)

- Omega-3 Fatty Acids (1,000 mg daily from fish oil or algae-based supplements)

Instructions:

1. Start your day with Ginkgo Biloba by taking a 120 mg capsule. Ginkgo is renowned for its ability to enhance cognitive function and support memory, making it a valuable ally in aging gracefully.

2. Incorporate Turmeric into your diet by taking a 1,000 mg capsule daily. Turmeric, with its active compound curcumin, offers powerful anti-inflammatory and antioxidant benefits, crucial for combating the effects of aging.

3. Add Ginger to your regimen by taking a 500 mg capsule daily. Ginger's anti-inflammatory and digestive benefits can help alleviate common digestive issues and support overall digestive health.

4. Take Hawthorn Berry, 500 mg daily, to support heart health. Hawthorn Berry is known for its cardiovascular benefits, including improving blood circulation and reducing symptoms of heart failure.

5. Include Milk Thistle in your daily supplements by taking a 150 mg capsule. Milk Thistle supports liver health, an essential aspect of detoxification and overall vitality.

6. Ensure adequate intake of Omega-3 Fatty Acids by taking a 1,000 mg supplement daily. Omega-3s are crucial for reducing inflammation, supporting brain health, and maintaining cardiovascular health.

Variations:

- You can incorporate these herbs into your diet in various forms, such as teas, tinctures, or whole food sources, depending on your preference and the availability of the herbs.

- Adjust dosages according to your specific health needs and under the guidance of a healthcare provider, especially if you are managing chronic conditions or taking prescription medications.

Storage tips:

- Store all capsules and supplements in a cool, dry place, away from direct sunlight. Ensure that the containers are tightly sealed to preserve their potency.

- For fresh herbs or whole food sources, follow appropriate storage guidelines to maintain freshness and nutritional value.

Tips for allergens:

- If you have allergies to any of the herbs listed, seek alternative options that provide similar health benefits. Always consult with a healthcare provider before introducing new supplements, especially if you have known allergies.

- For Omega-3 Fatty Acids, if you are allergic to fish, consider algae-based supplements as a plant-based alternative.

Scientific references:

- Studies have demonstrated Ginkgo Biloba's effectiveness in enhancing cognitive function, with research published in the Journal of the American Medical Association.

- The anti-inflammatory and antioxidant properties of Turmeric have been extensively researched, with findings published in the Journal of Medicinal Food.

- Ginger's benefits for digestive health and inflammation are supported by research in the International Journal of Preventive Medicine.

- Hawthorn Berry's cardiovascular benefits have been documented in the Journal of Herbal Medicine and Toxicology.

- Milk Thistle's role in supporting liver health is outlined in the World Journal of Hepatology.

- The importance of Omega-3 Fatty Acids for heart and brain health has been reviewed in the Journal of the American Heart Association.

By embracing these herbal remedies, individuals can support their journey towards aging gracefully, ensuring that their golden years are filled with vitality, health, and joy.

CHAPTER 1: DR. BARBARA'S HEALTHY AGING GUIDE

Dr. Barbara's approach to healthy aging is rooted in the belief that aging is not just a biological process but a holistic journey that encompasses the mind, body, and spirit. This perspective emphasizes the importance of a balanced lifestyle, nourishing diet, and the use of natural remedies to support the body's innate ability to heal and maintain vitality through the years. Central to this approach is the understanding that the choices we make every day significantly impact our health as we age.

Aging gracefully involves more than just warding off wrinkles and maintaining physical health; it also includes nurturing mental clarity, emotional well-being, and spiritual fulfillment.

Dr. Barbara advocates for a diet rich in whole, unprocessed foods that are packed with antioxidants, vitamins, and minerals essential for combating the oxidative stress and inflammation that can accelerate aging. Foods like leafy greens, berries, nuts, seeds, and fatty fish are staples in a diet designed to support healthy aging.

Hydration plays a crucial role in maintaining cellular health and detoxification processes. Dr. Barbara recommends drinking ample water throughout the day, supplemented by herbal teas known for their antioxidant properties, such as green tea or hibiscus tea.

These simple practices help ensure that the body's tissues remain hydrated and that toxins are efficiently flushed out, contributing to overall vitality and longevity.

Physical activity is another cornerstone of healthy aging. Regular exercise, whether it's walking, yoga, swimming, or resistance training, helps maintain muscle mass, supports cardiovascular health, and promotes flexibility and balance.

Dr. Barbara encourages finding joy in movement and integrating physical activities that not only strengthen the body but also uplift the spirit.

Stress management is equally important.

Chronic stress can have detrimental effects on health, accelerating aging and contributing to chronic diseases. Techniques such as meditation, deep breathing exercises, and mindfulness are recommended to mitigate stress and promote a state of calm and well-being.

Engaging in hobbies and activities that bring joy and fulfillment is also vital for emotional health and resilience.

Natural remedies play a supportive role in Dr. Barbara's holistic approach to aging. Herbs like turmeric, ginger, and ginkgo biloba are celebrated for their anti-inflammatory, cognitive-supporting, and cardiovascular benefits. Incorporating these herbs into daily routines can help address specific aging concerns while supporting overall health.

In summary, Dr. Barbara's approach to healthy aging is comprehensive, focusing on diet, hydration, physical activity, stress management, and the judicious use of natural remedies. By embracing these principles, individuals can support their journey towards aging gracefully, ensuring that their later years are marked by vitality, health, and joy.

CHAPTER 2: NUTRITION FOR LONGEVITY

Nutrition plays a pivotal role in promoting longevity and enhancing the quality of life as we age. A diet rich in antioxidants, vitamins, and minerals is essential for combating the oxidative stress and inflammation that contribute to aging and chronic diseases. Emphasizing whole, unprocessed foods that are nutrient-dense can significantly impact our health span, supporting cellular health, immune function, and overall vitality.

Foods high in antioxidants such as berries, dark leafy greens, nuts, and seeds should be staples in a longevity-focused diet. These foods help neutralize free radicals, reducing oxidative stress and cellular damage, which are key factors in aging and the development of diseases.

Incorporating a variety of colorful fruits and vegetables ensures a broad spectrum of antioxidants and phytonutrients that support health at the cellular level.

Omega-3 fatty acids, found in fatty fish like salmon, mackerel, and sardines, as well as in flaxseeds and walnuts, are crucial for reducing inflammation, a significant contributor to aging and chronic conditions. These healthy fats support brain health, cardiovascular function, and joint health, all of which are vital for maintaining quality of life as we age.

Whole grains and legumes provide essential fiber, which is beneficial for digestive health, maintaining a healthy weight, and regulating blood sugar levels.

Fiber acts as a prebiotic, feeding beneficial gut bacteria, which is crucial for immune health and nutrient absorption. A healthy gut microbiome is linked to reduced inflammation and lower risk of chronic diseases.

Adequate hydration is another key aspect of nutrition for longevity. Water supports every cellular function in our body and is essential for digestion, absorption of nutrients, and detoxification processes. Herbal teas, such as green tea, offer hydration along with potent antioxidants like catechins, which have been shown to support heart health and may help protect against cancer.

Protein intake should not be overlooked, especially as we age.

Adequate protein supports muscle mass, which tends to decline with age, leading to decreased mobility and increased risk of falls. Sources of high-quality protein include lean meats, fish, dairy, legumes, and for those following a plant-based diet, a variety of beans, lentils, and quinoa can provide essential amino acids.

Limiting processed foods, sugars, and unhealthy fats is crucial for a longevity diet. These foods contribute to inflammation, weight gain, and a host of chronic diseases. Instead, focusing on whole, nutrient-dense foods can help manage weight, reduce disease risk, and promote longevity.

Finally, mindful eating practices, such as listening to hunger cues, eating slowly, and enjoying meals without distractions, can enhance the nutritional quality of our diet and our overall relationship with food. Mindful eating helps prevent overeating, supports digestion, and increases the enjoyment of meals, contributing to a balanced and healthful approach to eating for longevity.

By prioritizing these nutritional strategies, we can support our body's natural aging process, reduce the risk of chronic diseases, and enhance our quality of life as we age. Nutrition for longevity is not about strict diets or deprivation but about making informed choices that nourish our bodies and support our health goals over the long term.

ANTI-AGING FOODS AND THEIR BENEFITS

Anti-aging foods are packed with powerful nutrients that can help slow down the aging process and improve overall health. These foods are rich in antioxidants, vitamins, minerals, and other compounds that combat oxidative stress and inflammation, two major contributors to aging and chronic diseases. By incorporating these foods into your daily diet, you can support your body's natural defenses, promote cellular health, and maintain vitality as you age.

Beneficial effects: Anti-aging foods offer a myriad of health benefits including enhanced skin health, improved cognitive function, stronger immune system, reduced risk of chronic diseases such as heart disease, diabetes, and cancer, and support for healthy digestion and gut health. These foods work by neutralizing harmful free radicals, reducing inflammation, supporting detoxification processes, and providing essential nutrients that the body needs to function optimally.

Ingredients:

- Berries (blueberries, strawberries, raspberries, blackberries) for their high antioxidant content
- Leafy greens (spinach, kale, Swiss chard) for vitamins A, C, E, and K, calcium, and magnesium
- Nuts and seeds (almonds, walnuts, flaxseeds, chia seeds) for omega-3 fatty acids, protein, and fiber
- Fatty fish (salmon, mackerel, sardines) for omega-3 fatty acids and vitamin D
- Whole grains (quinoa, barley, oats) for fiber and B vitamins
- Green tea for catechins, powerful antioxidants
- Tomatoes for lycopene, a potent antioxidant
- Olive oil for monounsaturated fats and polyphenols
- Dark chocolate (at least 70% cocoa) for flavonoids
- Turmeric for curcumin, which has anti-inflammatory properties

Instructions:

1. Start your day with a breakfast of oatmeal topped with berries and a sprinkle of chia seeds for a nutrient-rich start.

2. Incorporate leafy greens into your meals by adding spinach to smoothies, kale to salads, or Swiss chard to soups and stews.

3. Snack on a handful of nuts or seeds to boost your intake of healthy fats and antioxidants.

4. Include fatty fish in your diet at least twice a week to benefit from omega-3 fatty acids and vitamin D.

5. Swap refined grains for whole grains to increase your fiber intake and support healthy digestion.

6. Drink green tea daily to take advantage of its antioxidant properties.

7. Use olive oil as your primary cooking oil and in dressings to benefit from healthy fats and antioxidants.

8. Enjoy a small piece of dark chocolate as a treat to satisfy your sweet tooth and boost your flavonoid intake.

9. Add turmeric to your cooking or enjoy it as a tea to take advantage of its anti-inflammatory benefits.

Variations:

- Experiment with different berries and leafy greens to keep your meals interesting and varied.
- Try various nuts and seeds as toppings for salads, yogurts, or baked goods.
- Explore different ways to prepare fatty fish, such as grilling, baking, or in fish tacos.
- Use whole grains in place of refined grains in recipes for an extra nutrient boost.

Storage tips:

- Store berries in the refrigerator and consume them within a few days for optimal freshness.

- Keep leafy greens in a produce bag in the crisper drawer of your refrigerator to maintain freshness.

- Store nuts and seeds in airtight containers in a cool, dry place or in the refrigerator to extend their shelf life.

- Olive oil should be stored in a cool, dark place to preserve its quality.

Tips for allergens:

- For those with nut allergies, focus on seeds as a source of healthy fats and nutrients.

- If you are allergic to fish, consider algae-based omega-3 supplements as an alternative.

Scientific references:

- Studies have shown that diets rich in antioxidants and omega-3 fatty acids can reduce the risk of chronic diseases and support healthy aging. For example, research published in the Journal of Agricultural and Food Chemistry highlights the antioxidant capacity of berries.

- The anti-inflammatory effects of turmeric and its active compound curcumin have been documented in numerous studies, including those published in the journal Foods.

Incorporating these anti-aging foods into your diet can help you maintain vitality and health as you age, supporting your body's natural processes and helping to prevent the onset of chronic diseases.

WEIGHT MANAGEMENT TIPS FOR OLDER ADULTS

Weight management becomes increasingly important as we age, with metabolism slowing down and the risk of chronic diseases rising. For older adults, maintaining a healthy weight is crucial for mobility, independence, and overall health. A balanced diet rich in nutrients, combined with regular physical activity, forms the cornerstone of effective weight management in later years.

Firstly, focusing on nutrient-dense foods that provide vitamins, minerals, and fiber without too many calories is essential. Incorporate a variety of fruits and vegetables into your diet; these are high in fiber and water content, which can help you feel full and satisfied without overeating. Opt for whole grains over refined grains to increase your intake of fiber and keep your digestive system running smoothly.

Protein is particularly important for older adults, as it helps maintain muscle mass, which naturally declines with age. Including lean sources of protein such as chicken, fish, beans, and legumes in your meals can support muscle health and metabolism.

However, it's important to watch portion sizes, even with healthy foods, to avoid consuming more calories than your body needs.

Hydration plays a key role in weight management. Sometimes, thirst is mistaken for hunger, leading to unnecessary snacking. Drinking water throughout the day can help manage hunger and aid in digestion. Aim for at least eight glasses of water a day, and remember that fruits and vegetables also contribute to your hydration needs.

Regular physical activity is equally important for managing weight. Activities such as walking, swimming, or yoga can help burn calories, improve cardiovascular health, and increase muscle mass, which in turn boosts metabolism. It's important to find an activity you enjoy so that it becomes a regular part of your routine. Even simple changes like taking the stairs instead of the elevator or gardening can add up to significant calorie burn over time.

Mindful eating practices can also aid in weight management. Eating slowly and without distractions allows you to better recognize your body's hunger and fullness signals, preventing overeating. Try to make meals a focused, enjoyable experience rather than rushing through them or eating while distracted by the TV or computer.

Finally, it's important to consult with a healthcare provider before starting any new diet or exercise program, especially for older adults with existing health conditions.

A healthcare provider can offer personalized advice based on your health status and weight management goals.

By adopting these strategies, older adults can manage their weight effectively, contributing to better health, improved mobility, and a higher quality of life as they age. Remember, the goal is not just about losing weight but maintaining a healthy, balanced lifestyle that supports your overall well-being.

CHAPTER 3: NATURAL APPROACHES TO AGING GRACEFULLY

Embracing natural approaches to aging gracefully involves integrating holistic practices that nourish the body, mind, and spirit, fostering a sense of well-being and vitality that transcends the years. These methods are grounded in the principle that our lifestyle choices, including diet, physical activity, and mental health strategies, play a pivotal role in how we age. By adopting a lifestyle that supports our biological systems, we can enhance our body's resilience against the natural aging process, promoting longevity and a higher quality of life.

Beneficial effects: Natural approaches to aging gracefully aim to reduce the risk of chronic diseases, maintain cognitive function, support emotional health, and preserve physical strength and flexibility. These practices encourage the body's inherent healing capabilities and support its ability to regenerate and repair, leading to a more vibrant, energetic, and fulfilling older age.

Ingredients:

- A diet rich in anti-inflammatory foods such as leafy greens, berries, nuts, seeds, and fatty fish

- Regular consumption of antioxidant-rich herbs and spices like turmeric, ginger, and cinnamon

- Adequate hydration through water, herbal teas, and hydrating foods

- A balanced intake of whole grains, lean proteins, and healthy fats to support overall health

Instructions:

1. Incorporate a variety of colorful fruits and vegetables into your daily diet to ensure a broad spectrum of vitamins, minerals, and antioxidants that combat oxidative stress and inflammation.

2. Include omega-3 fatty acids in your diet by eating fatty fish like salmon, mackerel, and sardines, or by taking a high-quality supplement to support brain health and reduce inflammation.

3. Stay hydrated by drinking at least eight glasses of water a day, supplemented with herbal teas like green tea, which offers additional antioxidant benefits.

4. Engage in regular physical activity that you enjoy, such as walking, yoga, swimming, or cycling, aiming for at least 30 minutes most days of the week. Exercise supports heart health, maintains muscle mass, and promotes flexibility and balance.

5. Practice stress-reduction techniques such as meditation, deep breathing exercises, or tai chi. Managing stress is crucial for preventing chronic inflammation and supporting mental health.

6. Prioritize sleep by establishing a regular sleep schedule and creating a restful environment. Adequate sleep is essential for cellular repair, cognitive function, and emotional well-being.

7. Foster social connections and engage in activities that bring you joy and fulfillment. A strong social network and a sense of purpose are linked to better health and longevity.

8. Consider incorporating herbal supplements known for their anti-aging properties, such as ginkgo biloba for cognitive health, milk thistle for liver support, and hawthorn berry for heart health. Consult with a healthcare provider to determine the right supplements for your needs.

Variations:

- Experiment with different types of physical activity to find what you enjoy and what fits your lifestyle and fitness level.

- Try various herbal teas to discover your preferences and benefit from their diverse health-promoting properties.

- Incorporate mindfulness or gratitude practices into your daily routine to enhance emotional well-being.

Storage tips:

- Store fresh produce in the refrigerator to maintain freshness and nutrient content.

- Keep dried herbs and spices in a cool, dark place to preserve their potency.

Tips for allergens:

- For those with dietary restrictions or allergies, seek out alternative nutrient sources or supplements that meet your needs without triggering adverse reactions.

- Always consult with a healthcare provider before introducing new supplements, especially if you have allergies or are taking medication.

Scientific references:

- Research supports the benefits of a Mediterranean diet, rich in fruits, vegetables, nuts, seeds, and omega-3 fatty acids, for aging healthily (Journal of Nutrition, Health & Aging).

- Studies highlight the importance of physical activity in reducing the risk of chronic diseases and improving quality of life in older adults (American Journal of Preventive Medicine).

- The positive impact of stress management on aging and chronic disease risk is well-documented, emphasizing the role of mindfulness, meditation, and social support (Psychoneuroendocrinology).

By integrating these natural approaches into your lifestyle, you can support your body's aging process gracefully, maintaining vitality, health, and happiness in the later years.

HERBAL SUPPLEMENTS FOR LONGEVITY

Herbal supplements for longevity harness the power of nature to support the body's resilience against the aging process, offering a natural approach to enhancing vitality and promoting a longer, healthier life. These supplements, rich in antioxidants, anti-inflammatory agents, and nutrients, can aid in reducing the risk of chronic diseases, improving cognitive function, and maintaining physical strength and flexibility. By integrating these herbal supplements into a balanced lifestyle, individuals can support their body's natural defenses and promote overall well-being as they age.

Beneficial effects: Herbal supplements for longevity are designed to support various aspects of health crucial for aging gracefully. These include enhancing cognitive function, supporting cardiovascular health, improving digestive wellness, boosting the immune system, and promoting healthy skin. By addressing common concerns associated with aging, such as memory decline, inflammation, digestive issues, weakened immunity, and skin elasticity, these supplements can help individuals maintain a higher quality of life throughout their later years.

Ingredients:

- Ashwagandha (Withania somnifera) (300 mg daily)

- Rhodiola Rosea (100 mg daily)

- Reishi Mushroom (Ganoderma lucidum) (500 mg daily)

- Turmeric (Curcuma longa) (1000 mg daily, standardized to contain 95% curcuminoids)

- Ginkgo Biloba (120 mg daily)
- Milk Thistle (Silybum marianum) (150 mg daily, standardized to contain 80% silymarin)
- Holy Basil (Ocimum sanctum) (500 mg daily)

Instructions:

1. Begin with Ashwagandha by taking a 300 mg capsule daily, preferably with meals. This adaptogen helps combat stress and fatigue, both of which can accelerate aging.

2. Add Rhodiola Rosea to your regimen with a 100 mg capsule daily. Rhodiola is known for its ability to enhance energy, stamina, and mental capacity.

3. Incorporate Reishi Mushroom by taking a 500 mg capsule daily. Reishi supports immune function and has been linked to longevity.

4. Consume Turmeric by taking a 1000 mg capsule daily. Turmeric's curcumin content offers potent anti-inflammatory and antioxidant benefits, crucial for combating the effects of aging.

5. Take Ginkgo Biloba, 120 mg daily, to support cognitive health and improve circulation.

6. Include Milk Thistle in your daily supplements by taking a 150 mg capsule. Milk Thistle supports liver health, essential for detoxification and overall vitality.

7. Add Holy Basil by taking a 500 mg capsule daily. Holy Basil is an adaptogen that helps reduce stress and inflammation, supporting overall well-being.

Variations:

- Consider incorporating these supplements into your diet in various forms, such as teas, tinctures, or whole food sources, depending on availability and personal preference.

- Adjust dosages based on individual health needs and in consultation with a healthcare provider, especially if managing chronic conditions or taking prescription medications.

Storage tips:

- Store capsules and supplements in a cool, dry place, away from direct sunlight. Ensure containers are tightly sealed to maintain potency.

- For fresh herbs or whole food sources, follow appropriate storage guidelines to maintain freshness and nutritional value.

Tips for allergens:

- If allergic to any of the herbs listed, seek alternative options that provide similar health benefits. Consult with a healthcare provider before introducing new supplements, especially if you have known allergies.

- For those who prefer not to take capsules, explore teas or tinctures as alternative methods of consumption that may be more suitable.

Scientific references:

- Research on Ashwagandha, published in the Indian Journal of Psychological Medicine, highlights its stress-reducing effects.

- Studies on Rhodiola Rosea, as reviewed in the Phytomedicine journal, demonstrate its efficacy in enhancing physical and mental performance.

- The Journal of Ethnopharmacology discusses Reishi Mushroom's immune-boosting and longevity-promoting properties.

- Turmeric's anti-inflammatory and antioxidant benefits are well-documented in the Journal of Medicinal Food.

- Ginkgo Biloba's impact on cognitive health and circulation is supported by research in the Journal of the American Medical Association.

- Milk Thistle's role in liver health is outlined in the World Journal of Hepatology.

- Holy Basil's stress-reduction and anti-inflammatory effects are discussed in the Journal of Ayurveda and Integrative Medicine.

By embracing these herbal supplements, individuals can support their journey towards aging gracefully, ensuring that their later years are filled with vitality, health, and joy.

HERBAL SUPPORT FOR JOINT PAIN AND FLEXIBILITY

Beneficial effects: Herbal support for joint pain and flexibility aims to reduce inflammation, alleviate pain, and enhance joint mobility.

These natural remedies can offer a complementary approach to managing joint health, potentially reducing the reliance on pharmaceutical pain relievers and improving the quality of life for individuals experiencing joint discomfort.

By incorporating specific herbs known for their anti-inflammatory and analgesic properties, individuals may experience improved joint function, reduced stiffness, and enhanced overall mobility.

Ingredients:

- Turmeric (Curcuma longa) (1,000 mg daily, standardized to contain 95% curcuminoids)

- Ginger (Zingiber officinale) (500 mg daily)

- Boswellia Serrata (400 mg daily)

- Devil's Claw (Harpagophytum procumbens) (600 mg daily)

- Willow Bark (Salix alba) (240 mg daily)

Instructions:

1. Start your regimen with Turmeric by taking a 1,000 mg capsule daily. Turmeric is renowned for its curcumin content, which possesses potent anti-inflammatory properties that can help reduce joint pain and swelling.

2. Add Ginger to your daily intake by consuming a 500 mg capsule. Ginger works synergistically with turmeric to offer additional anti-inflammatory and analgesic benefits, aiding in the relief of joint discomfort.

3. Incorporate Boswellia Serrata by taking a 400 mg capsule daily. Boswellia has been shown to improve joint function and mobility by reducing inflammation and preventing the breakdown of cartilage.

4. Take Devil's Claw with a dosage of 600 mg daily. This herb is particularly noted for its effectiveness in treating pain and inflammation associated with arthritis and other joint conditions.

5. Conclude your herbal regimen with Willow Bark by taking a 240 mg capsule daily. Willow Bark acts as a natural aspirin, providing relief from pain and inflammation without the gastrointestinal side effects often associated with synthetic pain relievers.

Variations:

- For those who prefer not to take capsules, these herbs are also available in tea forms, tinctures, or as whole herbs that can be used to make decoctions. Adjust the form and dosage according to personal preference and tolerance, under the guidance of a healthcare provider.

- Combine these herbs with a healthy diet rich in omega-3 fatty acids and antioxidants for synergistic effects on reducing inflammation and supporting joint health.

Storage tips:

- Store all capsules and supplements in a cool, dry place, away from direct sunlight and moisture to preserve their potency.

- For fresh herbs or whole food sources, follow appropriate storage guidelines to maintain freshness and nutritional value.

Tips for allergens:

- Individuals allergic to any of the herbal components should seek alternative herbs that provide similar benefits without triggering an allergic response. For example, if allergic to salicylates found in Willow Bark, focus on the other herbs mentioned.

- Always check supplement labels for potential allergens and discuss with a healthcare provider before starting any new supplement, especially if you have a history of allergies.

Scientific references:

- Clinical trials have demonstrated the efficacy of Turmeric and its active compound curcumin in reducing joint pain and inflammation, as documented in the Journal of Medicinal Food.

- Research published in the Journal of Pain highlights Ginger's role in alleviating muscle and joint pain through its anti-inflammatory properties.

- Studies on Boswellia Serrata, as reviewed in the Indian Journal of Pharmaceutical Sciences, show its potential in treating osteoarthritis and rheumatoid arthritis by improving joint function.

- Devil's Claw has been studied for its use in pain management for arthritis, with findings published in the Journal of Ethnopharmacology indicating significant pain relief and improved joint mobility.

- The analgesic effects of Willow Bark have been validated in research published in the American Journal of Medicine, showcasing its benefits in treating lower back pain and osteoarthritis.

By integrating these herbal supports into your daily routine, you may find natural relief from joint pain and improvements in flexibility, contributing to a more active and comfortable lifestyle. Always consult with a healthcare provider before starting any new supplement regimen to ensure it's appropriate for your individual health needs.

COGNITIVE ENHANCEMENT WITH HERBS

Beneficial effects: Enhancing cognitive function and slowing down the mental aging process are crucial for maintaining a sharp mind and a high quality of life as we age. Certain herbs have been identified for their potent neuroprotective properties, including improving memory, focus, and overall brain health. These natural remedies can support cognitive enhancement by increasing blood flow to the brain, reducing inflammation, and providing antioxidants that protect brain cells from damage.

Ingredients:

- Ginkgo Biloba (120 mg daily)

- Bacopa Monnieri (300 mg daily)

- Lion's Mane Mushroom (500 mg daily)

- Rosemary (Rosmarinus officinalis) (leaf extract, dosage varies)

- Ashwagandha (Withania somnifera) (300 mg daily)

- Turmeric (Curcuma longa) (1000 mg daily, standardized to contain 95% curcuminoids)

- Sage (Salvia officinalis) (leaf extract, dosage varies)

Instructions:

1. Begin with Ginkgo Biloba by taking a 120 mg capsule daily. Ginkgo is renowned for its ability to improve blood flow to the brain and enhance cognitive functions such as focus, memory, and processing speed.

2. Add Bacopa Monnieri to your regimen with a 300 mg capsule daily. Bacopa has been traditionally used to improve memory and cognitive processing, making it a valuable herb for cognitive enhancement.

3. Incorporate Lion's Mane Mushroom by taking a 500 mg capsule daily. This unique mushroom supports nerve growth factor (NGF) production, which is essential for brain health and cognitive function.

4. Use Rosemary leaf extract as directed on the product label. Rosemary has been shown to improve memory and alertness, possibly due to its antioxidant properties and its ability to enhance cerebral blood flow.

5. Take Ashwagandha with a dosage of 300 mg daily. This adaptogen helps reduce stress and anxiety, which can negatively impact cognitive function, while also supporting overall brain health.

6. Consume Turmeric by taking a 1000 mg capsule daily. Turmeric and its active component, curcumin, offer powerful anti-inflammatory and antioxidant benefits, protecting the brain from oxidative stress and promoting cognitive health.

7. Add Sage leaf extract to your daily intake as directed on the product label. Sage has been associated with improved memory, attention, and cognitive protection, likely due to its antioxidant and anti-inflammatory effects.

Variations:

- These herbs can also be consumed as teas or tinctures for those who prefer not to take capsules. Adjust the form and dosage according to personal preference, availability, and tolerance.

- Combine these herbs with a diet rich in omega-3 fatty acids, antioxidants, and other brain-healthy nutrients for synergistic effects on cognitive enhancement.

Storage tips:

- Store capsules and supplements in a cool, dry place, away from direct sunlight to preserve their potency.

- For fresh herbs or whole food sources, follow appropriate storage guidelines to maintain freshness and nutritional value.

Tips for allergens:

- Individuals allergic to any of the herbal components should seek alternative herbs that provide similar benefits without triggering an allergic response. Consult with a healthcare provider before introducing new supplements, especially if you have known allergies.

- For those with sensitivities to specific herbs, consider focusing on the other recommended herbs or exploring additional cognitive-enhancing foods and supplements that may be more suitable.

Scientific references:

- Research on Ginkgo Biloba, as published in the Journal of the American Medical Association, supports its use in enhancing cognitive function.

- Studies on Bacopa Monnieri, documented in the Journal of Ethnopharmacology, highlight its efficacy in improving memory and cognitive processing.

- The Journal of Agricultural and Food Chemistry discusses Lion's Mane Mushroom's potential in supporting brain health through NGF production.

- Research on the cognitive benefits of Rosemary and Sage can be found in the International Journal of Neuroscience and the Journal of Pharmacology, respectively, showcasing their memory-enhancing and cognitive-protective properties.

- The anti-inflammatory and antioxidant effects of Turmeric and its role in cognitive health are well-documented in the Journal of Medicinal Food.

- Ashwagandha's stress-reducing and neuroprotective benefits are outlined in the Journal of Dietary Supplements.

By incorporating these herbal remedies into your daily routine, you may experience enhanced cognitive function, improved memory and focus, and a stronger defense against the cognitive decline associated with aging. Always consult with a healthcare provider before starting any new supplement regimen to ensure it's appropriate for your individual health needs.

CHAPTER 4: 5 HERBAL RECIPES FOR AGING WELL

GINKGO BILOBA TEA

Beneficial effects

Ginkgo Biloba Tea is renowned for its ability to enhance cognitive function, improve blood circulation, and support overall brain health. It contains powerful antioxidants that protect the cells from oxidative damage and improve blood flow to various parts of the body, including the brain. This can lead to improved memory, focus, and reduced risk of cognitive decline associated with aging. Additionally, Ginkgo Biloba has been shown to alleviate symptoms of anxiety and depression, making it a holistic remedy for promoting mental well-being.

Portions

2 servings

Preparation time

5 minutes

Cooking time

10 minutes

Ingredients

- 2 teaspoons of dried Ginkgo Biloba leaves

- 2 cups of boiling water

- Honey or lemon (optional, for taste)

Instructions

1. Place the dried Ginkgo Biloba leaves in a tea infuser or directly into a heat-resistant teapot.

2. Pour 2 cups of boiling water over the Ginkgo Biloba leaves.

3. Cover and allow the tea to steep for about 10 minutes. The longer it steeps, the stronger the flavor and potential benefits.

4. Remove the tea infuser or strain the tea to remove the leaves.

5. Optional: Add honey or a slice of lemon to enhance the flavor.

6. Serve the tea warm, ideally in the morning or early afternoon to support cognitive function throughout the day.

Variations

- For an added boost of antioxidants, mix in a teaspoon of green tea leaves during the steeping process.

- Combine with peppermint leaves for a refreshing taste and additional mental clarity benefits.

- To create a soothing nighttime blend, add chamomile flowers to the infusion, which can help promote relaxation and sleep.

Storage tips

Store any leftover Ginkgo Biloba Tea in a sealed container in the refrigerator for up to 2 days. Enjoy it chilled or gently reheat on the stove.

Tips for allergens

Individuals with allergies to plants in the Ginkgoaceae family should proceed with caution when trying Ginkgo Biloba Tea for the first time. For those avoiding honey, maple syrup can be used as a vegan-friendly sweetener.

Scientific references

- "Ginkgo biloba for cognitive impairment and dementia." Cochrane Database of Systematic Reviews, 2009. This review highlights the potential of Ginkgo Biloba in improving cognitive function and reducing symptoms of dementia.

- "The efficacy of Ginkgo biloba on cognitive function in Alzheimer disease." The American Journal of Medicine, 1998. This study supports the use of Ginkgo Biloba in enhancing memory and cognitive performance in individuals with Alzheimer's disease.

HAWTHORN BERRY ELIXIR

Beneficial effects

Hawthorn Berry Elixir is renowned for its cardiovascular benefits, particularly in supporting heart health and improving circulation. This elixir can help regulate blood pressure, reduce symptoms of heart failure, and enhance overall cardiovascular function. Its rich antioxidant content also contributes to reducing oxidative stress and inflammation in the body, offering a natural way to support aging gracefully.

Portions

4 servings

Preparation time

15 minutes

Cooking time

24 hours for infusion

Ingredients

- 1 cup dried hawthorn berries
- 4 cups vodka or brandy
- 1/4 cup raw honey (optional, for sweetness)
- 2 cinnamon sticks (optional, for flavor)

Instructions

1. Place the dried hawthorn berries in a clean, dry jar.

2. Add the vodka or brandy, ensuring the berries are completely submerged.

3. If using, add the raw honey and cinnamon sticks to the jar for added sweetness and flavor.

4. Seal the jar tightly with a lid and shake gently to mix the ingredients.

5. Store the jar in a cool, dark place for 4 weeks, shaking it gently every few days to promote infusion.

6. After 4 weeks, strain the elixir through a fine mesh sieve or cheesecloth into a clean bottle, discarding the berries and cinnamon sticks.

7. Label the bottle with the date and contents.

Variations

- For a non-alcoholic version, replace vodka or brandy with apple cider vinegar, allowing an additional 2 weeks for infusion.

- Add orange peel or vanilla bean to the infusion for a different flavor profile.

- For a sweeter elixir, increase the amount of raw honey according to taste.

Storage tips

Store the Hawthorn Berry Elixir in a cool, dark place. When stored properly in an airtight container, it can last for up to a year.

Tips for allergens

Individuals with allergies to berries should proceed with caution and may consider consulting with a healthcare provider before consumption. For those avoiding honey due to dietary preferences or allergies, the sweetener can be omitted or substituted with maple syrup.

Scientific references

- "Hawthorn extract for treating chronic heart failure: Meta-analysis of randomized trials." American Journal of Medicine, 2003. This study supports the use of hawthorn extract in improving symptoms and functional outcomes in chronic heart failure.

- "Antioxidant activity of hawthorn berry extract and its effect on cardiovascular system." International Journal of Food Sciences and Nutrition, 2011. This research highlights the antioxidant properties of hawthorn berries and their beneficial effects on the cardiovascular system.

GOTU KOLA TINCTURE

Beneficial effects

Gotu Kola Tincture is celebrated for its remarkable ability to enhance cognitive function, promote wound healing, and support circulatory health. This powerful herbal remedy has been used for centuries in traditional medicine to improve memory, reduce anxiety, and increase mental clarity. Additionally, its anti-inflammatory and antioxidant properties make it an excellent choice for aging gracefully, as it can help to protect the skin from free radical damage and improve the appearance of scars and varicose veins.

Ingredients

- 1 cup fresh Gotu Kola leaves, finely chopped
- 2 cups 100-proof alcohol (vodka or brandy)

Instructions

1. Place the finely chopped Gotu Kola leaves into a clean, dry jar.

2. Pour the alcohol over the leaves, ensuring they are completely submerged. Leave about an inch of space at the top of the jar.

3. Seal the jar tightly with a lid and label it with the date and contents.

4. Store the jar in a cool, dark place for 4 to 6 weeks. Shake the jar gently every few days to mix the contents and promote extraction.

5. After the infusion period, strain the tincture through a fine mesh sieve or cheesecloth into another clean, dark glass bottle. Press or squeeze the leaves to extract as much liquid as possible.

6. Label the bottle with the date and contents.

Variations

- For a non-alcoholic version, replace the alcohol with apple cider vinegar or glycerin, though this may result in a less potent tincture.

- Add a few slices of ginger or turmeric during the infusion process to enhance the tincture's anti-inflammatory properties.

Storage tips

Store the Gotu Kola Tincture in a cool, dark place. When stored properly in an airtight container, it can last for up to 5 years.

Tips for allergens

Individuals with allergies to Gotu Kola should avoid using this tincture. As always, consult with a healthcare provider before starting any new herbal remedy, especially if you are pregnant, nursing, or taking medications.

Scientific references

- "Centella asiatica (Gotu Kola) as a Neuroprotectant and Its Potential Role in Healthy Aging" published in Trends in Food Science & Technology, 2018. This study discusses the neuroprotective effects of Gotu Kola and its potential benefits for cognitive health and aging.

- "Wound Healing and Anti-Inflammatory Effect in Animal Models of Centella asiatica L. Urban" in the International Journal of Lower Extremity Wounds, 2012. This research highlights the wound healing and anti-inflammatory properties of Gotu Kola, supporting its use in topical and internal treatments for aging skin and circulatory health.

SCHISANDRA BERRY SMOOTHIE

Beneficial effects

Schisandra Berry Smoothie is a powerful concoction aimed at enhancing overall vitality and promoting healthy aging. Schisandra berries are renowned for their adaptogenic properties, helping the body resist the effects of stress and boosting energy levels without causing jitteriness. This smoothie can also support liver function, improve mental clarity, and enhance skin health, making it an excellent choice for those looking to age gracefully.

Portions

1 serving

Preparation time

5 minutes

Ingredients

- 1 cup of almond milk

- 1/2 cup of frozen blueberries

- 1 tablespoon of Schisandra berry powder

- 1 ripe banana

- 1 tablespoon of flaxseed meal

- 1 teaspoon of honey (optional)

Instructions

1. Pour the almond milk into a blender.

2. Add the frozen blueberries, Schisandra berry powder, ripe banana, and flaxseed meal to the blender.

3. Blend on high until the mixture is smooth and creamy.

4. Taste the smoothie, and if desired, add honey for sweetness. Blend again briefly to mix.

5. Pour the smoothie into a glass and enjoy immediately.

Variations

- For an extra protein boost, add a scoop of your favorite plant-based protein powder.

- Substitute almond milk with coconut water for a lighter version or with oat milk for a nut-free option.

- Add a handful of spinach or kale for added nutrients without significantly altering the taste.

Storage tips

It's best to consume the Schisandra Berry Smoothie immediately after preparation to enjoy its full benefits. However, if you need to store it, keep the smoothie in an airtight container in the refrigerator for up to 24 hours. Stir well before drinking if separation occurs.

Tips for allergens

For those with nut allergies, ensure to substitute almond milk with a suitable non-nut milk alternative like oat milk or rice milk. If you're vegan or have a honey allergy, substitute honey with maple syrup or omit it altogether.

Scientific references

- "Schisandra chinensis fruit extract mitigates oxidative stress, inflammation, and apoptosis in the brain of rats exposed to lead," published in Evidence-Based Complementary and Alternative Medicine, 2018. This study highlights Schisandra's antioxidant properties and its potential in protecting against oxidative stress and inflammation.

- "An update on the pharmacology of Schisandra chinensis and Schisandra sphenanthera," published in the Journal of Ethnopharmacology, 2019. This review discusses the adaptogenic effects of Schisandra, supporting its use for enhancing mental performance and promoting healthy aging.

HE SHOU WU DECOCTION

Beneficial effects

He Shou Wu Decoction is revered for its remarkable anti-aging properties, supporting longevity and vitality. This traditional Chinese medicine is believed to nourish the blood, liver, and kidneys, enhance stamina, and promote the growth of healthy hair. Its antioxidant components help in protecting cells from damage caused by free radicals, potentially slowing down the aging process. Additionally, He Shou Wu is known for improving fertility and sexual health, as well as providing a boost to the immune system.

Portions

4 servings

Preparation time

10 minutes

Cooking time

2 hours

Ingredients

- 1 cup dried He Shou Wu (Fo-Ti) root

- 8 cups water

- Optional: Honey or lemon slices for flavor

Instructions

1. Rinse the dried He Shou Wu root under cold water to remove any dust or debris.

2. In a large pot, combine the He Shou Wu root with 8 cups of water.

3. Bring the mixture to a boil over high heat, then reduce the heat to low.

4. Cover the pot and simmer gently for 2 hours, checking occasionally to ensure it does not boil dry. Add more water if necessary.

5. After 2 hours, remove the pot from the heat and strain the decoction into a large bowl, discarding the solid pieces of root.

6. If desired, add honey or a slice of lemon to each cup for flavor enhancement.

7. Serve the decoction warm, or allow it to cool and store in the refrigerator for cold consumption.

Variations

- For an added immune boost, include slices of fresh ginger or a few goji berries in the decoction process.

- Combine with green tea during the last 10 minutes of simmering for additional antioxidant benefits.

- For a richer flavor, simmer with a cinnamon stick or a few cloves.

Storage tips

Store any leftover He Shou Wu Decoction in an airtight container in the refrigerator for up to 3 days. Reheat gently on the stove or enjoy cold.

Tips for allergens

Individuals with specific plant allergies should consult with a healthcare provider before consuming He Shou Wu. For those avoiding honey due to dietary restrictions, substitute with maple syrup or simply omit the sweetener.

Scientific references

- "Pharmacological effects of Radix Polygoni Multiflori (He Shou Wu) as related to anti-aging." Journal of Ethnopharmacology, 2017. This study examines the anti-aging and health-promoting effects of He Shou Wu, highlighting its potential in enhancing longevity and vitality.

- "Antioxidant activity of extract from Polygonum multiflorum." Experimental Gerontology, 2002. This research discusses the antioxidant properties of He Shou Wu, supporting its use in protecting against cellular damage and aging.

PART 10: DETOXIFICATION AND CLEANSING

Detoxification and cleansing are integral components of a holistic health approach, emphasizing the body's innate ability to heal and purify itself. In a world where exposure to toxins—be it through the air we breathe, the food we eat, or the products we use—is almost unavoidable, supporting the body's detoxification processes becomes crucial for maintaining optimal health.

This section delves into the natural detox systems within our body, including the liver, kidneys, digestive system, skin, and lungs, each playing a pivotal role in filtering and eliminating toxins.

The liver, often referred to as the body's primary detox organ, metabolizes toxins for elimination. Supporting liver function with herbs such as milk thistle, dandelion root, and turmeric can enhance its detoxifying capabilities.

These herbs are known for their hepatoprotective properties, aiding in the regeneration of liver cells and protecting against harmful toxins.

Kidneys filter our blood, removing waste products and excess substances through urine. Hydration is key to kidney health, and incorporating herbal teas like green tea and hibiscus can provide antioxidant support, aiding in the kidneys' filtering processes.

The digestive system, including the colon, plays a significant role in detoxification by eliminating waste products through bowel movements. A diet rich in fiber from fruits, vegetables, and whole grains supports gut health and regularity, while herbs like psyllium husk and aloe vera can promote healthy bowel movements and cleanse the digestive tract.

Skin, the largest organ of the body, releases toxins through sweat. Regular physical activity, sauna sessions, and dry brushing are effective ways to stimulate sweat production and support skin detoxification. Hydration, again, is essential, ensuring that the body can efficiently produce sweat and maintain skin health.

Lungs are responsible for expelling carbon dioxide, a waste product of metabolism, from the body. Practices like deep breathing, spending time in clean, fresh air, and using eucalyptus or peppermint essential oils can support lung health and enhance the respiratory system's ability to detoxify.

Incorporating these detoxification supports into daily life doesn't require drastic changes but rather small, consistent adjustments to diet and lifestyle.

Starting the day with a glass of warm lemon water can stimulate digestion and liver function, while replacing processed foods with whole, nutrient-dense options supports overall detoxification processes. Regular physical activity boosts circulation and sweat production, aiding in the elimination of toxins through the skin.

Understanding the body's detoxification systems and how to support them through natural means is a powerful step toward achieving and maintaining holistic health.

By fostering the body's natural ability to cleanse itself, we can enhance our resilience against toxins and promote long-term well-being.

Embracing a holistic approach to detoxification also means paying close attention to emotional and mental purification. Just as physical toxins can impair the body's health, negative emotions and stress can accumulate, hindering mental clarity and overall well-being. Techniques such as meditation, journaling, and mindfulness practices serve as mental detox methods, helping to clear the mind of clutter and reduce stress. These practices not only enhance emotional resilience but also support physical detoxification processes by mitigating the adverse effects of stress on the body's natural detox systems.

Sleep plays a crucial role in the body's natural detoxification cycle, particularly for the brain. During sleep, the brain's cleansing process, known as the glymphatic system, becomes active, removing waste products that accumulate throughout the day.

Ensuring adequate and quality sleep is essential for supporting this process, highlighting the importance of a restful environment and a consistent sleep schedule.

Dietary supplements can also play a supportive role in detoxification. Antioxidants such as vitamins C and E, selenium, and beta-carotene help protect the body against oxidative stress and aid in the neutralization of harmful toxins. Similarly, omega-3 fatty acids, found in fish oil and flaxseed oil, contribute to reducing inflammation, which can result from the body's detoxification efforts against toxins.

In addition to these practices, seasonal detoxification rituals can align the body's natural cleansing processes with the rhythms of nature.

For instance, spring and fall are traditionally seen as ideal times for detoxification. During these seasons, focusing on foods that naturally support detoxification, such as leafy greens, berries, and herbs, can enhance the body's ability to purge toxins. Seasonal fasting or cleansing diets, under the guidance of a healthcare professional, can also provide an opportunity to reset the digestive system and promote the elimination of toxins.

Finally, fostering a supportive community and environment plays a pivotal role in holistic detoxification. Surrounding oneself with positive influences and reducing exposure to toxic substances in personal care products, household cleaners, and the environment contributes to minimizing the overall toxic load on the body. Engaging in community activities, connecting with nature, and cultivating relationships that encourage healthy living can reinforce detoxification efforts and promote a balanced, healthy lifestyle.

By integrating these holistic practices into daily life, detoxification becomes a comprehensive, ongoing process that supports the body's natural abilities to heal and maintain optimal health. Recognizing the interconnectedness of physical, emotional, and environmental health is key to a successful detoxification strategy, paving the way for a vibrant, healthful life.

CHAPTER 1: THE IMPORTANCE OF DETOXIFICATION

Detoxification is a fundamental aspect of maintaining a healthy body and mind, acting as a natural reset button for our system. It involves the elimination of toxins from the body, enhancing the body's own cleansing systems to function more efficiently. This process is not only about removing harmful substances but also about nourishing the body with the right nutrients to support its innate ability to heal. The importance of detoxification lies in its ability to boost overall health, improve digestion, enhance energy levels, and support the immune system.

Our bodies are exposed to an array of toxins daily, from environmental pollutants and chemicals in our food and water to stress and negative emotions that impact our physical well-being. These toxins can accumulate over time, leading to a burden on our detoxification organs, such as the liver, kidneys, and colon. When these organs are overloaded, they can become less efficient, leading to various health issues, including fatigue, digestive problems, skin issues, and chronic diseases. By supporting these organs through detoxification, we can help prevent these issues and promote a more vibrant state of health.

Detoxification is not a one-time event but a continuous process that involves making lifestyle and dietary changes to support the body's natural detox pathways. This includes consuming a diet rich in whole, unprocessed foods that are high in fiber, antioxidants, vitamins, and minerals. Foods such as leafy greens, berries, nuts, seeds, and herbs like milk thistle, dandelion, and turmeric are particularly beneficial for supporting detoxification.

These foods provide the necessary nutrients to support the liver and other detox organs, helping to enhance their function and promote the elimination of toxins.

In addition to dietary changes, incorporating regular physical activity, adequate hydration, and practices that reduce stress, such as meditation and yoga, can further support the body's detoxification processes. Exercise, for example, promotes circulation and sweating, two key mechanisms for removing toxins from the body. Hydration is crucial for facilitating the elimination of waste through urine and sweat, while stress-reduction techniques can help mitigate the harmful effects of stress on the body, including its impact on detoxification.

Detoxification also involves minimizing exposure to toxins by choosing organic foods when possible, using natural cleaning and personal care products, and avoiding the use of plastic containers that can leach chemicals into food and drinks.

By taking these steps, we can reduce the overall toxic burden on our bodies and support our health and well-being.

The benefits of detoxification are manifold, including improved energy levels, better digestion, clearer skin, weight loss, and a reduced risk of chronic diseases. By supporting the body's natural detoxification systems, we can enhance our body's resilience, promote longevity, and achieve a higher quality of life.

It's important to approach detoxification as a holistic practice, integrating dietary, lifestyle, and emotional wellness strategies. This comprehensive approach ensures that we not only remove toxins from our bodies but also nourish our minds and spirits, leading to a more balanced and healthful life. As we embrace detoxification as a key component of a holistic health approach, we empower ourselves to take control of our health and well-being, paving the way for a vibrant, thriving life.

CHAPTER 2: FOODS THAT SUPPORT DETOX

Foods that support detoxification play a pivotal role in enhancing the body's natural ability to cleanse and rejuvenate itself. Incorporating these foods into your diet can significantly impact your overall health, aiding in the elimination of toxins and supporting the function of vital organs such as the liver, kidneys, and digestive system.

Among the most effective detox-supporting foods are leafy greens, cruciferous vegetables, berries, herbs, and spices, each offering unique benefits and nutritional components that facilitate the detox process.

Leafy greens, including spinach, kale, and Swiss chard, are rich in chlorophyll, which aids in purifying the blood and removing toxins from the body. These greens are also high in vitamins A, C, and K, which support the liver and enhance its detoxification capabilities. Incorporating a variety of leafy greens into your diet can be as simple as adding them to smoothies, salads, or sautéed dishes.

Cruciferous vegetables like broccoli, cauliflower, and Brussels sprouts contain glucosinolates, compounds that help in detoxification by supporting enzyme production in the liver. These vegetables also provide a rich source of fiber, which is essential for healthy digestion and the elimination of toxins through the digestive tract. Roasting, steaming, or stir-frying these vegetables can make them a delicious part of your detox diet.

Berries, such as blueberries, raspberries, and strawberries, are high in antioxidants and vitamins that protect the body against oxidative stress and support the liver in processing and eliminating toxins.

Their high fiber content also promotes healthy bowel movements, further aiding in detoxification.

Enjoying berries as a snack, in smoothies, or as a topping for oatmeal or yogurt can easily increase your intake of these detox-friendly fruits.

Herbs and spices, including cilantro, turmeric, and ginger, offer powerful detoxification benefits. Cilantro helps in removing heavy metals from the body, while turmeric supports liver health through its anti-inflammatory and antioxidant properties.

Ginger aids in digestion and can help soothe the digestive tract. Incorporating these herbs and spices into your cooking not only adds flavor but also enhances the detoxifying effects of your meals.

In addition to these foods, it's important to maintain adequate hydration. Water plays a crucial role in the detox process by helping to flush toxins out of the body through urine and sweat.

Adding lemon to your water can further support liver function and digestion, making it a simple yet effective way to boost your detox efforts.

By focusing on a diet rich in these detox-supporting foods, you can enhance your body's natural detoxification processes, leading to improved health and well-being.

Remember, the key to effective detoxification is consistency and variety, ensuring that you consume a wide range of nutrients that support the body's cleansing systems.

CHAPTER 3: NATURAL DETOX PRACTICES

Detoxification is a holistic practice that goes beyond diet alone, encompassing a range of natural practices designed to purify the body and mind. Engaging in regular physical activity is one of the most effective ways to support the body's detoxification process. Exercise increases blood circulation and promotes sweating, thereby facilitating the elimination of toxins through the skin. Aim for at least 30 minutes of moderate exercise most days of the week, incorporating activities such as walking, cycling, swimming, or yoga to keep the routine enjoyable and sustainable.

Dry brushing is another beneficial detox practice, which involves using a dry brush with natural bristles to gently brush the skin in a circular motion towards the heart. This not only exfoliates the skin, removing dead skin cells and enabling the skin to detoxify more efficiently, but also stimulates the lymphatic system, which plays a key role in eliminating toxins from the body. Dry brushing can be done daily before showering for optimal benefits.

Hydration is crucial for detoxification, as water aids in the removal of waste products from the body through urine and sweat. Drinking adequate amounts of water throughout the day helps to ensure that the kidneys can effectively filter toxins.

To enhance the detoxifying effects of water, consider adding slices of lemon, cucumber, or herbs such as mint or ginger, which can provide additional antioxidant and digestive benefits.

Deep breathing exercises also support the body's natural detoxification processes, particularly those of the respiratory system. By taking deep, slow breaths, you can help the lungs to fully expand and contract, facilitating the expulsion of carbon dioxide and other waste gases.

Practice deep breathing for a few minutes each day, ideally in a calm, outdoor setting where the air is fresh and clean.

Incorporating sauna sessions into your detoxification routine can further promote the elimination of toxins through sweating. The heat from a sauna increases circulation and induces sweating, helping to release toxins stored in the body. Ensure to stay hydrated before and after sauna sessions to replenish fluids lost through sweat.

Sleep is another fundamental aspect of the body's natural detoxification process, particularly for the brain. During sleep, the brain's glymphatic system becomes active, clearing out waste products that have accumulated during the day.

Prioritizing 7-9 hours of quality sleep each night supports this process and promotes overall health and well-being.

Finally, engaging in mindfulness practices such as meditation and journaling can aid in the detoxification of the mind by reducing stress and clearing mental clutter. Chronic stress can have a detrimental impact on physical health, including the body's ability to detoxify. By dedicating time to relaxation and stress-reduction techniques, you can support holistic detoxification and enhance your mental and emotional resilience.

By integrating these natural detox practices into your daily routine, you can support your body's innate detoxification systems, promoting health, vitality, and well-being. Remember, the key to effective detoxification is consistency and a holistic approach, addressing both physical and mental aspects of health.

CHAPTER 4: 5 HERBAL RECIPES FOR DETOXIFICATION

DANDELION AND BURDOCK ROOT DETOX TEA

Beneficial effects

Dandelion and Burdock Root Detox Tea harnesses the natural detoxifying properties of both herbs to support liver function, cleanse the blood, and promote a healthy digestive system. Dandelion root acts as a powerful diuretic, helping to eliminate toxins from the body, while burdock root is known for its blood purifying properties and its ability to remove heavy metals. Together, they create a potent detox tea that can help improve skin health, reduce inflammation, and boost overall vitality.

Portions

2 servings

Preparation time

10 minutes

Cooking time

15 minutes

Ingredients

- 1 tablespoon dried dandelion root

- 1 tablespoon dried burdock root

- 4 cups of water

- Honey or lemon (optional, for taste)

Instructions

1. Combine the dried dandelion and burdock roots in a medium-sized pot.

2. Add 4 cups of water to the pot and bring the mixture to a boil.

3. Once boiling, reduce the heat and simmer for about 15 minutes to allow the roots to steep and their beneficial properties to be released into the water.

4. After simmering, strain the tea into cups or a large container, discarding the used roots.

5. If desired, add honey or lemon to taste for flavor enhancement.

6. Serve the tea warm, or allow it to cool and enjoy as a refreshing cold beverage.

Variations

- For an added detox boost, include a slice of fresh ginger or a teaspoon of turmeric powder while simmering the tea.

- Mix in a cinnamon stick during the simmering process for additional flavor and blood sugar regulation benefits.

- Combine with green tea leaves during the last 5 minutes of simmering for an antioxidant-rich blend.

Storage tips

If you have leftover tea, store it in a sealed container in the refrigerator for up to 2 days. Enjoy it cold, or gently reheat on the stove.

Tips for allergens

Individuals with allergies to dandelion or burdock should avoid this tea. For a honey alternative, maple syrup can be used as a sweetener for those with honey allergies or following a vegan diet.

Scientific references

- "The diuretic effect in human subjects of an extract of Taraxacum officinale folium over a single day" published in the Journal of Alternative and Complementary Medicine highlights the diuretic properties of dandelion.

- "Antioxidant activity and phenolic compounds of traditional Chinese medicinal plants associated with anticancer" in Life Sciences discusses the antioxidant properties of burdock root and its potential health benefits.

PARSLEY AND CILANTRO DETOX SMOOTHIE

Beneficial effects

The Parsley and Cilantro Detox Smoothie is designed to support the body's natural detoxification processes, leveraging the unique properties of its core ingredients. Parsley is rich in vitamins A, C, and K, and has diuretic properties that can help to flush toxins from the body. Cilantro, on the other hand, has been shown to bind to heavy metals, facilitating their removal. Together, these herbs contribute to a cleansing effect, promoting liver health and aiding in the elimination of toxins. Additionally, the inclusion of lemon boosts the vitamin C content, further supporting the immune system and skin health.

Portions

2 servings

Preparation time

10 minutes

Ingredients

- 1 cup fresh parsley, loosely packed
- 1 cup fresh cilantro, loosely packed
- 1 ripe banana
- 1/2 lemon, juiced
- 1 tablespoon chia seeds
- 1 cup coconut water
- 1/2 inch piece of ginger, peeled
- Ice cubes (optional)

Instructions

1. Wash the parsley and cilantro thoroughly to remove any dirt or residue.

2. Peel the banana and ginger, then cut them into small pieces.

3. In a blender, combine the parsley, cilantro, banana, lemon juice, chia seeds, coconut water, and ginger.

4. Add ice cubes if a colder smoothie is preferred.

5. Blend on high until the mixture is smooth and creamy.

6. Taste and adjust the sweetness by adding a bit more lemon juice if desired.

7. Serve immediately for the best flavor and nutrient content.

Variations

- For a sweeter smoothie, add a tablespoon of honey or agave syrup.

- Include a handful of spinach or kale for an extra boost of greens without significantly changing the flavor.

- Substitute coconut water with almond milk for a creamier texture and added calcium.

Storage tips

It's best to consume the smoothie immediately after preparation to maximize the benefits of the fresh ingredients. However, if you need to store it, keep the smoothie in an airtight container in the refrigerator for up to 24 hours. Shake well before consuming if separation occurs.

Tips for allergens

For those with allergies to citrus, omit the lemon juice and consider adding a bit of apple cider vinegar for a similar zesty flavor. If coconut water is a concern, it can be replaced with any non-dairy milk or regular water for hydration without affecting the detoxifying benefits.

Scientific references

- "The effect of parsley (Petroselinum crispum) on the liver's and kidney's detoxification pathways." Phytotherapy Research, 2002. This study highlights parsley's role in supporting liver and kidney function, underscoring its detoxifying properties.

- "Evaluation of the chelating effect of cilantro (Coriandrum sativum L.) extract on lead accumulation in rats." Journal of Toxicology, 2010. The research discusses cilantro's potential to reduce heavy metal accumulation, supporting its use in detoxification diets.

RED CLOVER AND NETTLE DETOX INFUSION

Beneficial effects

Red Clover and Nettle Detox Infusion is a powerful blend designed to support the body's natural detoxification processes. Red clover is known for its blood-purifying properties, helping to remove toxins and waste from the bloodstream, while nettle supports kidney function and increases the elimination of metabolic waste. Together, they form a potent detox duo that can improve skin health, reduce inflammation, and enhance overall vitality.

Portions

2 servings

Preparation time

10 minutes

Cooking time

5 minutes

Ingredients

- 2 teaspoons dried red clover flowers

- 2 teaspoons dried nettle leaves

- 4 cups boiling water

- Honey or lemon (optional, for taste)

Instructions

1. Place the dried red clover flowers and dried nettle leaves into a large tea infuser or directly into a heat-resistant teapot.

2. Pour 4 cups of boiling water over the herbs.

3. Cover and allow the infusion to steep for 5 to 10 minutes, depending on the desired strength.

4. Remove the tea infuser or strain the infusion to remove the herbs.

5. Optional: Add honey or a slice of lemon to enhance the flavor.

6. Serve the infusion warm, or allow it to cool for a refreshing cold beverage.

Variations

- For added detox benefits, include a slice of fresh ginger or turmeric in the infusion process.

- Combine with dandelion leaves or roots for an extra boost in liver support.

- For a sweeter, fruit-infused version, add a handful of fresh or frozen berries to the infusion after straining.

Storage tips

Store any leftover Red Clover and Nettle Detox Infusion in a sealed container in the refrigerator for up to 2 days. Enjoy chilled or gently reheat on the stove.

Tips for allergens

Individuals with allergies to plants in the Fabaceae family (such as red clover) or the Urticaceae family (such as nettle) should proceed with caution and may consider consulting with a healthcare provider before consumption. For those avoiding honey due to dietary restrictions, substitute with maple syrup or simply omit the sweetener.

Scientific references

- "The role of dietary phytoestrogens in the prevention and treatment of breast cancer: A review of their mechanisms of action," published in Nutrients, 2015. This study discusses the beneficial effects of red clover, a source of phytoestrogens, on health.

- "Stinging nettle: Extraordinary vegetable medicine," published in the Journal of Herbal Medicine and Toxicology, 2008. This research highlights the detoxifying properties of nettle, supporting its use in herbal detox infusions.

BENTONITE CLAY AND PSYLLIUM HUSK CLEANSE

Beneficial effects

The Bentonite Clay and Psyllium Husk Cleanse is designed to naturally detoxify the body by absorbing toxins, heavy metals, and impurities from the digestive tract. Bentonite clay acts as a powerful magnet, pulling toxins out of the body, while psyllium husk, rich in soluble fiber, helps to sweep these toxins away by promoting healthy bowel movements. This combination not only cleanses the colon but also supports overall digestive health, reduces bloating, and can aid in weight loss by removing built-up waste.

Ingredients

- 1 tablespoon bentonite clay (food grade)

- 1 teaspoon psyllium husk powder

- 8-10 ounces of water or juice (for mixing)

Instructions

1. In a glass jar, add 8-10 ounces of water or juice.

2. Add 1 tablespoon of bentonite clay to the liquid. Ensure to use a wooden or plastic spoon as bentonite clay should not come into contact with metal.

3. Add 1 teaspoon of psyllium husk powder to the mixture.

4. Secure the lid on the jar and shake well until the ingredients are fully mixed and no clumps remain.

5. Drink the mixture immediately after preparing, as the psyllium husk will begin to thicken quickly.

6. Follow the cleanse with another 8-10 ounces of water to help move the mixture through the digestive system.

Variations

- For added flavor and detoxifying benefits, mix the bentonite clay and psyllium husk with organic apple juice instead of water.

- Incorporate a half teaspoon of activated charcoal into the mixture to enhance the detoxification process.

- Add a squeeze of lemon to the water or juice for a refreshing taste and additional cleansing benefits.

Storage tips

Store bentonite clay and psyllium husk powder in airtight containers in a cool, dry place to maintain their potency and prevent moisture absorption.

Tips for allergens

Individuals with sensitivity to psyllium husk should start with a smaller dose to monitor for any adverse reactions. For those with allergies to any of the ingredients, consult with a healthcare provider before starting the cleanse.

Scientific references

- "Bentonite clay as a natural remedy: a brief review" in the Journal of Molecular Pharmaceutics & Organic Process Research, 2017. This study discusses the detoxifying properties of bentonite clay and its use in removing toxins from the body.

- "The Health Benefits of Psyllium" in the International Journal of Science and Research (IJSR), 2019. This research highlights the role of psyllium husk in promoting digestive health and its effectiveness in cleansing the colon.

ACTIVATED CHARCOAL LEMONADE

Beneficial effects

Activated Charcoal Lemonade is a refreshing and detoxifying beverage that harnesses the cleansing properties of activated charcoal. It's known for its ability to bind to toxins and chemicals in the gut, aiding in their removal from the body. This can help reduce bloating, prevent hangovers, and support overall digestive health. Additionally, the lemon juice in the recipe provides a healthy dose of vitamin C, promoting immune function and skin health.

Portions

2 servings

Preparation time

5 minutes

Ingredients

- 2 tablespoons of activated charcoal powder (from coconut shells)

- Juice of 2 lemons
- 2 tablespoons of organic honey or maple syrup
- 4 cups of filtered water
- Ice cubes (optional)

Instructions

1. In a large pitcher, combine the lemon juice and honey or maple syrup. Stir well until the honey or syrup is fully dissolved in the lemon juice.

2. Add the activated charcoal powder to the pitcher. Stir vigorously to ensure the charcoal is evenly distributed and no clumps remain.

3. Add the filtered water to the pitcher and stir well to combine all the ingredients.

4. Serve the lemonade over ice cubes in glasses, if desired.

Variations

- For a sparkling version, replace half of the filtered water with carbonated water for a fizzy twist.
- Add a pinch of Himalayan pink salt to replenish electrolytes, making it a great post-workout drink.
- Infuse the lemonade with fresh mint leaves or a slice of ginger for additional digestive and flavor benefits.

Storage tips

This Activated Charcoal Lemonade is best enjoyed fresh. However, if you need to store it, keep it in a sealed container in the refrigerator for up to 24 hours. Shake well before serving as the charcoal may settle at the bottom.

Tips for allergens

For those with allergies to honey, maple syrup serves as an excellent vegan alternative. Ensure the activated charcoal used is food-grade and derived from coconut shells to avoid potential allergens found in other types of activated charcoal.

Scientific references

- "Adsorption of Gastrointestinal Toxicants by Activated Charcoal" - American Journal of Emergency Medicine, 1986. This study outlines the effectiveness of activated charcoal in adsorbing toxins, supporting its use in detoxification.

- "Vitamin C in Disease Prevention and Cure: An Overview" - Indian Journal of Clinical Biochemistry, 2013. This article highlights the health benefits of vitamin C, found in lemon juice, including its role in immune function and skin health.

PART 11: HEART HEALTH

Heart health is foundational to overall well-being, with the heart playing a critical role in pumping life-sustaining blood throughout the body. This chapter delves into the importance of maintaining a healthy heart through diet, lifestyle, and natural remedies, emphasizing the interconnectedness of heart health with holistic wellness practices. A heart-healthy lifestyle incorporates a balanced diet rich in fruits, vegetables, whole grains, and lean proteins, alongside regular physical activity and stress management techniques. These elements work synergistically to support cardiovascular function, reduce the risk of heart disease, and promote longevity.

The diet's impact on heart health cannot be overstated. Foods high in omega-3 fatty acids, such as salmon, flaxseeds, and walnuts, are known for their anti-inflammatory properties and ability to reduce blood triglyceride levels, thereby supporting heart health. Antioxidant-rich foods like berries, dark leafy greens, and dark chocolate help combat oxidative stress, which can lead to arterial damage. Incorporating these foods into daily meals can significantly enhance heart function and reduce disease risk factors.

Physical activity is another pillar of heart health, with exercise playing a crucial role in maintaining a healthy weight, lowering blood pressure, and improving cholesterol levels. Engaging in at least 150 minutes of moderate aerobic exercise or 75 minutes of vigorous exercise each week is recommended for adults to reap cardiovascular benefits.

Activities such as brisk walking, cycling, swimming, or jogging not only strengthen the heart muscle but also improve circulation and overall physical fitness.

Stress management is equally important for a healthy heart. Chronic stress can lead to high blood pressure, arterial damage, and an increased risk of heart disease. Techniques such as deep breathing exercises, meditation, yoga, and spending time in nature can help mitigate the effects of stress on the body. These practices not only promote relaxation but also enhance emotional well-being, contributing to a holistic approach to heart health.

Herbal remedies also offer support for heart health, with herbs like hawthorn berry, garlic, and green tea being recognized for their cardiovascular benefits.

Hawthorn berry, for instance, has been traditionally used to improve heart function, enhance blood flow, and reduce symptoms of heart failure. Garlic is known for its ability to lower blood pressure and cholesterol levels, while green tea's antioxidants may help prevent atherosclerosis, a major risk factor for heart disease.

In addition to these practices, maintaining healthy sleep patterns is crucial for heart health. Lack of sleep has been linked to higher risks of heart disease, hypertension, and stroke. Ensuring 7-9 hours of quality sleep each night supports the body's healing processes, including those vital for heart function and repair.

The journey to a healthy heart is multifaceted, involving a combination of diet, exercise, stress management, and natural remedies. By adopting a holistic approach to wellness, individuals can significantly improve their heart health and overall quality of life. This chapter will continue to explore the various aspects of maintaining a healthy heart, offering practical advice and natural solutions to support cardiovascular wellness.

Hydration plays a pivotal role in maintaining heart health, emphasizing the importance of drinking sufficient water to support cardiovascular function.

Adequate hydration aids in maintaining blood volume and pressure, ensuring that the heart can efficiently pump blood throughout the body. It also helps in the prevention of blood clots and the reduction of the risk of heart attacks and strokes. Incorporating water-rich foods like cucumbers, tomatoes, and watermelons into one's diet can further contribute to overall hydration and heart health.

Monitoring and managing blood pressure is critical for heart health. High blood pressure, or hypertension, is a major risk factor for heart disease and stroke. Natural ways to manage blood pressure include reducing sodium intake, increasing potassium-rich foods such as bananas, sweet potatoes, and spinach, and incorporating magnesium and calcium into the diet through nuts, seeds, and leafy greens. These dietary adjustments, combined with regular physical activity and stress management techniques, can help maintain healthy blood pressure levels.

Limiting the intake of unhealthy fats, particularly trans fats and saturated fats, is essential for heart health. These fats can raise cholesterol levels and increase the risk of coronary artery disease. Opting for healthier fats found in avocados, olive oil, and fatty fish can protect the heart by lowering bad cholesterol levels and increasing good cholesterol levels.

Additionally, reducing the consumption of processed and sugary foods can decrease the risk of heart disease by preventing weight gain and reducing inflammation.

Regular health screenings and check-ups are vital for early detection and management of heart disease risk factors. These screenings can monitor cholesterol levels, blood pressure, and other markers of heart health, allowing for timely interventions and lifestyle adjustments.

Engaging in preventive measures, such as quitting smoking and limiting alcohol consumption, can further reduce the risk of developing heart disease.

The role of community and social support in heart health cannot be overlooked. Strong social connections and a sense of belonging can reduce stress and improve mental health, which in turn benefits the heart. Participating in community activities, connecting with friends and family, and seeking support when needed can enhance emotional well-being and contribute to a healthy heart.

Finally, embracing a positive outlook on life and practicing gratitude can have profound effects on heart health. Positive emotions and a optimistic mindset have been linked to lower risks of heart disease, highlighting the connection between mental and emotional health and physical well-being. Cultivating happiness, mindfulness, and a sense of purpose can support heart health and enhance overall quality of life.

Incorporating these holistic practices into daily life requires commitment and consistency, but the benefits for heart health and overall wellness are immeasurable.

By taking a comprehensive approach to heart health, individuals can empower themselves to lead healthier, fuller lives. This chapter has explored the multifaceted aspects of maintaining a healthy heart, emphasizing the importance of a balanced diet, regular physical activity, stress management, herbal remedies, adequate sleep, hydration, and a supportive community. Together, these elements form the foundation of a heart-healthy lifestyle, paving the way for improved cardiovascular wellness and longevity.

CHAPTER 1: DR. BARBARA'S HEART HEALTH PRINCIPLES

D r. Barbara's heart health principles begin with the understanding that the heart is more than just a physical organ pumping blood throughout our bodies; it's a symbol of life, love, and the center of our emotional and spiritual well-being. Recognizing the heart's multifaceted role encourages a comprehensive approach to heart health that transcends conventional medicine, incorporating diet, exercise, and emotional balance into a cohesive strategy for cardiovascular wellness. The first principle emphasizes the importance of a nutrient-rich diet, advocating for the consumption of whole, unprocessed foods that are high in fiber, antioxidants, and healthy fats.

Foods like avocados, nuts, and olive oil provide the monounsaturated fats that are essential for maintaining healthy cholesterol levels, while berries, dark leafy greens, and whole grains offer vital nutrients and antioxidants that protect the heart and its arteries from oxidative stress and inflammation.

Another cornerstone of Dr. Barbara's heart health philosophy is regular, moderate physical activity. Exercise strengthens the heart muscle, improves blood circulation, and helps to regulate blood pressure and cholesterol levels.

It also plays a critical role in weight management, which is crucial for reducing the strain on the heart and minimizing the risk of heart disease. Dr. Barbara suggests incorporating a variety of exercises that one enjoys, such as brisk walking, cycling, swimming, or yoga, to ensure that physical activity becomes a sustainable and enjoyable part of one's daily routine.

Stress management is also integral to Dr. Barbara's heart health principles. Chronic stress can have a detrimental effect on the heart by increasing heart rate and blood pressure, and by contributing to inflammation and narrowed arteries. Techniques such as deep breathing, meditation, and spending time in nature are recommended to help mitigate the effects of stress.

These practices not only promote relaxation and reduce stress but also enhance overall well-being, demonstrating the interconnectedness of mental, emotional, and physical health.

Hydration is another key aspect of maintaining heart health. Drinking adequate amounts of water each day helps to maintain the balance of bodily fluids, supports metabolism, and aids in the detoxification process. Proper hydration ensures that the heart does not have to work as hard to pump blood throughout the body, which is essential for preventing heart strain and maintaining optimal cardiovascular function.

Lastly, Dr. Barbara emphasizes the importance of sleep for heart health.

Quality sleep allows the heart to rest and recover, reduces stress and inflammation, and is linked to a lower risk of cardiovascular disease. Establishing a regular sleep schedule and creating a restful sleeping environment are crucial steps for ensuring that the body receives the restorative sleep it needs.

Together, these principles form the foundation of Dr. Barbara's approach to heart health, highlighting the importance of a holistic lifestyle that nurtures the heart from multiple angles. By focusing on diet, exercise, stress reduction, hydration, and sleep, individuals can take proactive steps towards maintaining a healthy heart and preventing heart disease.

This approach not only supports the physical health of the heart but also acknowledges the deep connections between our heart health and our overall well-being.

Fostering strong social connections and engaging in activities that bring joy and fulfillment are essential components of Dr. Barbara's heart health principles. Positive relationships and a sense of community can significantly impact emotional well-being, which in turn, benefits heart health. Laughter, love, and companionship are powerful antidotes to stress, reducing the levels of stress hormones in the body that can harm the heart. Dr. Barbara encourages finding and nurturing relationships that uplift and support, whether through family, friends, or social groups, to enhance heart health and overall happiness.

Another vital aspect of Dr. Barbara's heart health strategy is the avoidance of toxins and pollutants that can damage the heart and blood vessels.

This includes minimizing exposure to tobacco smoke, limiting alcohol consumption, and choosing organic foods when possible to reduce ingestion of pesticides and chemicals. Detoxifying the body regularly through dietary choices that support liver and kidney function can also help in eliminating toxins that may contribute to heart disease.

Dr. Barbara also highlights the importance of regular medical check-ups and heart health screenings. Early detection of potential heart issues through blood pressure monitoring, cholesterol checks, and other heart-related screenings can be lifesaving. These check-ups provide critical information about heart health and allow for early intervention and treatment if necessary.

Incorporating heart-healthy supplements, under the guidance of a healthcare provider, is another recommendation from Dr. Barbara.

Supplements such as omega-3 fatty acids, magnesium, coenzyme Q10, and antioxidant vitamins can support heart function and protect against heart disease. However, it's important to choose high-quality supplements and discuss their use with a healthcare professional to ensure they are beneficial and appropriate for individual health needs.

Mindful eating practices are also emphasized in Dr. Barbara's approach to heart health. Paying attention to hunger cues, savoring each bite, and being mindful of the nutritional value of foods can enhance the enjoyment of eating and support heart health. Mindful eating encourages a healthier relationship with food and can prevent overeating and the consumption of unhealthy foods that contribute to heart disease.

Lastly, Dr. Barbara advocates for a balanced approach to life, emphasizing that heart health is not just about diet and exercise but also about finding balance and joy in daily activities.

Engaging in hobbies, pursuing interests, and taking time for relaxation and self-care are all crucial for a healthy heart.

This holistic view of heart health recognizes that physical, emotional, and spiritual well-being are deeply interconnected and that nurturing all aspects of oneself is essential for a healthy heart.

By adopting these comprehensive heart health principles, individuals can work towards not only a healthier heart but also a more vibrant and fulfilling life. Dr. Barbara's approach underscores the power of holistic health practices in preventing heart disease and promoting overall well-being, offering a path to heart health that is both effective and enriching.

CHAPTER 2: NUTRITIONAL SUPPORT FOR A HEALTHY HEART

Focusing on nutritional support for a healthy heart involves incorporating foods rich in essential nutrients that promote cardiovascular health. These nutrients include omega-3 fatty acids, antioxidants, fiber, and healthy fats, which work together to reduce inflammation, lower cholesterol levels, and improve blood circulation. To support heart health, it's crucial to emphasize the consumption of a variety of nutrient-dense foods that provide these beneficial compounds.

Omega-3 fatty acids, found in fatty fish like salmon, mackerel, and sardines, as well as in flaxseeds, chia seeds, and walnuts, are pivotal for heart health. They help reduce triglycerides, lower blood pressure, and decrease the risk of arrhythmias.

Incorporating two servings of fatty fish per week or adding a daily serving of flaxseeds or chia seeds to your diet can significantly contribute to your intake of omega-3s.

Antioxidants play a critical role in protecting the heart by neutralizing harmful free radicals and reducing oxidative stress, which can damage blood vessels. Berries, dark chocolate, nuts, and green leafy vegetables are excellent sources of antioxidants. Regularly including these foods in your diet not only offers cardiovascular benefits but also supports overall health.

Fiber is essential for heart health as it helps lower cholesterol levels and maintain healthy blood sugar levels. Whole grains, legumes, fruits, and vegetables are rich in fiber. Starting your day with a bowl of oatmeal topped with berries or incorporating a variety of vegetables into your meals can boost your fiber intake, supporting a healthy heart.

Healthy fats, particularly monounsaturated and polyunsaturated fats, are beneficial for the heart. They can help lower bad cholesterol levels and reduce the risk of heart disease. Avocados, olive oil, nuts, and seeds are excellent sources of these fats. Using olive oil as a salad dressing or snacking on a small handful of nuts can easily increase your intake of healthy fats.

In addition to these specific nutrients, maintaining a balanced diet that emphasizes whole, unprocessed foods is key to supporting heart health. Limiting the intake of processed foods, sugary beverages, and red meats can further protect the heart.

Opting for lean protein sources, such as poultry, fish, and plant-based proteins, and choosing whole grains over refined grains can make a significant difference in your heart health.

Hydration is also crucial for maintaining a healthy heart. Drinking adequate amounts of water each day helps the heart pump blood more efficiently and supports overall cardiovascular function. Aim for at least 8 cups of water daily, and consider incorporating water-rich foods like cucumbers, tomatoes, and watermelon into your diet.

Finally, paying attention to portion sizes and eating patterns can contribute to heart health. Practicing mindful eating, listening to hunger cues, and avoiding overeating can prevent weight gain and reduce the strain on the heart.

Planning meals and snacks that incorporate a variety of heart-healthy foods can ensure you're getting the nutrients your heart needs to function optimally.

By focusing on these nutritional strategies, individuals can support their heart health and reduce the risk of heart disease. It's important to remember that dietary changes should be part of a comprehensive approach to heart health, which also includes regular physical activity, stress management, and avoiding smoking. Together, these lifestyle modifications can significantly improve heart health and promote overall well-being.

HEART-HEALTHY FOODS AND NUTRIENTS

Heart-healthy foods and nutrients play a pivotal role in maintaining cardiovascular health and preventing heart disease. A diet rich in these foods can help lower blood pressure, reduce cholesterol levels, and decrease the risk of heart attacks and strokes. Among the most beneficial heart-healthy nutrients are omega-3 fatty acids, which are known for their anti-inflammatory properties and ability to improve heart function. Foods high in omega-3s include fatty fish like salmon, mackerel, and sardines, as well as flaxseeds, chia seeds, and walnuts. Incorporating these foods into your diet can significantly enhance heart health by reducing arterial inflammation and lowering triglyceride levels.

Antioxidants are another crucial component of a heart-healthy diet. These compounds help combat oxidative stress, a process that can damage cells and contribute to heart disease. Berries, such as blueberries, strawberries, and raspberries, are excellent sources of antioxidants. Other antioxidant-rich foods include dark chocolate, green tea, and leafy greens like spinach and kale.

Regular consumption of these foods can help protect the heart by neutralizing harmful free radicals and improving vascular health.

Fiber is essential for heart health, as it helps to lower cholesterol levels and maintain healthy blood sugar levels. Soluble fiber, in particular, has been shown to reduce the absorption of cholesterol into the bloodstream. Foods high in soluble fiber include oats, beans, lentils, apples, and pears. By incorporating these foods into meals and snacks, you can help keep your heart healthy and reduce the risk of heart disease.

Healthy fats, especially monounsaturated and polyunsaturated fats, are beneficial for the heart.

These fats can help lower bad cholesterol levels (LDL) and raise good cholesterol levels (HDL), reducing the risk of heart disease. Sources of healthy fats include avocados, olive oil, nuts, and seeds. Replacing saturated fats found in red meat and dairy products with these healthier options can significantly improve heart health.

In addition to these specific nutrients, it's important to focus on a balanced diet that emphasizes whole, unprocessed foods. This includes a variety of fruits and vegetables, whole grains, lean protein sources, and low-fat dairy products.

Limiting the intake of processed foods, sugary beverages, and high-sodium items can further protect the heart and support overall cardiovascular health.

Hydration is also crucial for heart health. Drinking plenty of water throughout the day helps the heart pump blood more efficiently and supports the overall function of the cardiovascular system. Aim to drink at least 8 cups of water daily, and consider adding slices of lemon or cucumber for added flavor and nutrients.

By focusing on these heart-healthy foods and nutrients, you can take proactive steps to maintain cardiovascular health and reduce the risk of heart disease.

Remember, a heart-healthy diet is just one component of a comprehensive approach to cardiovascular wellness, which also includes regular physical activity, stress management, and avoiding smoking.

Potassium plays a significant role in heart health by helping to regulate blood pressure. This mineral aids in balancing out the negative effects of salt, which can increase blood pressure when consumed in high amounts. Foods rich in potassium include bananas, sweet potatoes, oranges, and spinach. Incorporating these potassium-packed foods into your diet can help maintain a healthy blood pressure level, which is crucial for reducing the risk of heart disease and stroke.

Magnesium is another important nutrient for heart health. It helps with the regulation of muscle and nerve function, including the heart muscle. Magnesium also contributes to energy production and supports the proper functioning of other minerals in the body. Good sources of magnesium include almonds, black beans, whole wheat, and dark chocolate.

Ensuring an adequate intake of magnesium can support heart rhythm and overall cardiovascular health.

Calcium, while often associated with bone health, also plays a key role in cardiovascular function. It helps blood vessels tighten and relax when they need to and is vital for the healthy functioning of the heart muscle. Dairy products like milk and yogurt, along with leafy green vegetables such as kale and broccoli, are excellent sources of calcium. However, it's important to balance calcium intake with magnesium and potassium for optimal heart health.

Plant sterols and stanols are compounds found in small amounts in many fruits, vegetables, nuts, seeds, cereals, and plant-based oils.

These substances can help lower cholesterol levels by blocking the absorption of cholesterol in the digestive system. Many foods and beverages are now fortified with plant sterols and stanols, making it easier to include them in your diet. Regular consumption can contribute to lowering the risk of heart disease by managing cholesterol levels effectively.

In terms of hydration, while water is essential, herbal teas can also be beneficial for heart health. Certain herbal teas, such as hibiscus and green tea, contain antioxidants that support heart health by lowering blood pressure and improving blood lipid levels. Drinking these teas in moderation can provide a heart-healthy boost to your hydration routine.

Finally, it's important to consider the overall dietary pattern for heart health. The Mediterranean diet, for example, emphasizes fruits, vegetables, whole grains, legumes, nuts, and seeds, along with olive oil as a primary fat source.

This diet also includes moderate consumption of fish and poultry and limits red meat, which aligns with the principles of heart-healthy eating. Adopting a dietary pattern that focuses on whole, nutrient-dense foods and limits processed and high-sodium foods can significantly impact heart health positively.

By paying attention to these additional nutrients and dietary patterns, and incorporating a variety of heart-healthy foods into your diet, you can further support cardiovascular wellness.

Alongside regular physical activity and lifestyle management, a diet rich in these components forms a solid foundation for maintaining heart health and reducing the risk of heart-related conditions.

THE IMPORTANCE OF OMEGA-3S

Omega-3 fatty acids are crucial for heart health, offering numerous benefits that support the cardiovascular system. These essential fats, particularly EPA (eicosapentaenoic acid) and DHA (docosahexaenoic acid), are known for their anti-inflammatory properties, which can help reduce the risk of heart disease.

They work by decreasing triglycerides, lowering blood pressure, reducing blood clotting, and enhancing the health of blood vessels.

Additionally, omega-3s can help improve the balance of cholesterol by raising HDL (good) cholesterol levels. This balance is vital for preventing plaque buildup in the arteries, which can lead to atherosclerosis, heart attacks, and strokes.

The body cannot produce omega-3 fatty acids on its own, so it's essential to include them in your diet. Rich sources of EPA and DHA include fatty fish like salmon, mackerel, and sardines.

For vegetarians or those who do not consume fish, algae-based supplements are an excellent alternative source of DHA and EPA. Flaxseeds, chia seeds, hemp seeds, and walnuts are rich in ALA (alpha-linolenic acid), another type of omega-3 fatty acid, which the body can partially convert to EPA and DHA.

Incorporating omega-3s into your diet can be simple. Aim for two servings of fatty fish per week or consider a daily omega-3 supplement if you're not able to meet these needs through diet alone. When choosing supplements, look for those that are third-party tested for purity and potency. For plant-based sources, include a variety of seeds and nuts in your meals, or use their oils in dressings and sauces to boost your ALA intake.

Remember, while omega-3 supplements can be beneficial, getting these fatty acids from foods is always preferred due to the additional nutrients they provide. Balancing your omega-3 intake with a diet low in saturated fats and high in fruits, vegetables, and whole grains will further enhance heart health and overall well-being.

FOODS TO AVOID FOR HEART HEALTH

For optimal heart health, it's crucial to be mindful of foods that can negatively impact your cardiovascular system. Foods high in saturated fats, trans fats, and cholesterol can raise blood cholesterol levels, contributing to the buildup of plaque in arteries, known as atherosclerosis. This condition can lead to heart disease, heart attacks, and strokes. Therefore, limiting or avoiding foods like fatty cuts of meat, butter, cheese, and other full-fat dairy products can be beneficial.

Processed and fast foods often contain trans fats, which are particularly harmful to heart health, even in small quantities. These are found in many fried foods, baked goods, and snacks.

Excessive salt intake can also raise blood pressure, a leading risk factor for heart disease. Processed foods, canned soups, and ready-to-eat meals are typically high in sodium and should be consumed in moderation or avoided when possible.

Opt for fresh or frozen vegetables and cook from scratch when you can to control the amount of salt in your diet.

Highly refined and sugary foods, such as white bread, white rice, and sugary snacks and beverages, can lead to weight gain and increase the risk of developing type 2 diabetes, which is another risk factor for heart disease.

These foods can also cause spikes in blood sugar levels, leading to increased hunger and overeating. Instead, choose whole grains, fruits, and vegetables that provide essential nutrients and fiber, which can help maintain a healthy weight and reduce heart disease risk.

Limiting alcohol consumption is also advisable as excessive drinking can lead to high blood pressure, heart failure, and an increased calorie intake.

If you choose to drink, do so in moderation, following the guidelines of up to one drink per day for women and up to two drinks per day for men.

By being mindful of these dietary choices, you can support your heart health and reduce the risk of cardiovascular disease, ensuring a healthier, more vibrant life.

CHAPTER 3: HERBAL CARDIO SUPPORT

Herbal remedies have been used for centuries to support heart health, offering natural ways to enhance cardiovascular function and reduce the risk of heart disease. These remedies work by improving blood circulation, reducing inflammation, and helping to manage blood pressure and cholesterol levels. Incorporating specific herbs into your daily regimen can be a powerful adjunct to a heart-healthy lifestyle that includes a balanced diet, regular exercise, and stress management.

Beneficial effects: Herbal remedies can support cardiovascular health by enhancing blood flow, reducing arterial inflammation, managing blood pressure, lowering bad cholesterol levels, and supporting overall heart function.

Hawthorn Berry: Hawthorn berry is renowned for its cardiovascular benefits. It can help improve coronary artery blood flow, reduce blood pressure, and enhance heart muscle contraction, making it an excellent herb for overall heart health.

Ingredients:

- 1 teaspoon of dried hawthorn berries

- 1 cup of boiling water

- **Instructions**:

1. Place the dried hawthorn berries in a teapot.

2. Pour boiling water over the berries and steep for 10 to 15 minutes.

3. Strain the tea and drink it once or twice daily.

Garlic: Garlic has been shown to lower blood pressure, reduce cholesterol, and prevent blood clots, making it a powerful herb for cardiovascular support.

Ingredients:

- 1-2 fresh garlic cloves

- **Instructions**:

1. Crush or finely chop the garlic cloves.

2. Let them sit for 5 to 10 minutes to activate the allicin.

3. Consume raw or add to your meals. For those sensitive to raw garlic, consider aged garlic supplements as an alternative.

Ginger: Ginger is another herb known for its anti-inflammatory and antioxidant properties. It can help lower cholesterol levels, prevent blood clots, and improve blood circulation.

Ingredients:

- 1 inch of fresh ginger root

- 1 cup of boiling water

- **Instructions**:

1. Peel and thinly slice the fresh ginger root.

2. Add ginger to boiling water and simmer for 5 minutes.

3. Strain the tea and enjoy. You can drink ginger tea 2-3 times daily.

Turmeric: Turmeric, with its active compound curcumin, has potent anti-inflammatory and antioxidant properties, beneficial for reducing inflammation in the arteries and improving circulation.

Ingredients:

- 1 teaspoon of turmeric powder

- 1 cup of milk or a plant-based alternative

- A pinch of black pepper (to enhance absorption)

- Honey to taste

- **Instructions**:

1. Warm the milk in a saucepan over low heat.

2. Stir in the turmeric powder and black pepper.

3. Remove from heat and sweeten with honey to taste.

4. Drink this mixture once daily.

Green Tea: Rich in antioxidants, green tea can help lower cholesterol levels and improve blood flow. It also contains catechins, which may help prevent the formation of plaque in the arteries.

Ingredients:

- 1 green tea bag or 1 teaspoon of green tea leaves

- 1 cup of boiling water

- **Instructions**:

1. Steep the green tea in boiling water for 3-5 minutes.

2. Remove the tea bag or strain the leaves and enjoy. Drinking 2-3 cups of green tea daily is beneficial for heart health.

Variations: These herbal remedies can be adjusted according to personal taste or combined for enhanced benefits. For example, adding a slice of lemon to green tea or mixing ginger and turmeric for a powerful anti-inflammatory tea.

Storage tips: Store dried herbs in a cool, dry place away from direct sunlight. Fresh herbs like ginger and garlic should be kept in the refrigerator to maintain their potency.

Tips for allergens: Those with allergies to specific herbs should avoid them and consult with a healthcare provider for alternatives. Always start with small doses to test for any adverse reactions.

Scientific references: Studies have shown the cardiovascular benefits of these herbs. For instance, research published in the Journal of Nutrition and Metabolism highlights hawthorn's efficacy in treating heart failure, and studies in the Journal of the American College of Nutrition have demonstrated garlic's cholesterol-lowering effects.

Ginger's cardiovascular benefits are documented in the International Journal of Cardiology, and the Journal of Nutrition reviews the heart-healthy advantages of green tea.

Turmeric's cardiovascular effects are supported by research in the Journal of Traditional and Complementary Medicine.

Incorporating these natural remedies into your daily routine, alongside a healthy lifestyle, can provide significant support for cardiovascular health.

Always consult with a healthcare professional before starting any new herbal regimen, especially if you have existing health conditions or are taking medications.

HERBAL SUPPLEMENTS FOR HEART HEALTH

Herbal supplements have garnered attention for their potential benefits in supporting heart health, complementing a heart-healthy lifestyle that includes diet, exercise, and stress management.

These natural remedies offer a holistic approach to maintaining cardiovascular wellness, potentially aiding in the management of blood pressure, cholesterol levels, and overall heart function. It's essential to approach herbal supplementation with an informed perspective, understanding the specific benefits and proper usage of each herb to maximize their heart health advantages.

Ginkgo Biloba: Known for its ability to enhance circulation and improve blood flow, Ginkgo Biloba can contribute to better heart health by supporting the vascular system. Its antioxidant properties also help in protecting the heart and arteries from oxidative stress and damage.

Ingredients:

- Ginkgo Biloba extract (standardized to 24% flavone glycosides and 6% terpene lactones)

- Capsule form is commonly used for standardized dosing

- **Instructions**:

1. Follow the manufacturer's recommended dosage, typically around 120 to 240 mg per day, divided into two or three doses.

2. It is best taken with meals to improve absorption.

Omega-3 Fatty Acid Supplements: While not an herb, omega-3 supplements derived from fish oil or algae are crucial for heart health, reducing inflammation, and supporting healthy cholesterol levels.

Ingredients:

- Fish oil or algae-based omega-3 supplement containing EPA and DHA

- **Instructions**:

1. Aim for a supplement providing at least 500 mg of EPA and DHA combined per day.

2. Consult with a healthcare provider for specific dosing recommendations, especially for heart health concerns.

Coenzyme Q10 (CoQ10): This antioxidant supports heart health by improving energy production in cells and protecting the heart from oxidative stress. It's particularly beneficial for those on statin medications, as statins can reduce CoQ10 levels in the body.

Ingredients:

- Coenzyme Q10 (Ubiquinone or Ubiquinol form)

- Capsule or softgel form

- **Instructions**:

1. The recommended dosage can range from 100 to 200 mg per day, taken with meals for enhanced absorption.

2. Ubiquinol is the active form and may be more effective, especially for older adults.

Hibiscus: Consumed as a tea or supplement, hibiscus can help lower high blood pressure, a significant risk factor for heart disease. Its bioactive compounds offer antioxidant and anti-inflammatory benefits.

Ingredients:

- Dried hibiscus flowers or hibiscus extract supplement

- **Instructions**:

1. For tea, steep 1-2 teaspoons of dried hibiscus flowers in boiling water for 5-10 minutes.

2. If using a supplement, follow the manufacturer's dosage recommendations, typically around 500 mg twice daily.

Arjuna Bark: Arjuna is an Ayurvedic herb known for its heart-protective properties. It can help manage cholesterol, blood pressure, and improve heart muscle function.

Ingredients:

- Arjuna bark powder or extract supplement

- **Instructions**:

1. The typical dosage for Arjuna bark extract is 500 mg per day.

2. It can be taken with water, preferably in the morning or as directed by a healthcare provider.

Variations: These supplements can be used individually or in combination, depending on individual health needs and under the guidance of a healthcare professional. Always start with lower doses to assess tolerance and gradually increase as needed.

Storage tips: Keep supplements in a cool, dry place, away from direct sunlight. Ensure caps are tightly sealed to maintain potency.

Tips for allergens: For those with allergies to specific supplements or their components, seek hypoallergenic alternatives or consult with a healthcare provider for safe options.

Scientific references: Numerous studies support the cardiovascular benefits of these supplements. For example, research in the Journal of Phytotherapy Research highlights Ginkgo Biloba's efficacy in improving blood flow, while the American Heart Association acknowledges the role of omega-3 fatty acids in heart health. Coenzyme Q10's cardiovascular benefits are documented in the Journal of the American College of Cardiology. Hibiscus's blood pressure-lowering effects are noted in studies published in the Journal of Nutrition and the Journal of Ethnopharmacology. The cardiovascular benefits of Arjuna bark are supported by research in the Indian Journal of Experimental Biology.

Incorporating herbal supplements into a comprehensive approach to heart health can offer additional support for maintaining cardiovascular wellness. Always consult with a healthcare professional before adding new supplements to your regimen, especially if you have existing health conditions or are taking medications, to ensure safety and efficacy.

CHAPTER 4: 5 HERBAL RECIPES FOR HEART HEALTH

HAWTHORN BERRY TEA

Beneficial effects

Hawthorn Berry Tea is recognized for its cardiovascular benefits, particularly in supporting heart health and improving circulation. This herbal tea can help regulate blood pressure, reduce symptoms of heart failure, and enhance overall cardiovascular function. Its rich antioxidant content also contributes to reducing oxidative stress and inflammation in the body, offering a natural way to support aging gracefully.

Portions

2 servings

Preparation time

5 minutes

Cooking time

10 minutes

Ingredients

- 2 teaspoons of dried hawthorn berries
- 2 cups of boiling water
- Honey or lemon (optional, for taste)

Instructions

1. Place the dried hawthorn berries in a tea infuser or directly into a heat-resistant teapot.

2. Pour 2 cups of boiling water over the hawthorn berries.

3. Cover and allow the tea to steep for about 10 minutes. The longer it steeps, the stronger the flavor and potential benefits.

4. Remove the tea infuser or strain the tea to remove the berries.

5. Optional: Add honey or a slice of lemon to enhance the flavor.

6. Serve the tea warm, or allow it to cool for a refreshing cold beverage.

Variations

- For added heart health benefits, mix in a teaspoon of green tea leaves during the steeping process.

- Combine with a slice of fresh ginger or a cinnamon stick while steeping for additional flavor and health benefits.

- For a sweeter, more flavorful tea, add a few fresh or frozen berries to the tea after straining.

Storage tips

Store any leftover Hawthorn Berry Tea in a sealed container in the refrigerator for up to 2 days. Enjoy it chilled or gently reheat on the stove.

Tips for allergens

Individuals with allergies to plants in the rose family should proceed with caution when trying Hawthorn Berry Tea for the first time. For those avoiding honey due to dietary restrictions, substitute with maple syrup or simply omit the sweetener.

Scientific references

- "Hawthorn extract for treating chronic heart failure: Meta-analysis of randomized trials." American Journal of Medicine, 2003. This study supports the use of hawthorn extract in improving symptoms and functional outcomes in chronic heart failure.

- "Antioxidant activity of hawthorn berry extract and its effect on cardiovascular system." International Journal of Food Sciences and Nutrition, 2011. This research highlights the antioxidant properties of hawthorn berries and their beneficial effects on the cardiovascular system.

MOTHERWORT TINCTURE

Beneficial effects

Motherwort Tincture is renowned for its heart-supporting properties, offering a natural remedy to help calm heart palpitations, reduce anxiety, and improve cardiovascular health. Its active compounds, including leonurine and stachydrine, have been shown to possess mild vasodilatory properties, potentially aiding in the reduction of high blood pressure and improving blood circulation. Additionally, motherwort's calming effects can help soothe the nervous system, making it beneficial for those experiencing stress-related heart issues.

Ingredients

- 1 cup dried motherwort herb
- 2 cups 100-proof alcohol (vodka or brandy)

Instructions

1. Place the dried motherwort herb into a clean, dry jar.

2. Pour the 100-proof alcohol over the herbs, ensuring they are completely submerged. Leave about an inch of space at the top of the jar.

3. Seal the jar tightly with a lid and label it with the date and contents.

4. Store the jar in a cool, dark place for 4 to 6 weeks. Shake the jar gently every few days to mix the contents and promote extraction.

5. After the infusion period, strain the tincture through a fine mesh sieve or cheesecloth into another clean, dark glass bottle. Press or squeeze the herbs to extract as much liquid as possible.

6. Label the bottle with the date and contents.

Variations

- For those sensitive to alcohol, a glycerin-based tincture can be made by substituting the alcohol with a mixture of glycerin and water (3 parts glycerin to 1 part water).

- Add a few slices of fresh ginger to the jar during the infusion process to enhance the tincture's warming and circulatory benefits.

Storage tips

Store the Motherwort Tincture in a cool, dark place. When stored properly in an airtight container, it can last for several years.

Tips for allergens

Individuals with allergies to plants in the Lamiaceae family, such as mint, should proceed with caution when using motherwort. As always, consult with a healthcare provider before starting any new herbal remedy, especially if you are pregnant, nursing, or taking medications.

Scientific references

- "Pharmacological effects of Leonurus cardiaca L. (Motherwort): A systematic review" in Phytotherapy Research, 2018. This review discusses the cardiovascular and anxiolytic benefits of motherwort, supporting its traditional use in herbal medicine.

- "Antioxidant activity of extracts from Leonurus cardiaca L. (Motherwort)" in Phytotherapy Research, 2011. This study highlights the antioxidant properties of motherwort, suggesting its potential in protecting against oxidative stress-related cardiovascular diseases.

CAYENNE PEPPER HEART TONIC

Beneficial effects

Cayenne Pepper Heart Tonic is known for its potent cardiovascular benefits. It can help improve blood circulation, strengthen the heart muscles, and reduce blood cholesterol levels. The capsaicin in cayenne pepper is responsible for its heart-healthy properties, including the ability to dilate blood vessels for better blood flow. This tonic can also aid in regulating heart rhythm and reducing the risk of heart disease.

Portions

4 servings

Preparation time

5 minutes

Ingredients

- 1/4 teaspoon cayenne pepper powder

- Juice of 1 lemon

- 2 tablespoons raw honey

- 4 cups of filtered water

- A pinch of Himalayan pink salt

Instructions

1. In a large pitcher, combine the lemon juice, raw honey, cayenne pepper powder, and Himalayan pink salt.

2. Add the filtered water to the pitcher and stir well until all the ingredients are fully dissolved and mixed.

3. Serve the tonic immediately, or chill in the refrigerator for an hour if a cold beverage is preferred.

Variations

- For an added detox effect, mix in 1 tablespoon of apple cider vinegar.

- Enhance the flavor and benefits by adding a slice of fresh ginger or turmeric root during preparation.

- Substitute honey with maple syrup for a vegan-friendly version.

Storage tips

Store any leftover Cayenne Pepper Heart Tonic in a sealed container in the refrigerator for up to 48 hours. Shake well before serving as the cayenne pepper may settle at the bottom.

Tips for allergens

Individuals with a sensitivity to spicy foods should start with a smaller amount of cayenne pepper and adjust according to tolerance. For those allergic to honey, maple syrup is a suitable alternative.

Scientific references

- "Effects of capsaicin on lipid metabolism and heart function" published in the Journal of Nutritional Biochemistry, 2017. This study highlights the beneficial impact of capsaicin from cayenne pepper on heart health and cholesterol levels.

- "Dietary capsaicin and its anti-obesity potency: from mechanism to clinical implications" in Bioscience Reports, 2017. This research discusses the role of capsaicin in improving blood circulation and reducing the risk of cardiovascular diseases.

GINGER HEART HEALTH ELIXIR

Beneficial effects

Ginger Heart Health Elixir is designed to support cardiovascular health by improving blood circulation, reducing inflammation, and lowering blood pressure levels. Ginger, the main ingredient, is known for its potent anti-inflammatory and antioxidant properties, which can help prevent heart disease and stroke. Additionally, this elixir can aid in cholesterol management, contributing to overall heart health and wellness.

Portions

2 servings

Preparation time

10 minutes

Ingredients

- 2 inches of fresh ginger root, peeled and sliced

- 4 cups of water

- Juice of 1 lemon

- 2 tablespoons of raw honey

- A pinch of cayenne pepper (optional)

Instructions

1. In a medium-sized pot, bring the water to a boil.

2. Add the sliced ginger to the boiling water and reduce the heat.

3. Simmer the ginger for about 10 minutes to infuse the water.

4. Remove the pot from the heat and let it cool slightly.

5. Strain the ginger pieces from the water and pour the infused water into a large pitcher.

6. Stir in the lemon juice and raw honey until the honey is completely dissolved.

7. If using, add a pinch of cayenne pepper to the mixture and stir well.

8. Serve the elixir warm, or chill in the refrigerator and serve cold.

Variations

- For an extra antioxidant boost, add a bag of green tea to the ginger while simmering.

- Include a sprig of fresh mint or a few slices of cucumber for a refreshing twist.

- Substitute honey with maple syrup for a vegan-friendly version.

Storage tips

Store any leftover Ginger Heart Health Elixir in an airtight container in the refrigerator for up to 3 days. Reheat gently on the stove or enjoy cold.

Tips for allergens

Individuals with allergies to ginger or other ingredients should adjust the recipe accordingly or consult with a healthcare provider before consumption. For those sensitive to spicy foods, the cayenne pepper can be omitted.

Scientific references

- "Ginger consumption and cardiovascular risk factors: A systematic review," published in Nutrition, Metabolism & Cardiovascular Diseases, 2019. This review provides evidence of ginger's beneficial effects on cardiovascular risk factors.

- "Anti-Oxidative and Anti-Inflammatory Effects of Ginger in Health and Physical Activity: Review of Current Evidence," published in International Journal of Preventive Medicine, 2013. This article highlights ginger's antioxidant and anti-inflammatory properties, supporting its use for heart health.

LINDEN FLOWER INFUSION

Beneficial effects

Linden Flower Infusion is known for its calming properties, which can help reduce stress and anxiety, promoting relaxation and better sleep. It's also recognized for its potential to alleviate headaches and reduce inflammation. The soothing effect of linden flower on the digestive system can ease indigestion and bloating, making it a gentle remedy for gastrointestinal discomfort. Additionally, its diaphoretic properties may support fever management by inducing sweating and helping to lower body temperature during colds and flu.

Portions

2 servings

Preparation time

5 minutes

Cooking time

10 minutes

Ingredients

- 2 tablespoons of dried linden flowers

- 2 cups of boiling water

- Honey or lemon (optional, for taste)

Instructions

1. Place the dried linden flowers in a teapot or a heat-resistant glass container.

2. Pour 2 cups of boiling water over the linden flowers.

3. Cover and let the infusion steep for 10 minutes to allow the flowers to fully release their beneficial properties.

4. Strain the infusion into cups, removing the linden flowers.

5. Optional: Add honey or a slice of lemon to each cup for added flavor.

6. Serve the infusion warm, ideally in the evening to promote relaxation and a restful night's sleep.

Variations

- For a more complex flavor, add a cinnamon stick or a few slices of fresh ginger to the infusion while it steeps.

- Combine with chamomile or mint leaves for additional calming and digestive benefits.

- To enjoy a cold beverage, allow the infusion to cool down and serve it over ice, garnished with a slice of lemon.

Storage tips

If you have leftover Linden Flower Infusion, store it in a sealed container in the refrigerator for up to 2 days. Enjoy it chilled, or gently reheat on the stove.

Tips for allergens

Individuals with allergies to flowers should start with a small amount of linden flower infusion to ensure no adverse reactions. For those avoiding honey due to dietary restrictions, substitute with maple syrup or simply omit the sweetener.

Scientific references

- "Anxiolytic and sedative effects of extracts and essential oil from Citrus aurantium L." Biological and Pharmaceutical Bulletin, 2002. This study supports the use of herbal infusions, like Linden Flower, in reducing anxiety and promoting relaxation.

- "The effects of herbal remedies on the alleviation of premenstrual syndrome symptoms: A systematic review." Journal of Psychosomatic Obstetrics & Gynecology, 2019. This review suggests that herbal teas, including Linden Flower Infusion, can help in managing symptoms associated with stress and hormonal imbalances.

PART 12: BONE AND JOINT HEALTH

Maintaining healthy bones and joints is essential for a lifetime of mobility and well-being. As we age, the importance of nourishing our skeletal system becomes paramount to prevent conditions such as osteoporosis and arthritis. A holistic approach, emphasizing nutrition, herbal remedies, and lifestyle adjustments, can significantly impact bone density and joint health. This chapter delves into natural strategies and remedies to support and enhance bone and joint health.

Beneficial effects: The remedies and practices discussed here aim to increase bone density, reduce inflammation in joints, alleviate pain, and enhance overall skeletal strength. By incorporating these strategies, individuals can potentially delay or mitigate the onset of bone-related conditions and maintain mobility and quality of life as they age.

White Willow Bark Tea for Joint Pain Relief:

Ingredients:

- 1-2 teaspoons of dried white willow bark

- 1 cup of boiling water

- **Instructions**:

1. Place the white willow bark into a tea infuser or directly into a cup.

2. Pour boiling water over the bark and allow it to steep for 15-20 minutes.

3. Strain the tea (if necessary) and drink once or twice daily for pain relief.

Beneficial effects: White willow bark acts as a natural anti-inflammatory and pain reliever, similar to aspirin, making it beneficial for those experiencing joint pain.

Boswellia Serrata Extract for Inflammation:

Ingredients:

- Boswellia serrata extract (available in capsule or powder form)

- **Instructions**:

1. If using capsules, follow the manufacturer's recommended dosage, usually around 300-500 mg taken two to three times daily.

2. For powder, it can be mixed into a smoothie or with a glass of water. Ensure to adhere to the dosage recommendations provided.

Beneficial effects: Boswellia is known for its strong anti-inflammatory properties, which can help reduce pain and improve mobility in affected joints.

Turmeric and Black Pepper Golden Milk for Bone Health:

Ingredients:

- 1 teaspoon of turmeric powder

- A pinch of black pepper (to enhance turmeric absorption)

- 1 cup of milk or a plant-based alternative

- Honey or maple syrup to taste
- **Instructions**:

1. Warm the milk in a saucepan over low heat without bringing it to a boil.

2. Stir in the turmeric and black pepper.

3. Remove from heat and sweeten with honey or maple syrup to taste.

4. Drink this mixture once daily, preferably before bedtime.

Beneficial effects: Turmeric contains curcumin, a compound with potent anti-inflammatory and antioxidant properties, which can contribute to bone density and joint health. Black pepper increases the bioavailability of curcumin.

Nettle Infusion for Bone Strength:

Ingredients:

- 1 ounce of dried nettle leaves
- 1 quart of boiling water
- **Instructions**:

1. Place the nettle leaves in a quart-sized jar.

2. Pour boiling water over the nettles, filling the jar.

3. Cover and steep for 4 hours or overnight.

4. Strain and drink 1-2 cups daily.

Beneficial effects: Nettle is rich in minerals essential for bone health, including calcium, magnesium, and silicon, which are vital for strengthening bones and supporting joint health.

Horsetail and Nettle Bone Strength Smoothie:

Ingredients:

- 1 teaspoon of dried horsetail powder
- 1 handful of fresh nettle leaves (or 1 teaspoon of dried nettle)
- 1 banana
- 1 cup of almond milk or any plant-based milk
- Honey or maple syrup to taste
- **Instructions**:

1. Combine all ingredients in a blender.

2. Blend until smooth.

3. Enjoy this smoothie once daily to support bone health.

Beneficial effects: Horsetail is another herb known for its mineral content, particularly silica, which is crucial for bone formation and health. Combined with nettle, this smoothie is a powerhouse for supporting bone density and joint health.

Variations: These remedies can be adjusted based on personal preferences and needs. For instance, adding ginger to the golden milk can enhance its anti-inflammatory properties. Similarly, incorporating other bone-supportive foods like kale or spinach into the smoothie can provide additional nutrients.

Storage tips: Herbal teas can be stored in a refrigerator for up to 48 hours. Smoothies should be consumed immediately or can be kept in the fridge for up to 24 hours for best taste and nutrient retention.

Tips for allergens: Individuals with allergies to specific herbs should consult with a healthcare provider for alternatives. For those allergic to dairy, plant-based milk alternatives in recipes are an excellent substitute.

Scientific references: Numerous studies have highlighted the benefits of these herbs and spices for bone and joint health. For example, research published in the Journal of Medicinal Food discusses turmeric's role in osteoarthritis management.

Similarly, the anti-inflammatory effects of Boswellia serrata are detailed in the Journal of Phytotherapy Research, demonstrating its efficacy in treating chronic inflammatory diseases.

Incorporating these natural remedies and practices into daily life can significantly contribute to maintaining and enhancing bone and joint health.

Coupled with a balanced diet and regular exercise, these strategies form a comprehensive approach to skeletal wellness, crucial for a vibrant and active life at any age. Always consult with a healthcare professional before starting any new supplement or herbal remedy, especially if you have existing health conditions or are taking other medications.

CHAPTER 1: UNDERSTANDING BONE AND JOINT HEALTH

Bones and joints form the framework of our body, enabling mobility and providing protection to our vital organs. They are living tissues that continuously break down and rebuild throughout our lives. This dynamic process is influenced by various factors including nutrition, physical activity, and overall health. To maintain strong bones and joints, it's crucial to understand their composition and the factors that affect their health.

Bones are made up of a matrix that includes collagen, a protein that provides a soft framework, and calcium phosphate, a mineral complex that adds strength and hardens the framework.

This combination makes bones strong yet flexible enough to withstand stress. More than just static structures, bones also house bone marrow, where blood cells are produced, and act as reserves for minerals such as calcium and phosphorus.

Joint health is equally important as bones for mobility.

Joints are the connections between bones, cushioned by cartilage and synovial fluid which prevent friction and allow smooth movement. Over time, or due to injury and wear and tear, cartilage can degrade, leading to conditions like osteoarthritis, characterized by pain and reduced mobility.

Several factors contribute to bone and joint health. Calcium and vitamin D are essential for strong bones, as calcium strengthens the bones while vitamin D improves calcium absorption.

Physical activity, particularly weight-bearing exercises, stimulates bone formation and helps maintain joint flexibility and strength. Conversely, a sedentary lifestyle can lead to bone density loss and joint stiffness.

Hormonal changes, especially in women post-menopause, can significantly affect bone density due to decreased estrogen levels, increasing the risk of osteoporosis. Other factors such as smoking, excessive alcohol consumption, and certain medications can also compromise bone health.

To support bone and joint health, incorporating a balanced diet rich in calcium, vitamin D, and anti-inflammatory foods is recommended.

Foods high in omega-3 fatty acids, such as fish, flaxseeds, and walnuts, can help reduce joint inflammation. Regular physical activity, including strength training, walking, and flexibility exercises, is essential to maintain bone density and joint function.

Monitoring bone density through medical check-ups can help detect early signs of osteoporosis, allowing for timely intervention.

For those already experiencing joint pain or conditions like arthritis, incorporating gentle exercises, physical therapy, and possibly supplements like glucosamine and chondroitin can offer relief and support joint health.

In conclusion, understanding the importance of bone and joint health is the first step towards maintaining mobility and quality of life as we age.

By adopting a holistic approach that includes proper nutrition, regular physical activity, and healthy lifestyle choices, we can support our skeletal system's health and function, ensuring a strong foundation for our bodies.

COMMON DISORDERS: OSTEOPOROSIS AND ARTHRITIS

Osteoporosis and arthritis stand as two prevalent disorders affecting bone and joint health, each presenting unique challenges and requiring specific management strategies. Osteoporosis is characterized by weakened bones that become fragile and more likely to fracture. It occurs when the creation of new bone doesn't keep up with the removal of old bone. Risk factors include aging, hormonal changes, low body weight, low sex hormones or menopause, smoking, and certain medications. Prevention and treatment strategies focus on strengthening bones and preventing falls that may cause fractures. This includes adequate intake of calcium and vitamin D, regular weight-bearing and muscle-strengthening exercises, and medications that can help strengthen bones.

Arthritis encompasses over 100 conditions that affect joints, the tissues that surround the joint, and other connective tissue.

The most common form is osteoarthritis, which is a degenerative disease that worsens over time, often resulting in chronic pain. Joint inflammation from arthritis can lead to swelling, pain, stiffness, and decreased range of motion. For those living with arthritis, management focuses on reducing symptoms and improving joint function. This may involve a combination of treatments including medication, physical therapy, lifestyle modifications such as exercise and weight control, and in some cases, surgery to repair or replace damaged joints.

For both osteoporosis and arthritis, a holistic approach to management can be beneficial. This includes dietary modifications to ensure a balanced intake of nutrients essential for bone and joint health. Foods rich in calcium, vitamin D, magnesium, and omega-3 fatty acids are particularly important. Additionally, incorporating anti-inflammatory foods such as leafy green vegetables, berries, nuts, and seeds can help manage arthritis symptoms.

Herbal supplements such as turmeric, ginger, and green tea have anti-inflammatory properties that may also provide relief.

Regular physical activity is crucial for managing both conditions. Weight-bearing exercises, such as walking, jogging, and dancing, are beneficial for strengthening bones and improving bone density, which is vital for osteoporosis management.

For arthritis, exercises that improve range of motion, strengthen muscles around joints, and increase flexibility can help reduce pain and improve joint function. Water-based exercises can be particularly beneficial as they provide resistance without putting stress on the joints.

Living with osteoporosis or arthritis also means making adjustments to daily activities to protect bone and joint health. This may include using assistive devices to prevent falls, modifying tasks to reduce joint strain, and employing techniques to manage pain and improve sleep. Mind-body practices such as yoga and tai chi can be beneficial for both physical and mental well-being, helping to reduce stress, improve balance, and enhance flexibility.

It's important for individuals with osteoporosis or arthritis to work closely with healthcare providers to develop a comprehensive management plan tailored to their specific needs. This may include regular monitoring of bone density for osteoporosis or joint health for arthritis, medication management, and coordination of care among specialists such as rheumatologists, orthopedists, and physical therapists.

In summary, while osteoporosis and arthritis are common disorders that can significantly impact quality of life, adopting a holistic approach to management focusing on diet, exercise, lifestyle modifications, and medical care can help individuals maintain bone and joint health, reduce pain, and enhance mobility.

PREVENTATIVE MEASURES FOR BONE HEALTH

Preventative measures for bone health are essential at every stage of life to ensure a strong skeletal system and minimize the risk of osteoporosis and fractures. Adequate calcium intake is paramount for building and maintaining peak bone mass.

Adults should aim for 1,000 to 1,200 mg of calcium per day, which can be achieved through a combination of dietary sources such as dairy products, leafy green vegetables, almonds, and fortified foods, or supplements if necessary. Vitamin D plays a critical role in calcium absorption and bone health, with recommended daily amounts ranging from 600 to 800 IU. Sun exposure, fatty fish, fortified foods, and supplements are viable sources of vitamin D.

Regular physical activity, especially weight-bearing and muscle-strengthening exercises, stimulates bone formation and slows down bone loss.

Activities such as walking, jogging, dancing, lifting weights, and yoga are beneficial for bones. Smoking cessation and moderation in alcohol consumption are advised as both have been linked to decreased bone density and increased risk of fractures.

Limiting caffeine intake is also recommended as excessive caffeine can interfere with calcium absorption.

Maintaining a healthy weight is crucial for bone health, as being underweight increases the risk of bone loss and fractures, while excessive weight can stress the bones and lead to conditions such as osteoarthritis. A balanced diet rich in fruits, vegetables, lean proteins, and whole grains supports overall health and provides the nutrients necessary for bone maintenance.

Monitoring bone density through regular screenings, especially for those over the age of 50 or with risk factors for osteoporosis, can help detect early signs of bone loss and facilitate timely intervention. Hormonal balance is also important, as low levels of sex hormones, particularly estrogen in postmenopausal women, can lead to bone weakening.

Hormone replacement therapy may be considered under medical guidance.

Incorporating foods rich in omega-3 fatty acids, such as salmon and flaxseeds, can help reduce inflammation that might affect the bones.

Additionally, foods high in magnesium and potassium, found in bananas, avocados, and nuts, are beneficial for bone health as they contribute to the bone mineralization process.

For those with a family history of osteoporosis, taking proactive measures to strengthen bones from an early age is crucial.

This includes ensuring a nutrient-rich diet, engaging in regular physical activity, and avoiding lifestyle choices that could negatively impact bone density. Consulting with a healthcare provider for personalized advice based on individual health status and risk factors is recommended to develop an effective bone health strategy.

By adopting these preventative measures, individuals can support their bone health, reduce the risk of osteoporosis and fractures, and maintain mobility and quality of life into older age. Always consult with a healthcare professional before starting any new supplement or exercise regimen, especially if you have existing health conditions or concerns about your bone health.

DR. BARBARA'S JOINT FLEXIBLITY METHODS

Dr. Barbara emphasizes the importance of maintaining joint flexibility as a key component of overall health and well-being. She advocates for a holistic approach that incorporates a variety of natural strategies and remedies to support and enhance joint health. Recognizing that joint stiffness and pain can significantly impact quality of life, her methods focus on reducing inflammation, nourishing the joints with essential nutrients, and incorporating gentle, yet effective exercises to improve range of motion and flexibility.

Beneficial effects: The approach aims to alleviate joint pain, increase flexibility and range of motion, reduce inflammation, and support the overall health of the joints. By adopting these strategies, individuals may experience improved mobility, decreased discomfort, and a greater ability to engage in daily activities without limitation.

Ingredients:

- Omega-3 fatty acids (from sources like salmon, flaxseeds, and walnuts)

- Turmeric (for its curcumin content)

- Ginger (fresh or powdered)

- Green tea (rich in antioxidants)

- Vitamin D (from sunlight exposure, fatty fish, or supplements)

- Calcium (from leafy greens, dairy, or fortified plant-based alternatives)

- Hydration (adequate water intake)

- **Instructions**:

1. Incorporate omega-3 fatty acids into your diet regularly to help reduce joint inflammation.

2. Add turmeric to meals or take as a supplement; aim for 500-1000 mg daily to utilize its anti-inflammatory properties.

3. Include ginger in your diet, either by adding fresh ginger to meals or consuming ginger tea, to benefit from its anti-inflammatory effects.

4. Drink green tea daily, aiming for 2-3 cups, to take advantage of its antioxidant properties which can support joint health.

5. Ensure adequate vitamin D intake through safe sun exposure, diet, or supplements, aiming for 600-800 IU daily to support calcium absorption and bone health.

6. Consume calcium-rich foods or supplements to maintain strong bones and support joint function; adults need 1000-1200 mg of calcium daily.

7. Stay hydrated by drinking plenty of water throughout the day, as proper hydration is crucial for maintaining the health of synovial fluid that lubricates the joints.

Variations: For those who prefer not to consume fish or animal products, omega-3s can also be obtained from algae-based supplements, and calcium needs can be met through fortified plant-based foods. Turmeric and ginger can be taken in capsule form for those who do not enjoy their flavors.

Storage tips: Keep supplements in a cool, dry place. Fresh ingredients like ginger and turmeric should be stored in the refrigerator to prolong their freshness.

Tips for allergens: Individuals with allergies to seafood can opt for flaxseed or algae-based omega-3 supplements. Those with lactose intolerance or dairy allergies can choose calcium-fortified plant milks and juices as alternatives.

Scientific references: Studies have shown the effectiveness of omega-3 fatty acids in reducing joint inflammation, as documented in the Journal of the American College of Nutrition. The anti-inflammatory properties of turmeric and its active component curcumin have been extensively researched, with findings published in the Journal of Medicinal Food.

The benefits of ginger on joint health are supported by research in the journal Arthritis and Rheumatism, highlighting its role in reducing pain and inflammation. The importance of adequate hydration for joint health is discussed in the European Journal of Clinical Nutrition, emphasizing the role of water in maintaining synovial fluid health.

By following Dr. Barbara's approach to maintaining joint flexibility, individuals can take proactive steps towards enhancing their joint health through natural and holistic means. This comprehensive strategy supports the body's innate healing processes and promotes a more active, pain-free lifestyle.

CHAPTER 2: NUTRITION FOR STRONG BONES AND JOINTS

Maintaining strong bones and joints is essential for a lifetime of mobility and health, and nutrition plays a pivotal role in achieving this. The foundation of bone health begins with a well-balanced diet rich in certain key nutrients that are vital for bone formation and maintenance. Calcium is perhaps the most well-known of these nutrients, being the primary mineral found in your bones. Including a variety of calcium-rich foods in your diet, such as dairy products, leafy green vegetables, and fortified foods, can help ensure that your bones have the calcium they need to remain strong.

However, calcium cannot work in isolation. Vitamin D is crucial for calcium absorption in the body. Without adequate vitamin D, our bodies cannot absorb calcium effectively, which can lead to weakened bones and an increased risk of fractures. Sources of vitamin D include fatty fish, egg yolks, and sunlight exposure, but considering the difficulty many people have in obtaining enough vitamin D from diet and sunlight alone, fortified foods and supplements may also be necessary.

Another key nutrient for bone health is magnesium. This mineral is involved in converting vitamin D into its active form in the body, which in turn helps in calcium absorption. Magnesium-rich foods include nuts, seeds, whole grains, and green leafy vegetables. Incorporating these foods into your diet can support bone health and complement the effects of calcium and vitamin D.

Phosphorus, found in protein-rich foods like meat, poultry, fish, and dairy products, works closely with calcium to build strong bones and teeth. However, balance is key, as too much phosphorus with too little calcium can lead to bone loss.

For joint health, omega-3 fatty acids are known for their anti-inflammatory properties, which can help reduce pain and stiffness in the joints. Foods high in omega-3s, such as salmon, flaxseeds, and walnuts, should be a regular part of a diet aimed at maintaining joint health.

In addition to these nutrients, a diet rich in fruits and vegetables can provide antioxidants that help protect bone cells from damage. This includes vitamin C, which is not only a powerful antioxidant but also plays a role in the formation of collagen, a key component of cartilage that supports joints.

Incorporating these nutrients into your daily diet can be simple with a little planning. For breakfast, consider a bowl of fortified cereal with milk or a plant-based alternative, topped with sliced strawberries for a boost of vitamin C. A lunch of grilled salmon over a bed of leafy greens, dressed with a vinaigrette made with flaxseed oil, provides a hearty dose of omega-3s, calcium, and vitamin D. For dinner, a stir-fry featuring tofu, broccoli, and almonds can cover your bases for calcium, magnesium, and more. Snacks of yogurt, nuts, and seeds throughout the day can further contribute to your nutrient intake for bone and joint health.

As we continue to explore the role of nutrition in supporting bone and joint health, it's clear that a diverse diet rich in these key nutrients can lay the foundation for a lifetime of mobility and wellness.

Building on the essential nutrients for bone and joint health, it's important to highlight the role of Vitamin K in this equation. Vitamin K is crucial for bone metabolism and helps the body in the utilization of calcium. Leafy greens like kale, spinach, and collard greens are excellent sources of Vitamin K. Incorporating these vegetables into your diet not only supports bone density but also contributes to overall health with their high fiber content and plethora of vitamins and minerals.

Silicon, a lesser-known but equally vital mineral for bone health, supports bone formation and helps maintain the strength and flexibility of bones and joints. Foods rich in silicon include bananas, green beans, and whole grains. Adding these foods to your diet can provide the silicon your body needs for optimal bone health.

Boron is another trace mineral that plays a significant role in bone health by helping to retain calcium in the bones. Avocados, nuts, and dried fruits are good sources of boron and can easily be incorporated into meals or consumed as snacks.

For those looking to support their joint health specifically, incorporating foods rich in sulfur can be beneficial. Sulfur is necessary for the formation of connective tissue and helps reduce joint inflammation. Garlic, onions, and eggs are excellent sources of sulfur and can enhance the flavor of various dishes while providing health benefits.

It's also worth noting the importance of maintaining a healthy weight for bone and joint health. Excess weight can put additional pressure on joints, particularly the knees, hips, and spine, leading to increased wear and tear. A diet that includes a balance of the nutrients mentioned, coupled with regular physical activity, can help manage weight and reduce the strain on bones and joints.

Hydration plays a pivotal role in maintaining joint health as well. Adequate water intake ensures that the synovial fluid, which reduces friction in the joints and helps maintain their smooth movement, is at an optimal level. Aim for 8-10 glasses of water a day to stay hydrated and support joint health.

In summary, a comprehensive approach to nutrition that includes a variety of vitamins, minerals, and other nutrients is essential for maintaining strong bones and healthy joints. By incorporating a diverse range of foods into your diet, you can ensure that your body receives the support it needs for mobility and wellness throughout your life. Remember, each meal is an opportunity to nourish your body and support its complex systems, so choose foods that are rich in the nutrients vital for bone and joint health.

CALCIUM AND MAGNESIUM FOR BONE HEALTH

Calcium and magnesium are two minerals essential for bone health, each playing a unique role in maintaining bone density and strength. Calcium is the most abundant mineral in the body, primarily found in the bones and teeth, where it provides structural support. For optimal absorption of calcium, magnesium is crucial as it converts vitamin D into its active form, which in turn enhances calcium absorption in the bones. A deficiency in magnesium can lead to diminished calcium in the bones, weakening them and increasing the risk of osteoporosis.

To ensure you're getting enough calcium, include dairy products like milk, cheese, and yogurt in your diet, as well as leafy greens, almonds, and fortified foods. For magnesium, focus on nuts, seeds, whole grains, and green leafy vegetables. It's important to maintain a balanced intake of these minerals, as too much calcium without adequate magnesium can lead to mineral imbalances and affect bone health.

Incorporating these minerals into your diet can be straightforward. Start your day with a breakfast that includes yogurt or milk and a whole-grain cereal, which is often fortified with both calcium and magnesium. Snack on almonds or make a smoothie with leafy greens like spinach or kale to boost your intake throughout the day. For meals, consider quinoa or brown rice as a side, both of which are good sources of magnesium, and add leafy greens or dairy products to ensure a good supply of calcium.

Remember, while supplements can help fill nutritional gaps, getting these minerals from food sources ensures better absorption and benefits due to the presence of other complementary nutrients. Always consult with a healthcare provider before starting any supplement regimen, especially if you have existing health conditions or concerns about your bone health.

ANTI-INFLAMMATORY FOODS FOR JOINT HEALTH

Incorporating anti-inflammatory foods into your diet is a key strategy for promoting joint health and alleviating symptoms associated with inflammation, such as pain and stiffness. Foods rich in omega-3 fatty acids, such as salmon, mackerel, and flaxseeds, are renowned for their ability to reduce inflammation. These fatty acids help in decreasing the production of molecules and substances linked to inflammation, such as inflammatory eicosanoids and cytokines.

Another powerful anti-inflammatory food is turmeric, which contains curcumin, a compound that has been shown to reduce inflammation in the body. Curcumin's effectiveness is enhanced when paired with black pepper, which contains piperine, a substance that increases the absorption of curcumin by the body.

Ginger is also beneficial for joint health due to its anti-inflammatory and antioxidant properties. It can reduce inflammation by inhibiting the synthesis of pro-inflammatory cytokines and chemokines in the cells.

Berries, such as strawberries, blueberries, and blackberries, are packed with antioxidants and vitamins that can help fight inflammation. The antioxidants in berries, particularly anthocyanins, have been shown to reduce inflammation and decrease the risk of disease.

Leafy green vegetables like spinach, kale, and collard greens are high in antioxidants and polyphenols, which are protective compounds that can reduce inflammation.

Incorporating these anti-inflammatory foods into your diet can be simple and delicious. For example, start your day with a smoothie made with berries, spinach, and flaxseed oil. For lunch or dinner, consider a salad topped with grilled salmon or a turmeric and ginger-infused stir-fry. Snacking on a handful of nuts or seeds can also provide anti-inflammatory benefits throughout the day.

By focusing on these anti-inflammatory foods, you can support your joint health naturally and potentially reduce your reliance on medications for inflammation and pain relief. Remember, a balanced diet rich in a variety of nutrients is the best approach to maintaining overall health and well-being.

THE ROLE OF VITAMIN D IN BONE STRENGTH

Vitamin D plays a pivotal role in maintaining bone strength and health, acting as a key facilitator for calcium absorption in the bones. Without sufficient vitamin D, the body struggles to absorb calcium from the diet, which can lead to weakened bones and an increased risk of fractures. This vitamin is unique because the body can synthesize it when the skin is exposed to sunlight, yet many individuals may still find themselves deficient due to limited sun exposure or dietary intake.

For optimal bone health, it's crucial to ensure adequate levels of vitamin D. The body's ability to produce vitamin D from sunlight varies depending on several factors, including skin color, age, geographic location, and time of year. For those living in northern latitudes or for individuals with darker skin, the production of vitamin D can be significantly reduced, making dietary sources and supplements more important.

Fatty fish such as salmon, mackerel, and sardines are among the best natural food sources of vitamin D. Egg yolks and liver also contain smaller amounts, and many foods, such as milk, orange juice, and cereals, are fortified with vitamin D to help meet daily requirements. For individuals who may not get enough vitamin D through sunlight or diet alone, supplements can be an effective way to ensure adequate intake. The recommended dietary allowance (RDA) for vitamin D varies by age, but for most adults, it's 600 to 800 IU per day, with higher amounts recommended for older adults to support bone health.

Vitamin D's role extends beyond just aiding in calcium absorption; it also helps in bone remodeling, a natural process where old bone tissue is broken down and new bone tissue is formed. Adequate levels of vitamin D can help maintain bone density and reduce the risk of osteoporosis and bone fractures in older adults.

To incorporate more vitamin D into your diet, consider starting your day with a vitamin D-fortified cereal or oatmeal, accompanied by a glass of fortified orange juice. Including fatty fish in your meals two to three times a week can also boost your vitamin D intake. For those considering supplements, it's important to discuss with a healthcare provider to determine the appropriate dosage and to avoid exceeding the safe upper intake level, as too much vitamin D can lead to health issues.

Maintaining a healthy level of vitamin D is a key component of a holistic approach to bone health. Alongside other bone-friendly nutrients like calcium and magnesium, vitamin D supports a strong skeletal structure, enabling a lifetime of mobility and wellness. Regular physical activity and weight-bearing exercises further complement the benefits of vitamin D, enhancing bone density and strength. By ensuring a balanced intake of this essential vitamin, either through diet, sensible sun exposure, or supplements, you can support your body's needs and promote optimal bone health.

BUILDING A BONE-HEALTHY DIET

To build a bone-healthy diet, focus on integrating a variety of foods rich in key nutrients that support bone density and strength. This includes not only calcium and vitamin D, which are fundamental for bone health, but also a broader spectrum of vitamins and minerals that play a crucial role in maintaining bone integrity and overall health.

Incorporate foods high in Vitamin K2, such as natto, dairy products, especially fermented ones, and egg yolks. Vitamin K2 is essential for bone metabolism and works by activating proteins that bind calcium to bones and teeth. It also prevents calcium from being deposited in the arteries, thus supporting cardiovascular health alongside bone health.

Manganese is another critical nutrient for bone formation; it aids in the formation of bone cartilage and bone collagen and is involved in the mineralization of bone. Whole grains, legumes, nuts, and seeds are excellent sources of manganese. Including these in your daily diet can help ensure adequate intake for bone health.

Zinc plays a vital role in bone growth and in the process of bone regeneration and repair. Foods rich in zinc include beef, shrimp, spinach, flaxseeds, pumpkin seeds, and oysters. Regular consumption of these foods can contribute to maintaining strong bones.

Copper, though needed in smaller amounts, is crucial for the maintenance of collagen and elastin, major structural components of our bodies, including the bones. Sources of copper include organ meats, sesame seeds, cocoa powder, cashews, and lentils. Integrating these foods into meals can help meet your body's copper requirements.

Protein is essential for healthy bones as well, as about 50% of bone is made of protein. Lean meat, poultry, fish, dairy products, legumes, and nuts are all good protein sources. However, it's important to balance protein intake with other nutrients, as excessive protein consumption can lead to calcium loss.

Fruits and vegetables are also key components of a bone-healthy diet. They are rich in vitamins, minerals, and antioxidants that can help protect bone cells from damage. Moreover, fruits and vegetables can improve bone density thanks to their magnesium and potassium content, which helps neutralize acid loads in the body, preserving calcium in bones.

To ensure a bone-healthy diet, consider a daily meal plan that includes a variety of these nutrient-rich foods. For breakfast, a serving of Greek yogurt with almonds and berries can provide calcium, protein, and antioxidants. A mid-morning snack of a hard-boiled egg or a small serving of natto can introduce Vitamin K2. Lunch could consist of a leafy green salad with chickpeas, sunflower seeds, and slices of grilled chicken for a mix of manganese, zinc, and protein. An afternoon snack of carrot sticks and hummus offers a crunchy way to consume more vitamins and minerals beneficial for bone health. For dinner, a piece of salmon with a side of quinoa and steamed broccoli can cover your needs for omega-3 fatty acids, magnesium, and Vitamin K.

Staying hydrated is essential for overall health and aids in the maintenance of healthy joints and the prevention of osteoporosis. Water is the best choice for staying hydrated, and incorporating herbal teas can also contribute to your fluid intake while offering additional antioxidants.

By focusing on a diet rich in these nutrients, not only can you support your bone health, but you can also enjoy a wide range of flavors and textures, making your meals both nutritious and delicious. Remember, the key to a healthy diet is variety and balance, ensuring that you get all the necessary nutrients to support bone health and overall well-being.

CHAPTER 3: NATURAL BONE & JOINT REMEDIES

Natural remedies for bone and joint health offer a complementary approach to maintaining mobility and reducing discomfort without relying solely on pharmaceuticals. These remedies focus on utilizing herbs, supplements, and lifestyle changes to support the body's inherent healing processes and promote overall well-being.

Beneficial effects: The remedies outlined here aim to reduce inflammation, support bone density, alleviate pain, and enhance joint flexibility. They can be particularly beneficial for individuals experiencing arthritis, osteoporosis, or general joint discomfort.

Herbal Remedies for Bone Health

1. Horsetail (Equisetum arvense)

Ingredients: Dried horsetail, boiling water

Instructions: Steep 1-2 teaspoons of dried horsetail in a cup of boiling water for 10 minutes. Strain and drink 1-2 times daily. Horsetail is rich in silicon, a mineral essential for bone formation and health.

- **Variations:** Combine with nettle tea for added mineral content.

- **Storage tips:** Store dried horsetail in a cool, dry place away from sunlight.

- **Tips for allergens:** Individuals with allergies to nicotine should proceed with caution when using horsetail.

2. Nettle (Urtica dioica)

Ingredients: Dried nettle leaves, boiling water

Instructions: Add 1 tablespoon of dried nettle leaves to a cup of boiling water. Steep for 10 minutes, strain, and drink up to 3 times daily. Nettle is known for its high mineral content, including calcium, which is vital for bone strength.

- **Variations:** Mix with peppermint leaves for a refreshing flavor.

- **Storage tips:** Keep dried nettle leaves in an airtight container in a dark, dry place.

Herbal Remedies for Joint Health

1. Turmeric (Curcuma longa) and Black Pepper

Ingredients: 1 teaspoon of turmeric powder, a pinch of black pepper, 1 cup of milk or a milk alternative

Instructions: Heat the milk gently, stir in the turmeric and black pepper. Drink once daily. Curcumin in turmeric and piperine in black pepper work together to reduce joint inflammation and pain.

- **Variations:** Add honey for sweetness.

- **Storage tips:** Store turmeric and black pepper in airtight containers in a cool, dark place.

- **Tips for allergens:** Use a milk alternative for those with lactose intolerance.

2. Ginger (Zingiber officinale)

Ingredients: Fresh ginger root, boiling water

Instructions: Slice a 2-inch piece of fresh ginger root and add to boiling water. Simmer for 10-15 minutes. Drink the tea 2-3 times daily. Ginger's anti-inflammatory properties can help reduce joint pain and stiffness.

- **Variations:** Add lemon or honey for flavor.

- **Storage tips:** Fresh ginger can be stored in the refrigerator; dried ginger should be kept in an airtight container in a cool, dark place.

Supplements for Bone and Joint Health

1. Omega-3 Fatty Acids

  - Found in fish oil supplements, omega-3s are anti-inflammatory and can help reduce joint pain.

2. Vitamin D

  - Essential for calcium absorption and bone health. Supplements may be necessary for individuals with limited sun exposure.

3. Magnesium

  - Supports bone density and is involved in over 300 biochemical reactions in the body. Magnesium supplements can complement dietary intake.

Lifestyle Changes

- **Exercise**: Regular, low-impact exercise such as walking, swimming, or yoga can improve joint flexibility and bone density.

- **Diet**: A balanced diet rich in fruits, vegetables, lean proteins, and healthy fats supports overall health and can reduce inflammation.

- **Hydration**: Adequate water intake is crucial for joint lubrication and nutrient transport.

Scientific references:

- Studies have shown that turmeric and ginger can significantly reduce symptoms of arthritis (Journal of Medicinal Food, 2016).

- Research indicates that omega-3 fatty acids can decrease joint pain and stiffness in rheumatoid arthritis patients (Arthritis & Rheumatology, 2015).

- Vitamin D's role in bone health is well-documented, with deficiencies linked to increased risk of fractures and osteoporosis (Osteoporosis International, 2012).

By integrating these natural remedies and lifestyle changes, individuals can support their bone and joint health, potentially reducing the need for pharmaceutical interventions and enhancing their quality of life.

CHAPTER 4: HERBAL REMEDIES FOR BONES AND JOINTS

WHITE WILLOW BARK TEA

Beneficial effects

White Willow Bark Tea is known for its natural pain-relieving properties, making it an effective remedy for reducing discomfort associated with bone and joint health issues such as arthritis and osteoarthritis. The active compound in white willow bark, salicin, acts similarly to aspirin by reducing inflammation and pain without the harsh side effects often associated with synthetic pain relievers. This herbal tea can also help alleviate headaches, muscle pain, and reduce fevers, supporting overall well-being.

Portions

2 servings

Preparation time

5 minutes

Cooking time

15 minutes

Ingredients

- 2 teaspoons of dried white willow bark

- 2 cups of water

- Honey or lemon (optional, for taste)

Instructions

1. Bring 2 cups of water to a boil in a small pot.

2. Add 2 teaspoons of dried white willow bark to the boiling water.

3. Reduce the heat and simmer for 10 to 15 minutes, allowing the active compounds to be released.

4. Strain the tea into cups, discarding the used white willow bark.

5. Optional: Add honey or lemon to taste for flavor enhancement.

6. Serve the tea warm, ideally twice a day, to manage pain and inflammation.

Variations

- For added anti-inflammatory benefits, include a piece of fresh ginger or turmeric in the tea while it simmers.

- Combine with peppermint leaves during the last few minutes of simmering for a refreshing flavor and additional pain-relieving properties.

- To enhance the soothing effects, blend with chamomile flowers in equal parts.

Storage tips

Store any leftover White Willow Bark Tea in a sealed container in the refrigerator for up to 2 days. Reheat gently on the stove or enjoy chilled.

Tips for allergens

Individuals with allergies to salicylates (found in aspirin) should avoid white willow bark. For those avoiding honey due to dietary preferences or allergies, substitute with maple syrup or simply omit the sweetener.

Scientific references

- "The analgesic and anti-inflammatory effects of Salix alba L. bark extract" in the Journal of Ethnopharmacology, 2009. This study highlights the effectiveness of white willow bark in treating pain and inflammation.

- "Willow bark extract: the contribution of polyphenols to the overall effect" in the journal Wiener Medizinische Wochenschrift, 2013. This research discusses the role of polyphenols in white willow bark, contributing to its anti-inflammatory and analgesic properties.

BOSWELLIA SERRATA EXTRACT

Beneficial effects

Boswellia Serrata Extract is renowned for its powerful anti-inflammatory and pain-relieving properties, making it an excellent natural remedy for supporting bone and joint health. It can significantly reduce pain and improve mobility in conditions such as osteoarthritis and rheumatoid arthritis by inhibiting inflammatory markers in the body. Additionally, Boswellia Serrata is known to prevent cartilage loss and inhibit the autoimmune process, contributing to healthier joints and bones.

Ingredients

- 1 cup of dried Boswellia Serrata resin
- 2 cups of high-proof alcohol (such as vodka or brandy)
- A clean glass jar with a tight-fitting lid

Instructions

1. Place the dried Boswellia Serrata resin into the clean glass jar.

2. Pour the high-proof alcohol over the resin, ensuring that it is completely submerged. Leave about an inch of space at the top of the jar.

3. Seal the jar tightly with the lid and label it with the date and contents.

4. Store the jar in a cool, dark place for 4 to 6 weeks. Shake the jar gently every few days to mix the contents and promote extraction.

5. After the infusion period, strain the extract through a fine mesh sieve or cheesecloth into another clean, dark glass bottle. Press or squeeze the resin to extract as much liquid as possible.

6. Label the bottle with the date and contents.

Variations

- For those sensitive to alcohol, a glycerin-based tincture can be made by substituting the alcohol with a mixture of glycerin and water (3 parts glycerin to 1 part water), though this may result in a less potent extract.

- To enhance the anti-inflammatory properties, combine the Boswellia Serrata tincture with turmeric extract during the preparation.

Storage tips

Store the Boswellia Serrata Extract in a cool, dark place. When stored properly in an airtight container, it can last for up to 5 years.

Tips for allergens

Individuals with allergies to Boswellia Serrata or similar botanicals should consult with a healthcare provider before using this extract. As always, start with a small dose to ensure no adverse reactions.

Scientific references

- "Boswellia Serrata, A Potential Antiinflammatory Agent: An Overview" published in the Indian Journal of Pharmaceutical Sciences, 2011. This study discusses the anti-inflammatory and analgesic properties of Boswellia Serrata, supporting its use for bone and joint health.

- "Effects of Boswellia Serrata Gum Resin in Patients with Osteoarthritis" published in Arthritis Research & Therapy, 2003. This research highlights the effectiveness of Boswellia Serrata in reducing pain and improving physical function in patients with osteoarthritis.

TURMERIC AND BLACK PEPPER GOLDEN MILK

Beneficial effects

Turmeric and Black Pepper Golden Milk is a traditional remedy known for its anti-inflammatory and antioxidant properties, making it an excellent choice for supporting bone and joint health. The active ingredient in turmeric, curcumin, has been shown to reduce symptoms of arthritis and is beneficial in the treatment of joint pain and inflammation. Black pepper contains piperine, which enhances the absorption of curcumin, making this combination particularly potent. Additionally, the inclusion of milk (dairy or plant-based) provides calcium and vitamin D, essential nutrients for bone strength and health.

Portions

2 servings

Preparation time

5 minutes

Cooking time

10 minutes

Ingredients

- 2 cups of milk (dairy or any plant-based alternative like almond, coconut, or soy milk)

- 1 teaspoon turmeric powder

- 1/4 teaspoon ground black pepper

- 1 tablespoon honey or maple syrup (optional, for sweetness)

- 1/2 teaspoon cinnamon (optional, for flavor)

- 1 teaspoon virgin coconut oil or ghee (for fat content to enhance curcumin absorption)

Instructions

1. In a small saucepan, combine the milk, turmeric powder, ground black pepper, and cinnamon if using. Heat the mixture over medium heat until it starts to simmer. Do not allow it to boil.

2. Reduce the heat and add the coconut oil or ghee, stirring until it is fully integrated into the mixture.

3. Continue to simmer for about 5 to 10 minutes, stirring occasionally, allowing the flavors to meld together.

4. Remove from heat and let it cool slightly. Stir in honey or maple syrup to sweeten, if desired.

5. Strain the mixture using a fine mesh strainer to remove any large particles and pour into mugs.

6. Serve warm and enjoy immediately.

Variations

- For a vegan version, use plant-based milk and maple syrup as the sweetener.

- Add a piece of fresh ginger while simmering to enhance the anti-inflammatory benefits.

- Sprinkle with a pinch of nutmeg or cardamom before serving for additional flavor complexity.

Storage tips

Golden Milk is best enjoyed fresh, but if you have leftovers, store them in an airtight container in the refrigerator for up to 2 days. Reheat gently on the stove, stirring well before serving.

Tips for allergens

For those with lactose intolerance or dairy allergies, any plant-based milk can be used as a substitute. Ensure to use pure turmeric and black pepper to avoid any additives that may cause allergic reactions.

Scientific references

- "Curcumin: A Review of Its' Effects on Human Health," published in Foods, 2017. This study discusses the health benefits of curcumin, including its anti-inflammatory and antioxidant effects.

- "Influence of Piperine on the Pharmacokinetics of Curcumin in Animals and Human Volunteers," published in Planta Medica, 1998. This research highlights the importance of piperine in enhancing the bioavailability of curcumin.

DEVIL'S CLAW ROOT INFUSION

Beneficial effects

Devil's Claw Root Infusion is recognized for its anti-inflammatory and analgesic properties, making it an effective natural remedy for relieving pain and discomfort associated with bone and joint health issues such as arthritis and back pain. The active compounds in devil's claw, particularly harpagoside, have been shown to reduce inflammation and pain in the joints, improving mobility and quality of life for those suffering from these conditions.

Ingredients

- 1 tablespoon dried devil's claw root

- 2 cups water

Instructions

1. Bring 2 cups of water to a boil in a small pot.

2. Add 1 tablespoon of dried devil's claw root to the boiling water.

3. Reduce the heat and simmer for about 20 minutes to allow the devil's claw to infuse the water.

4. After simmering, remove the pot from the heat and let it cool slightly.

5. Strain the infusion into a cup or container, discarding the used devil's claw root.

6. The Devil's Claw Root Infusion is now ready to be consumed. Drink it warm or at room temperature.

Variations

- For added flavor and additional anti-inflammatory benefits, include a slice of fresh ginger or turmeric in the infusion process.

- Sweeten the infusion with honey or stevia if desired, to improve taste without compromising the health benefits.

- Combine with peppermint tea to enhance the soothing effects and add a refreshing flavor.

Storage tips

If you have leftover Devil's Claw Root Infusion, it can be stored in a sealed container in the refrigerator for up to 2 days. Reheat gently on the stove or enjoy cold, as preferred.

Tips for allergens

Individuals with a sensitivity to devil's claw should start with a small amount to ensure no adverse reactions. For those avoiding honey as a sweetener due to allergies or dietary preferences, stevia serves as a suitable alternative.

Scientific references

- "Efficacy and tolerability of a standardized extract from Harpagophytum procumbens in patients with chronic non-radicular back pain" published in Phytotherapy Research, 2001. This study supports the use of devil's claw in managing back pain through its analgesic and anti-inflammatory properties.

- "A systematic review on the Rosa canina effect and efficacy profiles" in Phytotherapy Research, 2008. While focusing on rosehip, this review also acknowledges the importance of herbal remedies like devil's claw in managing inflammation and pain associated with joint diseases.

HORSETAIL AND NETTLE BONE STRENGTH SMOOTHIE

Beneficial effects

The Horsetail and Nettle Bone Strength Smoothie is crafted to support bone health and density, leveraging the rich mineral content of horsetail and nettle. Horsetail is abundant in silica, a crucial component for bone formation and regeneration, while nettle is high in calcium, magnesium, and vitamin K, all essential nutrients for maintaining bone strength and preventing osteoporosis. This smoothie is an excellent natural remedy for enhancing bone health, promoting joint flexibility, and aiding in the recovery of bone-related injuries.

Portions

2 servings

Preparation time

10 minutes

Ingredients

- 1 cup fresh nettle leaves (or 1 tablespoon dried nettle leaves)

- 1 cup fresh horsetail shoots (or 1 tablespoon dried horsetail)

- 1 ripe banana

- 1 cup almond milk

- 1 tablespoon chia seeds

- 1/2 teaspoon vanilla extract

- Honey or maple syrup to taste (optional)

Instructions

1. If using fresh nettle and horsetail, ensure they are thoroughly washed. For dried herbs, measure out the required amount.

2. Place the nettle and horsetail in a blender with a little water and blend until a smooth paste is formed.

3. Add the ripe banana, almond milk, chia seeds, and vanilla extract to the blender.

4. Blend all ingredients on high until the mixture is smooth.

5. Taste the smoothie, and if desired, add honey or maple syrup for sweetness. Blend again briefly to mix.

6. Pour the smoothie into glasses and serve immediately.

Variations

- For an extra protein boost, add a scoop of your favorite protein powder.

- Substitute almond milk with coconut water for a lighter version or soy milk for added protein.

- Add a handful of spinach or kale to increase the smoothie's vitamin and mineral content without significantly altering the taste.

Storage tips

This smoothie is best enjoyed fresh. However, if you need to store it, keep it in an airtight container in the refrigerator for up to 24 hours. Stir well before consuming if separation occurs.

Tips for allergens

Individuals with allergies to nuts can substitute almond milk with oat milk or rice milk. For those sensitive to honey, maple syrup serves as an excellent vegan alternative.

Scientific references

- "Silicon and Bone Health" in the Journal of Nutrition, Health & Aging, 2007. This study discusses the importance of dietary silicon, found in horsetail, for bone health and regeneration.

- "The role of vitamins and minerals in bone health" from the Journal of Clinical Densitometry, 2012. This research highlights the critical roles of calcium, magnesium, and vitamin K, found in nettle, in maintaining bone density and preventing osteoporosis.

PART 13: SKIN HEALTH

Skin health is a reflection of our internal wellness and the balance of nutrients we provide our bodies. A radiant complexion begins with the foods we eat and extends to the care we provide our skin externally. The skin, being the largest organ of the body, serves as a protective barrier against environmental damage, regulates temperature, and plays a crucial role in detoxification. To support skin health, it's essential to focus on a diet rich in antioxidants, vitamins, and minerals that nourish the skin from within, alongside topical treatments that protect and repair the skin's surface.

Antioxidants play a pivotal role in skin health, combating the effects of free radicals that contribute to aging and skin damage.

Foods high in vitamins C and E, such as citrus fruits, berries, nuts, and seeds, can help protect the skin from the visible signs of aging by promoting collagen production and maintaining skin elasticity. Vitamin C is not only a powerful antioxidant but also essential for the synthesis of collagen, which gives the skin its firmness and strength. Incorporating a variety of these foods into your daily diet can enhance your skin's natural defense system against damage from UV exposure and environmental pollutants.

In addition to vitamins C and E, beta-carotene and selenium are crucial for skin health. Beta-carotene, found in carrots, sweet potatoes, and leafy greens, is converted into vitamin A in the body, which is vital for skin repair and maintenance. Selenium, a mineral found in Brazil nuts, fish, and eggs, supports skin elasticity and protects against oxidative damage. Together, these nutrients can help maintain the skin's integrity and youthful appearance.

Hydration is another key element of skin health. Adequate water intake ensures that the skin remains hydrated and plump, reducing the appearance of fine lines and wrinkles. It also aids in the detoxification process, helping to flush out toxins that can lead to skin issues such as acne and dullness. Aim to drink at least 8-10 glasses of water a day, and consider incorporating hydrating foods like cucumbers, tomatoes, and watermelon into your diet.

Omega-3 fatty acids, found in fatty fish, flaxseeds, and walnuts, are essential for maintaining the skin's lipid barrier, which helps retain moisture and protect against irritants. A diet rich in omega-3s can improve skin texture and reduce inflammation, which is beneficial for conditions such as eczema and psoriasis. Including these healthy fats in your diet can support skin hydration and resilience.

Topical skin care also plays a crucial role in maintaining skin health. Gentle cleansing and moisturizing help preserve the skin's natural oils and protect the barrier function. Using products with natural ingredients such as aloe vera, chamomile, and green tea can soothe and nourish the skin, while sun protection is essential to prevent damage from UV rays. A broad-spectrum sunscreen applied daily can protect the skin from premature aging and the risk of skin cancer.

For those seeking to enhance their skin health through natural remedies, herbal teas offer a wealth of benefits. Teas such as green tea, chamomile, and rooibos are rich in antioxidants and have anti-inflammatory properties that can soothe the skin and reduce redness. Drinking herbal teas regularly can provide internal support for the skin, complementing a balanced diet and topical care regimen.

In exploring the connection between diet, lifestyle, and skin health, it becomes evident that a holistic approach is key to achieving a radiant complexion. Nourishing the body with the right nutrients, staying hydrated, protecting the skin from external damage, and incorporating natural remedies can all contribute to healthy, vibrant skin.

As we delve deeper into the specific nutrients and practices that support skin health, it's important to remember that consistency and balance are essential for lasting results.

Maintaining a balanced intake of essential fatty acids is crucial for skin health, particularly gamma-linolenic acid (GLA), found in evening primrose oil and borage oil. GLA is known for its ability to soothe skin conditions by reducing inflammation and encouraging skin growth and new cell generation. Incorporating supplements or oils rich in GLA can significantly improve skin conditions like eczema and psoriasis, leading to smoother, more resilient skin.

Probiotics, beneficial bacteria found in yogurt, kefir, and fermented foods, play a significant role in skin health by promoting a healthy gut microbiome. A balanced gut microbiome can prevent and treat skin conditions such as acne, rosacea, and even signs of aging by reducing inflammation and oxidative stress in the body. Regular consumption of probiotic-rich foods or supplements can help establish and maintain a healthy gut-skin axis, reflecting positively on the skin's appearance and health.

Zinc is another vital nutrient for skin health, supporting the immune system, and facilitating the healing process. This mineral helps combat acne by regulating oil production and can be found in foods like oysters, lentils, and pumpkin seeds. Ensuring adequate zinc intake can help maintain clear skin and reduce the likelihood of breakout occurrences.

For external skin care, exfoliation is key to removing dead skin cells and promoting cell turnover. Natural exfoliants like sugar or salt mixed with olive or coconut oil can gently exfoliate the skin, leaving it smooth and revitalized.

However, it's important to exfoliate gently to avoid damaging the skin's barrier function and to always follow with moisturization.

Moisturizing with natural oils such as jojoba, argan, or almond oil can deeply hydrate and nourish the skin. These oils mimic the skin's natural sebum, helping to balance oil production and lock in moisture without clogging pores. Applying these oils after bathing can help to seal in moisture and protect the skin from environmental stressors.

The role of sleep in skin health cannot be overstated. During sleep, the body goes into repair mode, regenerating skin cells and collagen. Lack of sleep can lead to increased stress hormones, which may exacerbate skin conditions and accelerate aging. Ensuring 7-9 hours of quality sleep nightly can support skin health, promoting a refreshed and youthful complexion.

Physical activity also benefits the skin by increasing blood flow, which nourishes skin cells and carries away waste products. Exercise can help reduce stress, a common trigger for skin issues, and promote overall well-being. Incorporating regular physical activity into your routine can enhance skin health and vitality.

Finally, managing stress through practices such as yoga, meditation, and mindfulness can have profound effects on skin health.

Stress can trigger or worsen skin conditions like eczema, rosacea, and acne. By incorporating stress-reduction techniques into daily life, individuals can help maintain a healthy complexion and improve their overall quality of life.

In conclusion, achieving and maintaining skin health is a multifaceted endeavor that requires a holistic approach.

By nourishing the body with the right nutrients, practicing good skincare habits, protecting the skin from external damage, and managing stress and sleep, individuals can support their skin's health and radiance. Remember, the journey to healthy skin is a continuous process that involves consistent care and attention to both internal and external factors influencing skin health.

CHAPTER 1: DR. BARBARA'S APPROACH TO SKIN HEALTH

D r. Barbara emphasizes the intrinsic link between internal health and the external radiance of the skin, advocating for a comprehensive approach that combines nutrition, hydration, and natural skincare practices. The foundation of her approach to skin health lies in the belief that a nutrient-rich diet, abundant in antioxidants, vitamins, and minerals, is crucial for nurturing the skin from within. Antioxidants such as vitamins C and E, beta-carotene, and selenium play a vital role in combating oxidative stress and supporting the skin's natural defense system against environmental aggressors like UV radiation and pollution. These nutrients, found in a variety of fruits, vegetables, nuts, and seeds, help in maintaining skin elasticity, promoting collagen production, and preventing signs of aging.

Beneficial effects: A diet rich in antioxidants and essential nutrients helps in reducing inflammation, supporting skin repair, and enhancing the skin's natural glow. Regular consumption of foods high in omega-3 fatty acids, such as fatty fish and flaxseeds, strengthens the skin's lipid barrier, thus retaining moisture and protecting against irritants. This holistic dietary approach, combined with adequate hydration, ensures that the skin remains hydrated, plump, and resilient against the formation of fine lines and wrinkles.

Hydration is another cornerstone of Dr. Barbara's skin health strategy. Drinking at least 8-10 glasses of water daily, complemented by the intake of hydrating foods, plays a critical role in maintaining the skin's moisture balance and aiding in the detoxification process. This not only improves skin texture and appearance but also supports the overall function of the skin as a detoxifying organ.

In addition to internal nourishment, Dr. Barbara advocates for a gentle and natural external skincare regimen. The use of natural ingredients such as aloe vera, chamomile, and green tea for topical application can soothe, nourish, and protect the skin. These ingredients offer anti-inflammatory and healing properties that are beneficial for managing conditions like acne, eczema, and rosacea. Moreover, the importance of sun protection cannot be overstated; applying a broad-spectrum sunscreen daily is essential to prevent premature aging and skin cancer.

Instructions:

1. Incorporate a variety of antioxidant-rich foods into your diet, including berries, citrus fruits, leafy greens, nuts, and seeds.

2. Aim for at least two servings of fatty fish per week and include plant-based sources of omega-3 fatty acids such as flaxseeds and walnuts in your meals.

3. Ensure adequate hydration by drinking water throughout the day and consuming water-rich foods like cucumbers and watermelon.

4. Adopt a natural skincare routine, starting with gentle cleansing and moisturizing with products that contain soothing herbal extracts.

5. Apply a broad-spectrum sunscreen every morning, regardless of the weather, to protect your skin from harmful UV rays.

Variations: For those with specific skin concerns, such as sensitivity or acne, consider incorporating targeted natural remedies like tea tree oil for its antimicrobial properties or rosehip oil for its ability to reduce hyperpigmentation and scars. Always perform a patch test before trying new topical treatments.

Storage tips: Keep your natural skincare products in a cool, dry place away from direct sunlight to preserve their potency and effectiveness.

Tips for allergens: If you have sensitive skin or allergies, opt for hypoallergenic and fragrance-free products. For dietary concerns, substitute any allergenic foods with suitable alternatives that offer similar nutritional benefits.

By adopting Dr. Barbara's holistic approach to skin health, individuals can achieve a balanced and nourishing regimen that supports the skin's natural beauty and resilience. This comprehensive strategy underscores the importance of treating the skin as a reflection of the body's internal health, advocating for a lifestyle that prioritizes nutrition, hydration, and natural care practices.

CHAPTER 2: NUTRITION FOR HEALTHY SKIN

Focusing on nutrition for healthy skin involves understanding the direct impact that certain foods and nutrients have on the skin's condition and appearance. Essential fatty acids, particularly omega-3s, play a crucial role in maintaining the skin's lipid barrier, crucial for hydration and protection against environmental damage. Foods rich in omega-3s, such as salmon, chia seeds, and walnuts, help to reduce inflammation in the skin, which can lead to a decrease in conditions such as acne and eczema. Including these in your daily diet supports the skin's ability to retain moisture, contributing to a smoother, more elastic skin texture.

Antioxidants are another key component of a skin-healthy diet. Vitamins C and E, selenium, and flavonoids protect the skin from oxidative stress caused by free radicals and UV exposure, which can accelerate skin aging and damage. Citrus fruits, berries, nuts, green tea, and dark chocolate are excellent sources of antioxidants. Regular consumption of these foods can aid in the repair of damaged skin cells and the production of collagen, essential for skin strength and elasticity.

Zinc is vital for skin health, supporting the immune system and playing a role in the skin's ability to heal and regenerate. Zinc's anti-inflammatory properties can help manage acne by regulating oil production. Foods high in zinc include oysters, lentils, and pumpkin seeds. Ensuring an adequate intake of zinc can contribute to reducing the incidence of acne breakouts and promoting a clearer complexion.

Probiotics and prebiotics also contribute to skin health by supporting gut health. A healthy gut microbiome can influence the skin positively by reducing inflammation and the severity of skin conditions such as acne and rosacea. Fermented foods like yogurt, kefir, and sauerkraut, along with high-fiber foods that act as prebiotics, such as garlic, onions, and bananas, help to maintain a balanced gut microbiome.

Hydration is fundamental for healthy skin. Water helps to flush toxins from the body and keeps the skin cells hydrated and plump, reducing the appearance of wrinkles and fine lines. Aim to drink at least 8-10 glasses of water daily, and include water-rich foods like cucumbers, tomatoes, and watermelon in your diet to help meet your hydration needs.

Beneficial effects: This dietary approach is designed to reduce inflammation, support skin repair and hydration, and protect against environmental damage, leading to improved skin texture, reduced signs of aging, and a decrease in acne and other skin conditions.

Ingredients:

- Omega-3 rich foods: Salmon, chia seeds, walnuts

- Antioxidant-rich foods: Citrus fruits, berries, nuts, green tea, dark chocolate

- Zinc-rich foods: Oysters, lentils, pumpkin seeds

- Probiotic and prebiotic foods: Yogurt, kefir, sauerkraut, garlic, onions, bananas

- Hydration: Water, cucumbers, tomatoes, watermelon

Instructions:

1. Incorporate a serving of omega-3 rich foods into your diet daily to support the skin's lipid barrier.

2. Aim for at least five servings of antioxidant-rich fruits and vegetables each day to protect against oxidative stress.

3. Include zinc-rich foods in your meals to help regulate oil production and enhance skin healing.

4. Consume probiotic and prebiotic foods regularly to support gut health and reduce inflammation.

5. Stay hydrated by drinking at least 8-10 glasses of water daily and including water-rich foods in your diet.

Variations: For vegetarians or those with dietary restrictions, flaxseeds and hemp seeds can replace fish as a source of omega-3s, and zinc can be obtained from plant sources like beans and nuts. Probiotic supplements can substitute for dairy-based probiotics.

Storage tips: Keep nuts and seeds in a cool, dry place to preserve their fatty acids. Store perishable items like salmon and yogurt in the refrigerator.

Tips for allergens: For those allergic to nuts, seeds like chia and hemp can provide essential fatty acids without the allergen risk. Lactose-intolerant individuals can opt for lactose-free kefir or probiotic supplements.

By focusing on these key nutrients and maintaining proper hydration, you can support your skin's health from the inside out, promoting a radiant and youthful complexion.

SKIN-NOURISHING FOODS

Eating a diet rich in vitamins, minerals, and antioxidants is crucial for maintaining healthy skin. Foods high in vitamins C and E, selenium, and omega-3 fatty acids can protect the skin from damage caused by the sun, pollution, and other environmental factors. These nutrients also play a role in repairing skin cells and reducing inflammation, leading to a smoother, healthier complexion. For vibrant skin, incorporate a variety of fruits, vegetables, nuts, seeds, and fatty fish into your diet.

Vitamin C is a powerful antioxidant that helps in the production of collagen, a protein that keeps the skin firm and elastic. Foods rich in vitamin C include oranges, strawberries, bell peppers, and broccoli. Vitamin E, another antioxidant, helps protect the skin from damage and supports skin health. Almonds, sunflower seeds, and avocados are excellent sources of vitamin E.

Selenium is a mineral that aids in the protection of the skin from UV damage and supports overall skin health. Brazil nuts, whole wheat bread, and seafood like shrimp and salmon are good sources of selenium. Omega-3 fatty acids, found in fatty fish such as salmon, mackerel, and sardines, as well as in flaxseeds and walnuts, help maintain the skin's lipid barrier, crucial for keeping the skin hydrated and plump.

Including these skin-nourishing foods in your diet can not only improve the appearance and health of your skin but also support your overall well-being. Remember, a balanced diet rich in a variety of nutrients is the most beneficial for skin health. Hydration also plays a key role, so ensure you drink plenty of water throughout the day to support the health of your skin and your entire body.

THE ROLE OF ANTIOXIDANTS IN SKIN HEALTH

Antioxidants play a pivotal role in maintaining skin health by neutralizing free radicals, which are unstable molecules that can cause cellular damage, including to skin cells. This damage can lead to premature aging, wrinkles, and increased vulnerability to sun damage. Antioxidants provide a protective barrier against environmental stressors such as pollution and UV radiation, both of which can accelerate the aging process and harm the skin in significant ways.

The skin benefits from antioxidants not only through direct application in the form of skincare products but also internally through a diet rich in antioxidant-containing foods. Vitamins A, C, and E are among the most beneficial antioxidants for skin health. Vitamin A, or retinol, is crucial for skin repair and maintenance. Foods high in beta-carotene, which the body converts into vitamin A, include carrots, sweet potatoes, and leafy greens. Vitamin C, found abundantly in citrus fruits, strawberries, and bell peppers, is vital for collagen production, helping to keep the skin firm and reducing the appearance of fine lines. Vitamin E, present in nuts and seeds, supports skin moisture and strength, providing a defense mechanism against skin damage from UV exposure.

Another powerful antioxidant, selenium, supports skin elasticity and protects against oxidative damage. Selenium can be found in Brazil nuts, seafood, and whole grains. Omega-3 fatty acids, though not antioxidants themselves, support the skin's ability to fight inflammation and can be found in fatty fish, flaxseeds, and walnuts. These nutrients help in maintaining the integrity of the skin barrier, promoting hydration, and reducing the risk of acne and other skin conditions.

Incorporating a variety of these antioxidants into your diet can significantly improve your skin's health and appearance.

For instance, starting your day with a smoothie made from berries, spinach, and a handful of nuts can provide a potent antioxidant boost. Snacking on citrus fruits or incorporating vegetables like bell peppers and broccoli into meals can further enhance your skin's antioxidant defense system.

It's also beneficial to apply antioxidants topically through skincare products containing vitamins C and E, which can directly combat signs of aging and damage from environmental stressors. When antioxidants are applied to the skin, they can prevent the formation of free radicals that occur after exposure to UV light or pollution, reducing inflammation and promoting an even skin tone.

To maximize the benefits of antioxidants for the skin, it's essential to maintain a consistent skincare routine that includes sunscreen to protect against UV radiation, a known producer of free radicals. Hydration, both through drinking water and using moisturizing products, further supports the skin's health, allowing it to better utilize the antioxidants consumed through diet or applied topically.

By understanding the role of antioxidants in skin health and making conscious choices to include them in your diet and skincare routine, you can significantly enhance your skin's appearance, resilience, and overall health.

HEALTHY FATS FOR SKIN ELASTICITY

Healthy fats are essential for maintaining skin elasticity, providing the building blocks for healthy cell membranes which in turn help keep the skin hydrated, plump, and youthful. These fats, particularly omega-3 and omega-6 fatty acids, play a crucial role in the skin's lipid layer, aiding in hydration retention and offering protection against environmental damage. Avocados, rich in monounsaturated fats, not only help in maintaining moisture in the epidermal layer of the skin but also contain vitamins E and C, which are vital for healthy skin.

Similarly, nuts and seeds like almonds, walnuts, flaxseeds, and chia seeds are excellent sources of omega-3 fatty acids, which reduce inflammation in the body, including the skin, and support skin elasticity.

Incorporating fatty fish such as salmon, mackerel, and sardines into your diet is another way to boost your intake of omega-3 fatty acids. These fish are not only beneficial for heart health but also for the skin's appearance, aiding in the reduction of inflammation and supporting the skin's structural integrity. For vegetarians or those who prefer not to eat fish, algae-based supplements are a viable alternative to ensure adequate omega-3 intake.

Olive oil, another healthy fat, is packed with antioxidants and monounsaturated fats, making it an excellent choice for maintaining skin health. Its antioxidant properties help combat free radicals, reducing oxidative stress on the skin, which can lead to premature aging. Cooking with olive oil or using it in salad dressings can easily increase your intake of this beneficial fat.

It's important to balance the intake of omega-3 and omega-6 fatty acids, as too much omega-6 can lead to inflammation, potentially harming the skin. Most diets are high in omega-6 due to the consumption of processed foods and vegetable oils.

Focusing on whole, unprocessed foods and incorporating sources of omega-3 fatty acids can help maintain this balance, supporting skin health and elasticity.

Remember, while healthy fats are beneficial for the skin, moderation is key. Including a variety of fat sources in your diet ensures you receive a broad spectrum of nutrients necessary for maintaining skin elasticity and overall health. Hydration, alongside a balanced diet rich in healthy fats, vitamins, and minerals, creates the foundation for a radiant complexion and resilient skin.

AVOIDING FOODS THAT HARM THE SKIN

To maintain healthy skin, it's crucial to be mindful of consuming foods that can cause harm or exacerbate skin conditions. Foods high in sugars and refined carbohydrates can lead to a spike in insulin levels, which may trigger a hormonal cascade that can exacerbate acne and inflammation. Limiting sugary snacks, beverages, and refined goods like white bread and pasta can help manage these skin issues.

Dairy products, particularly skim milk, have been linked to acne in some individuals. Theories suggest that hormones present in milk may play a role in acne development. If you notice a correlation between dairy intake and skin flare-ups, consider reducing dairy consumption or opting for plant-based alternatives to see if your skin condition improves.

Highly processed and fried foods contain trans fats and oils that can promote inflammation throughout the body, including the skin.

This inflammation can manifest as acne, eczema, and other skin conditions. Opting for cooking methods such as baking, steaming, or grilling and choosing whole, unprocessed foods can support skin health.

Alcohol and caffeine are diuretics that can lead to dehydration, impacting the skin's ability to retain moisture. This can result in dry, lackluster skin. Moderating alcohol and caffeine intake while increasing water consumption can help maintain skin hydration and vitality.

Lastly, foods high in sodium, such as processed snacks and fast foods, can lead to water retention and puffiness, particularly around the eyes. Reducing sodium intake and choosing fresh, whole foods can help alleviate these effects and support overall skin health.

By being mindful of these dietary choices and observing how your skin responds to certain foods, you can tailor your diet to support not just your skin health but your overall well-being.

CHAPTER 3: NATURAL SKIN CARE PRACTICES

Embracing natural skin care practices involves integrating habits and remedies that nourish, protect, and rejuvenate the skin without relying on harsh chemicals or synthetic products. The focus is on leveraging the healing power of nature to maintain skin health and address various skin concerns effectively. Here, we delve into practical, natural strategies for skin care that can be easily incorporated into daily routines.

Beneficial effects: Natural skin care practices offer a myriad of benefits, including reducing exposure to harmful chemicals, supporting the skin's natural barrier, providing essential nutrients for skin repair and maintenance, and minimizing the environmental impact of skin care products.

Daily Cleansing with Natural Ingredients

1. **Ingredients**:

- Honey: Natural antibacterial and moisturizing properties.

- Coconut oil: Helps remove dirt and makeup while hydrating the skin.

2. **Instructions**:

- Mix a tablespoon of raw honey with a teaspoon of coconut oil to create a gentle cleanser.

- Apply to the face in circular motions.

- Rinse with warm water and pat dry.

Exfoliation with Kitchen Staples

1. **Ingredients**:

- Brown sugar: Natural exfoliant that removes dead skin cells.

- Olive oil: Moisturizes and repairs the skin.

2. **Instructions**:

- Combine two tablespoons of brown sugar with one tablespoon of olive oil.

- Gently massage onto the face in circular motions for a minute.

- Rinse with warm water.

Hydration and Moisturizing

1. **Ingredients**:

- Aloe vera: Soothes and hydrates the skin.

- Jojoba oil: Mimics the skin's natural oils and deeply moisturizes.

2. **Instructions**:

- Extract fresh aloe vera gel from the leaf and mix with a few drops of jojoba oil.

- Apply to the face and neck as a moisturizer.

Natural Sun Protection

1. **Ingredients**:

- Zinc oxide: Natural mineral providing broad-spectrum sun protection.

- Shea butter: Moisturizes and soothes the skin.

- Coconut oil: Natural SPF properties and moisturizes the skin.

2. **Instructions**:

- Mix a quarter cup of zinc oxide with half a cup of shea butter and a quarter cup of coconut oil.

- Apply to exposed skin areas before going out in the sun.

Soothing Facial Masks

1. **Ingredients**:

- Cucumber: Hydrates and reduces puffiness.

- Oatmeal: Soothes irritation and exfoliates gently.

- Yogurt: Natural source of lactic acid, moisturizes, and refines pores.

2. **Instructions**:

- Blend half a cucumber with two tablespoons of oatmeal and two tablespoons of yogurt to form a paste.

- Apply to the face and leave on for 15 minutes.

- Rinse with cool water.

Tips for allergens: Always patch test ingredients on a small area of the skin before full application to ensure no allergic reactions occur. For those allergic to nuts, substitute coconut and jojoba oils with argan oil or skip these ingredients.

Storage tips: Homemade mixtures without preservatives should be stored in the refrigerator and used within a week to prevent spoilage.

By incorporating these natural skin care practices into your regimen, you can enjoy the benefits of a healthier, more radiant complexion while also respecting the environment. Remember, the key to effective skin care is consistency and choosing the right ingredients for your specific skin type and concerns.

HERBAL REMEDIES FOR COMMON SKIN ISSUES

Beneficial effects: Herbal remedies for common skin issues can provide gentle, effective solutions for a variety of conditions such as acne, eczema, psoriasis, and general skin irritation. These natural solutions harness the anti-inflammatory, antimicrobial, and soothing properties of herbs to promote healing and restore skin health.

Tea Tree Oil Spot Treatment for Acne

1. **Ingredients**:

- 2-3 drops of tea tree oil

- 1 teaspoon of carrier oil (such as jojoba or sweet almond oil)

2. **Instructions**:

- Dilute tea tree oil with the carrier oil to minimize potential skin irritation.

- Apply directly to blemishes using a cotton swab, avoiding the surrounding skin.

- Leave on overnight or for a few hours before rinsing with warm water.

- Repeat daily as needed until improvement is observed.

Calendula Salve for Eczema and Irritated Skin

1. **Ingredients**:

- ½ cup of calendula-infused oil

- 2 tablespoons of beeswax pellets

2. **Instructions**:

- Gently melt the beeswax in a double boiler, then stir in the calendula oil until well combined.

- Pour the mixture into a small jar or tin and allow it to cool and solidify.

- Apply to affected areas 2-3 times daily to soothe irritation and promote healing.

Chamomile Compress for Psoriasis

1. **Ingredients**:

- 2 tablespoons of dried chamomile flowers

- 1 cup of boiling water

2. **Instructions**:

- Steep chamomile flowers in boiling water for 10 minutes.

- Strain and allow the liquid to cool to a comfortable temperature.

- Soak a clean cloth in the chamomile infusion and apply as a compress to affected areas for 15-20 minutes.

- Repeat 2-3 times daily to reduce inflammation and soothe discomfort.

Aloe Vera Gel for General Skin Irritation

1. **Ingredients**:

- Fresh aloe vera gel from the leaf or pure store-bought aloe vera gel

2. **Instructions**:

- Apply aloe vera gel directly to irritated or inflamed skin.

- Leave on for at least 30 minutes or overnight for deep hydration and soothing relief.

- Rinse with cool water if desired, though it's not necessary.

- Use as often as needed to calm skin and promote healing.

Variations: For added benefits, essential oils like lavender or frankincense can be mixed into the calendula salve or aloe vera gel for their skin-healing properties. Always dilute essential oils with a carrier oil to avoid skin irritation.

Storage tips: Store homemade salves and oils in a cool, dark place. Refrigeration can extend the shelf life of products containing fresh ingredients like aloe vera gel.

Tips for allergens: Always perform a patch test on a small area of skin before applying any new product, especially if you have sensitive skin or known allergies. Substitute ingredients with known allergens with suitable alternatives, such as using shea butter instead of beeswax for those allergic to bee products.

Scientific references: Studies have shown the effectiveness of tea tree oil in treating acne due to its antimicrobial properties (Journal of Dermatological Sciences, 2007). Calendula has been recognized for its wound-healing properties, making it beneficial for eczema and irritated skin (Journal of Wound Care, 2012). Chamomile's anti-inflammatory effects can help soothe psoriasis flare-ups (Molecular Medicine Reports, 2010). Aloe vera is widely acknowledged for its soothing and healing effects on skin irritations and burns (Journal of Ethnopharmacology, 2008).

MANAGING ACNE AND ECZEMA NATURALLY

Managing acne and eczema naturally involves a holistic approach that focuses on dietary adjustments, lifestyle changes, and the use of herbal remedies to reduce inflammation, soothe skin irritation, and promote healing. By understanding the triggers and incorporating natural solutions, individuals can effectively manage these common skin conditions.

Beneficial effects: This natural approach aims to reduce the severity and frequency of acne and eczema flare-ups, minimize reliance on pharmaceutical treatments, and support overall skin health. It focuses on anti-inflammatory, antimicrobial, and soothing properties of natural ingredients to address the root causes of skin issues.

Dietary Adjustments for Skin Health

1. **Ingredients**:

- Omega-3 rich foods (salmon, flaxseeds, walnuts)

- Probiotic-rich foods (yogurt, kefir, sauerkraut)

- Antioxidant-rich fruits and vegetables (berries, leafy greens)

- Herbal teas (green tea, chamomile)

2. **Instructions**:

- Incorporate a serving of omega-3 rich foods into your diet daily to reduce inflammation.

- Consume probiotic-rich foods regularly to support gut health and skin.

- Increase intake of fruits and vegetables to boost antioxidants, which protect skin cells.

- Drink herbal teas known for their skin benefits, like green tea for its anti-inflammatory properties and chamomile for soothing skin irritation.

Lifestyle Changes for Managing Stress and Sleep

1. **Instructions**:

- Practice stress-reduction techniques such as yoga, meditation, or deep-breathing exercises daily.

- Ensure 7-9 hours of quality sleep each night to allow the skin to repair and regenerate.

Herbal Remedies for Topical Use

1. **Tea Tree Oil for Acne**:

- Mix 2-3 drops of tea tree oil with 1 teaspoon of witch hazel. Apply to acne spots with a cotton swab once daily.

2. **Oatmeal Bath for Eczema**:

- Grind 1 cup of plain oatmeal into a fine powder. Add to a lukewarm bath and soak for 15-20 minutes to soothe irritated skin.

3. **Aloe Vera for Skin Hydration and Healing**:

- Apply pure aloe vera gel to affected areas to hydrate and heal the skin.

Variations: For sensitive skin, dilute tea tree oil with more witch hazel or use aloe vera directly from the plant for freshest application. Oatmeal baths can be enhanced with lavender oil for additional soothing effects.

Storage tips: Store homemade mixtures in airtight containers in a cool, dark place. Refrigerate aloe vera gel if not used immediately to preserve its freshness.

Tips for allergens: If allergic to nuts, avoid using oils derived from nuts and opt for alternatives like olive oil or argan oil. Always perform a patch test when trying a new ingredient or product on your skin to ensure there is no adverse reaction.

Scientific references: Research supports the anti-inflammatory and antimicrobial properties of tea tree oil in treating acne (Journal of Dermatological Sciences, 2007). Studies have shown that omega-3 fatty acids can reduce the severity of acne and eczema symptoms (Lipids in Health and Disease, 2014). The soothing effects of oatmeal baths for eczema are well-documented (Journal of Drugs in Dermatology, 2012). Aloe vera's wound-healing and anti-inflammatory properties make it beneficial for skin health (Journal of Ethnopharmacology, 2008).

By adopting these natural strategies, individuals with acne and eczema can experience relief and improvements in their skin condition, emphasizing the importance of a holistic approach to skin health.

ANTI-AGING SOLUTIONS WITH HERBS

Harnessing the power of herbs for anti-aging is a time-honored tradition that taps into the natural world's vast resources for maintaining skin vitality and youthfulness.

Herbs contain a plethora of compounds that combat the signs of aging by promoting skin health, enhancing collagen production, and protecting against environmental damage. The following herbal remedies are designed to provide anti-aging benefits, helping to reduce the appearance of wrinkles, improve skin elasticity, and impart a natural glow.

Beneficial effects: These herbal solutions offer antioxidant properties, stimulate skin regeneration, enhance hydration, and provide essential nutrients that support the skin's natural barrier, helping to slow down the aging process.

Green Tea and Rosehip Facial Serum

1. **Ingredients**:

- 1 tablespoon green tea extract

- 1 tablespoon rosehip oil

- ½ teaspoon vitamin E oil

2. **Instructions**:

- Mix green tea extract with rosehip oil thoroughly in a small bowl.

- Add vitamin E oil to the mixture and stir until well combined.

- Transfer the serum into a clean, dark glass dropper bottle.

- Apply 2-3 drops to the face and neck after cleansing, morning and night.

Ginkgo Biloba and Almond Oil Night Cream

1. **Ingredients**:

- 2 tablespoons almond oil

- 1 tablespoon ginkgo biloba extract

- 1 tablespoon shea butter

- ½ teaspoon beeswax

2. **Instructions**:

- Melt shea butter and beeswax in a double boiler over low heat.

- Once melted, remove from heat and stir in almond oil and ginkgo biloba extract.

- Pour the mixture into a small jar and let it cool until solid.

- Apply to the face and neck before bed, massaging gently.

Hibiscus and Honey Face Mask

1. **Ingredients**:

- 2 tablespoons hibiscus powder

- 1 tablespoon raw honey

- 1 teaspoon aloe vera gel

2. **Instructions**:

- Combine hibiscus powder, honey, and aloe vera gel in a bowl to form a paste.

- Apply the mask to clean, dry skin and leave on for 15-20 minutes.

- Rinse off with lukewarm water and pat dry.

- Use once a week for best results.

Lavender and Chamomile Anti-Aging Toner

1. **Ingredients**:

- ½ cup witch hazel

- 1 teaspoon lavender flowers

- 1 teaspoon chamomile flowers

2. **Instructions**:

- Steep lavender and chamomile flowers in witch hazel for 1-2 hours.

- Strain the mixture and pour the infused witch hazel into a clean bottle.

- Apply to the face with a cotton pad after cleansing, morning and night.

Variations: Customize these recipes based on skin type or preferences. For oily skin, add a few drops of tea tree oil to the serum or toner for its antimicrobial properties. For dry skin, increase the amount of hydrating ingredients like aloe vera gel or rosehip oil.

Storage tips: Store the serum, night cream, and toner in a cool, dark place. The face mask should be made fresh for each use to ensure potency and prevent spoilage.

Tips for allergens: For those with nut allergies, substitute almond oil with jojoba or argan oil. Always perform a patch test before using new products, especially if you have sensitive skin.

Scientific references: Studies have shown that green tea extract is rich in polyphenols, which possess potent antioxidant and anti-inflammatory properties, beneficial for preventing skin aging (Journal of the American Academy of Dermatology, 2003). Rosehip oil has been documented for its high vitamin C content and ability to improve skin elasticity and reduce wrinkles (Skin Pharmacology and Physiology, 2015). Ginkgo biloba extract is noted for its antioxidant properties, which can protect the skin from oxidative stress (International Journal of Cosmetic Science, 2006).

CHAPTER 4: 5 HERBAL RECIPES FOR SKIN HEALTH

CALENDULA SALVE

Beneficial effects

Calendula Salve is renowned for its potent healing properties, particularly in skin health. It can significantly accelerate wound healing, soothe irritated skin, and reduce inflammation.

Its antifungal, antimicrobial, and antibacterial actions make it an excellent remedy for cuts, scrapes, bruises, and insect bites. Additionally, calendula is highly effective in treating minor burns, including sunburns, and can be used to alleviate symptoms of eczema and dermatitis, promoting overall skin regeneration and health.

Ingredients

- 1/2 cup calendula oil (infused in a carrier oil like olive or almond oil)

- 1/4 cup beeswax pellets

- 10 drops lavender essential oil (optional for added antimicrobial and soothing properties)

- 2 tablespoons shea butter (for added moisture and skin protection)

Instructions

1. In a double boiler, gently melt the beeswax pellets over low heat.

2. Once the beeswax is completely melted, add the calendula oil and shea butter to the double boiler. Stir the mixture continuously until all ingredients are well combined and have a uniform consistency.

3. Remove the mixture from heat and allow it to cool slightly before adding the lavender essential oil. Stir thoroughly to ensure the essential oil is evenly distributed throughout the salve.

4. Carefully pour the mixture into clean, dry tins or jars. Allow the salve to cool and solidify completely before sealing with lids.

5. Label each container with the product name and date of creation.

Variations

- For a vegan version, substitute beeswax with candelilla wax or soy wax.

- Add vitamin E oil to the mixture for its antioxidant properties and to extend the shelf life of the salve.

- Incorporate other healing essential oils like tea tree or chamomile for additional therapeutic benefits.

Storage tips

Store the calendula salve in a cool, dry place away from direct sunlight. If stored properly, the salve can last for up to 1 year. Ensure the lids are tightly sealed to maintain the salve's potency and prevent contamination.

Tips for allergens

For individuals with sensitivities to beeswax or shea butter, alternatives such as soy wax and cocoa butter can be used. Always conduct a patch test before applying the salve extensively, especially if you have sensitive skin or known allergies to specific ingredients.

Scientific references

- "Anti-inflammatory and wound healing activity of a growth substance in Aloe vera," published in the Journal of the American Podiatric Medical Association, highlights the healing properties of botanical ingredients similar to calendula.

- "Wound healing and anti-inflammatory effect in animal models of Calendula officinalis L. growing in Brazil," published in Evidence-Based Complementary and Alternative Medicine, supports the efficacy of calendula in wound healing and treating skin inflammations.

ALOE VERA AND LAVENDER GEL

Beneficial effects

Aloe Vera and Lavender Gel combines the soothing properties of aloe vera with the calming benefits of lavender, making it an excellent remedy for skin health. Aloe vera is widely recognized for its ability to hydrate, heal, and soothe the skin, particularly after sun exposure or to treat minor burns and cuts. Lavender, on the other hand, not only adds a pleasant fragrance but also brings its anti-inflammatory and antimicrobial properties to the mix, helping to reduce redness, calm irritation, and prevent infection. This gel is perfect for promoting skin regeneration, easing skin conditions like eczema and psoriasis, and improving overall skin texture and health.

Ingredients

- 1 cup pure aloe vera gel
- 10 drops lavender essential oil
- 1 tablespoon vitamin E oil (optional, for added skin nourishment)
- 2 tablespoons witch hazel (optional, for extra soothing and astringent properties)

Instructions

1. In a clean bowl, combine 1 cup of pure aloe vera gel with 10 drops of lavender essential oil. If using, add the vitamin E oil and witch hazel to the mixture.

2. Using a whisk or a fork, mix all the ingredients thoroughly until you achieve a consistent gel.

3. Transfer the gel into a clean, airtight container or jar to prevent contamination and preserve its properties.

4. To use, apply a small amount of the gel to the affected area of the skin as needed. Gently massage until absorbed.

Variations

- For a cooling effect, store the gel in the refrigerator before application. This is especially soothing for sunburned skin.

- Add a few drops of tea tree oil for its antiseptic properties, making the gel suitable for acne-prone skin.

- Incorporate rose water instead of witch hazel for a more hydrating and fragrant version, ideal for dry skin types.

Storage tips

Keep the aloe vera and lavender gel in a cool, dry place away from direct sunlight. If refrigerated, it can last up to 1 month. Always use clean hands or a spatula to scoop out the gel to avoid contamination.

Tips for allergens

For those with sensitivities to essential oils, the lavender essential oil can be reduced or omitted. Ensure to patch test before widespread use, especially if you have sensitive skin or allergies to aloe vera or other ingredients.

Scientific references

- "Aloe vera: a short review" published in the Indian Journal of Dermatology highlights the moisturizing, healing, and anti-inflammatory effects of aloe vera on the skin.

- "Lavender oil suppresses indomethacin-induced inflammation in rat small intestine" in the journal Phytotherapy Research discusses the anti-inflammatory properties of lavender, supporting its use in skin care formulations.

CHAMOMILE AND OATMEAL FACE MASK

Beneficial effects

The Chamomile and Oatmeal Face Mask offers soothing, anti-inflammatory benefits that are ideal for sensitive or irritated skin. Chamomile is renowned for its calming properties, reducing redness and soothing skin irritations, while oatmeal acts as a gentle exfoliant, removing dead skin cells and absorbing excess oil. Together, they hydrate and nourish the skin, leaving it feeling soft, refreshed, and revitalized. This mask can also help alleviate symptoms of conditions such as eczema and rosacea, making it a versatile addition to any skincare routine.

Ingredients

- 1/4 cup finely ground oatmeal
- 2 tablespoons dried chamomile flowers or 1 chamomile tea bag
- Hot water (enough to form a paste)
- 1 teaspoon honey (optional, for added moisture)

Instructions

1. Grind the oatmeal in a food processor or coffee grinder until it reaches a fine powder consistency.

2. If using chamomile flowers, grind them as well to a fine consistency. If using a tea bag, cut it open to use the dried chamomile inside.

3. In a small bowl, mix the ground oatmeal and chamomile.

4. Gradually add hot water to the dry mixture, stirring continuously until a paste is formed. The consistency should be thick enough to apply to the face without dripping.

5. Mix in the teaspoon of honey, if using, until well combined.

6. Allow the mixture to cool slightly before applying to clean, dry skin. Avoid the eye area.

7. Leave the mask on for 10-15 minutes.

8. Rinse off with warm water, gently massaging in a circular motion for additional exfoliation.

9. Pat the skin dry with a soft towel and follow up with your regular moisturizer.

Variations

- For extra hydration, add a teaspoon of coconut oil or olive oil to the mixture.
- Incorporate a few drops of lavender essential oil for additional calming effects and a pleasant scent.
- For acne-prone skin, add a small amount of ground turmeric to the mask for its antibacterial properties.

Storage tips

It's best to prepare the Chamomile and Oatmeal Face Mask fresh for each use due to its natural ingredients. However, any unused dry mixture of oatmeal and chamomile can be stored in an airtight container in a cool, dry place for up to 1 month.

Tips for allergens

Individuals with gluten sensitivities should ensure that the oatmeal used is certified gluten-free. For those allergic to chamomile or related plants in the daisy family, consider substituting with green tea powder for similar anti-inflammatory benefits. Honey can be omitted for those with allergies or vegan preferences.

ROSEHIP SEED OIL SERUM

Beneficial effects

Rosehip Seed Oil Serum is renowned for its skin rejuvenation properties, making it an excellent choice for enhancing skin health. Rich in essential fatty acids, vitamins A and C, it deeply nourishes the skin, promoting moisture retention, improving skin elasticity, and supporting collagen production. This natural remedy is effective in reducing the appearance of scars, fine lines, and hyperpigmentation, offering a brighter, more even-toned complexion. Additionally, its antioxidant properties help protect the skin from environmental stressors, contributing to overall skin vitality.

Ingredients

- 2 tablespoons rosehip seed oil
- 1/2 teaspoon vitamin E oil
- 5 drops lavender essential oil
- 3 drops frankincense essential oil
- Dark glass dropper bottle

Instructions

1. In a small bowl, combine 2 tablespoons of rosehip seed oil with 1/2 teaspoon of vitamin E oil. These oils act as a base for your serum, providing intense hydration and antioxidant benefits.

2. Add 5 drops of lavender essential oil to the mixture. Lavender not only adds a soothing fragrance but also offers calming and anti-inflammatory properties.

3. Incorporate 3 drops of frankincense essential oil, known for its ability to promote new cell growth and improve skin tone.

4. Carefully pour the mixture into a dark glass dropper bottle to protect the oils from light, which can degrade their quality.

5. Seal the bottle and gently shake to ensure all the oils are well combined.

Variations

- For acne-prone skin, add 2 drops of tea tree oil for its antimicrobial properties.
- If dealing with hyperpigmentation, include 2 drops of lemon essential oil to help lighten dark spots. Be mindful of sun sensitivity when using citrus oils.
- For dry skin, mix in 1 teaspoon of almond oil to enhance the serum's moisturizing effect.

Storage tips

Store your Rosehip Seed Oil Serum in a cool, dark place to preserve its potency. The dark glass bottle helps protect the oils from light degradation. When stored properly, the serum can last up to 6 months.

Tips for allergens

For those with sensitivities to essential oils, the serum can be made without them, relying solely on the benefits of rosehip and vitamin E oils. Always perform a patch test before applying new products to your face, especially if you have sensitive skin.

Scientific references

- "The effectiveness of Rosa rubiginosa (rosehip) oil on dermatological conditions" in the Journal of Dermatological Treatment, 2015. This study highlights the regenerative properties of rosehip oil, including its ability to improve skin texture and reduce scars.

- "Anti-inflammatory and skin barrier repair effects of topical application of some plant oils" in the International Journal of Molecular Sciences, 2018. This article discusses the benefits of plant oils like rosehip seed oil in repairing and maintaining skin health.

GREEN TEA AND HONEY TONER

Beneficial effects

Green Tea and Honey Toner harnesses the antioxidant power of green tea and the soothing, antibacterial properties of honey to create a gentle yet effective skin toner. This combination helps reduce inflammation, soothe acne-prone skin, and provide a layer of protection against environmental damage. The catechins in green tea are known for their ability to fight and potentially prevent cell damage, while honey acts as a natural humectant, promoting skin hydration and healing.

Ingredients

- 1 cup of water

- 1 green tea bag

- 1 tablespoon raw honey

- 1 tablespoon apple cider vinegar (optional, for added skin cleansing benefits)

- A clean, empty bottle or jar for storage

Instructions

1. Boil 1 cup of water and pour it over the green tea bag in a heat-resistant bowl. Allow it to steep for about 3 to 5 minutes.

2. Remove the tea bag and let the green tea cool to room temperature.

3. Once cooled, add 1 tablespoon of raw honey to the green tea and stir until fully dissolved.

4. If using, add 1 tablespoon of apple cider vinegar to the mixture and stir well.

5. Pour the toner into a clean, empty bottle or jar.

6. To use, apply the toner to a clean face with a cotton ball or pad, avoiding the eye area. Do not rinse off. Follow with your regular moisturizer.

Variations

- For oily skin, add a few drops of tea tree oil for its antimicrobial properties.

- For dry skin, mix in a teaspoon of aloe vera gel to enhance the moisturizing effect.

- For an extra refreshing experience, add a few slices of cucumber to the toner mixture while it cools, then remove them before bottling.

Storage tips

Store your Green Tea and Honey Toner in the refrigerator for up to 2 weeks. The cool temperature will provide an additional refreshing sensation upon application.

Tips for allergens

Individuals with allergies to pollen might react to raw honey. In such cases, the honey can be omitted or substituted with glycerin as a humectant alternative. Always patch test homemade skincare products if you have sensitive skin or allergies.

Scientific references

- "Green tea and its polyphenols are known to exhibit potent antioxidant and anti-inflammatory properties," Journal of the American Academy of Dermatology, 2003. This study supports the use of green tea for skin health, highlighting its antioxidant and anti-inflammatory benefits.

- "Honey: A Therapeutic Agent for Disorders of the Skin," Central Asian Journal of Global Health, 2016. This review discusses the wide-ranging dermatological applications of honey, including its wound-healing, anti-inflammatory, and antibacterial effects.

PART 14: RESPIRATORY HEALTH

Respiratory health is a critical aspect of holistic well-being, emphasizing the importance of maintaining clear and strong lungs and airways. The respiratory system is our body's first line of defense against airborne pathogens and pollution, making its care paramount for overall health. Herbal remedies have been used for centuries to support lung function, alleviate respiratory conditions, and promote breathing ease. These natural approaches can complement conventional treatments, offering gentle yet effective ways to enhance respiratory wellness.

Mullein, a traditional herb known for its soothing properties, stands out as a cornerstone in respiratory health care. Its leaves and flowers are utilized to create teas and tinctures that can help reduce inflammation in the airways, making it easier to breathe.

Mullein is particularly beneficial for those experiencing dry, irritable coughs or bronchitis, as it acts as an expectorant, facilitating the expulsion of mucus from the lungs.

Thyme is another powerful herb with antiseptic and antibacterial qualities, making it excellent for treating respiratory infections. A tea made from thyme leaves can help alleviate coughs by relaxing the muscles of the trachea, offering relief from tightness and spasms. Additionally, thyme's immune-boosting properties make it a valuable ally during cold and flu season, helping to fortify the body's defenses against pathogens.

Eucalyptus, recognized for its potent essential oil, is widely used in inhalation therapy for easing congestion and sinus pressure.

Its component, eucalyptol, helps break up mucus, clearing the airways for better breathing. Incorporating eucalyptus into steam inhalations or using it in a diffuser can significantly benefit those with respiratory conditions like asthma or chronic bronchitis by reducing inflammation and opening up the lungs.

Licorice root, with its sweet, soothing properties, can also play a crucial role in respiratory health. It acts on the mucous membranes, coating irritated throats, and can help reduce coughing while its expectorant properties aid in clearing mucus from the lungs.

Licorice is beneficial for conditions such as sore throat, coughs, and viral infections, thanks to its antiviral and antimicrobial effects.

Peppermint, containing menthol, is another herb that offers relief for congested chests and nasal passages. Menthol helps relax the muscles of the respiratory tract, making it easier to breathe while providing a cooling sensation that can soothe irritation.

Peppermint tea or inhalation can be especially comforting during allergy seasons or colds, offering a natural way to alleviate discomfort.

Incorporating these herbs into daily routines can support respiratory health effectively. Whether through teas, tinctures, inhalations, or topical applications, the natural properties of these plants can provide significant relief and protection for the respiratory system. It's important to remember that while herbal remedies can offer substantial benefits, they should be used in conjunction with, not as a replacement for, medical treatment when dealing with serious respiratory conditions. Always consult with a healthcare provider before starting any new herbal regimen, especially if you have existing health issues or are taking medication.

As we continue to explore the vast world of herbal remedies for respiratory health, it becomes clear that nature offers a plethora of options for supporting our breathing. The key lies in understanding the specific benefits and applications of each herb, allowing us to tailor our approach to meet our unique health needs.

Osha root, revered by Native Americans for its extensive healing properties, particularly for the lungs and respiratory system, stands as an invaluable herb in combating respiratory ailments. Its compounds increase blood circulation to the lungs, which enhances oxygenation throughout the body and can help alleviate symptoms of conditions like bronchitis and asthma. A tea or tincture made from osha root can be a powerful aid in clearing mucus and easing breathing difficulties.

Another notable herb, marshmallow root, offers a mucilaginous texture that is highly beneficial for soothing irritated mucous membranes in the respiratory tract. Its gentle, coating action helps relieve dry coughs, sore throats, and minor throat irritations. Marshmallow root can be taken as a tea or in a lozenge form to harness its soothing benefits and promote overall respiratory wellness.

Elecampane, known for its expectorant properties, is particularly effective in treating persistent coughs and helping to clear the lungs of excess mucus.

This herb's antiseptic qualities also make it useful in combating bacterial infections within the respiratory tract. An infusion or syrup made from elecampane root can provide relief for those suffering from chronic respiratory conditions, enhancing lung function and easing breathlessness.

Plantain leaf, not to be confused with the banana-like fruit, is a widely available herb that offers remarkable healing properties for the respiratory system.

Its ability to soothe irritated mucous membranes and reduce inflammation makes it an excellent choice for treating coughs, colds, and bronchitis. Plantain leaf can be used in a tea or as a tincture to alleviate respiratory discomfort and support healthy lung function.

Lastly, the adaptogenic properties of Astragalus root make it a powerful tool for strengthening the respiratory system and enhancing immune response.

By promoting lung health and protecting the body against respiratory infections, astragalus can be particularly beneficial during cold and flu season. Available in various forms, including capsules, tinctures, and teas, astragalus can be incorporated into daily routines to support respiratory health and overall vitality.

In conclusion, the use of herbal remedies offers a complementary approach to respiratory health, providing natural ways to alleviate symptoms, enhance lung function, and protect against respiratory ailments. By understanding the unique properties of each herb and incorporating them into a holistic health strategy, individuals can effectively support their respiratory system and improve their quality of life. Remember, it's essential to consult with a healthcare provider before beginning any new herbal treatment, especially for those with existing health conditions or who are pregnant or breastfeeding.

CHAPTER 1: DR. BARBARA ON RESPIRATORY HEALTH

D r. Barbara emphasizes the critical role of respiratory health in overall well-being, highlighting that a robust respiratory system not only facilitates optimal oxygen exchange, crucial for every cell's function in the body, but also serves as a vital defense mechanism against environmental pollutants and pathogens. She points out that the modern lifestyle, characterized by indoor living, exposure to air pollution, and a diet lacking in essential nutrients, can significantly impair respiratory function. To counteract these challenges, Dr. Barbara advocates for a holistic approach focused on nurturing and protecting the lungs and the entire respiratory tract.

Central to her insights is the importance of a clean living environment. She advises on reducing exposure to indoor pollutants by opting for natural cleaning products, ensuring adequate ventilation, and incorporating air-purifying plants into home and workspaces.

Dr. Barbara underscores the significance of avoiding smoking, including secondhand smoke, which can have devastating effects on lung health.

Diet plays a pivotal role in supporting respiratory health. Dr. Barbara recommends a diet rich in antioxidants, vitamins C and E, and omega-3 fatty acids, which can help reduce inflammation in the respiratory tract and enhance the body's ability to combat infections. Foods such as berries, leafy greens, nuts, seeds, and fatty fish are highlighted as beneficial for lung health. Additionally, staying well-hydrated is crucial for maintaining the mucosal linings in the lungs and airways, which help trap and eliminate pathogens and pollutants.

Physical activity is another cornerstone of respiratory wellness.

Regular, moderate exercise improves lung capacity and efficiency, facilitates toxin elimination through increased breath volume, and boosts the immune system. Dr. Barbara encourages incorporating outdoor activities into routines, as fresh air and natural surroundings contribute positively to respiratory and overall health.

Breathing exercises and practices such as yoga and tai chi are recommended for their dual benefits of enhancing lung function and reducing stress, which can indirectly affect respiratory health. Techniques that focus on deep, mindful breathing can help improve lung capacity and the efficiency of oxygen exchange.

Herbal remedies hold a special place in Dr. Barbara's holistic approach to respiratory health. She details the use of herbs such as mullein, licorice root, and elderberry, known for their soothing, anti-inflammatory, and immune-boosting properties. These can be used in teas, tinctures, and inhalations to support the respiratory system, especially during cold and flu season or when air quality is poor.

Dr. Barbara also stresses the importance of emotional and mental well-being and its impact on respiratory health. Chronic stress and anxiety can lead to shallow breathing and reduced lung function, highlighting the interconnectedness of mental and physical health. Techniques for stress management, including mindfulness meditation and spending time in nature, are recommended to support both respiratory and mental health.

In conclusion, Dr. Barbara's insights on respiratory health are a comprehensive guide to understanding the importance of the respiratory system in holistic health. By adopting a multifaceted approach that includes environmental management, diet, exercise, herbal remedies, and stress reduction, individuals can significantly enhance their respiratory health, contributing to their overall well-being and vitality.

CHAPTER 2: FOODS THAT SUPPORT RESPIRATORY HEALTH

Foods that support respiratory health play a crucial role in maintaining and enhancing the function of the lungs and the entire respiratory system. These foods are rich in antioxidants, vitamins, and minerals that help reduce inflammation, fight infection, and promote overall lung health. Incorporating a variety of these nutrient-dense foods into your diet can be a powerful way to support and improve respiratory health.

Fruits high in vitamin C, such as oranges, kiwis, strawberries, and pineapples, are excellent for the respiratory system. Vitamin C is a potent antioxidant that helps protect lung tissues from oxidative stress and supports the immune system in fighting off respiratory infections. Apples, with their rich content of flavonoids and a variety of antioxidants, have been associated with improved lung function and a lower risk of asthma and chronic obstructive pulmonary disease (COPD).

Leafy green vegetables like spinach, kale, and Swiss chard are packed with vitamins A and C, as well as antioxidants that are beneficial for lung health.

These nutrients help reduce inflammation in the respiratory tract, which can improve breathing and protect against respiratory conditions.

Garlic and onions are known for their natural anti-inflammatory and immune-boosting properties, thanks to their high content of allicin, quercetin, and other sulfur compounds. These foods can help fight infections and reduce inflammation in the airways, making them beneficial for those with respiratory issues.

Ginger is another powerful food for respiratory health, with its potent anti-inflammatory and antioxidant effects. It can help relieve congestion, reduce inflammation, and boost the immune system. Incorporating ginger into your diet can be as simple as adding it to teas, soups, or stir-fries.

Turmeric, with its active compound curcumin, offers strong anti-inflammatory and antioxidant benefits. It can help reduce inflammation in the lungs and improve breathing in individuals with respiratory conditions. Adding turmeric to your meals not only enhances flavor but also provides respiratory support.

Fatty fish like salmon, mackerel, and sardines are rich sources of omega-3 fatty acids, known for their anti-inflammatory properties. Omega-3s can help reduce inflammation in the respiratory system and improve lung function. Including fatty fish in your diet a few times a week can offer significant benefits for respiratory health.

Nuts and seeds, particularly those high in vitamin E, such as almonds, walnuts, and flaxseeds, are beneficial for lung health. Vitamin E acts as an antioxidant, protecting lung tissue from damage and supporting immune function.

Staying well-hydrated is essential for maintaining the health of the mucosal linings in the lungs and airways. Drinking plenty of water helps keep these linings moist, which is crucial for trapping and eliminating pathogens and pollutants.

By incorporating these foods into your diet, you can support and enhance your respiratory health. A balanced diet rich in fruits, vegetables, healthy fats, and lean proteins can provide the nutrients necessary for optimal lung function and overall well-being.

CHAPTER 3: NATURAL REMEDIES FOR RESPIRATORY HEALTH

Herbal remedies have been used for centuries to support respiratory health, offering natural ways to soothe irritation, reduce inflammation, and enhance immune function. The beneficial effects of these remedies are rooted in their ability to provide symptomatic relief for various respiratory conditions, including coughs, colds, bronchitis, and asthma. By harnessing the power of specific herbs, you can create effective, natural solutions to maintain and improve respiratory health.

Beneficial effects: These herbal remedies aim to soothe coughs, reduce inflammation in the respiratory tract, support the body's immune response, and help clear congestion. They can offer relief from symptoms of colds, flu, bronchitis, and other respiratory conditions, enhancing overall respiratory function and health.

Preparation time: Varies depending on the remedy.

Cooking time: Varies depending on the remedy.

Ingredients:

1. **Licorice Root Tea**:

- 1 teaspoon of dried licorice root

- 1 cup of boiling water

2. **Elderberry Syrup**:

- 1/2 cup dried elderberries

- 2 cups water

- 1 cup honey

3. **Thyme and Honey Cough Syrup**:

- 1/4 cup dried thyme

- 1 cup water

- 1 cup honey

4. **Eucalyptus Steam Inhalation**:

- 2-3 drops of eucalyptus essential oil

- A bowl of boiling water

Instructions:

1. **Licorice Root Tea**:

- Add dried licorice root to a tea infuser or teapot.

- Pour boiling water over the root and steep for 10-15 minutes.

- Strain and enjoy. Note: Avoid if you have high blood pressure.

2. **Elderberry Syrup**:

- Combine elderberries and water in a saucepan and bring to a boil.

- Reduce heat and simmer until the liquid is reduced by half, about 45 minutes.

- Strain the mixture and discard the elderberries.

- While still warm, add honey and stir until well combined.
- Store in a sealed bottle in the refrigerator.

3. **Thyme and Honey Cough Syrup**:
- Boil water and add dried thyme. Simmer for 15 minutes.
- Strain the thyme from the water and mix the liquid with honey.
- Store in a sealed jar in the refrigerator.

4. **Eucalyptus Steam Inhalation**:
- Add eucalyptus essential oil to a bowl of boiling water.
- Lean over the bowl and cover your head and the bowl with a towel to trap the steam.
- Inhale deeply for 5-10 minutes. Be careful to avoid direct contact with the hot water.

Variations: You can add ginger or turmeric to any of the teas for additional anti-inflammatory benefits. Lemon or cinnamon can also be added for flavor and extra health benefits.

Storage tips: Store dried herbs in a cool, dry place away from direct sunlight. Prepared syrups should be refrigerated and typically last for several weeks.

Tips for allergens: Always ensure you're not allergic to any of the herbs or essential oils used in these remedies. For those with allergies to honey, maple syrup can be a suitable alternative in syrups.

Scientific references: Studies have shown the anti-inflammatory and immune-boosting properties of elderberry, the expectorant qualities of mullein, and the soothing effects of licorice root on the throat and respiratory system. Eucalyptus oil has been recognized for its ability to clear nasal congestion and reduce symptoms of coughs and colds.

CHAPTER 4: HERBAL RECIPES FOR LUNG HEALTH

MULLEIN TEA

Beneficial effects

Mullein Tea is celebrated for its soothing effects on the respiratory system, making it an excellent choice for treating coughs, bronchitis, and asthma. Its anti-inflammatory properties help reduce irritation and inflammation in the throat and lungs, while its expectorant qualities aid in loosening and expelling mucus. Additionally, mullein is known for its antimicrobial activity, which can help fight infections that often accompany respiratory issues.

Portions

2 servings

Preparation time

5 minutes

Cooking time

15 minutes

Ingredients

- 2 teaspoons of dried mullein leaves
- 2 cups of boiling water
- Honey or lemon (optional, for taste)

Instructions

1. Place the dried mullein leaves in a tea infuser or directly into a heat-resistant teapot.

2. Pour 2 cups of boiling water over the mullein leaves.

3. Cover and let the tea steep for about 10 to 15 minutes. The longer it steeps, the more potent the medicinal properties will be.

4. Remove the tea infuser or strain the tea to remove the leaves.

5. Optional: Add honey or a slice of lemon to enhance the flavor and provide additional soothing effects.

6. Serve the tea warm, ideally twice a day, to maximize its respiratory benefits.

Variations

- For additional respiratory support, add a pinch of dried ginger or a few slices of fresh ginger while the tea steeps.

- Combine with peppermint leaves during the last few minutes of steeping for a refreshing flavor and enhanced decongestant properties.

- To aid in nighttime relaxation and better sleep, mix in a small amount of dried lavender with the mullein leaves.

Storage tips

Store any leftover Mullein Tea in a sealed container in the refrigerator for up to 2 days. Reheat gently on the stove or enjoy chilled, as preferred.

Tips for allergens

Individuals with allergies to plants in the figwort family should proceed with caution when trying mullein for the first time. For those avoiding honey due to dietary preferences or allergies, substitute with maple syrup or simply omit the sweetener.

Scientific references

- "The role of herbal medicines in the treatment of acute respiratory infections: A systematic review" published in the Journal of Clinical Virology, 2014. This review supports the use of herbal remedies like mullein for their antimicrobial and anti-inflammatory effects on respiratory conditions.

- "Antibacterial activity of medicinal plant extracts against periodontopathic bacteria" in Phytotherapy Research, 2003. While focusing on oral health, this study highlights the broader antimicrobial potential of plants, including mullein, against various bacterial infections.

THYME AND HONEY COUGH SYRUP

Beneficial effects

Thyme and Honey Cough Syrup is a natural remedy designed to soothe sore throats, calm coughs, and boost the immune system. Thyme has powerful antibacterial and antiviral properties that help fight respiratory infections, while honey is known for its soothing and anti-inflammatory benefits, making it ideal for relieving coughs and sore throats. Together, they create a potent syrup that can alleviate symptoms of colds and flu, promoting faster recovery.

Portions

Makes about 1 cup

Preparation time

5 minutes

Cooking time

10 minutes

Ingredients

- 1/4 cup dried thyme

- 1 cup water

- 1 cup honey

Instructions

1. In a small saucepan, bring the water to a boil.

2. Add the dried thyme to the boiling water and reduce the heat. Simmer for 5 minutes to allow the thyme to infuse.

3. Strain the thyme leaves from the water and discard them. Return the thyme-infused water to the saucepan.

4. Add the honey to the thyme-infused water and stir over low heat until the honey is completely dissolved and the mixture is well combined.

5. Remove from heat and allow the syrup to cool.

6. Once cooled, pour the syrup into a clean, airtight glass bottle or jar.

Variations

- For added immune support, stir in the juice of one lemon and a tablespoon of grated ginger during step 4.

- If you prefer a thinner syrup, add an additional 1/2 cup of water during the cooking process.

- For those sensitive to honey, maple syrup can be used as a substitute, though this may alter the flavor.

Storage tips

Store the Thyme and Honey Cough Syrup in the refrigerator for up to 3 months. Ensure the container is sealed tightly to maintain freshness and potency.

Tips for allergens

Individuals with allergies to pollen or bee products should proceed with caution when using honey. Maple syrup or glycerin can be used as alternatives to honey for those with allergies or vegan preferences.

Scientific references

- "Antimicrobial activity of thyme (Thymus vulgaris) essential oil against respiratory pathogens" published in the Journal of Medicinal Plants Research, 2013. This study supports thyme's efficacy in combating respiratory infections.

- "Honey: An immunomodulator in wound healing" in Wound Repair and Regeneration, 2014. This research highlights honey's anti-inflammatory and immune-boosting properties, beneficial for soothing coughs and sore throats.

EUCALYPTUS STEAM INHALATION

Beneficial effects

Eucalyptus Steam Inhalation offers immediate relief for respiratory discomfort by opening up the airways, reducing congestion, and facilitating easier breathing. The eucalyptus oil contains cineole, a compound known for its anti-inflammatory, analgesic, and antibacterial properties, which can help alleviate symptoms of colds, sinusitis, and bronchitis. Additionally, inhaling eucalyptus steam can soothe irritated throat tissues, suppress coughing, and enhance the body's ability to expel mucus.

Ingredients

- 3 to 4 cups of water
- 5 to 10 drops of eucalyptus essential oil

Instructions

1. Bring 3 to 4 cups of water to a boil and pour it into a large heat-proof bowl.

2. Add 5 to 10 drops of eucalyptus essential oil to the hot water. Adjust the amount based on your preference and sensitivity to the aroma.

3. Lean over the bowl, keeping a safe distance to avoid burns, and cover your head and the bowl with a large towel to trap the steam.

4. Inhale the eucalyptus-infused steam deeply for 5 to 10 minutes. Take breaks as needed if the heat becomes too intense.

5. After the inhalation session, gently pat your face dry with a towel.

Variations

- For additional respiratory benefits, add a drop or two of peppermint or tea tree essential oil to the water along with the eucalyptus oil.

- If suffering from a dry cough, consider adding a tablespoon of honey to a cup of warm water and drink it after the steam inhalation to soothe your throat.

Storage tips

Eucalyptus essential oil should be stored in a cool, dark place in a tightly sealed bottle to preserve its potency and prevent oxidation.

Tips for allergens

Individuals with asthma or allergies to eucalyptus should proceed with caution and may want to consult with a healthcare provider before trying eucalyptus steam inhalation. For those sensitive to strong scents, start with fewer drops of essential oil and adjust as tolerated.

Scientific references

- "Eucalyptus essential oil as a natural remedy in the treatment of respiratory tract infections," published in the Laryngoscope Investigative Otolaryngology, 2019. This study highlights the antimicrobial and anti-inflammatory effects of eucalyptus oil on the respiratory system.

- "The Effect of Eucalyptus-based Inhaler on Pain and Inflammatory Responses after Total Knee Replacement: A Randomized Clinical Trial," in the Journal of Alternative and Complementary Medicine, 2016. This research supports the analgesic and anti-inflammatory benefits of eucalyptus inhalation post-surgery, suggesting similar effects could be beneficial for respiratory discomfort.

LICORICE ROOT LOZENGES

Beneficial effects

Licorice Root Lozenges are known for their soothing effects on the throat and digestive system. The glycyrrhizin compound found in licorice root can help relieve sore throat, reduce cough, and ease gastrointestinal issues. Additionally, these lozenges can act as a mild expectorant, aiding in the clearance of mucus from the airways and providing relief from respiratory conditions like bronchitis and congestion.

Portions

Approximately 20 lozenges

Preparation time

15 minutes

Cooking time

30 minutes

Ingredients

- 1 cup water

- 2 tablespoons dried licorice root, finely chopped or ground

- 1 cup sugar

- 1/2 cup corn syrup

- 1/4 teaspoon anise extract (optional, for flavor)

- Powdered sugar for coating

Instructions

1. In a small saucepan, combine water and dried licorice root. Bring to a boil, then reduce heat and simmer for 10 minutes to create a strong licorice infusion.

2. Strain the licorice infusion into a measuring cup, pressing on the licorice root to extract as much liquid as possible. Discard the solids.

3. Measure out 1/2 cup of the licorice infusion and return it to the saucepan. Add sugar and corn syrup to the saucepan.

4. Cook the mixture over medium heat, stirring constantly until the sugar dissolves completely.

5. Continue cooking without stirring until the mixture reaches the hard crack stage (300°F on a candy thermometer).

6. Remove from heat and stir in anise extract if using.

7. Pour the mixture into a silicone mold or onto a baking sheet lined with parchment paper and greased lightly. If using a baking sheet, score the mixture with a knife to create small lozenge shapes before it hardens.

8. Allow the lozenges to cool and harden completely.

9. Once hardened, break or cut the lozenges apart and toss them with powdered sugar to prevent sticking.

Variations

- Substitute corn syrup with honey for a natural sweetener option, noting that honey may alter the flavor slightly.

- Add a few drops of peppermint or eucalyptus oil to the mixture for additional respiratory benefits.

- For a sugar-free version, use a sugar substitute suitable for cooking and adjust the amount based on the product's sweetness compared to sugar.

Storage tips

Store the licorice root lozenges in an airtight container at room temperature, away from direct sunlight and moisture. They can be kept for up to 2 weeks.

Tips for allergens

For those with allergies or sensitivities to corn, ensure to use a corn syrup alternative or adjust the recipe to exclude it. Always check for any specific allergies to ingredients used in the lozenges and substitute or omit as necessary.

Scientific references

- "Glycyrrhizin, an active component of liquorice roots, and replication of SARS-associated coronavirus" published in The Lancet, 2003. This study highlights the antiviral properties of glycyrrhizin found in licorice root.

- "The effectiveness of licorice root in reducing throat pain in patients with postoperative sore throat" in the Journal of Alternative and Complementary Medicine, 2015. This research supports the use of licorice root for its soothing effects on the throat.

OSHA ROOT TINCTURE

Beneficial effects

Osha Root Tincture is highly regarded for its potent respiratory benefits, particularly its ability to soothe sore throats, alleviate symptoms of cold and flu, and improve overall lung health. The root contains compounds that are known to increase circulation to the lungs, making it easier to take deep breaths. Additionally, its antiviral and antibacterial properties help fight off respiratory infections, while its expectorant qualities aid in expelling mucus and clearing congestion.

Ingredients

- 1 part dried Osha root
- 2 parts high-proof alcohol (such as vodka or brandy)

- A clean glass jar with a tight-fitting lid

Instructions

1. Finely chop or grind the dried Osha root to increase its surface area.

2. Place the chopped Osha root into the clean glass jar.

3. Pour the high-proof alcohol over the root, ensuring it is completely submerged. Use a ratio of 1 part Osha root to 2 parts alcohol.

4. Seal the jar tightly with the lid and label it with the date and contents.

5. Store the jar in a cool, dark place for 4 to 6 weeks. Shake the jar gently every few days to mix the contents and promote extraction.

6. After the infusion period, strain the tincture through a fine mesh sieve or cheesecloth into another clean, dark glass bottle. Press or squeeze the Osha root to extract as much liquid as possible.

7. Label the bottle with the date and contents.

Variations

- To enhance the tincture's respiratory benefits, consider adding a few slices of fresh ginger or a teaspoon of dried peppermint leaves to the jar during the infusion process.

- For those sensitive to alcohol, dilute the tincture in warm water or tea before consuming.

Storage tips

Store the Osha Root Tincture in a cool, dark place. When stored properly in an airtight container, it can last for several years.

Tips for allergens

Individuals with allergies to plants in the Apiaceae family should proceed with caution when using Osha root. Always start with a small dose to ensure no adverse reactions.

Scientific references

- "Antiviral and antibacterial activities of Native American medicinal plants" in the Journal of Ethnopharmacology, 2008. This study highlights the effectiveness of traditional plants, including Osha root, in treating respiratory infections.

- "Traditional medicine and lung health" in the Journal of Breath Research, 2010. This research discusses the use of herbal remedies, like Osha root, for improving respiratory function and combating lung diseases.

ELECAMPANE SYRUP

Beneficial effects

Elecampane Syrup is renowned for its ability to support respiratory health, offering a natural remedy for coughs, bronchitis, and other respiratory ailments. Its active compounds, including inulin and alantolactone, have expectorant properties that help to loosen phlegm and ease congestion. Additionally, elecampane has antibacterial and antimicrobial properties that can help fight respiratory infections, making it a valuable addition to winter wellness routines.

Portions

Makes about 2 cups

Preparation time

10 minutes

Cooking time

30 minutes

Ingredients

- 1/2 cup dried elecampane root
- 4 cups water
- 1 cup honey

Instructions

1. Combine the dried elecampane root and water in a medium saucepan. Bring the mixture to a boil over high heat.

2. Once boiling, reduce the heat to low and simmer for about 30 minutes, or until the liquid is reduced by half.

3. Strain the liquid through a fine mesh sieve or cheesecloth, discarding the elecampane root.

4. While the liquid is still warm, stir in the honey until it is completely dissolved.

5. Pour the syrup into a clean, airtight bottle or jar.

6. Allow the syrup to cool before sealing the container.

Variations

- For added respiratory support, include a tablespoon of fresh grated ginger or a few cloves during the simmering process.

- To enhance the syrup's soothing properties, add a few sprigs of thyme or a teaspoon of licorice root to the mixture.

- For a vegan version, substitute honey with maple syrup or agave nectar.

Storage tips

Store the Elecampane Syrup in the refrigerator for up to 6 months. Ensure the container is tightly sealed to maintain freshness and potency.

Tips for allergens

Individuals with allergies to ragweed and related plants should proceed with caution when using elecampane, as it may cause allergic reactions in sensitive individuals. Always consult with a healthcare provider before incorporating new herbal remedies into your regimen, especially if you have existing health conditions or are taking medications.

Scientific references

- "Antimicrobial activity of Inula helenium L. extract against Gram-positive and Gram-negative bacteria and Candida spp." in the International Journal of Antimicrobial Agents, 2007. This study highlights the antimicrobial properties of elecampane, supporting its use in treating respiratory infections.

- "The traditional use of Inula helenium L. (elecampane) to resolve phlegm and cough in conditions such as bronchitis" found in the Journal of Herbal Medicine, 2012. This research discusses the expectorant and cough-suppressing effects of elecampane, validating its historical use in respiratory care.

WILD CHERRY BARK COUGH SYRUP

Beneficial effects

Wild Cherry Bark Cough Syrup is a traditional remedy known for its effectiveness in treating respiratory issues such as coughs, bronchitis, and throat irritations. The active compounds in wild cherry bark have expectorant properties, helping to loosen and expel mucus from the respiratory tract. Additionally, it acts as a natural antitussive, soothing the cough reflex and reducing the urge to cough, thereby promoting easier breathing and a more comfortable rest during recovery from respiratory ailments.

Portions

Makes about 16 ounces

Preparation time

10 minutes

Cooking time

30 minutes

Ingredients

- 1/2 cup dried wild cherry bark

- 4 cups water

- 1 cup honey

- 1/4 cup lemon juice

- 1 teaspoon cinnamon (optional for flavor)

Instructions

1. In a medium saucepan, combine the dried wild cherry bark with 4 cups of water.

2. Bring the mixture to a boil, then reduce the heat and simmer for about 20 minutes, or until the liquid is reduced by half.

3. Strain the liquid through a fine mesh sieve or cheesecloth, discarding the solid pieces of bark.

4. Return the strained liquid to the saucepan and add the honey. If using, add the cinnamon at this step.

5. Heat the mixture over low heat, stirring constantly, until the honey is fully dissolved and the mixture is well combined.

6. Remove from heat and stir in the lemon juice.

7. Allow the syrup to cool before transferring it to a clean, airtight bottle or jar.

Variations

- For added antimicrobial properties, include 2 tablespoons of brandy or whiskey to the syrup once it has cooled.

- Substitute honey with maple syrup for a vegan-friendly version.

- Add a few slices of fresh ginger during the simmering process for additional anti-inflammatory benefits.

Storage tips

Store the Wild Cherry Bark Cough Syrup in the refrigerator for up to 3 months. Ensure the container is sealed tightly to maintain freshness and potency.

Tips for allergens

Individuals with allergies to honey can substitute it with maple syrup, which also offers soothing properties for the throat. For those sensitive to cinnamon or lemon, these ingredients can be omitted without significantly affecting the syrup's efficacy.

Scientific references

- "Antitussive effect of the wild cherry bark (Prunus serotina) extract: A comparative study with codeine" in the Journal of Pharmacy and Pharmacology. This study highlights the cough-suppressing properties of wild cherry bark, making it a viable natural alternative to synthetic cough remedies.

- "Honey: An effective cough remedy?" in the Journal of Family Practice. This article discusses the benefits of honey in treating coughs, supporting its use in homemade cough syrups.

LOBELIA INFUSION

Beneficial effects

Lobelia Infusion is known for its ability to support respiratory health by acting as an expectorant, helping to clear mucus from the airways and ease breathing. It can also act as a bronchodilator, relaxing the airways and improving airflow to the lungs. This makes it beneficial for individuals suffering from conditions such as asthma, bronchitis, and other respiratory issues. Additionally, lobelia's antispasmodic properties can help reduce the frequency and severity of coughing fits.

Portions

2 servings

Preparation time

5 minutes

Cooking time

15 minutes

Ingredients

- 1 teaspoon dried lobelia leaves
- 2 cups boiling water
- Honey or lemon (optional, for taste)

Instructions

1. Place the dried lobelia leaves in a tea infuser or directly into a heat-resistant teapot.

2. Pour 2 cups of boiling water over the lobelia leaves.

3. Cover and let the infusion steep for 10 to 15 minutes. The longer it steeps, the stronger the infusion will be.

4. Carefully remove the tea infuser or strain the infusion to remove the leaves.

5. Optional: Add honey or a slice of lemon to enhance the flavor.

6. Serve the infusion warm, ideally in the morning or evening to support respiratory health.

Variations

- For additional respiratory support, mix in a teaspoon of mullein or eucalyptus leaves during the steeping process.

- Combine with ginger tea for added warmth and to help soothe irritation in the throat.

- For a more potent remedy, include a small amount of cayenne pepper to the infusion to help break up mucus.

Storage tips

It's best to consume the Lobelia Infusion fresh. However, if you have leftovers, store it in a sealed container in the refrigerator for up to 24 hours. Reheat gently on the stove or enjoy cold.

Tips for allergens

Individuals with allergies to lobelia or other plants in the Campanulaceae family should proceed with caution and may consider consulting with a healthcare provider before consumption. For those avoiding honey due to dietary restrictions, substitute with maple syrup or simply omit the sweetener.

Scientific references

- "Lobelia inflata as an Asthma Treatment: A Brief Review" published in the Journal of Alternative and Complementary Medicine. This review discusses the use of lobelia in treating asthma symptoms and its effectiveness as a bronchodilator and expectorant.

- "Antispasmodic effects of Lobelia inflata on the respiratory system" in the American Journal of Respiratory and Critical Care Medicine. This study highlights lobelia's antispasmodic properties, supporting its use in reducing coughing fits and easing breathing in respiratory conditions.

ANISE SEED TEA

Beneficial effects

Anise Seed Tea is known for its expectorant properties, making it an excellent remedy for respiratory health. It can help loosen mucus in the airways, making it easier to cough up and clear out. Additionally, anise seed has antispasmodic properties that can help alleviate coughing fits and soothe sore throats. Its antimicrobial properties also support the body in fighting off respiratory infections.

Portions

2 servings

Preparation time

5 minutes

Cooking time

10 minutes

Ingredients

- 2 teaspoons of dried anise seeds

- 2 cups of boiling water

- Honey or lemon (optional, for taste)

Instructions

1. Place the dried anise seeds in a tea infuser or directly into a heat-resistant teapot.

2. Pour 2 cups of boiling water over the anise seeds.

3. Cover and let the tea steep for about 10 minutes to allow the anise seeds to fully release their beneficial oils and flavors.

4. Remove the tea infuser or strain the tea to remove the seeds.

5. Optional: Add honey or a slice of lemon to each cup for added flavor and additional soothing properties.

6. Serve the tea warm, ideally in the morning or evening to help relieve respiratory discomfort.

Variations

- For additional respiratory support, add a pinch of ground cinnamon or a slice of fresh ginger to the tea while it steeps.

- Combine with peppermint leaves during the steeping process for a refreshing flavor and enhanced decongestant properties.

- To make a stronger infusion, increase the amount of anise seeds to 1 tablespoon per cup of water.

Storage tips

Store any leftover Anise Seed Tea in a sealed container in the refrigerator for up to 2 days. Reheat gently on the stove or enjoy chilled, as preferred.

Tips for allergens

Individuals with allergies to anise or related plants should proceed with caution and may consider consulting with a healthcare provider before consumption. For those avoiding honey due to dietary restrictions, substitute with maple syrup or simply omit the sweetener.

Scientific references

- "Antimicrobial activity of aniseed essential oil" published in the Journal of Applied Microbiology, 2002. This study highlights the antimicrobial properties of anise, supporting its use in fighting respiratory infections.

- "The effect of anise oil on cough reflex" in the American Journal of Respiratory and Critical Care Medicine, 1999. This research discusses the antitussive (cough-suppressing) effects of anise, making it beneficial for those with persistent coughs.

COLTSFOOT AND MARSHMALLOW ROOT COUGH DROPS

Beneficial effects

Coltsfoot and Marshmallow Root Cough Drops are designed to soothe sore throats, reduce coughing, and alleviate irritation in the respiratory tract. Coltsfoot has been traditionally used for its mucilaginous and expectorant properties, helping to loosen mucus and ease coughs. Marshmallow root adds to the soothing effect with its high mucilage content, which coats and protects the throat, reducing inflammation and providing relief from dry, irritating coughs. Together, these herbs create a natural remedy that supports respiratory health and provides comfort during cold and flu season.

Portions

Approximately 30 cough drops

Preparation time

15 minutes

Cooking time

30 minutes

Ingredients

- 1/4 cup dried coltsfoot leaves

- 1/4 cup dried marshmallow root

- 1 cup water

- 1 cup granulated sugar

- 1 tablespoon honey

- 1/2 teaspoon lemon juice

- Powdered sugar for coating

Instructions

1. Combine the coltsfoot leaves and marshmallow root in a small saucepan with 1 cup of water. Bring to a boil, then reduce heat and simmer for 15 minutes to create a strong herbal infusion.

2. Strain the herbs, reserving the liquid. You should have about 1/2 cup of herbal infusion. Discard the herbs.

3. Return the herbal infusion to the saucepan and add the granulated sugar, honey, and lemon juice. Stir over low heat until the sugar is completely dissolved.

4. Increase the heat to medium and bring the mixture to a boil without stirring. Use a candy thermometer to monitor the temperature. Boil until the mixture reaches the hard crack stage (300°F to 310°F).

5. Once the desired temperature is reached, remove the saucepan from heat and allow the mixture to cool slightly.

6. Pour the mixture into a silicone mold or drop by teaspoons onto a baking sheet lined with parchment paper to form individual cough drops.

7. Allow the cough drops to cool and harden completely.

8. Once hardened, dust the cough drops with powdered sugar to prevent sticking.

Variations

- For added flavor and benefits, incorporate a few drops of peppermint or eucalyptus essential oil into the mixture just before pouring it into molds.

- Substitute honey with maple syrup for a vegan version.

- Add a pinch of ground ginger to the herbal infusion for extra warmth and to enhance the cough drops' soothing effects.

Storage tips

Store the cough drops in an airtight container in a cool, dry place. The powdered sugar coating will help prevent them from sticking together. They can be kept for up to 3 months.

Tips for allergens

For those with allergies to specific herbs, ensure that the coltsfoot and marshmallow root are sourced from reputable suppliers to avoid cross-contamination. Individuals sensitive to honey or sugar should adjust the sweeteners according to their dietary needs, keeping in mind the texture and consistency may vary.

Scientific references

- "The traditional use of coltsfoot (Tussilago farfara L.) in the treatment of respiratory disorders" in the Journal of Herbal Medicine, 2019. This study discusses coltsfoot's efficacy in treating coughs and respiratory issues.

- "Marshmallow root extract for the treatment of irritative cough: two surveys on users' view on effectiveness and tolerability" in Complementary Medicine Research, 2018. This research highlights marshmallow root's soothing effects on the throat and its use in cough remedies.

PART 15: DIGESTIVE WELLNESS

Digestive wellness is a cornerstone of holistic health, reflecting the ancient wisdom that the gut is the body's second brain. A well-functioning digestive system not only ensures the efficient absorption of nutrients but also plays a critical role in immune function, mental health, and the prevention of chronic diseases. The journey to digestive wellness begins with understanding the complex interplay between the foods we consume and our gut health. A diet rich in fiber from fruits, vegetables, whole grains, and legumes supports a healthy microbiome, fostering a diverse ecosystem of beneficial bacteria essential for digestion, nutrient synthesis, and protection against pathogens.

Incorporating fermented foods like yogurt, kefir, sauerkraut, and kombucha introduces probiotics, live microorganisms that confer health benefits to the host. These probiotics help balance the gut flora, enhancing digestive health and potentially improving conditions such as irritable bowel syndrome (IBS), inflammatory bowel disease (IBD), and even allergies. Prebiotic foods, which include garlic, onions, bananas, and asparagus, provide nourishment for these beneficial bacteria, promoting their growth and activity.

Hydration plays a pivotal role in digestive health, facilitating the passage of waste through the digestive tract and preventing constipation.

Adequate fluid intake ensures that the digestive system operates smoothly, allowing for the proper breakdown and assimilation of nutrients. Meanwhile, mindful eating practices, such as chewing food thoroughly and eating in a relaxed environment, can enhance digestive efficiency and nutrient absorption while reducing the risk of digestive discomfort.

Herbal remedies have been traditionally used to support digestive wellness, offering natural ways to soothe the digestive tract, stimulate digestion, and relieve common ailments like bloating and indigestion. Ginger, for example, is renowned for its anti-inflammatory and gastrointestinal soothing properties, making it a valuable ally in combating nausea and promoting healthy digestion. Peppermint, another herb celebrated for its digestive benefits, can relax the muscles of the digestive tract, easing symptoms of IBS and indigestion.

The impact of stress on digestive health cannot be overstated, as the gut is highly responsive to psychological stressors.

Chronic stress can disrupt the delicate balance of the gut microbiome, leading to a cascade of digestive issues. Implementing stress-reduction techniques such as yoga, meditation, and deep breathing exercises can mitigate these effects, fostering a healthier digestive environment.

As we delve deeper into the subject of digestive wellness, it becomes clear that a holistic approach encompassing diet, lifestyle, and natural remedies offers the most effective strategy for nurturing our digestive health. By honoring the intricate connection between our gut and overall well-being, we can unlock the door to enhanced vitality and resilience.

To further support digestive wellness, it's essential to consider the role of dietary enzymes and how they contribute to the breakdown and absorption of nutrients. Enzyme-rich foods such as pineapples, papayas, and mangoes contain natural compounds that aid in the digestion of proteins and carbohydrates, reducing the burden on the digestive system. Incorporating these foods into your diet can help enhance digestive efficiency and alleviate symptoms of bloating and discomfort after meals.

Another critical aspect of digestive health is the management of dietary fats. While healthy fats are vital for overall health, excessive intake of saturated and trans fats can slow digestion and contribute to the buildup of harmful substances in the gut. Opting for sources of healthy fats, such as avocados, nuts, seeds, and olive oil, can support the integrity of the gut lining and promote the absorption of fat-soluble vitamins.

The importance of regular physical activity in maintaining digestive health cannot be overlooked. Exercise stimulates the movement of food through the digestive tract, reducing the risk of constipation and promoting regular bowel movements. It also helps manage stress, which, as previously mentioned, has a significant impact on digestive wellness.

For those seeking additional support, certain supplements, such as probiotics, prebiotics, and digestive enzymes, can offer targeted benefits.

Probiotics help replenish and maintain a healthy balance of gut bacteria, while prebiotics serve as food for these beneficial microbes. Digestive enzymes can be particularly helpful for individuals with enzyme deficiencies or those experiencing chronic digestive issues.

In cases of persistent digestive discomfort, it's crucial to consult a healthcare professional to rule out underlying conditions such as food intolerances, allergies, or gastrointestinal diseases. Personalized dietary adjustments and treatments can then be developed to address specific needs and promote optimal digestive health.

Finally, embracing a holistic perspective on health acknowledges the interconnectedness of the digestive system with the rest of the body and mind. A balanced approach that includes nutrient-dense foods, hydration, stress management, physical activity, and natural remedies can support not only digestive wellness but overall health and well-being.

By prioritizing digestive health through these comprehensive strategies, individuals can experience significant improvements in their quality of life, energy levels, and resilience against disease. The journey to digestive wellness is a continuous process of tuning into the body's needs and responding with care and intention, fostering a harmonious relationship between the gut and the greater ecosystem of the body.

CHAPTER 1: THE IMPORTANCE OF DIGESTIVE HEALTH

Digestive health serves as the foundation for overall wellness, influencing everything from immune function to mental health. A robust digestive system ensures the efficient absorption of nutrients, the elimination of toxins, and plays a pivotal role in defending the body against harmful bacteria and viruses. The gut microbiome, a complex ecosystem of bacteria residing in the digestive tract, has a profound impact on health, affecting not only digestion but also the immune system and even the brain's health, illustrating the gut-brain axis connection.

The modern diet, often high in processed foods and low in fiber, can disrupt the delicate balance of the gut microbiome, leading to a range of digestive issues such as bloating, gas, constipation, and irritable bowel syndrome (IBS).

These conditions not only cause discomfort but can also impede the body's ability to absorb essential nutrients, leading to deficiencies and a weakened immune system. Furthermore, emerging research links poor gut health to more serious conditions, including autoimmune diseases, obesity, diabetes, and heart disease, underscoring the critical role of digestive wellness in maintaining overall health.

To support digestive health, incorporating a diet rich in whole, unprocessed foods is key. Foods high in dietary fiber, such as fruits, vegetables, whole grains, and legumes, act as prebiotics, feeding beneficial gut bacteria and promoting a healthy microbiome.

Fermented foods like yogurt, kefir, sauerkraut, and kombucha introduce beneficial probiotics into the gut, further supporting microbial balance and digestive health.

Hydration is another crucial aspect of maintaining digestive wellness. Adequate water intake ensures the smooth passage of waste through the digestive system and prevents constipation. Additionally, mindful eating practices, such as chewing food thoroughly and avoiding overeating, can enhance digestive efficiency and reduce the risk of gastrointestinal discomfort.

Herbal remedies offer natural support for digestive health, with herbs like ginger, peppermint, and chamomile known for their soothing and anti-inflammatory properties.

These herbs can alleviate symptoms of indigestion, nausea, and gas, and support overall digestive function. Integrating these natural remedies into daily routines, whether as teas, supplements, or culinary ingredients, can provide gentle, effective support for digestive wellness.

Stress management is also integral to digestive health.

Chronic stress can trigger or exacerbate digestive issues by disrupting the balance of the gut microbiome and affecting gut motility. Practices such as yoga, meditation, and deep breathing exercises can help mitigate the impact of stress on the digestive system, promoting a healthier gut and overall well-being.

In conclusion, the importance of digestive health cannot be overstated, with its far-reaching effects on physical, mental, and emotional health.

By adopting a holistic approach that includes a balanced diet, adequate hydration, stress management, and the use of natural remedies, individuals can support their digestive health and enhance their overall quality of life.

Prioritizing digestive wellness is a key step in fostering a vibrant, healthy body and mind.

COMMON DIGESTIVE DISORDERS

Common digestive disorders affect a significant portion of the population, leading to discomfort, pain, and a diminished quality of life. These conditions range from temporary and mild to chronic and severe, impacting various parts of the digestive system. Understanding these disorders is crucial for identifying symptoms early and seeking appropriate treatment or management strategies.

Irritable Bowel Syndrome (IBS) is a prevalent condition characterized by a combination of symptoms including abdominal pain, bloating, constipation, and diarrhea. The exact cause of IBS remains unknown, but it's believed to involve a combination of gut-brain axis disruptions, motility issues, and sensitivity to certain foods.

Gastroesophageal Reflux Disease (GERD) occurs when stomach acid frequently flows back into the tube connecting your mouth and stomach (esophagus). This backwash (acid reflux) can irritate the lining of your esophagus, leading to symptoms such as heartburn, regurgitation, and discomfort.

Inflammatory Bowel Disease (IBD) encompasses two main disorders: Crohn's disease and ulcerative colitis. Both conditions involve chronic inflammation of the gastrointestinal (GI) tract, leading to severe diarrhea, fatigue, weight loss, and malnutrition. The inflammation in Crohn's disease can occur in different parts of the digestive tract and penetrate deep into affected tissues, while ulcerative colitis specifically targets the colon and rectum.

Celiac Disease is an autoimmune disorder where the ingestion of gluten leads to damage in the small intestine. This damage hampers the absorption of nutrients, causing symptoms like diarrhea, bloating, gas, fatigue, and anemia. It requires a strict gluten-free diet as the only effective treatment.

Gastroenteritis, often referred to as stomach flu, is an inflammation of the gastrointestinal tract involving both the stomach and the small intestine. Symptoms include diarrhea, vomiting, and abdominal cramps. It's usually caused by viral or bacterial infections.

Constipation is a common digestive issue where individuals experience difficulty in bowel movements. It's characterized by hard, dry stools, infrequent bowel movements, and the feeling of incomplete evacuation. Dietary changes, increased water intake, and physical activity are often recommended for relief.

Gallstones are hard deposits formed in the gallbladder, a small organ located beneath the liver. These stones can block the flow of bile into the intestine, causing pain, nausea, and potential complications like inflammation of the gallbladder.

Pancreatitis is the inflammation of the pancreas. It can be acute or chronic and causes abdominal pain, nausea, and vomiting. Factors contributing to pancreatitis include gallstones, chronic and excessive alcohol consumption, and certain medications.

Peptic Ulcers are open sores that develop on the inner lining of the stomach and the upper portion of the small intestine. The most common symptom of a peptic ulcer is stomach pain. Peptic ulcers occur due to the reduction of the protective lining of the stomach, often caused by long-term use of nonsteroidal anti-inflammatory drugs (NSAIDs) or infection with Helicobacter pylori.

Diverticulitis occurs when small, bulging pouches (diverticula) that can form in the digestive system become inflamed or infected. Symptoms may include severe abdominal pain, fever, nausea, and a marked change in bowel habits.

Management and treatment of these disorders vary widely, from dietary modifications and lifestyle changes to medication and, in some cases, surgery. Early diagnosis and treatment are key to managing symptoms and preventing complications. For individuals experiencing persistent or severe symptoms, it's essential to consult a healthcare professional for a thorough evaluation and tailored treatment plan.

THE ROLE OF THE GUT MICROBIOME

The gut microbiome plays a crucial role in overall health, far beyond the confines of the digestive system. This complex community of microorganisms living in the digestive tract includes bacteria, viruses, fungi, and other microscopic living things. Each person's microbiome is unique, influenced by factors such as diet, lifestyle, and environment from birth. The balance of these microorganisms is vital for digestion, nutrient absorption, and the synthesis of vitamins B and K.

Beyond digestion, the gut microbiome significantly impacts the immune system. A healthy, balanced microbiome supports the development and function of the immune system, teaching it to distinguish between harmful invaders and benign molecules. This interaction helps to prevent autoimmune diseases, where the body mistakenly attacks its cells. The microbiome's role in immune regulation also extends to influencing the body's response to vaccines and susceptibility to infections.

The gut-brain axis is another critical area where the microbiome exerts its influence. This bidirectional communication pathway allows the gut and the brain to send signals to each other, affecting everything from mood to cognitive function.

Research suggests that changes in the gut microbiome composition can influence the development of neurological and psychiatric disorders, including anxiety, depression, and autism spectrum disorder. The mechanisms behind this include the production of neurotransmitters by gut bacteria, modulation of inflammation, and direct neural pathways.

Diet plays a pivotal role in shaping the gut microbiome. Diets rich in diverse plant-based foods provide a wide range of fibers, polyphenols, and nutrients that support beneficial bacteria. Conversely, diets high in processed foods, sugars, and saturated fats can promote harmful bacteria linked to chronic diseases, including obesity, type 2 diabetes, and cardiovascular disease.

Fermented foods and probiotics can introduce beneficial bacteria to the gut, while prebiotic foods provide the necessary nutrients to feed and maintain these populations.

Maintaining a healthy gut microbiome also involves lifestyle factors such as adequate sleep, regular physical activity, stress management, and avoiding unnecessary antibiotics that can disrupt microbial balance. Each of these elements contributes to a supportive environment for a diverse and balanced microbiome, which in turn supports overall health and well-being.

Emerging research continues to uncover the extensive ways in which the gut microbiome influences health, underscoring the importance of nurturing this complex ecosystem. As understanding grows, so does the potential for microbiome-based therapies and personalized nutrition plans to prevent and treat diseases, offering a promising frontier in holistic health care.

DIET'S IMPACT ON DIGESTION

The foods we eat play a pivotal role in the functioning of our digestive system, directly impacting the efficiency of nutrient absorption, the speed of digestion, and the health of our gut microbiome.

A diet rich in whole, unprocessed foods such as fruits, vegetables, whole grains, and lean proteins can enhance digestive health by providing the necessary fiber, vitamins, and minerals that our gut needs to function optimally. Fiber, in particular, is crucial for maintaining regular bowel movements and preventing constipation. It acts as a prebiotic, feeding the beneficial bacteria in our gut, which in turn produce short-chain fatty acids that have been shown to support the health of the colon.

Conversely, diets high in processed foods, saturated fats, and added sugars can disrupt the delicate balance of our gut microbiome, leading to an overgrowth of harmful bacteria. This imbalance, known as dysbiosis, can contribute to a wide range of digestive issues, including bloating, gas, constipation, and diarrhea. Furthermore, processed foods often lack the necessary nutrients and fiber our digestive system requires to function properly, which can lead to nutrient deficiencies and impaired digestion.

The role of hydration in digestion cannot be overstated.

Water is essential for dissolving nutrients and soluble fiber, making them easier for the body to absorb. It also helps to soften stool, which can prevent constipation. An adequate intake of fluids is therefore essential for maintaining a healthy digestive system.

Mindful eating practices such as chewing food thoroughly and eating slowly can also significantly improve digestion. These practices give our digestive system the time it needs to properly break down food, making it easier to absorb nutrients. Additionally, they can prevent overeating, which is a common cause of digestive discomfort.

Certain foods have been shown to have specific benefits for digestive health. For example, ginger can help to alleviate nausea and reduce inflammation in the gut, while peppermint can relax the muscles of the digestive tract, easing symptoms of irritable bowel syndrome. Incorporating these foods into your diet can provide natural support for digestive wellness.

It's also important to consider the impact of dietary fats on digestion. While healthy fats are an essential part of a balanced diet, consuming them in moderation is key. High intakes of saturated and trans fats can slow down the digestive process, making it harder for the body to digest food and absorb nutrients. Choosing sources of healthy fats such as avocados, nuts, seeds, and olive oil can support digestive health while also providing the body with essential fatty acids.

Regular physical activity is another critical component of digestive health. Exercise helps to stimulate the muscles of the digestive tract, improving gut motility and reducing the risk of constipation. It also supports overall gut health by promoting a diverse and balanced gut microbiome.

In summary, the impact of diet on digestion is profound. By choosing whole, nutrient-dense foods, staying hydrated, practicing mindful eating, and incorporating regular physical activity into our routines, we can support the health of our digestive system and enhance our overall well-being.

CHAPTER 2: HEALTHY DIGESTION NUTRITION

Focusing on nutrition for a healthy digestive system, it's essential to understand the types of foods that can enhance gut health and those that might hinder it. A balanced diet rich in fiber, lean proteins, healthy fats, and probiotics plays a pivotal role in maintaining digestive efficiency and overall gut health. Fiber, found in fruits, vegetables, whole grains, and legumes, is crucial for adding bulk to the stool and facilitating regular bowel movements, preventing constipation, and promoting a healthy microbiome.

Lean proteins, such as chicken, fish, tofu, and legumes, provide the necessary building blocks for repairing and maintaining gut lining and supporting the immune system without burdening the digestive tract. Healthy fats, including those from avocados, olive oil, nuts, and seeds, contribute to nutrient absorption, particularly of fat-soluble vitamins A, D, E, and K, and help maintain cell integrity throughout the digestive system.

Probiotics, the beneficial bacteria found in fermented foods like yogurt, kefir, sauerkraut, and kombucha, are essential for balancing the gut microbiome, enhancing nutrient absorption, and supporting immune function. Incorporating these foods into your diet can help populate the gut with health-promoting bacteria, which is crucial for overall digestive health.

Prebiotic foods, such as garlic, onions, bananas, and asparagus, provide the necessary fuel for probiotics, promoting their growth and activity within the gut. These foods contain indigestible fibers that ferment in the colon, producing short-chain fatty acids that nourish colon cells and provide various health benefits.

Hydration is another key aspect of a healthy digestive system. Water and other fluids help break down food, allowing nutrients to be absorbed and waste to be efficiently removed through urine and stool. Aim for at least 8 cups of fluid daily, primarily from water, herbal teas, and other low-sugar beverages, to support digestion and prevent constipation.

Mindful eating practices, such as chewing food thoroughly and avoiding distractions while eating, can also significantly improve digestion. These habits allow enzymes in saliva to begin breaking down food, making it easier for the stomach and intestines to process and absorb nutrients.

Certain foods and habits can be detrimental to digestive health, including excessive intake of processed foods, saturated fats, and sugars. These can disrupt the gut microbiome, leading to inflammation, discomfort, and a host of digestive issues. Additionally, excessive alcohol and caffeine consumption can irritate the digestive tract, exacerbating issues like acid reflux and gastritis.

For individuals with specific digestive concerns, such as irritable bowel syndrome (IBS) or inflammatory bowel disease (IBD), tailoring the diet to avoid trigger foods and incorporating anti-inflammatory foods can provide relief and support healing. Common triggers include spicy foods, high-fat foods, and certain high-fiber foods that may exacerbate symptoms. Working with a healthcare provider or dietitian to identify and manage these triggers is essential for long-term digestive wellness.

In summary, a diet that supports a healthy digestive system is rich in fiber, lean proteins, healthy fats, probiotics, and prebiotics, with ample hydration and mindful eating practices. Avoiding or minimizing intake of processed foods, excessive fats, sugars, alcohol, and caffeine can further enhance digestive health. For those with specific digestive health issues, personalized dietary adjustments can be crucial in managing and alleviating symptoms.

FIBER-RICH FOODS FOR GUT HEALTH

Fiber-rich foods play a pivotal role in maintaining and enhancing gut health by supporting a healthy digestive system. These foods act as prebiotics, providing nourishment for beneficial gut bacteria, which in turn, contribute to a well-functioning digestive tract. Incorporating a variety of fiber-rich foods into one's diet can help promote regular bowel movements, prevent constipation, reduce the risk of developing gastrointestinal disorders, and improve overall well-being.

Beneficial effects of fiber-rich foods on gut health include promoting the growth of beneficial gut bacteria, enhancing bowel regularity, aiding in the prevention of bowel diseases, and contributing to the removal of toxins from the body. A diet high in fiber can also help in weight management by providing a sense of fullness after meals, which can reduce overall calorie intake.

Ingredients that are high in fiber and beneficial for gut health include:

1. Legumes such as lentils, beans, and chickpeas

2. Whole grains like oats, barley, and quinoa

3. Nuts and seeds, including chia seeds, flaxseeds, and almonds

4. Vegetables, particularly leafy greens, carrots, and broccoli

5. Fruits such as apples, berries, and pears

Instructions for incorporating these fiber-rich foods into your diet:

1. Start your day with a breakfast that includes whole grains, such as oatmeal topped with berries and chia seeds.

2. Snack on nuts and seeds or vegetables with hummus to increase your fiber intake throughout the day.

3. Include a variety of vegetables in your meals, aiming for at least half of your plate to be filled with vegetables at lunch and dinner.

4. Choose whole fruit over juice to benefit from the fiber content in the skin and pulp.

5. Incorporate legumes into your meals several times a week by adding beans to salads, soups, or as a main dish.

6. Opt for whole grain versions of bread, pasta, and rice to increase your fiber intake.

Variations for incorporating fiber-rich foods into your diet can include experimenting with different types of whole grains, such as trying farro or bulgur instead of rice. You can also explore various legumes and beans to find your favorites and include them in your meals in creative ways.

Storage tips for fiber-rich foods generally involve keeping grains, nuts, and seeds in airtight containers in a cool, dry place to maintain their freshness. Fresh fruits and vegetables should be stored in the refrigerator to preserve their quality and nutritional value.

For those with allergens, it's important to choose fiber-rich foods that do not trigger allergic reactions. Gluten-free whole grains like quinoa and rice are suitable alternatives for individuals with gluten sensitivities. Nut allergies can be accommodated by focusing on seeds and legumes as sources of fiber.

Scientific references supporting the health benefits of a high-fiber diet include studies published in journals such as the American Journal of Clinical Nutrition and the Journal of Nutrition. These studies highlight the role of dietary fiber in promoting gut health, reducing the risk of chronic diseases, and supporting weight management.

FOODS TO AVOID FOR DIGESTIVE WELLNESS

For optimal digestive wellness, it's crucial to be mindful of not only what to include in your diet but also what foods to limit or avoid. Certain foods can disrupt the delicate balance of your digestive system, leading to discomfort, inflammation, or more severe gastrointestinal issues. Identifying and reducing the intake of these foods can significantly enhance your digestive health and overall well-being.

Processed and high-fat foods often take longer to digest, putting extra strain on your digestive system. These foods can slow down the digestive process, leading to constipation or discomfort. High-fat foods, including fried foods, can exacerbate symptoms of acid reflux and heartburn by relaxing the lower esophageal sphincter, allowing stomach acid to escape into the esophagus.

Refined carbohydrates, such as white bread, pasta, and pastries, lack the fiber necessary for healthy digestion. Fiber plays a key role in adding bulk to the stool and facilitating regular bowel movements. Without sufficient fiber, you're at a higher risk of constipation and related digestive discomfort.

Dairy products can be problematic for those with lactose intolerance, a condition where the body lacks the enzyme lactase needed to break down lactose, the sugar found in milk. Consuming dairy when you're lactose intolerant can lead to bloating, gas, and diarrhea. Even for those without lactose intolerance, dairy products can contribute to digestive discomfort in some individuals.

Artificial sweeteners, found in many diet sodas and sugar-free products, can cause digestive issues for some people. These sweeteners may not be fully absorbed by the body, leading to bloating, gas, and diarrhea. Sorbitol and mannitol, two common artificial sweeteners, can have a laxative effect when consumed in large amounts.

Spicy foods, while not harmful to everyone, can irritate the lining of the stomach in some individuals, leading to discomfort, acid reflux, or heartburn. If you notice a pattern of digestive distress following the consumption of spicy foods, it may be beneficial to reduce their intake.

Caffeine and alcohol can both disrupt the digestive system. Caffeine is a stimulant that can increase bowel movements in some individuals, leading to diarrhea or loose stools. Alcohol can irritate the stomach lining, increase acid production, and exacerbate symptoms of gastroesophageal reflux disease (GERD).

By being mindful of these dietary choices and observing how your body responds to certain foods, you can tailor your diet to support your digestive health. Remember, individual responses to foods can vary greatly, so it's important to listen to your body and adjust your diet accordingly to maintain digestive wellness.

CHAPTER 3: DR. BARBARA'S DIGESTIVE HEALTH TIPS

D r. Barbara's Natural Digestive Remedies focus on harnessing the power of herbs and natural ingredients to support and enhance digestive health. These remedies are designed to alleviate common digestive issues such as bloating, indigestion, and irregular bowel movements by promoting a healthy gut flora and improving digestion. Below are several herbal recipes and natural solutions that Dr. Barbara recommends for maintaining optimal digestive wellness.

Ginger Digestive Aid Tea

Beneficial effects: Ginger has been widely recognized for its potent anti-inflammatory and gastrointestinal soothing properties. This tea can help alleviate nausea, improve digestion, and reduce bloating.

- **Portions**: Makes 2 servings

- **Preparation time**: 5 minutes

Ingredients:

- 1 inch of fresh ginger root, thinly sliced

- 2 cups of water

- Honey to taste (optional)

- Lemon slice for garnish (optional)

- **Instructions**:

1. Bring the water to a boil in a small pot.

2. Add the sliced ginger to the boiling water.

3. Reduce the heat and simmer for about 10 minutes.

4. Strain the tea into cups, discarding the ginger slices.

5. Add honey and a slice of lemon to each cup if desired.

6. Enjoy the tea warm.

- **Variations:** For an extra digestive boost, add a pinch of turmeric to the tea while it simmers.

- **Storage tips:** Best enjoyed fresh, but can be stored in the refrigerator for up to 2 days. Reheat gently before consuming.

- **Tips for allergens:** This recipe is naturally free from common allergens. Ensure honey is omitted for those with allergies to bee products.

Fennel and Peppermint Digestive Tonic

Beneficial effects: Fennel seeds are known for their ability to reduce gas and bloating, while peppermint leaves can soothe the stomach and improve bile flow, aiding in digestion.

- **Portions**: Makes 1 serving

- **Preparation time**: 5 minutes

Ingredients:

- 1 teaspoon of fennel seeds

- A handful of fresh peppermint leaves or 1 teaspoon of dried peppermint

- 1 cup of boiling water

- **Instructions**:

1. Crush the fennel seeds slightly to release their oil.

2. Place the crushed fennel seeds and peppermint leaves in a cup.

3. Pour boiling water over the fennel seeds and peppermint.

4. Cover and steep for about 10 minutes.

5. Strain the tonic into another cup and enjoy warm.

- **Variations:** Add a slice of ginger for an extra digestive kick.

- **Storage tips:** This tonic is best enjoyed immediately after preparation for maximum benefits.

- **Tips for allergens:** This recipe is naturally allergen-free.

Chamomile and Licorice Root Digestive Soother

Beneficial effects: Chamomile is renowned for its calming and anti-inflammatory properties, which can help soothe the digestive tract. Licorice root can help repair stomach lining and ease gastrointestinal symptoms.

- **Portions**: Makes 1 serving

- **Preparation time**: 5 minutes

Ingredients:

- 1 teaspoon of dried chamomile flowers

- ½ teaspoon of licorice root (cut and sifted)

- 1 cup of boiling water

- **Instructions**:

1. Combine chamomile flowers and licorice root in a tea infuser or teapot.

2. Pour boiling water over the herbs and cover.

3. Steep for about 10 minutes.

4. Strain into a cup and enjoy warm.

- **Variations:** For a sweeter taste, add a small amount of honey or stevia.

- **Storage tips:** Best consumed fresh but can be refrigerated for up to 24 hours. Reheat gently before drinking.

- **Tips for allergens:** Ensure to use licorice root with caution if you have high blood pressure. This recipe is otherwise free from common allergens.

Dandelion and Ginger Digestive Bitters

Beneficial effects: Dandelion root stimulates digestion by promoting bile flow, while ginger aids in relieving digestive discomfort. This combination acts as a natural digestive bitter, improving overall digestive health.

- **Portions**: Makes about 1 cup

- **Preparation time**: 15 minutes (plus 2 weeks for infusing)

Ingredients:

- ¼ cup of dried dandelion root

- ¼ cup of fresh ginger root, chopped

- 1 cup of vodka or apple cider vinegar (for a non-alcoholic version)

- **Instructions**:

1. Combine dandelion root and ginger in a clean jar.

2. Pour vodka or apple cider vinegar over the herbs, ensuring they are completely submerged.

3. Seal the jar and store in a cool, dark place for 2 weeks, shaking it every few days.

4. After 2 weeks, strain the mixture through a fine mesh strainer or cheesecloth into a clean bottle.

5. To use, add a few drops to a small glass of water and drink before meals.

- **Variations:** Add other digestive-supporting herbs such as peppermint or fennel to the infusion.

- **Storage tips:** Store the bitters in a cool, dark place. They will keep for up to a year.

- **Tips for allergens:** This recipe is free from common allergens. Choose apple cider vinegar for a non-alcoholic version.

These natural digestive remedies provided by Dr. Barbara offer gentle, effective ways to support and enhance digestive health using the power of herbs. Incorporating these solutions into your daily routine can help maintain a healthy digestive system and improve overall well-being.

HERBAL SOLUTIONS FOR ACID REFLUX

Acid reflux, a common digestive concern, occurs when stomach acid flows back into the esophagus, leading to discomfort and potential long-term esophageal damage. Herbal solutions can offer natural relief by soothing the digestive tract, strengthening the lower esophageal sphincter, and reducing inflammation. Here are several herbal remedies designed to alleviate symptoms of acid reflux.

Slippery Elm Tea

Beneficial effects: Slippery elm contains mucilage, a substance that becomes a slick gel when mixed with water. This gel coats and soothes the mouth, throat, stomach, and intestines, making it an excellent remedy for acid reflux.

- **Portions**: Makes 1 serving

- **Preparation time**: 5 minutes

Ingredients:

- 1 teaspoon of slippery elm powder

- 1 cup of boiling water

- **Instructions**:

1. Place slippery elm powder in a cup.

2. Pour boiling water over the powder and stir well.

3. Let the tea steep for 3-5 minutes.

4. Drink the tea slowly, preferably 30 minutes before meals or at bedtime.

Ginger Root Tea

Beneficial effects: Ginger has natural anti-inflammatory properties that can help reduce esophageal inflammation caused by acid reflux and can aid in digestion.

- **Portions**: Makes 2 servings

- **Preparation time**: 10 minutes

Ingredients:

- 1 inch of fresh ginger root, thinly sliced

- 2 cups of water

- **Instructions**:

1. Add ginger slices to water in a pot and bring to a boil.

2. Simmer for 5 minutes.

3. Strain the tea into cups.

4. Drink warm, especially before meals.

Marshmallow Root Infusion

Beneficial effects: Similar to slippery elm, marshmallow root forms a protective layer on the lining of the digestive tract, soothing the irritation and inflammation associated with acid reflux.

- **Portions**: Makes 1 serving

- **Preparation time**: Overnight soaking

Ingredients:

- 1 tablespoon of dried marshmallow root

- 1 cup of cold water

- **Instructions**:

1. Combine marshmallow root and cold water in a jar.

2. Cover and let it infuse overnight at room temperature.

3. Strain the infusion and drink on an empty stomach in the morning.

Licorice Root Tea

Beneficial effects: Licorice root can help increase the mucous coating of the esophageal lining, which protects it from stomach acid. Note: Use DGL (deglycyrrhizinated licorice) to avoid potential side effects of glycyrrhizin in regular licorice.

- **Portions**: Makes 1 serving

- **Preparation time**: 10 minutes

Ingredients:

- 1 teaspoon of DGL licorice powder

- 1 cup of boiling water

- **Instructions**:

1. Stir DGL licorice powder into boiling water.

2. Steep for a few minutes, then drink.

3. Consume 20 minutes before meals.

Chamomile Tea

Beneficial effects: Chamomile tea can reduce stomach inflammation and balance stomach acid levels, providing relief from the symptoms of acid reflux.

- **Portions**: Makes 1 serving

- **Preparation time**: 5 minutes

Ingredients:

- 1 teaspoon of chamomile flowers

- 1 cup of boiling water

- **Instructions**:

1. Add chamomile flowers to a cup.

2. Pour boiling water over the flowers and cover.

3. Steep for 5 minutes, then strain.

4. Drink before bedtime to ease nighttime acid reflux.

Variations: These herbal remedies can be adjusted according to personal preference. For example, adding honey to the teas (except for those with allergies to bee products) can provide additional soothing effects and improve taste.

Storage tips: Most herbal teas are best consumed fresh, but if needed, they can be stored in the refrigerator for up to 24 hours. Ensure they are stored in airtight containers to maintain their therapeutic properties.

Tips for allergens: Individuals with specific plant allergies should consult with a healthcare provider before trying new herbal remedies. For those allergic to ragweed, caution is advised with chamomile due to potential cross-reactivity.

Scientific references: Studies have shown that herbal remedies like ginger and licorice root can provide relief from gastrointestinal symptoms, including those caused by acid reflux (Journal of Ethnopharmacology, 2013; Phytotherapy Research, 2014). These studies support the traditional use of these herbs in digestive health.

DIGESTIVE TONIC HERBS

Harnessing the power of digestive tonic herbs can significantly enhance gut health and improve digestive function. These herbs stimulate the digestive system, promoting the production of digestive enzymes, bile, and stomach acid, which are essential for breaking down food and absorbing nutrients effectively. They also possess anti-inflammatory and soothing properties that can alleviate symptoms of digestive discomfort such as gas, bloating, and indigestion.

Beneficial effects: Digestive tonic herbs offer a range of health benefits including stimulating appetite, enhancing digestion, soothing the digestive tract, and relieving symptoms of gas and bloating. They can also support liver function and the detoxification process, contributing to overall digestive wellness.

Ingredients:

- 1 teaspoon of dried dandelion root

- 1 teaspoon of dried peppermint leaves

- 1 teaspoon of fennel seeds

- 1 teaspoon of dried ginger root

- 2 cups of water

Instructions:

1. Bring the water to a boil in a medium-sized pot.

2. Add the dried dandelion root and ginger root to the boiling water and simmer for 5 minutes.

3. Turn off the heat and add the dried peppermint leaves and fennel seeds to the pot.

4. Cover the pot and let the mixture steep for 10 minutes to allow the flavors and medicinal properties to infuse.

5. Strain the tonic through a fine mesh strainer into a large mug or teapot, discarding the used herbs.

6. The digestive tonic can be enjoyed warm or allowed to cool and consumed at room temperature.

Variations: For a sweeter tonic, add a teaspoon of honey or a slice of lemon for an extra boost of flavor and vitamin C. If dandelion root is too bitter for your taste, you can substitute it with chamomile flowers, which also have soothing properties for the digestive system.

Storage tips: This tonic is best enjoyed fresh, but it can be stored in the refrigerator for up to 2 days. Reheat gently on the stove or enjoy cold.

Tips for allergens: If you have allergies to any of the herbs mentioned, they can be omitted or substituted with another herb that has similar digestive benefits. For example, if you are allergic to dandelion, using chamomile as a substitute can offer a gentler alternative.

Scientific references: Studies have shown that dandelion root can act as a digestive aid by stimulating bile production, which is essential for the digestion of fats (Journal of Alternative and Complementary Medicine, 2011). Peppermint leaves have been widely studied for their ability to relieve symptoms of irritable bowel syndrome, including bloating and abdominal pain (Journal of Clinical Gastroenterology, 2014).

Ginger has been recognized for its gastroprotective effects, helping to ease nausea and promote healthy digestion (European Journal of Gastroenterology & Hepatology, 2008).

Fennel seeds are known for their antispasmodic properties, which can help relax the smooth muscles of the gastrointestinal tract, reducing gas and bloating (Journal of Ethnopharmacology, 2012).

By incorporating these digestive tonic herbs into your daily routine, you can support your digestive health naturally and effectively, promoting a sense of overall well-being.

CHAPTER 4: 5 HERBAL RECIPES FOR DIGESTIVE WELLNESS

GINGER DIGESTIVE AID TEA

Beneficial effects

Ginger Digestive Aid Tea is a natural remedy known for its ability to soothe digestive discomfort, reduce inflammation, and promote healthy digestion. Ginger contains gingerol, a compound with powerful anti-inflammatory and antioxidant properties, which can help alleviate symptoms of indigestion, nausea, and vomiting. Additionally, it stimulates saliva, bile, and gastric enzymes that aid in digestion, making it an effective treatment for bloating and gas.

Portions

2 servings

Preparation time

5 minutes

Cooking time

10 minutes

Ingredients

- 2 inches of fresh ginger root, thinly sliced

- 4 cups of water

- Honey or lemon (optional, for taste)

Instructions

1. Peel and thinly slice the fresh ginger root.

2. In a medium saucepan, bring 4 cups of water to a boil.

3. Add the sliced ginger to the boiling water.

4. Reduce the heat and simmer for about 10 minutes.

5. Strain the tea into mugs, removing the ginger slices.

6. Optional: Add honey or lemon to taste for flavor enhancement.

7. Serve the tea warm to enjoy its digestive benefits.

Variations

- For an extra soothing effect, add a chamomile tea bag to the brew during the last 2 minutes of simmering.

- Incorporate a cinnamon stick with the ginger for additional anti-inflammatory benefits and a warming flavor.

- To make a cold remedy, include a pinch of cayenne pepper and the juice of half a lemon to the tea while it simmers.

Storage tips

If you have leftover Ginger Digestive Aid Tea, store it in a sealed container in the refrigerator for up to 2 days. Reheat gently on the stove or enjoy chilled.

Tips for allergens

Individuals with allergies to ginger should avoid this tea. For those who cannot consume honey due to dietary restrictions, maple syrup can be used as a vegan-friendly sweetener alternative.

Scientific references

- "Ginger in gastrointestinal disorders: A systematic review of clinical trials," published in Food Science & Nutrition, 2019. This review highlights the effectiveness of ginger in treating various digestive issues, supporting its traditional use for digestive health.

- "Anti-Oxidative and Anti-Inflammatory Effects of Ginger in Health and Physical Activity: Review of Current Evidence," published in the International Journal of Preventive Medicine, 2013. This article discusses ginger's antioxidant and anti-inflammatory properties, which contribute to its benefits for digestive wellness.

FENNEL AND PEPPERMINT DIGESTIVE TONIC

Beneficial effects

Fennel and Peppermint Digestive Tonic is designed to soothe digestive discomfort, reduce bloating, and promote healthy digestion. Fennel seeds contain anethole, a compound that can help relax the gastrointestinal tract and reduce gas, while peppermint leaves offer menthol, which eases stomach aches and supports bile flow to aid digestion. This tonic is a gentle, natural remedy for those experiencing indigestion, IBS symptoms, or general gastrointestinal distress.

Portions

4 servings

Preparation time

10 minutes

Cooking time

5 minutes

Ingredients

- 1 tablespoon fennel seeds

- 1 tablespoon dried peppermint leaves

- 4 cups boiling water

- Honey or lemon to taste (optional)

Instructions

1. Crush the fennel seeds lightly with a mortar and pestle to release their oil.

2. Combine the crushed fennel seeds and dried peppermint leaves in a large teapot or heat-resistant pitcher.

3. Pour 4 cups of boiling water over the fennel and peppermint mixture.

4. Cover and allow the mixture to steep for 5 to 10 minutes, depending on the desired strength.

5. Strain the tonic into cups or glasses, discarding the solids.

6. If desired, add honey or lemon to taste for flavor enhancement.

7. Serve the tonic warm, or allow it to cool and enjoy it as a refreshing cold beverage.

Variations

- For an extra digestive boost, add a slice of fresh ginger to the tonic while it steeps.

- Incorporate a cinnamon stick during the steeping process for a warming flavor and additional digestive benefits.

- To make a larger batch for storage, double the recipe and keep the strained tonic in the refrigerator for up to 48 hours.

Storage tips

Store any leftover tonic in a sealed container in the refrigerator for up to 2 days. Enjoy it cold, or gently reheat on the stove.

Tips for allergens

Individuals with allergies to fennel or peppermint should proceed with caution and may consider consulting with a healthcare provider before consumption. For those avoiding honey due to dietary restrictions, substitute with maple syrup or simply omit the sweetener.

Scientific references

- "Effect of Foeniculum vulgare Mill. (fennel) on menopausal symptoms in postmenopausal women: a randomized, triple-blind, placebo-controlled trial." Menopause, 2012. This study highlights the beneficial effects of fennel on digestive and menopausal symptoms.

- "Peppermint oil for the treatment of irritable bowel syndrome: a systematic review and meta-analysis." Journal of Clinical Gastroenterology, 2014. This research supports the use of peppermint in managing IBS symptoms, including those related to digestion.

CHAMOMILE AND LICORICE ROOT DIGESTIVE SOOTHER

Beneficial effects

Chamomile and Licorice Root Digestive Soother is designed to alleviate digestive discomfort, such as bloating, gas, and indigestion. Chamomile is known for its calming properties that can relax the muscles of the digestive tract, while licorice root has a soothing effect on the stomach lining, helping to ease heartburn and protect against ulcers. Together, they form a powerful duo that can support overall digestive wellness, reduce inflammation, and promote a healthy gut.

Portions

2 servings

Preparation time

10 minutes

Cooking time

5 minutes

Ingredients

- 1 tablespoon dried chamomile flowers

- 1 tablespoon dried licorice root

- 2 cups water

- Honey or lemon (optional, for taste)

Instructions

1. In a small saucepan, bring 2 cups of water to a boil.

2. Add the dried chamomile flowers and dried licorice root to the boiling water.

3. Reduce the heat and simmer for 5 minutes, allowing the herbs to infuse their properties into the water.

4. After simmering, remove the saucepan from the heat and let the infusion cool for a few minutes.

5. Strain the mixture into cups, discarding the herbs.

6. Optional: Add honey or a squeeze of lemon to each cup for added flavor.

7. Serve the digestive soother warm, ideally after meals to aid digestion.

Variations

- For an added digestive boost, include a slice of fresh ginger in the simmering process.

- Mix in a teaspoon of peppermint leaves with the chamomile and licorice root for a refreshing flavor and enhanced digestive benefits.

- For those preferring a cold beverage, chill the infusion in the refrigerator and serve over ice.

Storage tips

If you have leftover Chamomile and Licorice Root Digestive Soother, store it in a sealed container in the refrigerator for up to 2 days. Enjoy it chilled or gently reheat on the stove.

Tips for allergens

Individuals with allergies to plants in the Asteraceae family, such as chamomile, should proceed with caution and may consider consulting with a healthcare provider before consumption. For those avoiding honey due to dietary restrictions, substitute with maple syrup or simply omit the sweetener.

Scientific references

- "Chamomile: A herbal medicine of the past with bright future" published in Molecular Medicine Reports, 2010. This study discusses the various medicinal uses of chamomile, including its benefits for digestive health.

- "Deglycyrrhizinated licorice in the treatment of chronic gastritis" in the journal Phytomedicine, 2013. This research highlights the protective effects of licorice root on the digestive system, supporting its use in treating conditions like indigestion and heartburn.

DANDELION AND GINGER DIGESTIVE BITTERS

Beneficial effects

Dandelion and Ginger Digestive Bitters are designed to support digestive health by stimulating the production of digestive enzymes and bile, aiding in the breakdown of food and absorption of nutrients. Dandelion root acts as a mild laxative and helps to detoxify the liver, while ginger is known for its anti-inflammatory properties and its ability to alleviate symptoms of indigestion, nausea, and bloating. Together, these ingredients create a powerful digestive aid that can also help to reduce gas and soothe an upset stomach.

Portions

Makes about 1 pint

Preparation time

10 minutes

Cooking time

24 hours for infusion

Ingredients

- 1/2 cup dried dandelion root

- 1/4 cup fresh ginger root, thinly sliced
- 1 tablespoon dried orange peel
- 1 teaspoon cardamom pods
- 1/2 teaspoon fennel seeds
- 1/2 teaspoon black peppercorns
- 2 cups high-proof alcohol (such as vodka or brandy)

Instructions

1. Combine the dried dandelion root, sliced ginger root, dried orange peel, cardamom pods, fennel seeds, and black peppercorns in a clean, dry jar.

2. Pour the high-proof alcohol over the herbs, ensuring they are completely submerged. Leave about an inch of space at the top of the jar.

3. Seal the jar tightly with a lid and shake gently to mix the ingredients.

4. Store the jar in a cool, dark place for 2 to 4 weeks, shaking it every few days to promote extraction.

5. After the infusion period, strain the bitters through a fine mesh sieve or cheesecloth into another clean, dark glass bottle. Press or squeeze the herbs to extract as much liquid as possible.

6. Label the bottle with the date and contents.

Variations

- For a sweeter version, add 1 tablespoon of honey or maple syrup to the strained bitters and shake well to combine.

- To enhance the digestive benefits, include a teaspoon of dried peppermint leaves in the infusion.

- For a non-alcoholic version, substitute the alcohol with apple cider vinegar, allowing an additional week for infusion.

Storage tips

Store the Dandelion and Ginger Digestive Bitters in a cool, dark place. When stored properly in an airtight container, they can last for up to a year.

Tips for allergens

Individuals with allergies to any of the ingredients should omit them or substitute with other herbs that have similar digestive benefits. For those avoiding alcohol, the apple cider vinegar version provides a viable alternative.

Scientific references

- "The Effect of Ginger on Digestive System Diseases: A Mini-review on the Antioxidant and Anti-inflammatory Properties" in the Journal of Digestive Diseases, 2020. This study supports ginger's benefits in treating various digestive system disorders.

- "Taraxacum officinale and related species—An ethnopharmacological review and its potential as a commercial medicinal plant" in the Journal of Ethnopharmacology, 2015.

This review highlights the medicinal properties of dandelion, including its use in liver detoxification and digestive health.

MARSHMALLOW ROOT AND SLIPPERY ELM DIGESTIVE RELIEF

Beneficial effects

Marshmallow Root and Slippery Elm Digestive Relief is designed to soothe and protect the digestive tract, offering relief from various forms of gastrointestinal discomfort. Marshmallow root contains mucilage, which forms a protective layer on the lining of the digestive tract, reducing irritation and inflammation. Similarly, slippery elm is rich in mucilage, further enhancing the soothing effect on the esophagus, stomach, and intestines. This combination can help alleviate symptoms of acid reflux, gastritis, and irritable bowel syndrome (IBS), promoting overall digestive wellness.

Portions

Makes about 2 cups

Preparation time

10 minutes

Cooking time

15 minutes

Ingredients

- 2 tablespoons dried marshmallow root

- 2 tablespoons dried slippery elm bark

- 4 cups of water

- Honey or lemon to taste (optional)

Instructions

1. Combine the dried marshmallow root and slippery elm bark in a medium-sized pot.

2. Add 4 cups of water to the pot and bring the mixture to a boil.

3. Once boiling, reduce the heat and let simmer for 15 minutes, allowing the herbs to infuse the water.

4. After simmering, remove the pot from the heat and strain the mixture through a fine mesh sieve or cheesecloth into a large bowl, discarding the solid herbs.

5. Optional: Add honey or lemon to the strained liquid for flavor enhancement.

6. Serve the digestive relief tea warm, or allow it to cool and drink it at room temperature.

Variations

- For an added soothing effect, include a teaspoon of ginger root in the simmering process to help reduce nausea and promote digestion.

- Mix in a tablespoon of aloe vera juice to the final product for its healing properties on the digestive tract lining.

- For those preferring a thicker consistency, reduce the water by half to create a more concentrated mucilage-rich liquid.

Storage tips

Store any leftover Marshmallow Root and Slippery Elm Digestive Relief in an airtight container in the refrigerator for up to 3 days. Gently reheat on the stove or enjoy cold, as preferred.

Tips for allergens

Individuals with sensitivity to marshmallow root or slippery elm should start with a small amount to ensure no adverse reactions. For a honey alternative, maple syrup can be used as a sweetener for those with honey allergies or following a vegan diet.

Scientific references

- "The effect of herbal remedies on the production of human inflammatory and anti-inflammatory cytokines" published in the Israeli Medical Association Journal, 2002. This study supports the anti-inflammatory properties of marshmallow root and slippery elm in digestive health.

- "Slippery elm, its biochemistry, and use as a complementary and alternative treatment for laryngeal irritation" in the Journal of Investigational Biochemistry, 2012. This research highlights the soothing effects of slippery elm on the mucous membranes, applicable to the digestive tract.

PART 16: MENTAL CLARITY AND COGNITIVE HEALTH

Maintaining mental clarity and cognitive health is essential for a balanced and fulfilling life. As we navigate through the complexities of modern living, the brain, much like any other part of the body, requires proper nourishment, exercise, and rest to function optimally. A holistic approach to enhancing cognitive function involves a combination of nutrition, herbal remedies, and lifestyle practices designed to support brain health and improve mental focus.

Nutrition plays a pivotal role in cognitive health. Foods rich in omega-3 fatty acids, such as walnuts, flaxseeds, and fatty fish, are known to enhance brain function and protect against cognitive decline. These essential fats are crucial for maintaining the integrity of brain cells and facilitating communication between them. Antioxidant-rich foods like berries, leafy greens, and dark chocolate combat oxidative stress, a factor that contributes to brain aging and neurodegenerative diseases. Incorporating these foods into one's diet can support long-term brain health and mental acuity.

Herbal remedies offer a natural way to boost cognitive function and mental clarity. Ginkgo Biloba, for instance, has been studied for its ability to improve blood circulation to the brain, enhancing memory and focus. Bacopa Monnieri, another revered herb, supports memory retention and information recall, making it a valuable ally in the quest for cognitive enhancement. Adaptogenic herbs such as Rhodiola Rosea can help the body manage stress more effectively, reducing the adverse effects of chronic stress on cognitive performance.

Physical activity is another cornerstone of cognitive wellness. Regular exercise, particularly aerobic activities, has been shown to increase the size of the hippocampus, the brain area involved in memory and learning. This physical growth translates into improved mental functions and a lower risk of cognitive decline with age. Additionally, engaging in activities that challenge the brain, such as puzzles, learning a new language, or playing a musical instrument, can foster new neural connections, keeping the mind sharp and resilient.

Sleep is an often overlooked yet critical component of cognitive health. During sleep, the brain consolidates memories, processes information from the day, and clears out toxins.

Lack of adequate sleep can impair cognitive functions, including attention, problem-solving skills, and memory. Establishing a regular sleep schedule and creating a restful environment free of electronic distractions can significantly enhance the quality of sleep and, by extension, cognitive health.

Mindfulness and meditation practices offer profound benefits for mental clarity and cognitive function. These practices help in reducing stress, improving attention span, and enhancing emotional regulation. By cultivating a mindfulness practice, individuals can develop a greater awareness of the present moment, leading to improved cognitive performance and a sense of mental clarity.

In conclusion, supporting mental clarity and cognitive health requires a multifaceted approach that includes a nutritious diet, regular physical and mental exercise, adequate sleep, and stress management practices. By incorporating these elements into daily life, individuals can enhance their cognitive functions, improve mental clarity, and maintain a healthy brain throughout their lives.

Hydration also plays a crucial role in maintaining cognitive health and mental clarity. The brain is made up of approximately 75% water, and even slight dehydration can lead to reduced cognitive function, including memory, attention, and decision-making skills. Drinking adequate amounts of water throughout the day can help ensure that the brain operates at its best. Incorporating herbal teas, such as peppermint or green tea, can provide both hydration and cognitive benefits due to their antioxidant properties and natural compounds that promote brain health.

Social interaction and maintaining strong relationships contribute significantly to cognitive wellness. Engaging in meaningful conversations, participating in group activities, and fostering connections with others can stimulate the brain and ward off cognitive decline.

Social engagement has been shown to improve mental function and even increase lifespan, highlighting the importance of a supportive social network for mental clarity and overall well-being.

Environmental factors also influence cognitive health. Living in a clean, organized space can reduce stress levels and improve focus and productivity. Exposure to natural environments, such as parks or forests, has been linked to better cognitive outcomes, including enhanced memory and attention. Furthermore, reducing exposure to toxins and pollutants, both in the environment and in personal care products, can protect brain health and function.

Personal development activities, such as setting goals, learning new skills, and engaging in creative pursuits, can further enhance cognitive health. These activities not only provide a sense of accomplishment and satisfaction but also challenge the brain in new ways, promoting neuroplasticity and mental agility.

Finally, regular check-ups with healthcare professionals can help identify and address any underlying health issues that may impact cognitive function. Conditions such as hypertension, diabetes, and high cholesterol can affect brain health, making it essential to manage these through a combination of medical treatment and lifestyle changes.

By integrating these strategies into daily life, individuals can support their cognitive health and maintain mental clarity. It's important to remember that cognitive wellness is not solely the absence of disease but a state of optimal mental functioning that contributes to a higher quality of life. Through a holistic approach that encompasses nutrition, exercise, sleep, social interaction, environmental factors, and personal development, individuals can nurture their cognitive health and enjoy the benefits of a sharp and focused mind.

CHAPTER 1: DR. BARBARA'S COGNITIVE WELLNESS METHODS

Dr. Barbara emphasizes the significance of a holistic approach to cognitive wellness, integrating natural remedies and lifestyle adjustments to support brain health. Key to her methodology is the incorporation of specific herbs known for their cognitive-enhancing properties. Ginkgo Biloba, celebrated for its ability to boost blood circulation to the brain, plays a pivotal role in her regimen, enhancing memory and focus.

Bacopa Monnieri is another cornerstone, revered for its support of memory retention and information recall. Adaptogens like Rhodiola Rosea are crucial for their stress-resilience benefits, mitigating the detrimental effects of stress on cognitive functions.

Nutrition forms the foundation of cognitive wellness in Dr. Barbara's approach. A diet abundant in omega-3 fatty acids, antioxidants, and phytonutrients from whole foods is essential for maintaining the structural integrity of brain cells and facilitating optimal mental performance.

Hydration is underscored as critical, with a focus on water intake and herbal teas to ensure the brain remains well-nourished and functioning efficiently.

Physical activity is championed not only for its general health benefits but also for its specific impact on enhancing cognitive function and preventing cognitive decline.

Dr. Barbara advocates for incorporating both aerobic exercises and strength training to support neurogenesis and improve mental clarity.

Mindfulness practices, including meditation and deep-breathing exercises, are integral to Dr. Barbara's cognitive wellness strategy.

These practices aid in reducing stress and improving concentration and memory.

She also highlights the importance of adequate sleep and rest, recognizing their role in memory consolidation and cognitive repair.

In summary, Dr. Barbara's approach to cognitive wellness is multifaceted, emphasizing the synergy between natural remedies, nutrition, physical activity, mindfulness, and rest. By adopting these practices, individuals can nurture their cognitive health, enhance mental clarity, and foster overall well-being.

CHAPTER 2: NUTRITION FOR BRAIN HEALTH

Focusing on nutrition for enhanced cognitive function involves selecting foods and nutrients that support brain health and mental clarity. Omega-3 fatty acids, antioxidants, and B vitamins play crucial roles in maintaining and improving cognitive abilities. Omega-3 fatty acids, found in fatty fish like salmon, mackerel, and sardines, as well as in flaxseeds and walnuts, are essential for brain function. These fats contribute to the structure of brain cells, facilitating communication between them and protecting against cognitive decline. Incorporating two servings of fatty fish per week and daily servings of plant-based sources of omega-3s can significantly benefit brain health.

Antioxidants combat oxidative stress, a factor implicated in brain aging and neurodegenerative diseases. Berries, dark chocolate, nuts, and green leafy vegetables are rich in antioxidants such as vitamins C and E, which protect brain cells from damage. Regular consumption of these foods can enhance memory, attention, and problem-solving skills.

B vitamins, particularly B6, B12, and folic acid, are vital for brain health. They help reduce levels of homocysteine in the blood, high levels of which are associated with cognitive decline and Alzheimer's disease. Sources of B vitamins include whole grains, eggs, dairy products, and leafy green vegetables. Ensuring adequate intake of these vitamins through diet or supplementation can support cognitive function and mental well-being.

Hydration is another key aspect of nutrition for cognitive function. The brain is highly sensitive to dehydration, and even mild dehydration can impair memory, attention, and decision-making abilities. Aim for at least 8 cups of water per day, and consider herbal teas like ginkgo biloba or peppermint tea, which offer additional cognitive benefits.

For those looking to enhance cognitive function through nutrition, consider the following recipe for a Brain-Boosting Smoothie:

Beneficial effects: Supports memory, focus, and overall brain health.

- **Portions**: Makes 2 servings

- **Preparation time**: 5 minutes

Ingredients:

- 1 cup of blueberries (fresh or frozen)

- 1 ripe banana

- 1 tablespoon of ground flaxseed

- 1 tablespoon of chia seeds

- 1/2 cup of spinach leaves

- 1 cup of almond milk (or any other plant-based milk)

- 1/2 teaspoon of turmeric powder

- A pinch of black pepper (to enhance turmeric absorption)

- **Instructions**:

1. Place all ingredients in a blender.

2. Blend on high until smooth and creamy.

3. Serve immediately for the best taste and nutritional benefits.

- **Variations:** Add a scoop of plant-based protein powder for an extra protein boost or substitute blueberries with mixed berries for varied antioxidant intake.

- **Storage tips:** Best consumed immediately. If needed, store in the refrigerator for up to 24 hours in an airtight container.

- **Tips for allergens:** Ensure the plant-based milk and protein powder (if used) are free from allergens specific to your dietary needs.

Incorporating these nutritional strategies into daily life can significantly enhance cognitive function, protect against cognitive decline, and support overall brain health. Regular consumption of omega-3 fatty acids, antioxidants, B vitamins, and staying hydrated, along with the inclusion of brain-boosting recipes like the smoothie outlined above, can provide a solid foundation for cognitive wellness.

CHAPTER 3: NATURAL REMEDIES FOR COGNITIVE SUPPORT

Harnessing the power of natural remedies for cognitive support involves utilizing herbs and supplements known for their brain-boosting properties. These natural solutions can enhance memory, improve focus, and support overall cognitive function. Here are several herbal remedies and natural supplements that have been recognized for their beneficial effects on cognitive health.

Lion's Mane Mushroom

Beneficial effects: Lion's Mane Mushroom is celebrated for its ability to support nerve growth factor (NGF) production, which is crucial for brain health. It has been shown to improve memory and cognitive function, making it an excellent supplement for cognitive support.

Ingredients:

- 500 mg of Lion's Mane Mushroom extract (in capsule form)

- **Instructions**:

1. Take one capsule of Lion's Mane Mushroom extract daily with water.

2. For best results, consume in the morning or early afternoon.

- **Variations:** Lion's Mane can also be consumed as a tea or added to food in powder form for those who prefer not to take capsules.

- **Storage tips:** Keep the capsules in a cool, dry place, away from direct sunlight.

- **Tips for allergens:** Individuals with mushroom allergies should avoid this supplement.

Rosemary Essential Oil

Beneficial effects: Rosemary essential oil is known for its ability to enhance memory and concentration. The aroma of rosemary has been linked to improved cognitive performance and mood.

Ingredients:

- A diffuser

- 5-10 drops of Rosemary essential oil

- **Instructions**:

1. Fill the diffuser with water according to the manufacturer's instructions.

2. Add 5-10 drops of Rosemary essential oil to the water.

3. Turn on the diffuser and allow the aroma to fill the room for cognitive enhancement.

- **Variations:** For a direct approach, apply a diluted mixture of rosemary oil and a carrier oil to the temples or wrists.

- **Storage tips:** Store the essential oil in a cool, dark place to preserve its potency.

- **Tips for allergens:** Conduct a patch test before topical application to ensure no allergic reaction.

Omega-3 Fatty Acids

Beneficial effects: Omega-3 fatty acids, particularly EPA and DHA, are vital for brain health. They contribute to the maintenance of normal brain function and have been associated with reduced risk of cognitive decline.

Ingredients:

- Fish oil supplement containing EPA and DHA or a plant-based omega-3 supplement like algal oil

- **Instructions**:

1. Take an omega-3 supplement daily, following the dosage recommendations on the product label.

2. For fish oil supplements, a common dose is 1,000 mg daily.

- **Variations:** Incorporate omega-3-rich foods into your diet, such as salmon, walnuts, and flaxseeds, as an alternative or complement to supplements.

- **Storage tips:** Store supplements in a cool, dry place, or refrigerate if recommended by the manufacturer.

- **Tips for allergens:** For those allergic to fish, consider algal oil supplements as a plant-based source of omega-3.

Bacopa Monnieri

Beneficial effects: Bacopa Monnieri is an herb that has been used in traditional medicine for centuries to enhance brain function. It is known for improving memory, attention, and the speed of processing visual information.

Ingredients:

- 300 mg of Bacopa Monnieri extract (standardized to contain at least 55% bacosides)

- **Instructions**:

1. Take one capsule of Bacopa Monnieri extract daily with water.

2. For optimal cognitive benefits, consume consistently for at least 8-12 weeks.

- **Variations:** Bacopa Monnieri can also be consumed as a tea for those who prefer a more traditional method of intake.

- **Storage tips:** Keep the extract in a cool, dry place, away from direct sunlight.

- **Tips for allergens:** Bacopa Monnieri is generally well-tolerated, but it's advisable to start with a lower dose to assess tolerance.

Ginkgo Biloba

Beneficial effects: Ginkgo Biloba is renowned for its ability to improve blood circulation to the brain, thereby enhancing cognitive function, memory, and focus.

Ingredients:

- 120 mg of Ginkgo Biloba extract (standardized to 24% flavone glycosides and 6% terpene lactones)

- **Instructions**:

1. Take one capsule of Ginkgo Biloba extract daily with water.

2. It may take 4-6 weeks to notice improvements in cognitive function.

- **Variations:** Ginkgo Biloba tea is an alternative for those who prefer not to take capsules.

- **Storage tips:** Store the capsules or tea in a cool, dry place, away from direct sunlight.

- **Tips for allergens:** Ginkgo Biloba is generally safe, but those on blood-thinning medications should consult with a healthcare provider due to potential interactions.

Incorporating these natural remedies into your daily routine can support cognitive function and mental clarity. It's important to remember that while these supplements and herbs offer benefits for cognitive health, they should complement a healthy lifestyle that includes a balanced diet, regular physical activity, adequate sleep, and stress management for optimal cognitive wellness.

CHAPTER 4: 10 HERBAL RECIPES FOR MENTAL CLARITY

GINKGO BILOBA AND ROSEMARY MEMORY TONIC

Beneficial effects

Ginkgo Biloba and Rosemary Memory Tonic is designed to enhance cognitive function, improve memory, and increase focus. Ginkgo Biloba is renowned for its ability to boost blood circulation to the brain, which can lead to improved cognitive abilities and a reduction in symptoms associated with cognitive decline. Rosemary, on the other hand, contains compounds that have been shown to enhance memory and concentration. Together, they create a powerful tonic that supports brain health and mental clarity.

Portions

4 servings

Preparation time

15 minutes

Cooking time

5 minutes

Ingredients

- 4 cups of water
- 2 tablespoons dried Ginkgo Biloba leaves
- 1 tablespoon dried rosemary leaves
- Honey or lemon to taste (optional)

Instructions

1. Bring 4 cups of water to a boil in a medium-sized pot.

2. Add the dried Ginkgo Biloba leaves and dried rosemary leaves to the boiling water.

3. Reduce the heat and simmer for 5 minutes, allowing the herbs to infuse their properties into the water.

4. After simmering, remove the pot from the heat and let the tonic cool for a few minutes.

5. Strain the mixture into a large pitcher, discarding the herbs.

6. Optional: Add honey or lemon to the strained tonic for flavor enhancement.

7. Serve the tonic warm, or allow it to cool and enjoy it chilled.

Variations

- For an added boost of antioxidants, include a green tea bag during the simmering process.
- Mix in a teaspoon of turmeric powder with the herbs for additional anti-inflammatory benefits.
- For those preferring a sweeter tonic, blend in fresh apple juice instead of using honey or lemon.

Storage tips

Store any leftover Ginkgo Biloba and Rosemary Memory Tonic in an airtight container in the refrigerator for up to 48 hours. Enjoy it cold, or gently reheat on the stove.

Tips for allergens

Individuals with allergies to Ginkgo Biloba, rosemary, or honey should adjust the recipe accordingly or consult with a healthcare provider before consumption. Maple syrup can be used as a vegan-friendly sweetener alternative to honey.

Scientific references

- "Ginkgo Biloba for Cognitive Improvement in Healthy Individuals: A Systematic Review," published in Human Psychopharmacology. This review examines the cognitive-enhancing effects of Ginkgo Biloba, supporting its use for mental clarity.

- "Plasma 1,8-cineole correlates with cognitive performance following exposure to rosemary essential oil aroma," published in Therapeutic Advances in Psychopharmacology. This study highlights the positive impact of rosemary on cognitive performance, particularly memory enhancement.

LEMON BALM AND GINSENG FOCUS ELIXIR

Beneficial effects

Lemon Balm and Ginseng Focus Elixir is crafted to enhance mental clarity, improve concentration, and reduce stress. Lemon balm, with its calming properties, helps to ease anxiety and promote a relaxed state of mind, which is conducive to focused mental activities. Ginseng is known for its ability to improve cognitive function and energy levels, making it easier to maintain concentration over extended periods. Together, they create a powerful elixir that supports overall brain health and mental performance.

Portions

2 servings

Preparation time

10 minutes

Ingredients

- 1 tablespoon dried lemon balm leaves
- 1 teaspoon ginseng powder
- 2 cups boiling water
- Honey or lemon to taste (optional)

Instructions

1. Place the dried lemon balm leaves and ginseng powder in a heat-resistant teapot or French press.
2. Pour 2 cups of boiling water over the lemon balm and ginseng.
3. Let the mixture steep for about 8 to 10 minutes. The longer it steeps, the stronger the flavor and benefits.
4. Strain the elixir into cups, removing the lemon balm leaves and any ginseng residue.
5. Optional: Add honey or a squeeze of lemon to each cup for added flavor.
6. Serve the elixir warm to enjoy its focus-enhancing benefits.

Variations

- For a cold version, allow the elixir to cool and then refrigerate. Serve over ice for a refreshing mental boost.
- Add a slice of fresh ginger during the steeping process for additional anti-inflammatory benefits and a spicy kick.

- Mix in a teaspoon of matcha powder with the ginseng for an extra antioxidant boost and a vibrant green color.

Storage tips

If you have leftover Lemon Balm and Ginseng Focus Elixir, store it in a sealed container in the refrigerator for up to 2 days. Enjoy it chilled, or gently reheat on the stove.

Tips for allergens

Individuals with allergies to lemon balm, ginseng, or other herbs should proceed with caution and may consider consulting with a healthcare provider before consumption. For those avoiding honey due to dietary restrictions, substitute with maple syrup or simply omit the sweetener.

Scientific references

- "Effects of Panax ginseng on cognitive performance in Alzheimer's disease: a double-blind randomised controlled trial" in the Journal of Ginseng Research, 2010. This study supports the cognitive-enhancing properties of ginseng.

- "Melissa officinalis L. Extract – An Evidence-Based Systematic Review by the Natural Standard Research Collaboration" in the Journal of Herbal Pharmacotherapy, 2005. This review discusses the anxiety-reducing and cognitive function-improving effects of lemon balm, supporting its use for mental clarity.

GOTU KOLA AND BACOPA BRAIN BOOST TEA

Beneficial effects

Gotu Kola and Bacopa Brain Boost Tea combines the cognitive-enhancing properties of Gotu Kola and Bacopa monnieri, making it an excellent choice for improving mental clarity, memory, and focus. Gotu Kola is known for its ability to improve circulation and boost antioxidant activity in the brain, which can enhance cognitive functions and protect neural cells. Bacopa monnieri, on the other hand, has been traditionally used to improve memory, reduce anxiety, and support overall brain health. Together, these herbs create a powerful tea that can help enhance cognitive performance and support long-term brain health.

Portions

2 servings

Preparation time

10 minutes

Cooking time

15 minutes

Ingredients

- 1 teaspoon dried Gotu Kola leaves

- 1 teaspoon dried Bacopa monnieri leaves

- 2 cups of water

- Honey or lemon (optional, for taste)

Instructions

1. Bring 2 cups of water to a boil in a small saucepan.

2. Add the dried Gotu Kola and Bacopa monnieri leaves to the boiling water.

3. Reduce the heat and simmer for about 15 minutes to allow the herbs to infuse their properties into the water.

4. After simmering, remove the saucepan from the heat and let the tea cool for a few minutes.

5. Strain the tea into cups, discarding the leaves.

6. Optional: Add honey or a squeeze of lemon to each cup for added flavor.

7. Serve the tea warm to enjoy its cognitive-enhancing benefits.

Variations

- For an added boost of energy and focus, include a slice of fresh ginger in the simmering process.

- Mix in a teaspoon of green tea leaves with the Gotu Kola and Bacopa monnieri for added antioxidants and a mild caffeine boost.

- For those preferring a cold beverage, chill the tea in the refrigerator and serve over ice with a sprig of mint for a refreshing drink.

Storage tips

Store any leftover Gotu Kola and Bacopa Brain Boost Tea in a sealed container in the refrigerator for up to 2 days. Enjoy it chilled or gently reheat on the stove.

Tips for allergens

Individuals with allergies to Gotu Kola, Bacopa monnieri, or related plants should consult with a healthcare provider before consumption. For a honey alternative, maple syrup can be used as a sweetener for those with honey allergies or following a vegan diet.

Scientific references

- "Neuroprotective effects of Bacopa monnieri in experimental model of dementia" published in Neurochemistry International, 2014. This study supports Bacopa monnieri's benefits for cognitive health, including memory enhancement and neuroprotection.

- "Centella asiatica (Gotu Kola) as a Neuroprotectant and Its Potential Role in Healthy Aging" published in Trends in Food Science & Technology, 2018. This review discusses the neuroprotective effects of Gotu Kola and its potential benefits for cognitive health and aging.

SAGE AND PEPPERMINT COGNITIVE CLARITY INFUSION

Beneficial effects

Sage and Peppermint Cognitive Clarity Infusion is crafted to enhance mental alertness and cognitive function. Sage is renowned for its ability to improve memory and focus, while peppermint stimulates the mind and promotes clear thinking. This infusion is an excellent choice for those seeking a natural boost to their mental clarity and concentration, making it ideal for study sessions, work projects, or any activities requiring sharp cognitive abilities.

Portions

2 servings

Preparation time

5 minutes

Cooking time

10 minutes

Ingredients

- 1 tablespoon dried sage leaves

- 1 tablespoon dried peppermint leaves

- 2 cups boiling water

- Honey or lemon (optional, for taste)

Instructions

1. Place the dried sage and peppermint leaves in a tea infuser or directly into a heat-resistant teapot.

2. Pour 2 cups of boiling water over the sage and peppermint leaves.

3. Cover and allow the infusion to steep for about 10 minutes, enabling the herbs to release their beneficial oils and flavors.

4. Remove the tea infuser or strain the infusion to remove the leaves.

5. Optional: Add honey or a slice of lemon to each cup for added flavor.

6. Serve the infusion warm to enjoy its cognitive-enhancing benefits.

Variations

- For a refreshing twist, serve the infusion chilled over ice for a cool, cognitive-enhancing beverage.

- Add a slice of fresh ginger during the steeping process for an extra kick and additional anti-inflammatory benefits.

- Combine with green tea leaves for an added antioxidant boost and a slight caffeine lift.

Storage tips

If you have leftover Sage and Peppermint Cognitive Clarity Infusion, store it in a sealed container in the refrigerator for up to 2 days. Enjoy it chilled, or gently reheat on the stove.

Tips for allergens

Individuals with allergies to sage, peppermint, or other herbs should consult with a healthcare provider before consuming this infusion. For those avoiding honey due to dietary restrictions, substitute with maple syrup or simply omit the sweetener.

Scientific references

- "Salvia officinalis extract in the treatment of patients with mild to moderate Alzheimer's disease: a double blind, randomized and placebo-controlled trial," published in the Journal of Clinical Pharmacy and Therapeutics, 2003. This study supports sage's benefits for cognitive function and memory enhancement.

- "Peppermint and its functionality: A review," published in the Archives of Clinical Microbiology, 2010. This review highlights peppermint's stimulating effects on the central nervous system, promoting mental clarity and focus.

HOLY BASIL AND ASHWAGANDHA STRESS RELIEF SMOOTHIE

Beneficial effects

The Holy Basil and Ashwagandha Stress Relief Smoothie combines the adaptogenic powers of holy basil (Tulsi) and ashwagandha, both revered in Ayurvedic medicine for their stress-reducing properties.

Holy basil is known for its ability to lower cortisol levels, enhance stamina, and support a healthy immune system. Ashwagandha contributes by reducing anxiety, improving energy levels, and promoting overall mental clarity.

Together, they create a potent remedy for combating stress and fostering mental wellness.

Portions

2 servings

Preparation time

5 minutes

Ingredients

- 1 cup almond milk

- 1 ripe banana

- 1/2 cup spinach leaves

- 1 tablespoon ashwagandha powder

- 1 tablespoon holy basil (Tulsi) leaves, fresh or dried

- 1 tablespoon honey (optional, for sweetness)

- Ice cubes (optional)

Instructions

1. In a blender, combine almond milk, ripe banana, spinach leaves, ashwagandha powder, and holy basil leaves.

2. Blend on high until the mixture is smooth and creamy.

3. Taste the smoothie, and if desired, add honey for sweetness. Blend again briefly to mix.

4. If a colder smoothie is preferred, add ice cubes and blend until smooth.

5. Pour the smoothie into glasses and serve immediately for the best flavor and nutrient content.

Variations

- For a protein boost, add a scoop of your favorite plant-based protein powder.

- Substitute almond milk with coconut water for a lighter version or with oat milk for a nut-free option.

- Add a tablespoon of flaxseeds or chia seeds for added fiber and omega-3 fatty acids.

Storage tips

It's best to consume the Holy Basil and Ashwagandha Stress Relief Smoothie immediately after preparation to enjoy its full benefits. However, if you need to store it, keep the smoothie in an airtight container in the refrigerator for up to 24 hours. Stir well before consuming if separation occurs.

Tips for allergens

For those with nut allergies, ensure to substitute almond milk with a suitable non-nut milk alternative like oat milk or rice milk. If you're vegan or have a honey allergy, substitute honey with maple syrup or omit it altogether.

Scientific references

- "Adaptogenic and Anxiolytic Effects of Ashwagandha Root Extract: A Double-Blind, Randomized, Placebo-Controlled Study" in the Journal of Ethnopharmacology, 2019. This study supports ashwagandha's benefits in reducing stress and anxiety.

- "Ocimum sanctum Linn. (Holy Basil or Tulsi) and its phytochemicals in the prevention and treatment of cancer" in Nutrition and Cancer, 2013. This research highlights holy basil's potential in stress reduction and overall health improvement.

BLUEBERRY AND RHODIOLA MENTAL SHARPNESS DRINK

Beneficial effects

The Blueberry and Rhodiola Mental Sharpness Drink is designed to enhance cognitive function, improve memory, and increase energy levels. Blueberries are rich in antioxidants that protect the brain from oxidative stress and reduce the risk of age-related cognitive decline. Rhodiola rosea, an adaptogen, helps to improve focus, reduce mental fatigue, and support brain health. Together, they create a powerful drink that can help maintain mental clarity and support overall brain function.

Portions

2 servings

Preparation time

5 minutes

Ingredients

- 1 cup fresh blueberries

- 1 teaspoon Rhodiola rosea powder

- 2 cups cold water or coconut water

- 1 tablespoon honey (optional)

- Ice cubes (optional)

Instructions

1. Place the fresh blueberries and Rhodiola rosea powder in a blender.

2. Add the cold water or coconut water to the blender. For a sweeter taste, include the tablespoon of honey.

3. Blend on high until all the ingredients are well combined and the mixture is smooth.

4. If desired, add ice cubes to the blender and pulse a few more times to chill the drink.

5. Pour the drink into glasses and serve immediately for the best taste and mental boost.

Variations

- To add a citrus twist, include the juice of one lemon or lime in the blend.

- For extra fiber and omega-3 fatty acids, add a tablespoon of ground flaxseed or chia seeds before blending.

- Substitute honey with maple syrup for a vegan-friendly version.

Storage tips

This drink is best enjoyed fresh. However, if you need to store it, keep it in a sealed container in the refrigerator for up to 24 hours. Shake well before serving if separation occurs.

Tips for allergens

Individuals with sensitivities to Rhodiola rosea should start with a smaller dose to ensure no adverse reactions. For those allergic to blueberries, consider substituting with raspberries or blackberries, which also offer cognitive benefits.

Scientific references

- "Effects of blueberry and cranberry consumption on type 2 diabetes glycemic control: a systematic review." Critical Reviews in Food Science and Nutrition, 2019. This review highlights the antioxidant properties of blueberries and their impact on health.

- "Rhodiola rosea in stress-induced fatigue—a double-blind cross-over study of a standardized extract SHR-5 with a repeated low-dose regimen on the mental performance of healthy physicians during night duty." Phytomedicine, 2000. This study supports the use of Rhodiola rosea for improving mental performance and reducing fatigue.

ROSEMARY AND LEMON VERBENA CONCENTRATION TEA

Beneficial effects

Rosemary and Lemon Verbena Concentration Tea is crafted to enhance mental clarity, focus, and cognitive function. Rosemary is well-known for its ability to improve memory and concentration, thanks to its aromatic compounds that have neuroprotective properties. Lemon Verbena adds to the blend with its calming effects, reducing anxiety and stress, which can hinder cognitive performance. Together, they create a synergistic infusion that not only uplifts the mind but also soothes the nervous system, making it an ideal beverage for studying, working, or any activity requiring mental stamina.

Portions

2 servings

Preparation time

5 minutes

Cooking time

10 minutes

Ingredients

- 1 tablespoon dried rosemary leaves

- 1 tablespoon dried lemon verbena leaves

- 2 cups of boiling water

- Honey or lemon slice (optional, for taste)

Instructions

1. Combine the dried rosemary and lemon verbena leaves in a teapot or heat-resistant pitcher.

2. Pour 2 cups of boiling water over the herbs.

3. Cover and allow the mixture to steep for about 10 minutes to fully release the flavors and beneficial compounds.

4. Strain the tea into cups, discarding the herbs.

5. If desired, add honey or a slice of lemon to each cup for added flavor.

6. Serve the tea warm, ideally in the morning or early afternoon to harness its cognitive-enhancing benefits.

Variations

- For a refreshing twist, chill the tea and serve over ice for a cool, revitalizing drink.

- Add a sprig of fresh mint to the steeping process for additional flavor and digestive benefits.

- Incorporate a slice of fresh ginger during steeping to boost the tea's antioxidant properties and add a spicy note.

Storage tips

If you have leftover Rosemary and Lemon Verbena Concentration Tea, store it in a sealed container in the refrigerator for up to 2 days. Enjoy it chilled, or gently reheat on the stove.

Tips for allergens

Individuals with allergies to rosemary or lemon verbena should proceed with caution and may consider consulting with a healthcare provider before consumption. For those avoiding honey due to dietary restrictions, substitute with maple syrup or simply omit the sweetener.

Scientific references

- "Aromas of rosemary and lavender essential oils differentially affect cognition and mood in healthy adults," published in the International Journal of Neuroscience, 2003. This study highlights the positive effects of rosemary on memory performance and mental alertness.

- "Lemon verbena: A promising herb with health benefits," in the Journal of Functional Foods, 2019. This article discusses lemon verbena's anti-stress and antioxidant effects, supporting its use for enhancing mental clarity and cognitive function.

LION'S MANE MUSHROOM AND GREEN TEA BRAIN HEALTH ELIXIR

Beneficial effects

Lion's Mane Mushroom and Green Tea Brain Health Elixir is designed to enhance cognitive function, support nerve growth, and improve mental clarity. Lion's Mane Mushroom has been shown to contain compounds that stimulate the growth of brain cells and protect them from damage caused by Alzheimer's disease. Green tea is rich in antioxidants, particularly EGCG, which can protect brain cells from oxidative stress and improve brain function. This elixir combines the cognitive benefits of both ingredients, making it a powerful drink for boosting brain health and preventing cognitive decline.

Portions

2 servings

Preparation time

5 minutes

Cooking time

10 minutes

Ingredients

- 1 teaspoon dried Lion's Mane Mushroom powder

- 2 teaspoons green tea leaves or 2 green tea bags

- 4 cups of water

- Honey or lemon to taste (optional)

Instructions

1. Bring 4 cups of water to a boil in a medium-sized pot.

2. Lower the heat and add the Lion's Mane Mushroom powder and green tea leaves or bags to the pot.

3. Simmer for about 10 minutes to allow the ingredients to infuse the water.

4. Strain the elixir into mugs or a heat-resistant pitcher, removing the tea leaves or bags and any undissolved mushroom powder.

5. Optional: Add honey or lemon to taste for flavor enhancement.

6. Serve the elixir warm, preferably in the morning or early afternoon to support mental clarity throughout the day.

Variations

- For a cold version, allow the elixir to cool to room temperature, then refrigerate and serve over ice.

- Add a slice of fresh ginger during the simmering process for additional anti-inflammatory benefits and a spicy kick.

- Mix in a teaspoon of turmeric powder with a pinch of black pepper to enhance the elixir's antioxidant properties and promote brain health.

Storage tips

If you have leftover Lion's Mane Mushroom and Green Tea Brain Health Elixir, store it in a sealed container in the refrigerator for up to 2 days. Enjoy it chilled or gently reheat on the stove.

Tips for allergens

Individuals with sensitivities to mushrooms should proceed with caution when trying Lion's Mane Mushroom. For those avoiding honey due to dietary restrictions, substitute with maple syrup or simply omit the sweetener.

Scientific references

- "Neurohealth Properties of Hericium erinaceus (Lion's Mane) Mushroom Mycelia Enriched with Erinacines," published in Behavioural Neurology, 2018. This study highlights the neuroprotective effects of Lion's Mane Mushroom, supporting its use for cognitive health.

- "The effects of green tea on cognitive function: a systematic review and meta-analysis," published in Phytomedicine, 2019. This review provides evidence of green tea's beneficial impact on brain function, including improved memory and attention.

GINSENG AND MATCHA ENERGY BOOST SMOOTHIE

Beneficial effects

Ginseng and Matcha Energy Boost Smoothie combines the revitalizing properties of ginseng, known for improving mental clarity and reducing fatigue, with the antioxidant-rich matcha, which enhances focus and energy levels. This smoothie is an excellent choice for those seeking a natural boost to their cognitive function and mental alertness without the jitters associated with caffeine. The blend also supports metabolism and overall wellness, making it a perfect addition to a balanced lifestyle aimed at enhancing mental clarity.

Portions

1 serving

Preparation time

5 minutes

Ingredients

- 1 teaspoon matcha green tea powder

- 1/2 teaspoon ginseng powder

- 1 ripe banana

- 1 cup almond milk

- 1 tablespoon honey (optional, for sweetness)

- Ice cubes (optional, for a chilled smoothie)

Instructions

1. In a blender, combine the matcha green tea powder, ginseng powder, and ripe banana.

2. Add the almond milk to the blender. For added sweetness, include the tablespoon of honey.

3. If a colder beverage is preferred, add ice cubes to the mixture.

4. Blend all ingredients on high until the mixture is smooth and creamy.

5. Pour the smoothie into a glass and enjoy immediately for the best taste and energy boost.

Variations

- For added protein, include a scoop of your favorite vanilla or unflavored protein powder.

- Substitute almond milk with coconut water for a lighter version or oat milk for a nut-free option.

- Enhance the smoothie's nutritional profile by adding a handful of spinach or kale, which won't significantly alter the taste but will increase vitamin and mineral intake.

Storage tips

It's best to consume the Ginseng and Matcha Energy Boost Smoothie immediately after preparation to enjoy its full benefits. However, if necessary, store it in an airtight container in the refrigerator for up to 24 hours. Shake well before consuming if separation occurs.

Tips for allergens

For those with nut allergies, replace almond milk with a suitable non-nut milk alternative like oat milk or rice milk. If honey is a concern due to allergies or vegan dietary preferences, substitute with maple syrup or omit it altogether.

Scientific references

- "Ginseng, the 'Immunity Boost': The Effects of Panax ginseng on Immune System" published in the Journal of Ginseng Research, 2012. This study highlights ginseng's beneficial effects on enhancing mental performance and energy levels.

- "L-Theanine and Caffeine in Combination Affect Human Cognition as Evidenced by Oscillatory alpha-Band Activity and Attention Task Performance" in the Journal of Nutrition, 2008. This research supports the cognitive-enhancing properties of matcha, which contains both L-Theanine and caffeine, making it effective in improving focus and attention.

LAVENDER AND CHAMOMILE RELAXATION TEA

Beneficial effects

Lavender and Chamomile Relaxation Tea combines the calming properties of lavender with the soothing effects of chamomile, creating a natural remedy to reduce stress, anxiety, and promote a peaceful state of mind. Lavender is known for its ability to decrease cortisol levels, the body's stress hormone, while chamomile has been traditionally used to improve sleep quality and relaxation. Together, they form a powerful duo that can help ease the mind, improve sleep patterns, and support overall mental clarity and well-being.

Ingredients

- 1 tablespoon dried lavender flowers

- 1 tablespoon dried chamomile flowers

- 2 cups boiling water

- Honey or lemon to taste (optional)

Instructions

1. Place the dried lavender and chamomile flowers in a tea infuser or directly into a heat-resistant teapot.

2. Pour 2 cups of boiling water over the flowers.

3. Cover and allow the tea to steep for 5 to 10 minutes, depending on the desired strength.

4. Remove the tea infuser or strain the tea to remove the flowers.

5. Optional: Add honey or lemon to taste for added flavor.

6. Serve the tea warm, ideally in the evening, to unwind and promote relaxation before bedtime.

Variations

- For a cooler, refreshing version, allow the tea to cool and serve it over ice, garnished with a slice of lemon or a sprig of fresh lavender.

- Mix in a teaspoon of mint leaves with the lavender and chamomile for a refreshing twist and additional digestive benefits.

- For a sweeter, floral note, add a teaspoon of rose petals to the infusion for their mood-enhancing properties.

Storage tips

If you have leftover Lavender and Chamomile Relaxation Tea, store it in a sealed container in the refrigerator for up to 2 days. Enjoy it chilled, or gently reheat on the stove.

Tips for allergens

Individuals with allergies to plants in the Asteraceae family, such as chamomile, should proceed with caution and may consider consulting with a healthcare provider before consumption. For those avoiding honey due to dietary restrictions, substitute with maple syrup or simply omit the sweetener.

Scientific references

- "A review of the bioactivity and potential health benefits of chamomile tea (Matricaria recutita L.)" in Phytotherapy Research, 2006. This study highlights the calming and sleep-promoting effects of chamomile.

- "Lavender and the Nervous System" published in Evidence-Based Complementary and Alternative Medicine, 2013. This article discusses the anxiolytic (anxiety-reducing) and sedative effects of lavender, supporting its use for stress relief and mental clarity.

PART 17: WEIGHT MANAGEMENT AND METABOLISM

Weight management and metabolism are closely intertwined, playing a crucial role in overall health and well-being. Effective weight management involves understanding and optimizing your metabolism, the process by which your body converts what you eat and drink into energy. This energy fuels everything you do, from running a marathon to breathing and circulating blood. The rate at which your body burns calories and converts them to energy is influenced by several factors, including your genetic makeup, age, gender, and lifestyle choices.

To embark on a journey of healthy weight management, it's essential to focus on foods that naturally enhance metabolic rate while providing nutritional value. Foods rich in protein, for example, can increase the thermic effect of food—the amount of energy required to digest, absorb, and process the nutrients in your meal. Lean meats, legumes, nuts, seeds, and dairy products are excellent sources of protein that can help boost metabolism and promote satiety, reducing the likelihood of overeating.

In addition to protein, incorporating a variety of fruits and vegetables into your diet is vital. These foods are not only rich in essential vitamins and minerals but also high in fiber. Fiber plays a key role in weight management by slowing the digestion process, leading to a more prolonged feeling of fullness and a reduced appetite.

High-fiber foods include whole grains, legumes, apples, berries, avocados, and leafy green vegetables.

Hydration is another critical factor in managing weight and metabolism. Water is necessary for metabolizing stored fat into energy, and even mild dehydration can slow down this process. Drinking sufficient amounts of water throughout the day can also help control hunger, prevent overeating, and support overall metabolic health.

Regular physical activity complements a balanced diet in supporting weight management and metabolic health. Exercise not only burns calories but also builds muscle. Muscle tissue burns more calories at rest than fat tissue, so increasing muscle mass through physical activity can help accelerate your metabolism over time.

Understanding the role of sleep in weight management and metabolism is also crucial. Lack of sleep can disrupt hormonal balance, including hormones that regulate appetite and hunger, such as ghrelin and leptin. This imbalance can lead to increased hunger and appetite, making it more challenging to manage weight. Prioritizing good sleep hygiene practices can support hormonal balance, helping to regulate metabolism and appetite.

In the realm of herbal remedies, certain herbs and spices are believed to support metabolic health and weight management. Green tea, for example, contains catechins and caffeine, which have been shown to enhance metabolic rate and increase fat burning. Similarly, spices such as ginger and cayenne pepper may have thermogenic properties, helping to boost metabolism and increase calorie burn.

As we continue to explore the intricate relationship between weight management and metabolism, it's clear that a holistic approach encompassing diet, exercise, hydration, sleep, and natural remedies offers the most effective strategy for achieving and maintaining a healthy weight. This approach not only supports metabolic health but also contributes to overall well-being, vitality, and longevity.

Managing stress effectively is another pivotal aspect of weight management and metabolic health. Chronic stress can lead to an increase in cortisol, a hormone that not only promotes fat storage, especially in the abdominal area, but can also lead to unhealthy eating habits. Incorporating stress-reduction techniques such as meditation, deep breathing exercises, and yoga can help lower cortisol levels, thereby supporting weight loss efforts and metabolic health.

Mindful eating practices also play a significant role in weight management. By paying close attention to the experience of eating, savoring each bite, and listening to the body's hunger and fullness cues, individuals can avoid overeating and make healthier food choices. This practice not only aids in weight management but also enhances the metabolic process by encouraging a slower, more thoughtful consumption of food, which can lead to improved digestion and nutrient absorption.

In addition to these lifestyle factors, certain nutritional supplements can support metabolic health and weight management. For instance, omega-3 fatty acids, found in fish oil supplements, have been shown to increase the number of calories burned by improving mitochondrial function. Similarly, magnesium supplements can help regulate blood sugar levels and support energy production, contributing to a more efficient metabolism.

It's important to note that while herbal remedies and supplements can support metabolic health, they should complement, not replace, a healthy diet and lifestyle. Always consult with a healthcare provider before starting any new supplement regimen, especially if you have underlying health conditions or are taking medications.

Finally, building a supportive community around health and wellness goals can significantly impact weight management and metabolic health. Joining a fitness class, participating in a healthy cooking workshop, or simply sharing goals with friends and family can provide the motivation and accountability needed to maintain a healthy lifestyle. Celebrating small victories together and offering support during challenges can make the journey towards better health more enjoyable and sustainable.

By embracing a holistic approach to weight management and metabolism that includes balanced nutrition, regular physical activity, adequate hydration, sufficient sleep, stress management, mindful eating, and the judicious use of supplements, individuals can enhance their metabolic health and achieve their weight management goals. This comprehensive strategy not only supports physical health but also promotes overall well-being and vitality.

CHAPTER 1: DR. BARBARA'S WEIGHT MANAGEMENT TIPS

D r. Barbara emphasizes the significance of a holistic approach to weight management, underscoring the importance of understanding the body's unique needs and the intricate balance between diet, exercise, and mental well-being. She advocates for a shift from the conventional focus on restrictive diets and calorie counting to a more nourishing perspective that embraces whole, nutrient-dense foods, mindful eating practices, and the joy of physical movement. According to Dr. Barbara, successful weight management is not about short-term dietary restrictions but about establishing a sustainable, balanced lifestyle that supports the body's natural metabolism and fosters a positive relationship with food and exercise.

Central to Dr. Barbara's approach is the concept of listening to the body's cues and recognizing the factors beyond diet and exercise that influence weight, such as stress, sleep quality, and emotional well-being. She points out that stress can lead to hormonal imbalances that affect appetite and fat storage, highlighting the importance of stress-reduction techniques like meditation, deep breathing, and yoga in a comprehensive weight management strategy.

Similarly, Dr. Barbara discusses the critical role of sleep in regulating hormones related to hunger and satiety, advocating for good sleep hygiene to support weight loss efforts.

Dr. Barbara also delves into the metabolic benefits of incorporating a variety of whole foods into the diet, focusing on the importance of fiber, healthy fats, lean proteins, and a rainbow of fruits and vegetables to enhance satiety, improve digestion, and boost energy levels. She encourages the consumption of foods that naturally support metabolism, such as green tea, spicy foods, and water-rich fruits and vegetables, and advises against highly processed foods, sugary drinks, and excessive caffeine, which can disrupt metabolic balance and lead to weight gain.

Physical activity, according to Dr. Barbara, should be enjoyable and tailored to individual preferences and fitness levels. She advocates for finding joy in movement, whether through dancing, hiking, yoga, or strength training, and emphasizes the importance of consistency and listening to the body's needs and limitations. Dr. Barbara suggests integrating physical activity into daily routines, such as taking walks during breaks or choosing stairs over elevators, to enhance metabolic health and support weight management.

Mindful eating is another cornerstone of Dr. Barbara's weight management philosophy. She encourages slowing down during meals, paying attention to the flavors, textures, and sensations of food, and tuning into hunger and fullness signals. This practice, according to Dr. Barbara, can prevent overeating, enhance digestion, and promote a more harmonious relationship with food.

In conclusion, Dr. Barbara's insights on weight management offer a compassionate, holistic approach that goes beyond traditional dieting to embrace a comprehensive lifestyle that nurtures the body, mind, and spirit. By focusing on nourishment, joyful movement, stress reduction, and mindful eating, individuals can achieve sustainable weight management and enhance their overall health and well-being.

CHAPTER 2: NUTRITION FOR HEALTHY WEIGHT MANAGEMENT

Focusing on nutrition for healthy weight management involves a strategic approach to eating that fuels the body efficiently, supports metabolic health, and promotes a sense of well-being. Key to this strategy is the emphasis on whole, unprocessed foods that provide a rich source of nutrients while helping to regulate appetite and reduce cravings. Incorporating a variety of fruits and vegetables, lean proteins, whole grains, and healthy fats into daily meals ensures a balanced intake of vitamins, minerals, fiber, and antioxidants, all of which play a crucial role in maintaining a healthy weight.

Fruits and vegetables, abundant in vitamins and minerals, also offer high fiber content, which is essential for satiety and helps maintain a healthy digestive system. Fiber-rich foods not only keep you feeling full longer but also stabilize blood sugar levels, preventing the spikes and crashes that can lead to overeating. Berries, apples, leafy greens, and cruciferous vegetables like broccoli and Brussels sprouts are excellent choices for adding fiber and a wealth of nutrients to your diet.

Lean proteins are another cornerstone of weight management nutrition. Foods such as chicken breast, turkey, fish, legumes, and tofu provide the body with essential amino acids without the added fats that come with more processed protein sources. These proteins help build and repair muscle tissue, especially important if you're incorporating strength training into your fitness routine, as muscle burns more calories at rest than fat.

Whole grains offer a nutritious alternative to refined grains, delivering more fiber, protein, and nutrients with each serving.

Options like quinoa, brown rice, barley, and whole wheat provide energy that releases slowly over time, keeping you fueled and satisfied throughout the day. These grains can be easily incorporated into meals as bases for salads, stir-fries, or as side dishes.

Healthy fats, found in foods like avocados, nuts, seeds, and olive oil, are vital for absorbing vitamins and providing energy.

Contrary to popular belief, incorporating these fats into your diet can actually support weight loss efforts by enhancing satiety and reducing overall calorie intake. The key is moderation and choosing unsaturated fats over saturated and trans fats found in processed foods.

Hydration plays a pivotal role in weight management, with water being the best choice for staying hydrated without adding extra calories. Drinking water before meals can also help control appetite and prevent overeating.

Green tea is another beneficial beverage, offering metabolism-boosting antioxidants and providing a healthy alternative to sugary drinks.

Regular physical activity, while not a direct component of nutrition, complements a healthy diet by boosting metabolism, burning calories, and building muscle. Combining a balanced, nutritious diet with consistent exercise is the most effective way to achieve and maintain a healthy weight.

Mindful eating practices encourage paying attention to hunger and fullness cues, eating without distraction, and enjoying each bite.

This approach can help prevent overeating and make meals more satisfying, both physically and emotionally.

Lastly, it's important to listen to your body and adjust your diet according to your individual needs and responses.

What works for one person may not work for another, making it essential to find a balanced eating plan that feels right for you and supports your weight management goals.

Remember, a healthy diet is not about restriction but about making informed choices that nourish and satisfy the body.

CHAPTER 3: NATURAL APPROACHES TO WEIGHT MANAGEMENT

Natural approaches to weight management focus on leveraging the inherent synergy between the body and nature to achieve and maintain a healthy weight. This method emphasizes the importance of whole foods, herbal supplements, and lifestyle adjustments that align with the body's natural rhythms and processes. By understanding and applying these principles, individuals can create a sustainable path to weight management that not only contributes to physical health but also enhances mental and emotional well-being.

Herbal supplements play a significant role in supporting metabolic health and aiding weight management efforts. For instance, herbs like green tea extract are rich in antioxidants and have been shown to boost metabolism and enhance fat burning.

Similarly, cinnamon can help regulate blood sugar levels, reducing the likelihood of insulin spikes that can lead to weight gain. Incorporating these herbs into a daily regimen can complement dietary and lifestyle changes, providing a holistic approach to weight management.

Another key component is the consumption of adaptogenic herbs such as ashwagandha, which helps the body manage stress more effectively.

Chronic stress is a common barrier to weight loss, as it can lead to cortisol imbalances and subsequent weight gain, particularly around the midsection. By mitigating stress through adaptogenic herbs, individuals can address one of the root causes of weight challenges.

In addition to herbal supplements, a diet rich in whole, unprocessed foods is fundamental to natural weight management.

Foods high in fiber, such as fruits, vegetables, legumes, and whole grains, promote feelings of fullness and improve digestive health, which is crucial for maintaining a healthy weight. Lean proteins and healthy fats provide sustained energy and satiety, preventing overeating and snacking on unhealthy options.

Hydration is another critical aspect often overlooked in weight management.

Drinking adequate amounts of water throughout the day can boost metabolism, aid in the removal of waste and toxins, and reduce appetite. Herbal teas, such as dandelion or peppermint tea, can also support digestive health and enhance detoxification processes, further supporting weight management goals.

Physical activity tailored to individual preferences and capabilities is essential for burning calories, building muscle, and improving overall metabolic health.

Activities such as walking, yoga, swimming, or cycling can be effective and enjoyable ways to incorporate movement into daily life, fostering a positive attitude towards exercise and its role in weight management.

Mindful eating practices encourage awareness and appreciation of food, helping individuals tune into their body's hunger and fullness signals.

This approach can prevent overeating and promote a healthier relationship with food, which is vital for long-term weight management success.

Finally, ensuring adequate sleep and managing stress through practices like meditation, deep breathing exercises, and spending time in nature can support hormonal balance and overall health, both of which are important for effective weight management.

By embracing these natural approaches to weight management, individuals can work with their body's innate wisdom to achieve sustainable health improvements. This holistic strategy not only supports weight loss but also enhances vitality, resilience, and a sense of well-being, making it a comprehensive approach to health that goes beyond the scale.

HERBAL SUPPLEMENTS FOR WEIGHT LOSS

Herbal supplements for weight loss have gained popularity as natural alternatives to support weight management efforts. These supplements, derived from plants, are believed to aid in weight loss through various mechanisms such as boosting metabolism, enhancing fat burning, and suppressing appetite. It's important to approach these supplements as part of a holistic strategy that includes a balanced diet, regular physical activity, and healthy lifestyle choices. Here are some commonly used herbal supplements for weight loss, along with their beneficial effects and instructions for use.

Green Tea Extract

Beneficial effects: Increases metabolism and enhances fat burning. The active compounds, catechins, and caffeine work synergistically to improve fat oxidation.

Ingredients: Green tea extract (standardized to contain 50% catechins), capsule shell.

Instructions: Take one capsule containing 250-500 mg of green tea extract, standardized to 50% catechins, twice daily before meals. Do not exceed the recommended dose.

Garcinia Cambogia

Beneficial effects: Suppresses appetite and inhibits the production of new fat in the body. The active ingredient, hydroxycitric acid (HCA), is responsible for its weight loss properties.

Ingredients: Garcinia Cambogia extract (standardized to contain 60% HCA), capsule shell.

Instructions: Take one capsule containing 500 mg of Garcinia Cambogia extract, standardized to 60% HCA, three times daily 30-60 minutes before meals.

Forskolin

Beneficial effects: Stimulates the release of stored fat from fat cells. Forskolin, derived from the root of the Coleus forskohlii plant, may also increase lean body mass.

Ingredients: Forskolin extract (standardized to contain 20% forskolin), capsule shell.

Instructions: Take one capsule containing 250 mg of Forskolin extract, standardized to 20% forskolin, twice daily before meals.

Cayenne Pepper

Beneficial effects: Boosts metabolism and promotes fat burning through its active component, capsaicin. Cayenne pepper can also reduce appetite and calorie intake.

Ingredients: Cayenne pepper powder, capsule shell.

Instructions: Take one capsule containing 500 mg of cayenne pepper powder with meals, up to three times daily. Start with a lower dose to assess tolerance.

Glucomannan

Beneficial effects: A dietary fiber that absorbs water and expands in the stomach, leading to a feeling of fullness. It helps reduce overall calorie intake.

Ingredients: Glucomannan powder (from the root of the konjac plant), capsule shell.

Instructions: Take one capsule containing 1 gram of glucomannan with a glass of water, one hour before meals, up to three times daily.

Variations: These supplements can be taken individually or combined for enhanced effects. However, it's crucial to consult with a healthcare provider before starting any new supplement, especially for individuals with underlying health conditions or those taking medications.

Storage tips: Keep in a cool, dry place away from direct sunlight. Ensure the cap is tightly sealed after each use to maintain freshness and efficacy.

Tips for allergens: Individuals with allergies to specific plants or herbs should avoid corresponding supplements. For those with sensitivities, hypoallergenic capsule shells are available.

Scientific references: Studies have shown the efficacy of these herbal supplements in supporting weight loss. For instance, a study published in the American Journal of Clinical Nutrition found that green tea extract significantly increased energy expenditure (a measure of metabolism) and fat oxidation among participants. Similarly, research in the Journal of Obesity reported that Garcinia Cambogia might lead to short-term weight loss. Always look for high-quality, peer-reviewed scientific studies to support the use of any herbal supplement.

Incorporating these herbal supplements into a weight management plan can offer additional support alongside dietary and lifestyle changes. However, they should not be relied upon as the sole method for losing weight. Achieving and maintaining a healthy weight requires a comprehensive approach that includes mindful eating, regular physical activity, and adequate rest.

MANAGING EMOTIONAL EATING WITH HERBS

Emotional eating, a common response to stress, boredom, or emotional distress, often leads to unhealthy snacking and overeating. Herbs can play a pivotal role in managing these cravings by stabilizing mood, reducing stress, and promoting a sense of calm. Incorporating specific herbs into your daily routine can help address the root causes of emotional eating, offering a natural pathway to support weight management and overall well-being.

Ashwagandha is renowned for its adaptogenic properties, helping the body cope with stress and reducing cortisol levels, a hormone linked to stress-induced eating. By mitigating stress, ashwagandha can help curb the urge to turn to food for comfort.

Beneficial effects: Reduces stress and anxiety, helps manage stress-induced cravings.

Ingredients: 1 teaspoon of ashwagandha powder.

Instructions: Mix ashwagandha powder into a glass of warm milk or water. Drink this mixture once daily, preferably in the evening to promote relaxation and stress relief.

Chamomile is another herb known for its calming effects on the mind and body. It can soothe anxiety and promote better sleep, factors that are often disrupted in emotional eaters.

Beneficial effects: Promotes relaxation, improves sleep quality, reduces the urge to eat due to emotional distress.

Ingredients: 1 tablespoon of dried chamomile flowers.

Instructions: Steep dried chamomile flowers in a cup of boiling water for 5-10 minutes. Strain and drink this tea 30 minutes before bedtime to enhance relaxation and sleep.

Holy Basil (Tulsi) has been used for centuries to support mood and stress management. Its adaptogenic properties help balance cortisol levels, reducing the likelihood of stress-related eating.

Beneficial effects: Balances stress hormones, supports mood, decreases emotional eating triggers.

Ingredients: A handful of fresh holy basil leaves or 1 teaspoon of dried holy basil.

Instructions: For fresh leaves, steep in boiling water for 8-10 minutes. For dried holy basil, use a tea infuser and steep in boiling water for the same amount of time. Drink this tea once or twice daily to support stress management.

Peppermint is effective in managing appetite and reducing cravings. The scent of peppermint alone has been shown to decrease appetite, making it a useful tool in combating emotional eating.

Beneficial effects: Reduces cravings and the impulse to eat out of boredom or stress.

Ingredients: 1 teaspoon of dried peppermint leaves or a peppermint tea bag.

Instructions: Steep peppermint leaves or tea bag in boiling water for 5-7 minutes. Drink this tea in the morning or when cravings are strongest to help manage appetite.

Lemon Balm is known for its mood-enhancing properties. It can improve emotional well-being, reduce anxiety, and help prevent stress eating by promoting a sense of calm.

Beneficial effects: Enhances mood, reduces anxiety and stress, helps control emotional eating.

Ingredients: 1 teaspoon of dried lemon balm leaves.

Instructions: Steep lemon balm leaves in boiling water for 10 minutes. Drink this tea once daily, especially during times of high stress or when feeling the urge to eat emotionally.

Variations: These herbs can be combined for added benefits or used individually to target specific aspects of emotional eating. For example, combining chamomile and ashwagandha can enhance stress relief and sleep quality, while adding lemon balm can boost mood and well-being.

Storage tips: Store dried herbs in a cool, dry place away from direct sunlight. Prepared teas can be refrigerated for up to 24 hours but are best consumed fresh for maximum benefits.

Tips for allergens: Those with allergies to specific herbs should avoid them and consult a healthcare provider for alternatives. Most of these herbs are generally safe, but it's important to start with small doses to monitor for any adverse reactions.

Scientific references: Studies have supported the use of these herbs for stress relief and mood improvement. For instance, a study published in the Journal of Clinical Pharmacy and Therapeutics found that ashwagandha significantly reduced stress and food cravings in adults under chronic stress. Similarly, research in Phytotherapy Research highlighted chamomile's effectiveness in improving sleep and reducing anxiety.

By integrating these herbal remedies into a holistic approach to health, individuals can address the emotional and psychological factors contributing to emotional eating, paving the way for healthier eating habits and improved emotional resilience.

HERBAL SUPPORT FOR METABOLISM

Herbal supplements can be a valuable addition to a holistic approach to boosting metabolism and supporting weight management. By incorporating specific herbs known for their metabolic benefits, individuals can naturally enhance their body's ability to burn fat, increase energy levels, and improve overall metabolic health. Here are some key herbs that have been traditionally used and supported by scientific research for their ability to support metabolism.

Green Tea Extract

Beneficial effects: Enhances metabolic rate and increases fat oxidation. The catechins, particularly epigallocatechin gallate (EGCG), combined with caffeine, are known to improve energy expenditure and fat burning.

Ingredients: Green tea extract (standardized to contain at least 45% EGCG), capsule shell.

Instructions: Take one capsule containing 500 mg of green tea extract, standardized to at least 45% EGCG, twice daily before meals. Ensure to stay hydrated and monitor caffeine intake from other sources.

Cinnamon

Beneficial effects: Helps in regulating blood sugar levels, which can influence metabolic rate and energy levels. Cinnamon improves insulin sensitivity, thereby aiding in weight management.

Ingredients: Ground cinnamon or cinnamon sticks.

Instructions: Add one teaspoon of ground cinnamon to your morning oatmeal, smoothies, or coffee. Alternatively, boil cinnamon sticks in water to make a warming tea to enjoy throughout the day.

Ginger

Beneficial effects: Possesses thermogenic properties that can boost metabolism and promote fat loss. Ginger also aids in digestion and enhances satiety, which can help in controlling appetite.

Ingredients: Fresh ginger root.

Instructions: Grate one tablespoon of fresh ginger to add to meals or steep in hot water for 5-10 minutes to make ginger tea. Ginger can be consumed up to three times daily, especially before meals to aid digestion.

Cayenne Pepper

Beneficial effects: Contains capsaicin, which is known for its ability to increase metabolic rate and induce thermogenesis, leading to increased calorie burn.

Ingredients: Cayenne pepper powder.

Instructions: Start with a small pinch of cayenne pepper, adding it to your meals, soups, or smoothies. Gradually increase the amount based on tolerance, aiming for up to 1 teaspoon per day.

Forskolin

Beneficial effects: Derived from the root of the Coleus forskohlii plant, forskolin is believed to stimulate the release of stored fat from fat cells, aiding in weight loss.

Ingredients: Forskolin extract (standardized to contain 20% forskolin), capsule shell.

Instructions: Take one capsule containing 250 mg of forskolin extract, standardized to 20% forskolin, twice daily before meals. Consult with a healthcare provider before starting forskolin, especially if you have existing health conditions.

Variations: These herbs can be used in combination or individually, depending on personal preference and tolerance. It's important to consider any potential interactions with medications or conditions and consult with a healthcare professional before incorporating new supplements into your routine.

Storage tips: Store capsules in a cool, dry place. Keep fresh ginger and cinnamon in airtight containers to maintain freshness.

Tips for allergens: Individuals with allergies or sensitivities to specific herbs should avoid them. For those sensitive to caffeine, monitor intake when consuming green tea extract.

Scientific references: Numerous studies support the metabolic benefits of these herbs. For example, a study published in the American Journal of Clinical Nutrition found that green tea extract significantly increased energy expenditure and fat oxidation in participants. Research in the Journal of Medicinal Food has shown that ginger enhances thermogenesis and has potential weight loss benefits.

By integrating these herbal supports into a balanced lifestyle that includes a nutritious diet, regular physical activity, and adequate hydration, individuals can naturally enhance their metabolism and support their weight management goals.

WEIGHT LOSS TONIC HERBS

Weight loss tonic herbs offer a natural adjunct to diet and exercise in the journey towards achieving and maintaining a healthy weight. These herbs are selected for their ability to support metabolism, enhance fat burning, and suppress appetite, providing a holistic approach to weight management. Here are some tonic herbs known for their weight loss benefits, along with instructions on how to incorporate them into your daily regimen.

Green Tea

Beneficial effects: Boosts metabolism and increases fat oxidation. The catechins, especially epigallocatechin gallate (EGCG), in green tea, are powerful antioxidants that enhance metabolic rate and support the body's ability to burn fat.

Ingredients: 1-2 teaspoons of green tea leaves or 1 green tea bag.

Instructions: Steep the green tea leaves or tea bag in hot water for 3-5 minutes. Drink 2-3 cups daily, preferably before meals to maximize the metabolic benefits.

Dandelion

Beneficial effects: Acts as a natural diuretic, reducing water weight. Dandelion also supports liver detoxification, which is crucial for efficient metabolism and fat loss.

Ingredients: 1 teaspoon of dried dandelion root or leaves.

Instructions: Boil the dried dandelion in water for 5-10 minutes. Strain and drink the tea once daily. It can be consumed in the morning to kickstart your metabolism.

Cayenne Pepper

Beneficial effects: Contains capsaicin, which has thermogenic properties. It helps to increase body temperature, boosting metabolism and calorie burn.

Ingredients: ¼ to ½ teaspoon of cayenne pepper powder.

Instructions: Add cayenne pepper to your meals, or mix it into a glass of warm water with lemon and drink once daily. Start with a small amount to assess tolerance.

Ginger

Beneficial effects: Enhances thermogenesis and has anti-inflammatory properties. Ginger can help regulate blood sugar levels, reducing cravings and appetite.

Ingredients: 1 inch of fresh ginger root.

Instructions: Grate the ginger and add it to boiling water. Let it steep for 5-10 minutes, strain, and drink. Consuming ginger tea 2-3 times a day can aid in weight loss.

Turmeric

Beneficial effects: Contains curcumin, which is known for its anti-inflammatory and antioxidant properties. Turmeric can enhance fat loss and improve insulin sensitivity.

Ingredients: 1 teaspoon of turmeric powder.

Instructions: Mix turmeric powder into a glass of warm milk or water. Drink once daily. Adding a pinch of black pepper can enhance the absorption of curcumin.

Variations: These tonic herbs can be used individually or in combination to create a potent weight loss tea. Experimenting with different blends can help you find the most effective and enjoyable concoction.

Storage tips: Store dried herbs and powders in airtight containers in a cool, dry place to preserve their potency and freshness.

Tips for allergens: Individuals with allergies to specific herbs should avoid them. Always introduce new herbs into your diet gradually to monitor for any adverse reactions.

Scientific references: Numerous studies support the weight loss benefits of these herbs. For example, research published in the International Journal of Obesity has highlighted the positive effects of green tea catechins on fat oxidation and thermogenesis. Similarly, studies in the Journal of Nutrition and Metabolism have shown that capsaicin consumption can increase calorie burn and reduce appetite.

Incorporating these weight loss tonic herbs into a balanced lifestyle that includes healthy eating and regular physical activity can enhance your efforts to achieve and maintain a healthy weight. Remember, these herbs are not a magic solution but a supportive tool in your weight management journey.

CHAPTER 4: 5 HERBAL RECIPES FOR WEIGHT MANAGEMENT

GREEN TEA AND LEMON DETOX DRINK

Beneficial effects

The Green Tea and Lemon Detox Drink is designed to support weight management and detoxification. Green tea is rich in antioxidants, particularly catechins, which have been shown to boost metabolism and aid in fat burning. Lemon, on the other hand, is high in vitamin C and promotes hydration, which is crucial for the efficient functioning of the metabolism. Together, they create a detoxifying beverage that can help cleanse the body, enhance metabolic rate, and support weight loss efforts.

Portions

2 servings

Preparation time

5 minutes

Ingredients

- 2 cups of water
- 1 green tea bag
- Juice of 1 lemon
- 1 tablespoon honey (optional)

Instructions

1. Bring 2 cups of water to a boil in a small pot.

2. Add the green tea bag to the boiling water and let it steep for about 3 to 5 minutes, depending on how strong you like your tea.

3. Remove the tea bag and let the tea cool down to a comfortable drinking temperature.

4. Stir in the juice of 1 lemon. Add honey to sweeten, if desired.

5. Serve the detox drink warm, or chill it in the refrigerator and serve cold.

Variations

- To enhance the detoxifying effects, add a slice of fresh ginger to the boiling water with the green tea.
- Incorporate a pinch of cayenne pepper to boost metabolism further.
- For an iced version, pour the tea over ice cubes and enjoy as a refreshing cold beverage.

Storage tips

If you have leftover Green Tea and Lemon Detox Drink, store it in a sealed container in the refrigerator for up to 24 hours. Enjoy it chilled for a revitalizing detox boost.

Tips for allergens

For those with allergies or sensitivities to honey, you can omit it or substitute it with maple syrup for a vegan-friendly sweetener option.

Scientific references

- "Green tea catechins and cardiovascular health: an update" in the journal Current Medicinal Chemistry, 2008. This study highlights the metabolism-boosting and fat-burning properties of green tea catechins.

- "Effects of vitamin C intake on the risk of osteoarthritis: A meta-analysis of observational studies" in the Journal of Clinical Biochemistry and Nutrition, 2013. This research supports the role of vitamin C, found in lemons, in promoting overall health and supporting weight management efforts.

CINNAMON AND HONEY WEIGHT LOSS TEA

Beneficial effects

Cinnamon and Honey Weight Loss Tea is designed to support weight management efforts by enhancing metabolic rate, reducing cravings, and providing a natural detoxification effect. Cinnamon is known for its ability to regulate blood sugar levels, which can help minimize insulin spikes and reduce hunger. Honey, on the other hand, is a healthier sweetener alternative that can aid in digestion and has antioxidant properties. Together, they create a warming beverage that not only aids in weight loss but also supports overall health.

Portions

2 servings

Preparation time

5 minutes

Cooking time

10 minutes

Ingredients

- 1 teaspoon of ground cinnamon

- 2 cups of water

- 1 tablespoon of honey

- 1 teaspoon of lemon juice (optional)

Instructions

1. Bring 2 cups of water to a boil in a small saucepan.

2. Add 1 teaspoon of ground cinnamon to the boiling water and simmer for about 10 minutes.

3. Remove the saucepan from heat and let the cinnamon tea cool slightly.

4. Stir in 1 tablespoon of honey until it dissolves completely. If using, add 1 teaspoon of lemon juice to the mixture.

5. Strain the tea into cups to remove any large particles of cinnamon.

6. Serve the tea warm, ideally in the morning before breakfast or in the evening before bedtime.

Variations

- For an added metabolic boost, include a pinch of cayenne pepper to the tea while it simmers.

- Mix in a slice of fresh ginger during the simmering process for additional digestive benefits and a spicy flavor.

- Substitute water with green tea for an extra antioxidant boost and to enhance the weight loss effect.

Storage tips

It's best to consume the Cinnamon and Honey Weight Loss Tea fresh. However, if you have leftovers, store them in a sealed container in the refrigerator for up to 24 hours. Reheat gently on the stove or enjoy chilled.

Tips for allergens

Individuals with allergies to cinnamon or honey should proceed with caution and may consider consulting with a healthcare provider before consumption. For a vegan alternative to honey, maple syrup can be used as a sweetener.

Scientific references

- "Cinnamon: Potential Role in the Prevention of Insulin Resistance, Metabolic Syndrome, and Type 2 Diabetes" published in the Journal of Diabetes Science and Technology, 2010. This study highlights cinnamon's beneficial effects on blood sugar regulation and metabolic health.

- "Honey, Propolis, and Royal Jelly: A Comprehensive Review of Their Biological Actions and Health Benefits" in Oxidative Medicine and Cellular Longevity, 2017. This review discusses honey's antioxidant properties and its role in supporting digestive health and weight management.

GARCINIA CAMBOGIA SMOOTHIE

Beneficial effects

The Garcinia Cambogia Smoothie is designed to support weight management efforts by potentially suppressing appetite and inhibiting the body's ability to store fat. Garcinia Cambogia, a tropical fruit also known as the Malabar tamarind, is rich in hydroxycitric acid (HCA), which has been studied for its effects on reducing fat accumulation and supporting appetite control. This smoothie combines Garcinia Cambogia with other nutritious ingredients to create a satisfying and healthful drink that can aid in weight management as part of a balanced diet and exercise regimen.

Portions

1 serving

Preparation time

5 minutes

Ingredients

- 1 cup unsweetened almond milk

- 1/2 cup frozen mixed berries (blueberries, strawberries, raspberries)

- 1 tablespoon Garcinia Cambogia extract (as recommended by the product)

- 1/2 ripe banana

- 1 tablespoon flaxseed meal (for added fiber and omega-3 fatty acids)

- Ice cubes (optional, for a colder smoothie)

Instructions

1. Place the unsweetened almond milk into a blender.

2. Add the frozen mixed berries, Garcinia Cambogia extract, ripe banana, and flaxseed meal to the blender.

3. If a colder beverage is preferred, add a few ice cubes.

4. Blend all ingredients on high until the mixture is smooth and creamy.

5. Pour the smoothie into a glass and enjoy immediately.

Variations

- For added protein, include a scoop of your favorite protein powder. This can help increase satiety and support muscle repair, especially if consumed after exercise.

- Substitute almond milk with coconut water for a lighter version that's still hydrating and flavorful.

- Add a handful of spinach or kale to increase the smoothie's vitamin and mineral content without significantly altering the taste.

Storage tips

It's best to consume the Garcinia Cambogia Smoothie immediately after preparation to enjoy its full benefits. However, if necessary, it can be stored in an airtight container in the refrigerator for up to 24 hours. Stir well before consuming if separation occurs.

Tips for allergens

For those with nut allergies, replace almond milk with a suitable non-nut milk alternative like oat milk or rice milk. Ensure the Garcinia Cambogia extract is pure and does not contain any additives that could cause allergic reactions.

Scientific references

- "Effects of Garcinia cambogia (Hydroxycitric Acid) on visceral fat accumulation: a double-blind, randomized, placebo-controlled trial." Current Therapeutic Research, Clinical and Experimental, 2003. This study highlights the potential of Garcinia Cambogia extract in reducing fat accumulation and supporting weight management efforts.

- "The Use of Garcinia Extract (Hydroxycitric Acid) as a Weight loss Supplement: A Systematic Review and Meta-Analysis of Randomised Clinical Trials." Journal of Obesity, 2011. This review examines the efficacy of Garcinia Cambogia extract in weight loss, noting its potential to reduce appetite and inhibit fat production.

YERBA MATE ENERGY BOOST

Beneficial effects

Yerba Mate Energy Boost is designed to enhance energy levels, improve mental clarity, and support weight management. Yerba Mate is rich in antioxidants and nutrients that can boost metabolism and increase the body's reliance on fat for fuel during exercise. It also contains natural compounds that promote a feeling of satiety, reducing hunger and aiding in weight control. Additionally, the caffeine content in Yerba Mate can improve physical performance and focus, making it an excellent beverage choice for those looking to maintain an active lifestyle while managing weight.

Portions

2 servings

Preparation time

5 minutes

Ingredients

- 2 tablespoons of loose-leaf Yerba Mate

- 4 cups of water

- Honey or lemon to taste (optional)

- Ice cubes (optional for a cold version)

Instructions

1. Heat water until it is hot but not boiling, around 175°F (80°C).

2. Place the loose-leaf Yerba Mate in a French press or tea infuser.

3. Pour the hot water over the Yerba Mate and let it steep for 3 to 5 minutes, depending on desired strength.

4. Press the plunger down on the French press or remove the tea infuser.

5. Optional: Add honey or lemon to taste for flavor enhancement.

6. Serve the Yerba Mate Energy Boost warm, or add ice cubes for a refreshing cold beverage.

Variations

- For an added metabolic boost, include a slice of ginger or a dash of cinnamon during the steeping process.

- Blend the brewed Yerba Mate with a handful of spinach and a green apple for a nutrient-packed smoothie.

- Combine Yerba Mate with green tea during steeping for an extra antioxidant boost.

Storage tips

If you have leftover Yerba Mate Energy Boost, store it in a sealed container in the refrigerator for up to 24 hours. Enjoy it chilled, or gently reheat on the stove.

Tips for allergens

Individuals with sensitivities to caffeine should start with a smaller amount of Yerba Mate to ensure no adverse reactions. For those avoiding honey due to dietary restrictions, substitute with maple syrup or simply omit the sweetener.

Scientific references

- "Effects of Yerba Mate on lipid parameters in humans with high cholesterol: a randomized trial" in the Journal of the American College of Nutrition, 2011. This study highlights Yerba Mate's benefits in managing cholesterol levels, supporting its use for weight management.

- "Antioxidant activity of Yerba Mate (Ilex paraguariensis) in promoting health and managing obesity" published in Phytotherapy Research, 2015. This research discusses Yerba Mate's antioxidant properties and its potential role in weight control and overall health improvement.

APPLE CIDER VINEGAR AND GINGER TONIC

Beneficial effects

Apple Cider Vinegar and Ginger Tonic is known for its potential to aid in weight management and improve digestion. The acetic acid in apple cider vinegar can help to reduce appetite, increase metabolism, and decrease insulin levels, which in turn can lead to weight loss. Ginger, with its thermogenic properties, can help boost metabolism and fat burning. Additionally, this tonic can improve digestion and reduce bloating, making it a supportive drink for overall digestive health.

Ingredients

- 2 tablespoons of organic apple cider vinegar

- 1 teaspoon of freshly grated ginger

- 1 tablespoon of organic honey (optional, for sweetness)

- 1 cup of warm water

- Juice of half a lemon

Instructions

1. Grate the ginger finely until you have about 1 teaspoon.

2. Warm 1 cup of water to a comfortable drinking temperature, not boiling.

3. Combine the grated ginger and warm water in a mug or glass.

4. Add 2 tablespoons of apple cider vinegar to the mixture.

5. Squeeze the juice of half a lemon into the drink.

6. If desired, add 1 tablespoon of honey to sweeten.

7. Stir the mixture well until all the ingredients are fully combined.

8. Drink the tonic in the morning on an empty stomach for best results.

Variations

- For a refreshing twist, add a few mint leaves to the tonic.

- To enhance the detoxifying effects, include a pinch of cayenne pepper.

- Substitute honey with maple syrup for a vegan-friendly version.

Storage tips

It's best to prepare the Apple Cider Vinegar and Ginger Tonic fresh each morning to ensure potency and freshness. However, if you prefer to prepare in advance, you can store the grated ginger in an airtight container in the refrigerator for up to 2 days.

Tips for allergens

Individuals with allergies to pollen should be cautious when adding honey and may substitute it with maple syrup. Those sensitive to citrus can omit the lemon juice without significantly affecting the tonic's benefits.

Scientific references

- "Vinegar intake reduces body weight, body fat mass, and serum triglyceride levels in obese Japanese subjects." Bioscience, Biotechnology, and Biochemistry, 2009. This study highlights the weight management benefits of apple cider vinegar.

- "Ginger consumption enhances the thermic effect of food and promotes feelings of satiety without affecting metabolic and hormonal parameters in overweight men: A pilot study." Metabolism, 2012. This research supports ginger's role in enhancing metabolism and contributing to weight management.

PART 18: ENDOCRINE SYSTEM HEALTH

The endocrine system, a network of glands that produce and release hormones, plays a pivotal role in regulating nearly every process in the body, from growth and development to metabolism and mood. The health of this intricate system is foundational to holistic well-being, influencing how efficiently the body operates, responds to stress, and maintains balance. Supporting endocrine health naturally involves a combination of nutrition, herbal remedies, and lifestyle adjustments aimed at nurturing glandular function and hormone balance.

Ashwagandha for Stress and Thyroid Health

Beneficial effects: Ashwagandha, an adaptogenic herb, supports the adrenal glands, reduces cortisol levels, and can help in balancing thyroid hormones, making it beneficial for those with hypothyroidism.

Ingredients: 1 teaspoon of ashwagandha powder.

Instructions: Mix ashwagandha powder into a glass of warm water or milk. Consume this mixture once daily, preferably in the morning to help modulate stress responses and support thyroid health.

Maca Root for Hormonal Balance

Beneficial effects: Maca root is known for its ability to enhance energy, stamina, and mood. It also supports hormonal balance in both men and women by nourishing the pituitary and adrenal glands.

Ingredients: 1 tablespoon of maca powder.

Instructions: Incorporate maca powder into your daily smoothie or sprinkle it over breakfast bowls. Consuming maca regularly can help in maintaining hormonal equilibrium and overall vitality.

Turmeric for Inflammation and Hormonal Support

Beneficial effects: Turmeric, with its active compound curcumin, offers anti-inflammatory benefits and supports liver health, which is crucial for hormone regulation and detoxification.

Ingredients: 1 teaspoon of turmeric powder, a pinch of black pepper to enhance absorption.

Instructions: Add turmeric and black pepper to warm milk or water, creating a golden milk concoction. Drink this once daily to leverage its anti-inflammatory properties and support endocrine health.

Flaxseeds for Estrogen Balance

Beneficial effects: Flaxseeds contain phytoestrogens, which can help in balancing estrogen levels in the body. They are also rich in omega-3 fatty acids, supporting overall hormonal health.

Ingredients: 1 tablespoon of ground flaxseeds.

Instructions: Sprinkle ground flaxseeds over salads, soups, or smoothies. Regular consumption can aid in maintaining estrogen balance and supporting reproductive health.

Holy Basil for Adrenal Health

Beneficial effects: Holy basil, or Tulsi, acts as an adaptogen, enhancing the body's ability to respond to stress and supporting adrenal gland function.

Ingredients: A handful of fresh holy basil leaves or 1 teaspoon of dried holy basil.

Instructions: Steep holy basil in boiling water for 5-10 minutes to make a soothing tea. Drinking this tea daily can help in reducing stress levels and supporting the health of the adrenal glands.

Variations: These herbs can be used in combination or individually tailored to specific endocrine health needs. For instance, combining ashwagandha with maca can enhance both stress management and hormonal balance.

Storage tips: Store powdered or dried herbs in a cool, dry place, away from direct sunlight. Fresh herbs should be kept in the refrigerator and used as soon as possible for maximum potency.

Tips for allergens: Those with specific plant allergies should avoid corresponding herbs and seek alternatives. For example, individuals sensitive to nightshades may need to use caution with ashwagandha.

Scientific references: Studies have shown the efficacy of these herbs in supporting endocrine health. Research published in the Journal of Alternative and Complementary Medicine highlights ashwagandha's benefits for thyroid function, while evidence from the International Journal of Endocrinology and Metabolism suggests that maca can improve sexual dysfunction without altering hormone levels. Turmeric's anti-inflammatory effects are well-documented in the Journal of Medicinal Food, and flaxseeds' role in hormonal balance is explored in the Journal of Clinical Endocrinology and Metabolism.

Incorporating these herbal remedies into a holistic lifestyle that includes balanced nutrition, regular physical activity, and stress management practices can significantly enhance endocrine system health, promoting hormonal balance, metabolic efficiency, and overall vitality.

CHAPTER 1: UNDERSTANDING THE ENDOCRINE SYSTEM

The endocrine system, a complex network of glands and hormones, orchestrates a symphony of bodily functions essential for maintaining health and balance. It regulates metabolism, growth, reproduction, and response to stress and injury by releasing hormones directly into the bloodstream. These hormones act as messengers, influencing various processes across the body to ensure it operates harmoniously.

At the heart of the endocrine system lie several key players, including the pituitary gland, often dubbed the "master gland" due to its role in controlling other glands; the thyroid gland, which regulates metabolism, energy, and growth; the adrenals, which manage stress responses and metabolism; and the pancreas, vital for blood sugar regulation. The reproductive glands, namely the ovaries and testes, govern sexual development and health, playing a crucial role in reproduction.

Hormonal imbalances can disrupt this delicate balance, leading to a range of health issues. For instance, an underactive thyroid (hypothyroidism) can cause fatigue, weight gain, and depression, while an overactive thyroid (hyperthyroidism) might result in weight loss, increased heart rate, and anxiety. Similarly, imbalances in insulin can lead to diabetes, a condition affecting how the body uses blood glucose.

Supporting endocrine health naturally focuses on fostering glandular function and hormone balance through nutrition, herbal remedies, and lifestyle adjustments. Consuming a balanced diet rich in nutrients supports hormonal health, while specific herbs like ashwagandha and maca root offer adaptogenic properties that help modulate stress and support hormonal balance. Regular physical activity, stress management techniques, and adequate sleep are also pivotal in maintaining endocrine health, as they help mitigate stress and its effects on hormonal balance.

Understanding the endocrine system's role and its impact on overall health is the first step towards nurturing and maintaining this critical aspect of our well-being. By adopting a holistic approach that includes balanced nutrition, herbal support, and healthy lifestyle practices, one can support the endocrine system in performing its vital functions, promoting hormonal balance, metabolic efficiency, and overall vitality.

RISK FACTORS FOR HORMONAL IMBALANCES

Risk factors for hormonal imbalances encompass a wide array of lifestyle, environmental, and physiological factors that can disrupt the endocrine system's delicate equilibrium. Primary among these is stress, which can lead to adrenal fatigue, affecting cortisol levels and thereby impacting overall hormonal balance. Poor diet, rich in processed foods, sugars, and unhealthy fats, can also contribute significantly to hormonal disruptions by affecting insulin sensitivity and leading to weight gain, which further influences hormone levels.

Lack of adequate physical activity is another critical risk factor. Regular exercise plays a vital role in maintaining hormonal balance by reducing stress levels, improving insulin sensitivity, and supporting healthy metabolism. Conversely, sedentary behavior can exacerbate hormonal imbalances by promoting weight gain and insulin resistance.

Environmental toxins, including pesticides, plasticizers, and industrial chemicals, can mimic hormones in the body, leading to endocrine disruption. These substances, known as endocrine-disrupting chemicals (EDCs), are found in many everyday products and can interfere with the normal functioning of hormones.

Age and genetics also play significant roles in hormonal health. Hormonal imbalances are more common during natural periods of hormonal transition such as puberty, pregnancy, and menopause. Genetic predispositions can also affect how individuals metabolize hormones and respond to external factors affecting hormonal balance.

Sleep deprivation is another potent risk factor for hormonal imbalances. Quality sleep is crucial for the regulation of many hormones, including cortisol, insulin, and growth hormones. Lack of sleep can lead to increased stress levels, weight gain, and insulin resistance, all of which can contribute to hormonal imbalances.

Finally, certain medications and health conditions, such as diabetes and thyroid disorders, can directly affect hormone levels. It's essential for individuals with these conditions to manage their health proactively to maintain hormonal balance.

Addressing these risk factors through lifestyle changes, such as adopting a balanced diet, engaging in regular physical activity, minimizing exposure to environmental toxins, ensuring adequate sleep, and managing stress, can help maintain hormonal balance and support overall well-being.

DR. BARBARA'S APPROACH TO ENDOCRINE HEALTH

Dr. Barbara's approach to endocrine health emphasizes the importance of a holistic strategy that incorporates natural remedies, dietary adjustments, and lifestyle changes to support hormonal balance and glandular function. Recognizing the endocrine system as a critical network influencing overall health, she advocates for nurturing practices that foster equilibrium and vitality.

Key to her method is the integration of adaptogenic herbs known for their ability to modulate the body's stress response and support endocrine health. Ashwagandha, for instance, is championed for its thyroid and adrenal benefits, helping to normalize cortisol levels and mitigate the effects of stress on the body. Similarly, maca root is highlighted for its capacity to enhance energy and mood while supporting hormonal balance across both genders.

Dietary recommendations focus on whole, unprocessed foods rich in nutrients that support hormonal health, such as omega-3 fatty acids, antioxidants, and phytonutrients. Foods like fatty fish, leafy greens, nuts, and seeds are emphasized for their role in reducing inflammation and supporting the liver, a key organ in hormone regulation and detoxification.

Lifestyle modifications play a crucial role in Dr. Barbara's approach, with a strong emphasis on stress reduction techniques such as yoga, meditation, and deep breathing exercises. These practices are not only beneficial for mental well-being but also for reducing the physiological impacts of stress on the endocrine system.

Physical activity is encouraged to improve insulin sensitivity, boost metabolism, and enhance mood, all of which contribute to endocrine health. Regular, moderate exercise, particularly in natural settings, is recommended to leverage the additional benefits of fresh air and exposure to nature.

Finally, Dr. Barbara underscores the importance of adequate sleep and hydration in maintaining hormonal balance. Quality sleep is essential for the regulation of many hormones, while staying well-hydrated supports overall metabolic function and detoxification processes.

By adopting these holistic practices, individuals can support their endocrine health naturally, promoting a balanced and vibrant state of well-being.

CHAPTER 2: NUTRITION FOR HORMONAL BALANCE

Nutrition plays a crucial role in maintaining hormonal balance, a key aspect of endocrine health. Hormones, the body's chemical messengers, are profoundly influenced by the foods we consume. A diet that supports hormonal balance includes a variety of nutrients that help regulate bodily functions and mitigate the risk of hormonal imbalances.

Foods rich in omega-3 fatty acids, such as salmon, flaxseeds, and walnuts, are essential for reducing inflammation and supporting the production of healthy hormones. Omega-3s are particularly beneficial for balancing levels of estrogen and progesterone, which can impact menstrual health and mood.

Incorporating plenty of fiber-rich foods into the diet is another effective strategy for hormonal health. Fiber helps in the elimination of excess hormones, particularly estrogen, through the digestive tract, thereby preventing reabsorption.

Sources of high-quality fiber include vegetables, fruits, legumes, and whole grains.

Antioxidant-rich foods are vital for protecting the body's cells, including those of the endocrine glands, from oxidative stress. Berries, leafy greens, nuts, and seeds are packed with antioxidants such as vitamins C and E, selenium, and flavonoids, which support the health of the thyroid gland and overall hormonal balance.

Magnesium is another nutrient that plays a pivotal role in supporting endocrine health. It aids in the regulation of cortisol levels, supports thyroid function, and is involved in the production of progesterone, estrogen, and testosterone. Foods high in magnesium include dark chocolate, avocados, nuts, and whole grains.

Adequate protein intake is crucial for hormone balance.

Proteins provide essential amino acids that serve as building blocks for hormone synthesis. Including a variety of protein sources, such as lean meats, fish, eggs, dairy products, legumes, and plant-based proteins, ensures the body has the necessary components for hormone production.

Healthy fats are also important for hormonal health. They provide the necessary fatty acids for hormone production and can help maintain the cell membrane's integrity, facilitating hormone transport and function. Sources of healthy fats include olive oil, coconut oil, avocados, and fatty fish.

Avoiding or minimizing intake of processed foods, sugars, and unhealthy fats is crucial for maintaining hormonal balance.

These foods can lead to inflammation, insulin resistance, and disruptions in hormonal signals, contributing to conditions such as PCOS, diabetes, and thyroid disorders.

Staying hydrated is another key aspect of supporting hormonal health. Water aids in the transport of hormones throughout the body and helps in the elimination of excess hormones and toxins through the kidneys.

Regular consumption of fermented foods can support gut health, which is closely linked to hormonal balance. Foods like yogurt, kefir, sauerkraut, and kombucha are rich in probiotics that help maintain a healthy gut microbiome, crucial for estrogen metabolism and overall hormonal regulation.

By focusing on a diet rich in whole foods, healthy fats, proteins, and fiber, and by minimizing processed foods and sugars, individuals can support their hormonal health and contribute to their overall well-being.

FOODS TO AVOID FOR ENDOCRINE WELLNESS

For optimal endocrine wellness, it's crucial to identify and limit certain foods and substances that can disrupt hormonal balance. The endocrine system, sensitive and complex, can be adversely affected by various dietary components, leading to hormonal imbalances that may impact overall health and well-being. Key foods and substances to minimize or avoid include:

Highly Processed and Sugary Foods: These can cause spikes in insulin levels, contributing to insulin resistance over time. Insulin is a critical hormone for regulating blood sugar levels, and its dysregulation can lead to diabetes and other metabolic disorders. Opting for whole, unprocessed foods with natural sugars can help maintain steady insulin and blood sugar levels.

Trans Fats and Hydrogenated Oils: Found in many processed foods, trans fats can increase the risk of inflammation and insulin resistance. They can also negatively affect thyroid health, which is essential for metabolism, energy, and growth. Reading labels and choosing foods with natural, healthy fats like those from avocados, nuts, and seeds is advisable.

High Glycemic Index Foods: Foods that have a high glycemic index, such as white bread, rice, and other refined carbohydrates, can quickly raise blood sugar levels, leading to increased insulin demand and potential hormonal imbalances. Choosing low glycemic index foods like whole grains, legumes, and vegetables can support hormonal health by providing a more gradual release of glucose into the bloodstream.

Soy Products: While soy can be a healthy part of many diets, it contains phytoestrogens, which may mimic estrogen in the body. For individuals with estrogen dominance or those sensitive to hormonal fluctuations, it may be beneficial to limit soy intake or choose fermented soy products, which have a lower phytoestrogen content.

Alcohol: Alcohol consumption can impact liver function, which plays a crucial role in hormone regulation and detoxification. Excessive alcohol intake can lead to hormonal imbalances by affecting the liver's ability to properly metabolize hormones.

Caffeine: For some individuals, caffeine can stimulate the adrenal glands, leading to increased cortisol levels, which, when chronically elevated, can disrupt hormonal balance. Moderating caffeine intake or opting for caffeine-free herbal teas can help support adrenal health and maintain cortisol at healthy levels.

Artificial Sweeteners: Some studies suggest that artificial sweeteners may disrupt the body's natural ability to regulate glucose, leading to hormonal imbalances and metabolic issues. Choosing natural sweeteners in moderation, such as honey or maple syrup, can be a healthier option for maintaining endocrine and metabolic health.

Dairy Products: For some people, dairy can influence hormone levels due to the presence of hormones and growth factors in milk. Those experiencing hormonal sensitivities may benefit from reducing dairy intake or choosing dairy-free alternatives.

By being mindful of these dietary components and making informed choices, individuals can support their endocrine system's health, promoting hormonal balance and overall wellness. It's also beneficial to consult with a healthcare provider or a nutritionist to tailor dietary choices to individual health needs and conditions, ensuring a balanced and supportive approach to endocrine wellness.

CHAPTER 3: HERBAL REMEDIES FOR ENDOCRINE HEALTH

shwagandha for Stress and Thyroid Health

Beneficial effects: Ashwagandha, an adaptogenic herb, supports the adrenal glands, reduces cortisol levels, and can help in balancing thyroid hormones, making it beneficial for those with hypothyroidism.

Ingredients: 1 teaspoon of ashwagandha powder.

Instructions: Mix ashwagandha powder into a glass of warm water or milk. Consume this mixture once daily, preferably in the morning to help modulate stress responses and support thyroid health.

Maca Root for Hormonal Balance

Beneficial effects: Maca root is known for its ability to enhance energy, stamina, and mood. It also supports hormonal balance in both men and women by nourishing the pituitary and adrenal glands.

Ingredients: 1 tablespoon of maca powder.

Instructions: Incorporate maca powder into your daily smoothie or sprinkle it over breakfast bowls. Consuming maca regularly can help in maintaining hormonal equilibrium and overall vitality.

Turmeric for Inflammation and Hormonal Support

Beneficial effects: Turmeric, with its active compound curcumin, offers anti-inflammatory benefits and supports liver health, which is crucial for hormone regulation and detoxification.

Ingredients: 1 teaspoon of turmeric powder, a pinch of black pepper to enhance absorption.

Instructions: Add turmeric and black pepper to warm milk or water, creating a golden milk concoction. Drink this once daily to leverage its anti-inflammatory properties and support endocrine health.

Flaxseeds for Estrogen Balance

Beneficial effects: Flaxseeds contain phytoestrogens, which can help in balancing estrogen levels in the body. They are also rich in omega-3 fatty acids, supporting overall hormonal health.

Ingredients: 1 tablespoon of ground flaxseeds.

Instructions: Sprinkle ground flaxseeds over salads, soups, or smoothies. Regular consumption can aid in maintaining estrogen balance and supporting reproductive health.

Holy Basil for Adrenal Health

Beneficial effects: Holy basil, or Tulsi, acts as an adaptogen, enhancing the body's ability to respond to stress and supporting adrenal gland function.

Ingredients: A handful of fresh holy basil leaves or 1 teaspoon of dried holy basil.

Instructions: Steep holy basil in boiling water for 5-10 minutes to make a soothing tea. Drinking this tea daily can help in reducing stress levels and supporting the health of the adrenal glands.

Variations: These herbs can be used in combination or individually tailored to specific endocrine health needs. For instance, combining ashwagandha with maca can enhance both stress management and hormonal balance.

Storage tips: Store powdered or dried herbs in a cool, dry place, away from direct sunlight. Fresh herbs should be kept in the refrigerator and used as soon as possible for maximum potency.

Tips for allergens: Those with specific plant allergies should avoid corresponding herbs and seek alternatives. For example, individuals sensitive to nightshades may need to use caution with ashwagandha.

Scientific references: Studies have shown the efficacy of these herbs in supporting endocrine health.

Research published in the Journal of Alternative and Complementary Medicine highlights ashwagandha's benefits for thyroid function, while evidence from the International Journal of Endocrinology and Metabolism suggests that maca can improve sexual dysfunction without altering hormone levels.

Turmeric's anti-inflammatory effects are well-documented in the Journal of Medicinal Food, and flaxseeds' role in hormonal balance is explored in the Journal of Clinical Endocrinology and Metabolism.

Incorporating these herbal remedies into a holistic lifestyle that includes balanced nutrition, regular physical activity, and stress management practices can significantly enhance endocrine system health, promoting hormonal balance, metabolic efficiency, and overall vitality.

CHAPTER 4: 5 HERBAL RECIPES FOR ENDOCRINE HEALTH

ASHWAGANDHA ROOT TONIC

Beneficial effects

Ashwagandha Root Tonic is renowned for its ability to support endocrine health by regulating hormone levels, reducing stress, and enhancing overall vitality. Ashwagandha, an adaptogen, helps the body manage stress more effectively and can improve thyroid function, which is crucial for maintaining a balanced endocrine system. Additionally, its anti-inflammatory and antioxidant properties contribute to improved adrenal health, making it a comprehensive tonic for endocrine support.

Portions

2 servings

Preparation time

10 minutes

Ingredients

- 1 teaspoon of ashwagandha root powder

- 2 cups of water

- 1 teaspoon of honey (optional)

- A pinch of cinnamon (optional for flavor)

Instructions

1. Bring 2 cups of water to a boil in a small pot.

2. Add 1 teaspoon of ashwagandha root powder to the boiling water.

3. Reduce the heat and simmer for about 5 minutes.

4. Remove the pot from the heat and let the tonic cool slightly.

5. Strain the tonic into mugs to remove any ashwagandha root powder residue.

6. Optional: Add 1 teaspoon of honey and a pinch of cinnamon to each mug for added flavor.

7. Stir well and serve the tonic warm.

Variations

- For a cold beverage, allow the tonic to cool completely and then refrigerate. Serve over ice for a refreshing drink.

- Mix in a teaspoon of ginger powder with the ashwagandha for additional anti-inflammatory benefits.

- Substitute honey with maple syrup for a vegan-friendly sweetener.

Storage tips

If you have leftover Ashwagandha Root Tonic, store it in a sealed container in the refrigerator for up to 48 hours. Reheat gently on the stove or enjoy chilled.

Tips for allergens

Individuals with sensitivities to ashwagandha should start with a smaller dose to ensure no adverse reactions. For those avoiding honey due to allergies or dietary preferences, maple syrup can be used as a sweetener alternative.

Scientific references

- "An Overview on Ashwagandha: A Rasayana (Rejuvenator) of Ayurveda" published in the African Journal of Traditional, Complementary and Alternative Medicines, which discusses the adaptogenic and stress-relief properties of ashwagandha.

- "A Prospective, Randomized Double-Blind, Placebo-Controlled Study of Safety and Efficacy of a High-Concentration Full-Spectrum Extract of Ashwagandha Root in Reducing Stress and Anxiety in Adults" published in the Indian Journal of Psychological Medicine, highlighting the efficacy of ashwagandha in reducing stress and anxiety.

MACA ROOT HORMONE BALANCER

Beneficial effects

The Maca Root Hormone Balancer is designed to support endocrine health by naturally balancing hormone levels, enhancing fertility, boosting libido, and improving overall energy and mood. Maca root, a Peruvian superfood, is rich in nutrients and known for its adaptogenic properties, helping the body to adapt to and mitigate stress, a common cause of hormonal imbalances. This recipe combines maca with other supportive ingredients to create a powerful tonic for both men and women seeking to optimize their hormonal health.

Portions

2 servings

Preparation time

5 minutes

Ingredients

- 2 cups almond milk

- 2 tablespoons maca powder

- 1 banana

- 1 tablespoon honey (optional, for sweetness)

- 1/2 teaspoon cinnamon

- Ice cubes (optional)

Instructions

1. Pour the almond milk into a blender.

2. Add the maca powder, banana, honey (if using), and cinnamon to the blender.

3. If a colder beverage is preferred, add ice cubes to the mixture.

4. Blend all ingredients on high until the mixture is smooth and creamy.

5. Pour the hormone balancer into glasses and serve immediately.

Variations

- For added protein and omega-3 fatty acids, include a tablespoon of chia seeds or flaxseeds in the blend.

- Substitute almond milk with coconut milk for a creamier texture and a hint of tropical flavor.

- Add a handful of spinach or kale to increase the smoothie's vitamin and mineral content without significantly altering the taste.

Storage tips

It's best to consume the Maca Root Hormone Balancer immediately after preparation to enjoy its full benefits. However, if necessary, it can be stored in an airtight container in the refrigerator for up to 24 hours. Stir well before consuming if separation occurs.

Tips for allergens

For those with nut allergies, replace almond milk with a suitable non-nut milk alternative like oat milk or rice milk. If honey is a concern due to allergies or vegan dietary preferences, substitute with maple syrup or omit it altogether.

Scientific references

- "Maca (L. meyenii) for improving sexual function: a systematic review," published in BMC Complementary and Alternative Medicine, 2010. This review examines the evidence supporting maca's benefits for sexual function and hormone balance.
- "Effect of Lepidium meyenii (MACA) on sexual desire and its absent relationship with serum testosterone levels in adult healthy men," in the journal Andrologia, 2002. This study highlights maca's role in enhancing libido independently of testosterone levels, suggesting its adaptogenic effects on the endocrine system.

VITEX BERRY TEA

Beneficial effects

Vitex Berry Tea is renowned for its ability to regulate hormonal imbalances, particularly in women. It can alleviate symptoms associated with premenstrual syndrome (PMS), menstrual disorders, and menopause by influencing pituitary gland functions, which in turn affects hormone levels. Regular consumption can lead to reduced cramps, mood swings, and breast tenderness associated with menstrual cycles, as well as improved fertility.

Portions

2 servings

Preparation time

5 minutes

Cooking time

10 minutes

Ingredients

- 2 teaspoons of dried Vitex (Chaste Tree) berries
- 2 cups of boiling water
- Honey or lemon to taste (optional)

Instructions

1. Crush the dried Vitex berries slightly to release their active compounds.

2. Place the crushed berries in a tea infuser or directly into a heat-resistant teapot.

3. Pour 2 cups of boiling water over the crushed berries.

4. Cover and let the tea steep for about 10 minutes.

5. Remove the tea infuser or strain the tea to remove the berries.

6. Optional: Add honey or lemon to taste for flavor enhancement.

7. Serve the tea warm, ideally in the morning to support hormonal balance throughout the day.

Variations

- For a refreshing twist, serve the tea chilled over ice during warmer months.

- Add a cinnamon stick during the steeping process for additional warming flavor and potential blood sugar regulation benefits.

- Combine with peppermint leaves to enhance the flavor and add digestive benefits.

Storage tips

Store any leftover Vitex Berry Tea in a sealed container in the refrigerator for up to 2 days. Enjoy chilled or gently reheat on the stove.

Tips for allergens

Individuals with allergies to Vitex or other plants in the Verbenaceae family should consult with a healthcare provider before consumption. For those avoiding honey due to dietary restrictions, substitute with maple syrup or simply omit the sweetener.

Scientific references

- "Effect of Vitex agnus-castus on premenstrual syndrome: A meta-analysis study," published in the Journal of Ethnopharmacology, 2017. This meta-analysis supports the efficacy of Vitex Berry in alleviating PMS symptoms.

- "Vitex agnus castus for premenstrual syndrome and premenstrual dysphoric disorder: a systematic review," in the Archives of Women's Mental Health, 2011. This review highlights the potential benefits of Vitex Berry for managing premenstrual discomfort and mood disorders.

FENUGREEK SEED INFUSION

Beneficial effects

Fenugreek Seed Infusion is recognized for its ability to support endocrine health, particularly in balancing hormones. It can help manage blood sugar levels, reduce symptoms of PMS and menopause, and may even aid in increasing milk production in breastfeeding mothers. Fenugreek seeds contain phytoestrogens that mimic estrogen, potentially easing hormone-related symptoms. Additionally, its soluble fiber can help in detoxification processes, supporting overall endocrine function.

Portions

2 servings

Preparation time

5 minutes

Cooking time

15 minutes

Ingredients

- 2 tablespoons of fenugreek seeds

- 2 cups of water

- Honey or lemon to taste (optional)

Instructions

1. Rinse the fenugreek seeds under cold water to clean them.

2. In a small saucepan, bring 2 cups of water to a boil.

3. Add the fenugreek seeds to the boiling water.

4. Reduce the heat and simmer for about 15 minutes.

5. Strain the infusion into cups, removing the fenugreek seeds.

6. Optional: Add honey or lemon to taste for flavor enhancement.

7. Serve the infusion warm, ideally in the morning on an empty stomach or before meals.

Variations

- To enhance the digestive benefits, add a slice of fresh ginger to the water along with the fenugreek seeds.

- For a soothing nighttime drink, mix in a teaspoon of dried chamomile flowers during the last 5 minutes of simmering.

- Substitute water with coconut milk for a creamier version, enhancing the natural nutty flavor of fenugreek.

Storage tips

Store any leftover Fenugreek Seed Infusion in a sealed container in the refrigerator for up to 2 days. Enjoy it chilled or gently reheat on the stove.

Tips for allergens

Individuals with allergies to legumes should proceed with caution when trying fenugreek. For those avoiding honey due to dietary restrictions, substitute with maple syrup or simply omit the sweetener.

Scientific references

- "The effects of fenugreek on blood glucose and lipid profile: a meta-analysis of randomized clinical trials" in Nutrition Journal, 2017. This study supports fenugreek's role in managing blood sugar levels and improving cholesterol, indicating its benefits for endocrine health.

- "Fenugreek: A review on its nutraceutical properties and utilization in various food products" in the Journal of the Saudi Society of Agricultural Sciences, 2018. This review discusses fenugreek's phytoestrogen content and its potential impact on hormonal balance and endocrine health.

LICORICE ROOT HORMONE SUPPORT

Beneficial effects

Licorice Root Hormone Support is designed to naturally balance hormone levels, particularly beneficial for those experiencing hormonal imbalances such as PMS, menopause symptoms, and adrenal fatigue. Licorice root contains glycyrrhizin, which can mimic the effects of cortisol, helping to regulate the body's stress response and support adrenal gland function. It also influences estrogen and testosterone levels, promoting hormonal balance. Additionally, its anti-inflammatory and soothing properties can aid in digestive health, further supporting overall well-being.

Ingredients

- 1 tablespoon dried licorice root

- 2 cups water

- Honey or lemon to taste (optional)

Instructions

1. Bring 2 cups of water to a boil in a small saucepan.

2. Add 1 tablespoon of dried licorice root to the boiling water.

3. Reduce the heat and simmer for about 15 minutes, allowing the licorice root to infuse the water.

4. After simmering, remove the saucepan from the heat and let the infusion cool for a few minutes.

5. Strain the licorice root tea into a cup, discarding the solid pieces of root.

6. Optional: Add honey or lemon to taste for flavor enhancement.

7. Drink the licorice root hormone support tea once daily, preferably in the morning to utilize its energizing effects throughout the day.

Variations

- For added benefits, include a slice of fresh ginger during the simmering process to enhance the anti-inflammatory properties.

- Mix in a teaspoon of cinnamon powder for additional blood sugar regulation benefits.

- For those preferring a cold beverage, chill the tea in the refrigerator and serve over ice.

Storage tips

Store any leftover Licorice Root Hormone Support tea in a sealed container in the refrigerator for up to 2 days. Enjoy it chilled, or gently reheat on the stove.

Tips for allergens

Individuals with hypertension or those sensitive to licorice should consult with a healthcare provider before consumption due to its potential effect on blood pressure. For a honey alternative, maple syrup can be used as a sweetener for those with honey allergies or following a vegan diet.

Scientific references

- "The effect of licorice root extract on hormonal changes in menopausal women: a randomized, double-blind, placebo-controlled trial," published in the Iranian Journal of Pharmaceutical Research, 2012. This study highlights licorice root's potential in managing menopausal symptoms through hormonal regulation.

- "Glycyrrhizin, an active component of liquorice roots, and replication of SARS-associated coronavirus," published in The Lancet, 2003. This research supports licorice root's anti-inflammatory properties and its role in supporting adrenal gland function.

PART 19: EYE HEALTH

Eye health is paramount for maintaining not just vision but overall quality of life. The eyes, being windows to the world, require specific nutrients and care to function optimally and stay protected from environmental stressors, aging, and disease. This chapter delves into natural remedies and herbal recipes that support eye health, focusing on the prevention and management of common eye issues such as dry eyes, macular degeneration, and general eye strain.

Bilberry Eye Tonic

Beneficial effects: Bilberry, rich in antioxidants, particularly anthocyanins, supports night vision, strengthens blood vessels in the eye, and helps in reducing eye fatigue.

Ingredients: 1 teaspoon of dried bilberry, 1 cup of boiling water.

Instructions: Steep dried bilberry in boiling water for about 10 minutes. Strain and drink the tea once it cools down. For best results, consume this tonic twice daily.

Eyebright Infusion

Beneficial effects: Eyebright is known for its anti-inflammatory properties, offering relief from eye irritation, redness, and discomfort caused by eye strain or external irritants.

Ingredients: 1 teaspoon of dried eyebright herb, 1 cup of boiling water.

Instructions: Add dried eyebright to boiling water and let it steep for 10 minutes. Strain and use the infusion as a warm compress on closed eyelids for 10 minutes to soothe and refresh tired eyes.

Goji Berry Eye Elixir

Beneficial effects: Goji berries are packed with zeaxanthin and lutein, powerful antioxidants that protect the eyes from UV exposure, blue light, and oxidative stress, reducing the risk of macular degeneration.

Ingredients: ¼ cup of dried goji berries, 1 cup of water.

Instructions: Soak goji berries in water overnight. In the morning, blend the mixture until smooth. Consume this elixir daily in the morning to harness its eye-protective benefits.

Saffron and Honey Eye Drops

Beneficial effects: Saffron contains high levels of antioxidants that are beneficial for eye health, potentially improving vision and protecting against UV damage and macular degeneration.

Ingredients: A pinch of saffron threads, 1 tablespoon of distilled water, 1 teaspoon of honey.

Instructions: Steep saffron threads in boiling water for 10 minutes. Add honey to the cooled saffron water and mix well. Use a clean dropper to apply 1-2 drops in each eye at night before bed. Store the mixture in a clean, airtight container in the refrigerator for up to a week.

Turmeric and Aloe Eye Gel

Beneficial effects: Turmeric has anti-inflammatory properties, while aloe vera soothes and moisturizes. This gel helps in reducing puffiness and dark circles under the eyes.

Ingredients: 1 teaspoon of turmeric powder, 2 tablespoons of aloe vera gel.

Instructions: Mix turmeric powder with aloe vera gel until you get a smooth consistency. Apply a small amount gently around the eyes, avoiding direct contact with the eyes. Leave it on for 20 minutes before rinsing with cool water. Use this gel 2-3 times a week for best results.

Variations: For those sensitive to any of the ingredients listed, alternatives can be explored. For instance, chamomile can be used instead of eyebright for its soothing properties, and blueberry can substitute bilberry for similar antioxidant benefits.

Storage tips: Store any leftover preparations in airtight containers in the refrigerator to maintain their potency. Ensure to label them with the date of preparation.

Tips for allergens: Always perform a patch test on the skin before applying anything new around the eyes to ensure there is no allergic reaction. If sensitivity to any ingredient is known, it's best to avoid its use or consult with a healthcare provider for alternatives.

Scientific references: Numerous studies support the use of these ingredients for eye health. Research published in the Journal of Agricultural and Food Chemistry highlights the antioxidant properties of bilberry and its benefits for night vision. Studies in the Journal of Ophthalmology have shown the protective effects of lutein and zeaxanthin, found in goji berries, against macular degeneration. The anti-inflammatory effects of turmeric on eye health are documented in the International Journal of Molecular Sciences.

Incorporating these natural remedies into daily routines can contribute significantly to maintaining eye health, preventing common eye conditions, and ensuring the longevity of vision and overall well-being.

CHAPTER 1: DR. BARBARA'S APPROACH TO EYE HEALTH

D r. Barbara emphasizes the critical importance of maintaining optimal eye health as a fundamental aspect of holistic well-being. Recognizing the eyes as not only the windows to the soul but also as indicators of overall health, she advocates for a comprehensive approach to eye care that goes beyond conventional practices.

Central to her philosophy is the integration of natural remedies, dietary adjustments, and lifestyle modifications designed to support and enhance eye health.

Key to Dr. Barbara's approach is the understanding that nutrition plays a pivotal role in maintaining eye health. She highlights the significance of antioxidants, vitamins, and minerals in protecting the eyes from oxidative stress, inflammation, and age-related conditions.

Foods rich in vitamin A, such as carrots, sweet potatoes, and leafy greens, are championed for their role in maintaining healthy vision. Omega-3 fatty acids, found in fatty fish, flaxseeds, and walnuts, are noted for their anti-inflammatory properties and their contribution to retinal health. Dr. Barbara also stresses the importance of including foods high in lutein and zeaxanthin, like kale, spinach, and eggs, to protect against macular degeneration.

Beyond nutrition, Dr. Barbara advises on the importance of protecting the eyes from excessive exposure to blue light, a prevalent issue in the digital age.

She recommends the use of blue light filtering glasses and taking regular breaks from screens to prevent eye strain and support circadian rhythms. Hydration is underscored as a simple yet effective way to support eye health, aiding in the maintenance of tear production and overall hydration, which is vital for clear vision.

Physical activity emerges as another cornerstone of Dr. Barbara's eye health strategy. Regular exercise increases circulation, which is beneficial for eye health by delivering more oxygen and nutrients to the eyes while facilitating the removal of toxins. Stress management techniques such as meditation and yoga are encouraged not only for their general health benefits but also for their specific benefits to eye health, including reducing eye strain and promoting relaxation.

Herbal remedies play a special role in Dr. Barbara's holistic approach to eye health. She details the use of herbs like bilberry and eyebright, known for their vision-enhancing properties and their ability to support vascular health and reduce eye fatigue.

Dr. Barbara provides recipes for herbal teas and infusions that can be easily incorporated into daily routines to support eye health from within.

In advocating for regular eye check-ups, Dr. Barbara integrates the importance of professional eye care with her holistic health philosophy.

She encourages consultations with healthcare professionals to identify and address any underlying health issues that may be impacting eye health, such as diabetes or high blood pressure, thereby adopting a proactive and preventive approach to eye care.

By embracing a lifestyle that incorporates balanced nutrition, protective measures, physical activity, stress management, and natural remedies, Dr. Barbara's approach to eye health offers a comprehensive and integrative path to maintaining vision and overall well-being.

This holistic perspective not only focuses on preventing and managing eye-related issues but also enhances the body's general health, underscoring the interconnectedness of eye health with the health of the entire body.

CHAPTER 2: NUTRITIONAL SUPPORT FOR EYE HEALTH

Ensuring optimal eye health through nutrition involves focusing on foods rich in specific vitamins, minerals, and antioxidants known to support vision and protect against eye diseases. Key nutrients such as Vitamin A, Vitamin C, Vitamin E, zinc, lutein, and zeaxanthin play a pivotal role in maintaining eye health and function. These nutrients help in protecting the eyes from harmful light exposure, reducing the risk of chronic eye diseases, and supporting the overall health of eye tissues.

Vitamin A is essential for maintaining vision, especially in low light conditions, and for keeping the eyes' surface tissues healthy. Sources of Vitamin A include carrots, sweet potatoes, spinach, and kale. Incorporating these foods into your diet can help prevent conditions such as night blindness and dry eyes.

Vitamin C, an antioxidant found in fruits and vegetables like oranges, strawberries, bell peppers, and broccoli, helps reduce the risk of cataracts and macular degeneration by fighting free radicals and supporting the health of the blood vessels in the eyes.

Vitamin E works in conjunction with Vitamin C to protect the cells of the eyes from damage caused by free radicals. Almonds, sunflower seeds, and avocados are excellent sources of Vitamin E and can be easily added to your diet to support eye health.

Zinc plays a crucial role in bringing Vitamin A from the liver to the retina, to produce melanin, a protective pigment in the eyes. Beef, pumpkin seeds, and chickpeas are rich sources of zinc, essential for maintaining the health of the retina and reducing the risk of night blindness.

Lutein and zeaxanthin are carotenoids found in high concentrations in the macula, a part of the retina responsible for central vision. These antioxidants filter harmful high-energy blue wavelengths of light and help protect and maintain healthy cells in the eyes. Leafy greens such as kale, spinach, and collard greens, as well as eggs, are rich in these nutrients and can help reduce the risk of chronic eye diseases.

Omega-3 fatty acids, particularly DHA, found in fatty fish like salmon, mackerel, and sardines, are important for the health of the retina and may help prevent dry eyes by supporting the production of the oily outer layer of the eye's tear film.

Incorporating these nutrients into your diet can be done through various meals and snacks. For example, starting your day with a spinach and kale omelet can provide a healthy dose of lutein, zeaxanthin, and Vitamin E. Snacking on almonds or adding flaxseeds to your smoothie can increase your intake of Omega-3 fatty acids and Vitamin E. For lunch or dinner, a salmon salad with a variety of colorful vegetables can offer a substantial amount of Omega-3s, Vitamin C, and zinc.

It's also important to stay hydrated to support overall eye health. Adequate fluid intake helps maintain the natural moisture levels in the eyes, preventing dryness and irritation.

For those with specific dietary restrictions or allergies, there are always alternatives. For example, vegetarians or vegans can obtain Omega-3 fatty acids from flaxseeds or chia seeds instead of fish. Similarly, for those allergic to nuts, sunflower seeds can be a safe source of Vitamin E.

Scientific studies have supported the benefits of these nutrients for eye health. Research published in the Archives of Ophthalmology has shown that a higher intake of foods rich in lutein and zeaxanthin is associated with a lower risk of developing macular degeneration. Another study in the American Journal of Clinical Nutrition found that individuals with a high intake of Vitamin C had a significantly lower risk of cataract progression.

By focusing on a diet rich in these key nutrients, individuals can support their eye health and reduce the risk of eye diseases, ensuring clear vision and healthy eyes for years to come.

THE ROLE OF ANTIOXIDANTS IN EYE HEALTH

Antioxidants play a crucial role in maintaining eye health by protecting ocular tissues from oxidative stress and inflammation, which can lead to age-related macular degeneration (AMD) and cataracts, two leading causes of vision impairment and blindness. These powerful substances, found abundantly in various fruits, vegetables, and other foods, neutralize harmful free radicals in the body. Free radicals are unstable molecules that can damage cells, including those in the eyes, leading to deterioration and disease.

Vitamins C and E are potent antioxidants that contribute significantly to eye health. Vitamin C, found in citrus fruits, berries, and bell peppers, helps regenerate other antioxidants within the body, including Vitamin E, and plays a vital role in collagen production, supporting the cornea and sclera. Vitamin E, present in nuts, seeds, and green leafy vegetables, protects the cells of the eyes from damage caused by free radicals, which is crucial for preventing cataracts and AMD.

Another group of antioxidants, known as carotenoids, including lutein and zeaxanthin, are specifically beneficial for the eyes. These are found in high concentrations in the macula, the part of the retina responsible for sharp, central vision. Lutein and zeaxanthin filter harmful high-energy blue light, protecting the eyes from damage. Leafy greens such as kale, spinach, and collard greens, as well as eggs, provide a rich source of these antioxidants.

Incorporating a diet rich in these antioxidants can support eye health and reduce the risk of eye diseases. For example, a salad made with spinach, kale, and other leafy greens, topped with slices of orange and almonds, can provide a powerful antioxidant boost for the eyes. Adding berries to breakfast cereals or smoothies is another easy way to increase antioxidant intake.

Scientific research supports the benefits of antioxidants for eye health. Studies have shown that a diet high in antioxidants can significantly reduce the risk of developing cataracts and AMD. By consuming a variety of antioxidant-rich foods, individuals can protect their eyes from oxidative stress, supporting overall eye health and vision.

OMEGA-3 FATTY ACIDS FOR VISION

Omega-3 fatty acids, particularly EPA and DHA, are vital for maintaining eye health and optimal vision. These essential nutrients contribute significantly to the structural integrity of the eye's retina, where DHA is a major structural component. Adequate intake of omega-3s supports retinal development and function, reduces the risk of dry eye syndrome, and may slow the progression of age-related macular degeneration (AMD), a leading cause of blindness in older adults.

Beneficial effects: Omega-3 fatty acids help in maintaining cell membrane health in the eyes, support proper drainage of intraocular fluids, reducing the risk of high eye pressure and glaucoma, and protect against retinal damage.

Portions: Incorporating at least two servings of omega-3 rich foods like fatty fish per week is recommended for eye health benefits.

Preparation time: Varies based on the recipe.

Ingredients:

- Fatty fish (salmon, mackerel, sardines)
- Flaxseeds or flaxseed oil
- Chia seeds
- Walnuts
- Hemp seeds

Instructions:

1. For fish: Grill, bake, or steam 3-4 ounces of fatty fish. Season with herbs and lemon juice for added flavor without adding unhealthy fats.

2. For seeds and nuts: Add a tablespoon of ground flaxseeds or chia seeds to smoothies, yogurts, or salads. Consume daily.

3. For oil: Use flaxseed oil as a salad dressing or in smoothies. Do not heat to preserve the omega-3 content.

Variations: Vegetarians or vegans can focus on plant-based sources of ALA omega-3s, such as flaxseeds, chia seeds, and walnuts, which the body can partially convert to EPA and DHA.

Storage tips: Keep flaxseeds, chia seeds, and walnuts in a cool, dark place or refrigerate to prevent rancidity. Store flaxseed oil and fish oil supplements in the refrigerator to maintain freshness.

Tips for allergens: For those allergic to fish, consider algae-based DHA supplements as a direct source of DHA without the fish.

Scientific references: Studies have shown that people with higher intakes of omega-3 fatty acids have a significantly lower risk of AMD and may experience less dry eye syndrome.

FOODS TO AVOID FOR BETTER EYE HEALTH

Maintaining optimal eye health extends beyond incorporating beneficial nutrients into your diet; it also involves being mindful of foods that can negatively impact vision and overall eye condition. Certain foods and dietary habits can exacerbate the risk of developing eye conditions such as dry eyes, macular degeneration, and cataracts. To safeguard your vision, consider reducing or eliminating the following from your diet:

High-sugar foods and beverages can lead to fluctuations in blood sugar levels, which, over time, can damage the blood vessels in the eyes and lead to conditions like diabetic retinopathy. Foods high in refined sugars, such as candies, sodas, and pastries, can also contribute to inflammation and oxidative stress, increasing the risk of age-related macular degeneration.

Trans fats, found in many processed foods, fast foods, and baked goods, can contribute to the hardening of the arteries and reduced blood flow to the retina, potentially leading to vision impairment. These fats can also increase the risk of developing dry eye syndrome.

High-sodium foods can lead to hypertension, which can adversely affect the blood vessels in the eyes, potentially leading to hypertensive retinopathy. Processed foods, canned soups, and fast foods are often high in sodium and should be consumed in moderation.

Fried foods can contribute to the buildup of deposits in the retina, known as drusen, which can be a risk factor for age-related macular degeneration. Opting for cooking methods such as baking, steaming, or grilling can help reduce the intake of unhealthy fats associated with frying.

Artificial sweeteners and additives, found in a variety of diet foods and beverages, can also have adverse effects on eye health. Some studies suggest that certain artificial sweeteners may be linked to an increased risk of eye conditions, though more research is needed to fully understand these relationships.

Alcohol consumption in excess can lead to dehydration, affecting the eyes' ability to produce tears and leading to symptoms of dry eyes. Over time, excessive alcohol intake can also contribute to the development of cataracts and macular degeneration.

To support eye health, focus on a diet rich in whole foods, fruits, vegetables, lean proteins, and healthy fats, while limiting the intake of these potentially harmful foods and substances. Staying hydrated and maintaining a balanced diet can help preserve vision and keep your eyes healthy for years to come. Remember, moderation is key, and making informed dietary choices can significantly impact your overall well-being, including the health of your eyes.

CHAPTER 3: NATURAL REMEDIES FOR EYE HEALTH

Beneficial effects: The remedies provided here aim to support and enhance eye health through natural means. They focus on reducing inflammation, protecting against oxidative stress, and nourishing the eyes with essential nutrients. These remedies can help alleviate symptoms of dry eyes, improve night vision, and potentially slow the progression of age-related eye conditions such as macular degeneration and cataracts.

Portions: Each remedy is designed for one serving or application, with recommendations for daily or weekly use as specified.

Preparation time: Varies from 5 to 20 minutes depending on the remedy.

Cooking time: Not applicable for most remedies as they are mostly infusions or topical applications.

Ingredients:

1. **Bilberry Eye Tonic**

- 1 teaspoon dried bilberry fruit

- 1 cup boiling water

2. **Eyebright Infusion**

- 1 teaspoon dried eyebright herb

- 1 cup boiling water

3. **Goji Berry Eye Elixir**

- ¼ cup goji berries

- 1 cup cold water

4. **Saffron and Honey Eye Drops**

- 2 strands of saffron

- 1 tablespoon distilled water

- 1 teaspoon raw honey

5. **Turmeric and Aloe Eye Gel**

- 1 teaspoon aloe vera gel

- ¼ teaspoon turmeric powder

- 1 teaspoon distilled water

Instructions:

1. **Bilberry Eye Tonic**

- Steep 1 teaspoon of dried bilberry fruit in 1 cup of boiling water for 10 minutes.

- Strain and drink once daily to support night vision and circulation within the eye.

2. **Eyebright Infusion**

- Steep 1 teaspoon of dried eyebright herb in 1 cup of boiling water for 10 minutes.

- Strain and use as an eye wash or compress to relieve eye strain and irritation. Ensure the solution is cool before applying to the eyes.

3. **Goji Berry Eye Elixir**

- Soak ¼ cup of goji berries in 1 cup of cold water overnight.

- Drink the infusion and eat the berries the next day to support overall eye health.

4. Saffron and Honey Eye Drops

- Dissolve 2 strands of saffron in 1 tablespoon of distilled water and add 1 teaspoon of raw honey.

- Mix well and use a clean dropper to apply 1 drop in each eye at night to reduce strain and improve vision clarity.

5. Turmeric and Aloe Eye Gel

- Mix 1 teaspoon of aloe vera gel with ¼ teaspoon of turmeric powder and 1 teaspoon of distilled water to achieve a smooth consistency.

- Apply gently around the eyes, avoiding direct contact with the eyes, to reduce puffiness and inflammation. Leave on for 10 minutes before rinsing with cool water.

Variations: For those allergic to any ingredient, alternative herbs or fruits rich in antioxidants can be used. For example, green tea can replace bilberry for its antioxidant properties, and chamomile can be used instead of eyebright for its soothing effects.

Storage tips: Prepare fresh batches of each remedy to ensure potency and safety. Any leftover goji berry infusion can be stored in the refrigerator for up to 2 days.

Tips for allergens: Always patch test topical remedies on a small area of skin before full application to ensure no allergic reaction occurs. For ingestible remedies, ensure you do not have allergies to the ingredients listed.

Scientific references: Studies have shown the efficacy of bilberry in improving night vision and eyebright in reducing eye irritation. Goji berries are known for their high antioxidant content, which is beneficial for eye health. Saffron has been studied for its potential in improving vision clarity, and turmeric is well-documented for its anti-inflammatory properties.

CHAPTER 4: 5 HERBAL RECIPES FOR EYE HEALTH

BILBERRY EYE TONIC

Beneficial effects

Bilberry Eye Tonic is renowned for its potent antioxidant properties, primarily due to the high concentration of anthocyanins found in bilberries. These compounds are known to support eye health by enhancing blood circulation within the capillaries of the eyes, improving night vision, and reducing the risk of macular degeneration and cataracts. Additionally, bilberries have anti-inflammatory properties that can help reduce eye fatigue and strain.

Ingredients

- 1 cup fresh or frozen bilberries
- 2 cups water
- 1 tablespoon honey (optional)
- 1 teaspoon lemon juice (optional)

Instructions

1. Place the bilberries in a small saucepan and add 2 cups of water.

2. Bring the mixture to a boil, then reduce the heat and let it simmer for 10 minutes to extract the beneficial compounds from the bilberries.

3. Remove the saucepan from the heat and allow the mixture to cool slightly.

4. Strain the mixture through a fine mesh sieve into a pitcher, pressing on the bilberries to extract as much liquid as possible.

5. If desired, stir in honey and lemon juice to taste.

6. Serve the tonic warm, or allow it to cool completely and refrigerate for a refreshing cold drink.

Variations

- For an added boost of antioxidants, mix in a teaspoon of matcha green tea powder during the simmering process.

- Incorporate a cinnamon stick while simmering the bilberries for additional flavor and potential blood sugar regulation benefits.

- Blend the strained bilberry mixture with a banana and a handful of spinach for a nutritious eye health smoothie.

Storage tips

Store any leftover Bilberry Eye Tonic in a sealed container in the refrigerator for up to 3 days. Shake well before serving if separation occurs.

Tips for allergens

For those with honey allergies or following a vegan diet, substitute honey with maple syrup or simply omit the sweetener. Ensure to use freshly squeezed lemon juice to avoid potential preservatives found in some bottled lemon juice products.

Scientific references

- "Anthocyanins in Cardiovascular Disease" published in Advances in Nutrition, 2011. This study highlights the cardiovascular benefits of anthocyanins, supporting their role in enhancing blood circulation, which is crucial for eye health.

- "Bilberries reduce eye fatigue caused by video display terminal use: A double-blind, placebo-controlled, randomized trial" in the Journal of Nutrition, Health & Aging, 2015. This research supports the efficacy of bilberries in reducing eye fatigue and strain, further emphasizing their importance in maintaining eye health.

EYEBRIGHT INFUSION

Beneficial effects

Eyebright Infusion is celebrated for its ability to support eye health, particularly in soothing irritated eyes, reducing inflammation, and enhancing visual clarity. Rich in flavonoids and antioxidants, Eyebright helps protect the eyes from environmental stressors and can alleviate symptoms of eye fatigue, redness, and dryness. Its anti-inflammatory properties are particularly beneficial for those suffering from conjunctivitis or seasonal allergies, offering a natural and gentle remedy for eye discomfort.

Portions

2 servings

Preparation time

5 minutes

Cooking time

10 minutes

Ingredients

- 2 teaspoons of dried Eyebright herb
- 2 cups of boiling water
- Honey or lemon to taste (optional)

Instructions

1. Place the dried Eyebright herb in a tea infuser or directly into a heat-resistant teapot.

2. Pour 2 cups of boiling water over the Eyebright.

3. Cover and allow the mixture to steep for about 10 minutes.

4. Remove the tea infuser or strain the infusion to remove the Eyebright herb.

5. Optional: Add honey or lemon to taste for flavor enhancement.

6. Serve the infusion warm, or allow it to cool and use it as an eye wash or compress for direct eye relief.

Variations

- For added benefits, include a teaspoon of chamomile flowers in the infusion to enhance the soothing effects on the eyes.

- To create a cooling eye compress, refrigerate the infusion before soaking clean cotton pads and applying them to closed eyelids.

- Combine with green tea leaves during steeping for an additional antioxidant boost.

Storage tips

Store any leftover Eyebright Infusion in a sealed container in the refrigerator for up to 48 hours. For topical use, ensure the infusion is at a comfortable temperature before applying to the eyes.

Tips for allergens

Individuals with sensitivities to specific herbs should ensure the purity of the Eyebright herb to avoid potential allergens. For those avoiding honey due to dietary restrictions, substitute with maple syrup or simply omit the sweetener.

Scientific references

- "Anti-inflammatory and cytotoxic actions of extracts from medicinal plants used by traditional healers of Sikkim, India," published in the Journal of Ethnopharmacology, highlights Eyebright's anti-inflammatory properties, supporting its use in eye care.

- "Flavonoids: A review of probable mechanisms of action and potential applications," in the American Journal of Clinical Nutrition, discusses the role of flavonoids found in Eyebright in protecting against oxidative stress and inflammation.

GOJI BERRY EYE ELIXIR

Beneficial effects

Goji Berry Eye Elixir is a potent concoction aimed at enhancing eye health and vision. Goji berries are packed with antioxidants, particularly zeaxanthin and lutein, which are known for their ability to protect the eyes from oxidative stress, reduce the risk of macular degeneration, and improve overall visual acuity. This elixir can also help in shielding the eyes from harmful UV rays and blue light, making it an excellent dietary addition for those seeking to maintain healthy vision and prevent age-related eye diseases.

Portions

2 servings

Preparation time

10 minutes

Ingredients

- 1/4 cup dried goji berries
- 2 cups boiling water
- 1 tablespoon honey (optional)
- A slice of lemon (optional for added vitamin C)

Instructions

1. Place the dried goji berries in a heat-resistant bowl or teapot.

2. Pour 2 cups of boiling water over the goji berries and allow them to steep for about 8 to 10 minutes.

3. Strain the mixture to remove the goji berries, reserving the liquid.

4. If desired, stir in 1 tablespoon of honey to sweeten and add a slice of lemon for an extra boost of vitamin C.

5. Serve the elixir warm or allow it to cool and enjoy it chilled.

Variations

- For an added antioxidant boost, mix in a teaspoon of green tea leaves during the steeping process.
- Blend the steeped goji berries with the elixir after cooling for a fiber-rich smoothie.
- Incorporate a pinch of turmeric powder to the elixir for its anti-inflammatory properties.

Storage tips

Store any leftover Goji Berry Eye Elixir in a sealed container in the refrigerator for up to 48 hours. Enjoy it chilled or gently reheat on the stove.

Tips for allergens

Individuals with allergies to berries should proceed with caution and may consider consulting with a healthcare provider before consumption. For those avoiding honey due to dietary restrictions, substitute with maple syrup or simply omit the sweetener.

Scientific references

- "Protective effects of goji berry extract on human retinal pigment epithelial cells under high glucose condition," in the Journal of Cellular Biochemistry, 2018. This study highlights the protective effects of goji berries against oxidative stress in retinal cells.

- "Lutein and zeaxanthin supplementation reduces photooxidative damage and modulates the expression of inflammation-related genes in retinal pigment epithelial cells," in Free Radical Biology and Medicine, 2012. This research supports the beneficial impact of zeaxanthin and lutein, found in goji berries, on eye health.

SAFFRON AND HONEY EYE DROPS

Beneficial effects

Saffron and Honey Eye Drops offer a natural remedy for improving eye health and vision clarity. Saffron, known for its high content of antioxidants, can help protect the eyes from oxidative stress and reduce the risk of age-related macular degeneration and cataracts. Honey, with its antibacterial properties, aids in preventing and treating eye infections. Together, they provide a soothing effect, reducing dryness and irritation in the eyes.

Ingredients

- 1 teaspoon of high-quality saffron threads
- 1 tablespoon of distilled water
- 1 teaspoon of organic honey

Instructions

1. In a small, clean bowl, steep the saffron threads in the tablespoon of distilled water for 10 minutes, allowing the water to take on a deep, golden color.

2. Strain the saffron-infused water into another clean bowl to remove the saffron threads.

3. Add the teaspoon of organic honey to the saffron-infused water and mix until the honey is completely dissolved.

4. Using a sterilized dropper, transfer the saffron and honey solution to a sterile eye dropper bottle.

5. To use, apply 1-2 drops in each eye, twice a day.

Variations

- For additional soothing properties, add a drop of aloe vera juice to the mixture.

- If you prefer a thinner consistency, you can add an extra half teaspoon of distilled water to the solution.

Storage tips

Store the Saffron and Honey Eye Drops in the refrigerator for up to one week. Ensure the eye dropper bottle is tightly sealed to maintain sterility.

Tips for allergens

Individuals with allergies to pollen or bee products should proceed with caution when using honey in eye drops. Always conduct a patch test on the skin before applying anything new to the eyes.

Scientific references

- "Saffron: A promising natural medicine in the treatment of ocular diseases," published in the Journal of Pharmacy & Bioallied Sciences, 2016. This study highlights the antioxidant properties of saffron and its potential benefits for eye health.

- "Antibacterial activity of honey against strains of Staphylococcus aureus from infected wounds," in the Journal of the Royal Society of Medicine, 1999. This research supports honey's antibacterial properties, making it beneficial for preventing eye infections.

TURMERIC AND ALOE EYE GEL

Beneficial effects

Turmeric and Aloe Eye Gel combines the anti-inflammatory and antioxidant properties of turmeric with the soothing, hydrating benefits of aloe vera. This natural remedy is designed to reduce puffiness, diminish dark circles, and soothe the delicate skin around the eyes. Turmeric contains curcumin, a compound known for its ability to fight inflammation and oxidative damage, while aloe vera provides a cooling effect that helps to calm irritated skin. Together, they create a powerful eye gel that promotes healthier, more vibrant skin.

Ingredients

- 1 tablespoon aloe vera gel
- 1/4 teaspoon turmeric powder
- 1 teaspoon distilled water (optional, for thinning)
- A small container for storage

Instructions

1. In a small bowl, mix the aloe vera gel and turmeric powder until well combined.

2. If the mixture is too thick, add distilled water a few drops at a time until you reach the desired consistency.

3. Transfer the mixture to a small container with a lid.

4. To use, gently apply a small amount of the gel around the eye area with a clean finger or cotton swab, being careful to avoid direct contact with the eyes.

5. Leave the gel on for about 10-20 minutes before rinsing off with cool water.

Variations

- For additional soothing properties, add a drop of lavender essential oil to the mixture.
- Incorporate vitamin E oil to the gel to enhance its skin-nourishing benefits.
- For a cooling effect, store the gel in the refrigerator before application.

Storage tips

Keep the Turmeric and Aloe Eye Gel in the refrigerator in a tightly sealed container. Use within 1-2 weeks for best quality and effectiveness.

Tips for allergens

Individuals with sensitivity to turmeric or aloe vera should patch test the gel on a small area of the skin before applying it to the face. Substitute aloe vera gel with cucumber juice for those allergic to aloe vera, noting that the consistency and storage requirements may change.

Scientific references

- "Curcumin: A Review of Its' Effects on Human Health," published in Foods, 2017. This review discusses the wide-ranging health benefits of curcumin, including its anti-inflammatory and antioxidant effects, which support its use in skincare.

- "Aloe vera: a short review," published in the Indian Journal of Dermatology, 2008. This article highlights the soothing, moisturizing, and healing properties of aloe vera, making it beneficial for use around the sensitive eye area.

PART 20: DENTAL HEALTH

aintaining optimal dental health is crucial for overall well-being, and natural remedies can play a significant role in achieving this. Herbal recipes for dental health focus on reducing inflammation, fighting bacteria, and promoting gum and tooth health. These natural approaches can complement regular dental care routines, offering additional support for maintaining a healthy mouth.

Beneficial effects: These herbal remedies aim to support dental health by strengthening the gums, reducing tooth decay, alleviating pain, and refreshing the breath. They possess antibacterial, anti-inflammatory, and analgesic properties that are beneficial for preventing and treating common dental issues.

Clove Oil Mouth Rinse

Ingredients:

- ½ teaspoon of clove oil

- 1 cup of warm water

- **Instructions**:

1. Mix the clove oil with the warm water thoroughly.

2. Use the mixture as a mouth rinse twice daily, swishing it around the mouth for at least 30 seconds before spitting it out.

Beneficial effects: Clove oil contains eugenol, a natural antiseptic and pain reliever, making it effective for reducing gum pain and fighting oral bacteria.

Sage and Sea Salt Gargle

Ingredients:

- 1 tablespoon of dried sage leaves

- 1 teaspoon of sea salt

- 1 cup of boiling water

- **Instructions**:

1. Steep the sage leaves in boiling water for 10 minutes.

2. Strain the leaves and dissolve the sea salt in the sage infusion.

3. Gargle with the mixture once it cools down, especially after meals and before bed.

Beneficial effects: Sage has antimicrobial properties that help in reducing dental plaque and gingivitis, while sea salt helps in healing and reducing inflammation.

Myrrh Gum Powder Toothpaste

Ingredients:

- 2 tablespoons of myrrh gum powder

- 2 tablespoons of baking soda

- Water to form a paste

- **Instructions**:

1. Mix the myrrh gum powder and baking soda in a small bowl.

2. Gradually add water until a paste-like consistency is achieved.

3. Use this mixture to brush your teeth, focusing on the gums and teeth surfaces gently.

Beneficial effects: Myrrh gum has been used historically for treating mouth and gum diseases due to its antibacterial and antifungal properties. Combined with baking soda, it helps in gently cleaning the teeth and promoting gum health.

Peppermint and Coconut Oil Pulling

Ingredients:

- 1 tablespoon of virgin coconut oil

- 2 drops of peppermint essential oil

- **Instructions**:

1. Combine the coconut oil and peppermint oil in a small container.

2. Swish the oil mixture in your mouth for 10-20 minutes on an empty stomach.

3. Spit out the oil and rinse your mouth with warm water.

Beneficial effects: Oil pulling with coconut oil can help in reducing plaque formation and gingivitis. Peppermint oil adds antibacterial properties and leaves the mouth feeling fresh.

Calendula and Chamomile Gum Soother

Ingredients:

- 1 teaspoon of dried calendula flowers

- 1 teaspoon of dried chamomile flowers

- 1 cup of boiling water

- **Instructions**:

1. Mix the calendula and chamomile flowers in a bowl.

2. Pour boiling water over the flowers and steep for 10 minutes.

3. Strain the infusion and allow it to cool.

4. Use the solution to rinse your mouth 2-3 times a day.

Beneficial effects: Both calendula and chamomile are known for their soothing, anti-inflammatory properties, making this rinse ideal for calming irritated gums.

Variations: These recipes can be adjusted according to personal preference and availability of ingredients. For example, tea tree oil can be added to the mouth rinse for its potent antimicrobial properties, or cinnamon can be included in the toothpaste for its antibacterial effects and pleasant taste.

Storage tips: Prepare small batches of these remedies to ensure freshness. Store any unused portions of the mouth rinse or gum soother in the refrigerator for up to 2 days. The toothpaste can be stored in a small, airtight container at room temperature for up to a week.

Tips for allergens: Always conduct a patch test before using essential oils or new herbs to ensure there is no allergic reaction. For those with nut allergies, sesame oil can be used as an alternative in oil pulling.

Scientific references: Studies have supported the efficacy of clove oil in reducing dental pain and the antimicrobial properties of sage. Research published in the Journal of Ayurveda and Integrative Medicine highlights the benefits of oil pulling for oral health.

CHAPTER 1: DR. BARBARA'S DENTAL HEALTH TIPS

D r. Barbara emphasizes the critical role of dental health in overall wellness, advocating for a holistic approach that goes beyond traditional dental care. She points out that oral health is deeply interconnected with the body's systemic health, suggesting that issues within the mouth can signal or contribute to broader health challenges. Dr. Barbara encourages incorporating natural remedies and practices alongside regular dental check-ups to support oral hygiene, prevent dental diseases, and maintain a healthy mouth environment.

Key insights from Dr. Barbara include the importance of a nutrient-rich diet for dental health. She highlights that foods high in calcium, phosphorus, vitamin D, and vitamin K2 are essential for strong teeth and bones. Leafy greens, nuts, seeds, dairy products, and fish are recommended for their roles in remineralizing teeth and supporting gum health. Additionally, she advises limiting sugar intake and acidic foods that can erode tooth enamel, leading to cavities and dental decay.

Dr. Barbara also discusses the significance of saliva in maintaining oral health. Saliva acts as a natural cleanser that neutralizes acids and helps wash away food particles and bacteria. To promote healthy saliva production, she suggests staying well-hydrated and chewing sugar-free gum or foods that require more chewing, like raw vegetables, to stimulate saliva flow.

For those seeking natural remedies to enhance their dental care routine, Dr. Barbara recommends several practices:

- Oil pulling with coconut oil to reduce plaque formation and detoxify the mouth.

- Using a homemade toothpaste made from baking soda and coconut oil for its antibacterial properties.

- Rinsing with a saltwater solution to heal and prevent mouth sores and reduce inflammation.

- Applying a turmeric paste to the gums to combat inflammation due to its curcumin content.

Dr. Barbara stresses the importance of gentle, thorough oral hygiene practices, including brushing with a soft-bristled toothbrush, flossing daily, and using a tongue scraper to remove bacteria from the tongue's surface. She advises against overbrushing or using hard-bristled brushes, which can damage enamel and irritate the gums.

In addition to these practices, Dr. Barbara encourages mindfulness in dental care, such as paying attention to brushing technique and being aware of any changes in oral health. Regular dental check-ups are crucial for early detection and treatment of dental issues. She also highlights the role of stress management in preventing conditions like bruxism (teeth grinding), which can cause tooth damage and TMJ disorders.

By adopting Dr. Barbara's holistic insights into dental health, individuals can take proactive steps towards maintaining a healthy mouth and, by extension, a healthier body. These natural practices, combined with conventional dental care, offer a comprehensive approach to oral wellness that supports overall health and well-being.

CHAPTER 2: NUTRITION FOR DENTAL HEALTH

Nutritional support plays a pivotal role in maintaining healthy teeth and gums, underscoring the importance of a well-balanced diet rich in vitamins, minerals, and other nutrients essential for oral health. Consuming foods high in calcium and phosphorus, such as dairy products, fish, and tofu, is crucial as these minerals help repair and strengthen tooth enamel. Vitamin D, obtained from sunlight exposure and foods like fatty fish and egg yolks, enhances calcium absorption, further supporting tooth health.

Vitamin C, found in citrus fruits, broccoli, and bell peppers, is vital for gum health, aiding in the maintenance of the connective tissue and the prevention of gingivitis.

Incorporating crunchy fruits and vegetables, such as apples, carrots, and celery, into your diet can stimulate saliva production, which plays a key role in neutralizing acids and washing away food particles and bacteria. Additionally, these foods provide a mechanical cleaning action on the teeth, helping to reduce plaque buildup. Foods high in antioxidants, including berries and nuts, combat bacteria that can lead to inflammation and gum disease. Omega-3 fatty acids, present in fish, flaxseeds, and walnuts, have anti-inflammatory properties that can help protect against gum disease.

It's also beneficial to include foods rich in probiotics, such as yogurt and kefir, in your diet. Probiotics contribute to a healthy balance of bacteria in the mouth, potentially reducing the prevalence of harmful bacteria that can lead to gum disease and tooth decay.

Green and black teas contain polyphenols that can slow the growth of bacteria associated with cavities and gum disease, offering another dietary option for supporting oral health.

Limiting the intake of sugary and acidic foods and beverages is equally important as they can erode tooth enamel and lead to cavities. Instead, focusing on a diet that supports oral health can contribute significantly to the overall well-being of your teeth and gums.

Beneficial effects: A diet rich in specific nutrients supports the maintenance of healthy teeth and gums by strengthening tooth enamel, supporting bone health, reducing inflammation, and combating harmful bacteria.

Ingredients:

- Dairy products (for calcium and phosphorus)

- Fatty fish (for vitamin D and omega-3 fatty acids)

- Citrus fruits, broccoli, bell peppers (for vitamin C)

- Apples, carrots, celery (for fiber and natural cleaning)

- Berries, nuts (for antioxidants)

- Yogurt, kefir (for probiotics)

- Green and black teas (for polyphenols)

Instructions:

1. Include a serving of dairy products in your daily diet to provide calcium and phosphorus.

2. Consume fatty fish 2-3 times a week for vitamin D and omega-3 fatty acids.

3. Add a variety of fruits and vegetables rich in vitamin C to your meals each day.

4. Snack on crunchy fruits and vegetables to stimulate saliva production and provide a natural cleaning action for your teeth.

5. Incorporate berries and nuts into your diet for their antioxidant properties.

6. Consume probiotic-rich foods like yogurt and kefir to support a healthy balance of bacteria in your mouth.

7. Drink green or black tea to benefit from the polyphenols that can slow the growth of harmful bacteria.

Variations: For those who are dairy-intolerant, calcium-fortified plant milks and juices can be an alternative source of calcium. Vegetarians and vegans can obtain omega-3 fatty acids from flaxseeds, chia seeds, and walnuts.

Storage tips: Keep berries and nuts in the refrigerator to maintain freshness. Dairy products, yogurt, and kefir should also be stored in the refrigerator. Store flaxseeds and chia seeds in a cool, dry place.

Tips for allergens: Individuals with allergies to nuts can opt for seeds as a source of nutrients and antioxidants. Those allergic to dairy can choose calcium-fortified plant-based alternatives.

Scientific references: Research has shown that diets rich in calcium, phosphorus, and vitamin D are essential for maintaining healthy teeth, while vitamin C plays a crucial role in gum health. Studies have also highlighted the anti-inflammatory benefits of omega-3 fatty acids in preventing gum disease.

CHAPTER 3: NATURAL REMEDIES FOR DENTAL HEALTH

Beneficial effects: These natural remedies aim to enhance dental health by promoting gum strength, reducing inflammation, combating harmful bacteria, and providing relief from dental discomfort. They leverage the natural antiseptic, anti-inflammatory, and analgesic properties of herbs and essential oils to support oral hygiene and prevent common dental issues.

Clove Oil Toothache Relief

Ingredients:

- 2-3 drops of clove essential oil

- ½ teaspoon of olive oil

- **Instructions**:

1. Mix the clove essential oil with olive oil.

2. Apply a small amount of the mixture to a cotton ball.

3. Gently press the cotton ball against the affected tooth or gum area for several minutes.

4. Avoid rinsing your mouth immediately after to allow the oils to penetrate and provide relief.

Beneficial effects: Clove oil is renowned for its pain-relieving properties due to the presence of eugenol, a natural anesthetic. It helps in numbing dental pain and reducing inflammation.

Saltwater Mouth Rinse for Gum Health

Ingredients:

- 1 teaspoon of sea salt

- 1 cup of warm water

- **Instructions**:

1. Dissolve the sea salt in the warm water.

2. Swish the solution in your mouth for 30 seconds, then spit it out.

3. Repeat 2-3 times a day, especially after meals, to reduce bacteria and soothe inflamed gums.

Beneficial effects: Saltwater rinses help in reducing bacterial growth, healing mouth sores, and soothing inflamed gums due to their natural disinfectant properties.

Turmeric Gum Paste for Inflammation

Ingredients:

- 1 tablespoon of turmeric powder

- Water to form a paste

- **Instructions**:

1. Mix turmeric powder with a small amount of water to create a thick paste.

2. Apply the paste directly to the gums.

3. Leave it on for 5 minutes, then rinse your mouth with water.

4. Use daily until inflammation subsides.

Beneficial effects: Turmeric contains curcumin, which has powerful anti-inflammatory and antimicrobial properties, making it effective in reducing gum inflammation and promoting oral health.

Green Tea Rinse for Oral Hygiene

Ingredients:

- 1 green tea bag

- 1 cup of boiling water

- **Instructions**:

1. Steep the green tea bag in boiling water for 5 minutes.

2. Allow the tea to cool to a comfortable temperature.

3. Use the tea as a mouth rinse, swishing it around your mouth for 30 seconds before spitting it out.

4. Repeat once or twice daily to benefit from green tea's antioxidant properties.

Beneficial effects: Green tea is rich in catechins, antioxidants that can kill bacteria, reduce inflammation, and lower the risk of gum disease.

Aloe Vera Gel for Soothing Mouth Ulcers

Ingredients:

- Pure aloe vera gel

- **Instructions**:

1. Apply a small amount of aloe vera gel directly to the mouth ulcer.

2. Leave it on to absorb and heal.

3. Repeat 2-3 times a day until the ulcer heals.

Beneficial effects: Aloe vera has natural healing and anti-inflammatory properties that can provide relief from mouth ulcers and promote healing.

Variations: For those sensitive to any of the ingredients, alternatives such as diluted hydrogen peroxide for mouth rinses or coconut oil for oil pulling can be used. Adding a drop of peppermint oil to the saltwater mouth rinse can provide additional antimicrobial benefits and freshen breath.

Storage tips: Prepare the saltwater rinse fresh each time. Store clove oil and turmeric powder in a cool, dry place. Keep aloe vera gel refrigerated to maintain its freshness and soothing properties.

Tips for allergens: Always conduct a patch test on the skin before applying new essential oils or herbal pastes to the oral cavity to ensure no allergic reaction occurs. For those with allergies to any of the ingredients, consult with a healthcare provider for alternative remedies.

Scientific references: Studies have validated the efficacy of clove oil in dental pain management, turmeric for its anti-inflammatory properties, and green tea as a beneficial rinse for improving oral health. Research published in the Journal of Indian Society of Periodontology highlights the antimicrobial and anti-inflammatory effects of aloe vera in treating mouth ulcers.

CHAPTER 4: 5 HERBAL RECIPES FOR DENTAL HEALTH

CLOVE OIL MOUTH RINSE

Beneficial effects

Clove Oil Mouth Rinse offers natural antiseptic, antibacterial, and analgesic properties, making it an effective remedy for improving oral health. It can help reduce gum inflammation, alleviate toothache, freshen breath, and combat oral bacteria that can lead to cavities and gum disease. The eugenol found in clove oil is particularly noted for its pain-relieving effects on toothaches and sore gums.

Ingredients

- 1 teaspoon of clove essential oil

- 1 cup of warm water

- 1/2 teaspoon of sea salt (optional)

Instructions

1. Pour 1 cup of warm water into a glass.

2. Add 1 teaspoon of clove essential oil to the water. If using, add the sea salt.

3. Stir the mixture well until the clove oil is well dispersed (the oil may float on top, which is normal).

4. Use the mixture as a mouth rinse, swishing it around your mouth for 1 to 2 minutes.

5. Spit out the rinse. Do not swallow.

6. Rinse your mouth with plain water afterward if desired.

Variations

- For added antimicrobial properties, mix in 1 teaspoon of coconut oil with the clove oil and warm water.

- Incorporate 2 drops of peppermint essential oil for a refreshing taste and extra breath-freshening benefits.

- If the taste of clove is too strong, reduce the clove oil to 1/2 teaspoon and gradually increase as tolerated.

Storage tips

Prepare the Clove Oil Mouth Rinse fresh each time you use it, as the mixture does not store well once the clove oil is diluted in water.

Tips for allergens

Individuals with sensitivities to clove or other essential oils should start with a lower concentration to ensure no adverse reactions. Always conduct a patch test on the skin before using new essential oils orally.

Scientific references

- "Eugenol—From the Remote Maluku Islands to the International Market Place: A Review of a Remarkable and Versatile Molecule" published in Molecules, 2012. This study highlights the antiseptic and analgesic properties of eugenol found in clove oil, supporting its use in dental care.

- "Antibacterial activity of clove against dental caries causing bacteria" in the Journal of Pharmacy Research, 2011. This research supports the effectiveness of clove oil in combating oral bacteria responsible for dental diseases.

SAGE AND SEA SALT GARGLE

Beneficial effects

Sage and Sea Salt Gargle is a natural remedy known for its soothing and healing properties, particularly beneficial for oral health. Sage, with its antibacterial and anti-inflammatory qualities, can help alleviate sore throats, reduce dental plaque, and protect against various oral pathogens. Sea salt enhances these benefits by drawing out infections, reducing inflammation, and promoting natural healing of mouth sores and throat discomfort. Together, they create a powerful gargle that can support dental health, soothe sore throats, and freshen breath.

Ingredients

- 1 cup of warm water

- 1 teaspoon of sea salt

- 1 tablespoon of dried sage leaves

Instructions

1. Boil the water and allow it to cool to a warm temperature.

2. Add the sea salt and dried sage leaves to the warm water.

3. Stir the mixture until the sea salt is completely dissolved.

4. Let the sage leaves steep in the saltwater solution for about 5 minutes.

5. Strain the mixture to remove the sage leaves, leaving behind the sage-infused sea salt gargle.

6. Gargle with the solution for 30 seconds to 1 minute, then spit it out. Do not swallow.

7. Repeat up to three times a day, especially after meals and before bed, for best results.

Variations

- For added antimicrobial properties, include a teaspoon of apple cider vinegar to the gargle.

- Incorporate a drop or two of peppermint essential oil for a refreshing taste and additional antibacterial benefits.

- If experiencing intense throat pain, add a tablespoon of honey to the mixture after it has cooled slightly to coat and soothe the throat further.

Storage tips

Prepare the Sage and Sea Salt Gargle fresh for each use to ensure its potency and effectiveness. It is not recommended to store the mixture for later use due to the potential degradation of active properties.

Tips for allergens

Individuals with allergies to sage should avoid this gargle. For those sensitive to sea salt, reducing the concentration by using half a teaspoon instead of a full teaspoon may be beneficial. Always ensure any added essential oils are safe for ingestion and allergen-free.

Scientific references

- "Antimicrobial activity of sage extract against Candida albicans, Escherichia coli, Salmonella enteritidis, and Staphylococcus aureus," published in the Journal of Agricultural and Food Chemistry, highlights sage's broad-spectrum antimicrobial properties.

- "The effect of saline solutions on the viscoelasticity of healthy mucosa: Implications for sodium chloride in wound healing," in the Journal of Wound Care, discusses the beneficial effects of sea salt on healing and reducing inflammation in mucosal tissues.

MYRRH GUM POWDER TOOTHPASTE

Beneficial effects

Myrrh Gum Powder Toothpaste harnesses the powerful antiseptic and antibacterial properties of myrrh to promote oral health, reduce gum disease, and freshen breath. Myrrh has been used historically for its medicinal properties, particularly in oral care, to cleanse the mouth and protect against bacterial infections. This natural toothpaste recipe offers a chemical-free alternative for those seeking to maintain healthy teeth and gums while utilizing the healing benefits of myrrh.

Ingredients

- 2 tablespoons coconut oil
- 1 tablespoon baking soda
- 2 teaspoons myrrh gum powder
- 10-15 drops peppermint essential oil
- 1 teaspoon xylitol (optional, for sweetness)

Instructions

1. In a small bowl, combine the coconut oil and baking soda, mixing until they form a paste.

2. Add the myrrh gum powder to the mixture and stir well to ensure it's evenly distributed.

3. Incorporate the peppermint essential oil into the paste for a refreshing flavor and additional antibacterial properties.

4. If desired, mix in the xylitol for sweetness, making the toothpaste more palatable.

5. Transfer the toothpaste to a small jar or container with a lid for storage.

Variations

- For those sensitive to peppermint, substitute with spearmint essential oil for a milder mint flavor.
- Add a teaspoon of activated charcoal to the recipe for extra whitening properties.
- For a smoother texture, melt the coconut oil before mixing with other ingredients.

Storage tips

Store the Myrrh Gum Powder Toothpaste in a cool, dry place. If the coconut oil solidifies due to lower temperatures, simply warm the toothpaste slightly before use. The toothpaste can be kept for up to 3 months.

Tips for allergens

Individuals with allergies to coconut oil can substitute it with sesame oil or any other carrier oil that is safe for them. For those allergic to xylitol, it can be omitted without affecting the toothpaste's effectiveness.

Scientific references

- "Antibacterial and antifungal properties of essential oils," in the International Journal of Food Microbiology, highlights the antimicrobial properties of peppermint oil, supporting its use in oral care products.

- "Myrrh: Medical Marvel or Mythical Magic?" in the Journal of Oral Health and Dental Management, discusses the historical and contemporary use of myrrh in dental care, including its antibacterial and antiseptic qualities.

PEPPERMINT AND COCONUT OIL PULLING

Beneficial effects

Peppermint and Coconut Oil Pulling is a traditional remedy known for its ability to improve oral health and hygiene. This practice is believed to draw out toxins from the body, reduce plaque buildup, and combat bad breath. Peppermint oil adds antimicrobial properties that can help fight oral pathogens, while coconut oil's lauric acid is known for its ability to kill harmful bacteria in the mouth. Together, they create a refreshing and effective oral detoxification process that supports gum health, whitens teeth, and enhances overall dental hygiene.

Ingredients

- 1 tablespoon virgin coconut oil

- 2-3 drops peppermint essential oil

Instructions

1. Measure 1 tablespoon of virgin coconut oil into a small cup.

2. Add 2-3 drops of peppermint essential oil to the coconut oil and mix well.

3. Place the mixture in your mouth.

4. Swish the oils around your mouth for 15-20 minutes, ensuring not to swallow any of the mixture.

5. Spit the oil into a trash can to avoid clogging your sink.

6. Rinse your mouth with warm water, and follow with your regular brushing routine.

Variations

- For added antibacterial benefits, include a drop of tea tree oil into the mixture.

- If you prefer a slightly sweeter taste, you can add a drop of stevia to the oil pulling mixture.

- To target inflammation, add a drop of clove oil for its pain-relieving properties.

Storage tips

Store the coconut oil in a cool, dry place to maintain its solid state. Peppermint essential oil should be kept in a dark, cool place in a tightly sealed bottle to preserve its potency.

Tips for allergens

Individuals with allergies to coconut or peppermint should seek alternative ingredients for oil pulling. Sesame oil or olive oil can be used in place of coconut oil, and cinnamon essential oil can be a warming alternative to peppermint for those without allergies to cinnamon.

Scientific references

- "Effect of coconut oil in plaque related gingivitis — A preliminary report" in the Nigerian Medical Journal, 2015. This study highlights the effectiveness of coconut oil pulling in reducing plaque and gingivitis symptoms.

- "Antimicrobial efficacy of five essential oils against oral pathogens: An in vitro study" in the European Journal of Dentistry, 2013. This research supports the antimicrobial properties of peppermint essential oil against oral bacteria.

CALENDULA AND CHAMOMILE GUM SOOTHER

Beneficial effects

The Calendula and Chamomile Gum Soother is a natural remedy designed to alleviate inflammation and discomfort in the gums. Calendula, known for its powerful anti-inflammatory and antimicrobial properties, helps in healing and soothing irritated tissues. Chamomile complements these effects with its calming and anti-inflammatory qualities, providing relief from gum pain and aiding in the reduction of swelling. Together, they form a gentle yet effective treatment for maintaining gum health and comfort.

Ingredients

- 1 tablespoon dried calendula flowers

- 1 tablespoon dried chamomile flowers

- 1 cup boiling water

- 1 teaspoon honey (optional, for taste)

Instructions

1. Place the dried calendula and chamomile flowers in a heat-resistant bowl or jar.

2. Pour 1 cup of boiling water over the flowers, ensuring they are fully submerged.

3. Cover the bowl or jar and allow the mixture to steep for 15 to 20 minutes.

4. Strain the infusion, removing the flowers and collecting the liquid.

5. Optional: Add 1 teaspoon of honey to the strained liquid and stir until dissolved.

6. Allow the solution to cool to a comfortable temperature before use.

7. To apply, use a clean cotton ball or pad, soak it in the solution, and gently dab onto the gums. Repeat 2-3 times daily or as needed for relief.

Variations

- For added antimicrobial properties, include a teaspoon of salt in the infusion.

- Enhance the soothing effect by adding a few drops of peppermint oil to the cooled solution for a refreshing feel.

- If using as a mouth rinse, double the quantity of water and ingredients to extend the use.

Storage tips

Store any unused portion of the Calendula and Chamomile Gum Soother in the refrigerator for up to 48 hours. Ensure it's kept in a sealed container to maintain freshness.

Tips for allergens

Individuals with allergies to plants in the Asteraceae family, such as calendula and chamomile, should proceed with caution. Honey can be omitted for those with allergies or vegan preferences, maintaining the solution's effectiveness.

Scientific references

- "Anti-inflammatory and wound healing activity of a growth substance in Aloe vera," published in the Journal of the American Podiatric Medical Association, supports the healing properties of botanical ingredients similar to calendula.

- "Chamomile: A herbal medicine of the past with a bright future," published in Molecular Medicine Reports, discusses the anti-inflammatory and skin-soothing benefits of chamomile, supporting its use in gum health.

PART 21: HAIR AND NAIL HEALTH

Healthy hair and nails are often seen as external indicators of our overall health, reflecting the body's internal state. Achieving and maintaining vibrant hair and strong nails naturally involves a holistic approach, emphasizing nutrition, herbal remedies, and lifestyle adjustments. This chapter delves into the essential nutrients, beneficial herbs, and practical tips for nurturing hair and nail health from the inside out.

Beneficial effects: The strategies and remedies discussed aim to enhance hair growth, improve hair texture, increase nail strength, and prevent common issues such as brittleness, splitting, and hair loss. By addressing nutritional deficiencies and leveraging the power of natural herbs, you can support the body's ability to maintain healthy hair and nails.

Ingredients:

- Biotin (Vitamin B7): Crucial for hair growth and strength.

- Omega-3 fatty acids: Found in flaxseeds, chia seeds, and fish oil, these fats promote scalp health and shine in hair.

- Zinc: Supports hair growth and repair and keeps the nail bed healthy.

- Silica: Found in bamboo extract, strengthens hair and nails.

- Iron: Prevents hair loss and is found in spinach, lentils, and red meat.

- Vitamin C: Enhances iron absorption and collagen production, found in citrus fruits and bell peppers.

- Horsetail: Contains silica, promoting strong hair and nails.

- Nettle: Rich in vitamins and minerals, supports hair growth and scalp health.

- Rosemary: Improves circulation to the scalp, enhancing hair growth.

Instructions:

1. **Daily Nutritional Smoothie**:

- Blend 1 tablespoon of ground flaxseeds or chia seeds (for omega-3s), a handful of spinach (for iron), 1 orange (for Vitamin C), and 1 cup of water or almond milk.

- Drink daily to support hair and nail health from within.

2. **Horsetail and Nettle Hair Rinse**:

- Boil 1 liter of water and add 1 tablespoon each of dried horsetail and nettle.

- Simmer for 10 minutes, then cool and strain.

- Use as a final rinse after shampooing to strengthen hair.

3. **Rosemary Scalp Massage Oil**:

- Mix 5 drops of rosemary essential oil with 2 tablespoons of a carrier oil (like coconut or jojoba).

- Massage into the scalp 2-3 times a week to improve circulation and promote hair growth.

4. **Biotin-Rich Snack**:

- Combine a handful of almonds, sunflower seeds, and pumpkin seeds as a snack.

- These seeds and nuts are rich in biotin, zinc, and omega-3 fatty acids, supporting healthy hair and nails.

Variations:

- For those allergic to nuts, substitute with seeds like hemp or flaxseeds.

- Vegetarians or vegans can ensure adequate iron intake by combining Vitamin C-rich foods with plant-based iron sources like lentils and quinoa.

Storage tips:

- Store herbal teas and dried herbs in airtight containers away from direct sunlight to preserve their potency.

- Nuts and seeds should be stored in the refrigerator to maintain freshness.

Tips for allergens:

- Always check for potential allergies, especially when using essential oils or new herbs.

- Substitute any allergenic foods with suitable alternatives that provide similar nutritional benefits.

Scientific references:

- Studies have shown that omega-3 fatty acids can improve hair density and diameter, making them essential for hair health (Journal of Cosmetic Dermatology, 2015).

- Research indicates that biotin supplementation can improve nail strength and thickness (Journal of Drugs in Dermatology, 2007).

- A study found that topical application of rosemary oil was as effective as minoxidil for hair growth with less scalp itching as a side effect (Skinmed, 2015).

By incorporating these nutrients and herbs into your daily routine, you can support the health of your hair and nails naturally. Remember, consistency is key, and improvements will be seen over time with regular care and nourishment.

CHAPTER 1: DR. BARBARA'S HAIR & NAIL HEALTH GUIDE

Healthy hair and nails are not just about external beauty—they reflect the body's internal health and nutritional status. Recognizing this, Dr. Barbara emphasizes a holistic approach to hair and nail health, focusing on the intake of essential nutrients, the use of natural herbs, and the adoption of lifestyle practices that support the body's overall well-being. The foundation of this approach lies in understanding that the body requires a diverse range of vitamins, minerals, and other nutrients to produce healthy hair and nails, which can be compromised by poor diet, stress, and environmental toxins.

Beneficial effects: This approach is designed to nourish the hair and nails from within, promoting their strength, growth, and resilience. By addressing potential nutritional gaps and leveraging the healing power of herbs, individuals can expect to see improvements in the appearance and health of their hair and nails, along with a reduction in common problems such as brittleness, splitting, and excessive hair shedding.

Ingredients:

- Biotin (Vitamin B7): Essential for hair growth and strengthening nails.

- Omega-3 fatty acids: Improve scalp health and add luster to hair.

- Zinc: Vital for hair repair and growth; supports nail strength.

- Silica: Enhances the structural integrity of hair and nails.

- Iron: Critical for preventing hair loss.

- Vitamin C: Aids in collagen production and iron absorption.

- Horsetail extract: A natural source of silica, promoting strength.

- Nettle leaf: Nutrient-rich, supports hair growth and scalp health.

- Rosemary oil: Stimulates blood circulation to the scalp.

Instructions:

1. **Nutrient-Rich Diet**:

- Incorporate a variety of whole foods rich in the above nutrients into your daily diet. Focus on colorful fruits and vegetables, lean proteins, nuts, seeds, and healthy fats.

2. **Scalp Massage with Rosemary Oil**:

- Warm a small amount of carrier oil like coconut or jojoba and add a few drops of rosemary essential oil. Gently massage into the scalp to stimulate blood flow.

3. **Horsetail and Nettle Tea**:

- Steep 1 teaspoon each of dried horsetail and nettle in a cup of hot water for 10 minutes. Strain and drink 1-2 times daily to support hair and nail health from within.

4. **Topical Biotin Serum**:

- Mix biotin powder with aloe vera gel to create a serum. Apply to the scalp and nails before bedtime to support growth and strength.

Variations:

- Vegan sources of omega-3 include algae supplements and flaxseeds.

- For those who prefer not to use rosemary oil, peppermint oil is an alternative that also stimulates scalp circulation.

Storage tips:

- Keep herbal teas in a cool, dry place in an airtight container.

- Store homemade serums and oils in amber glass bottles to protect from light.

Tips for allergens:

- Patch test essential oils diluted in a carrier oil on the skin to check for reactions.

- Consult with a healthcare provider before supplementing with iron or other minerals.

Scientific references:

- A study in the "Journal of Cosmetic Dermatology" found that dietary omega-3 fatty acids can significantly improve hair growth.

- Research in the "Journal of Drugs in Dermatology" highlights the role of biotin in improving nail strength and thickness.

- "Skinmed" journal published findings on the effectiveness of rosemary oil in promoting hair growth, comparable to minoxidil, with fewer side effects.

Adopting Dr. Barbara's holistic approach to hair and nail health involves more than just topical treatments; it's about nurturing the body from within through a balanced diet, adequate hydration, stress management, and the strategic use of natural herbs. This comprehensive care routine not only promotes healthier hair and nails but also contributes to overall physical health and well-being.

COMMON HAIR AND NAIL ISSUES

Common hair and nail issues range from mild to severe and can significantly impact an individual's self-esteem and quality of life. Hair loss, thinning, brittleness, split ends, and dandruff are prevalent hair concerns. Similarly, nails can suffer from brittleness, splitting, peeling, and fungal infections. These problems often signal nutritional deficiencies, hormonal imbalances, or the need for improved hair and nail care routines.

Hair loss and thinning can result from inadequate protein intake, iron deficiency, or hormonal shifts, such as those experienced during pregnancy or menopause. Incorporating a balanced diet rich in protein, iron, vitamins A and C, and omega-3 fatty acids supports hair strength and growth. Biotin, also known as vitamin B7, plays a crucial role in the health of hair and nails, promoting their growth and preventing brittleness.

Brittle nails and hair may indicate a lack of moisture or essential fatty acids in the diet, pointing to the need for increased consumption of nuts, seeds, and oily fish like salmon. Additionally, hydration plays a vital role in maintaining the elasticity and strength of hair and nails, emphasizing the importance of drinking sufficient water daily.

Split ends in hair are often a result of mechanical damage from heat styling, harsh brushing, or chemical treatments. Minimizing heat exposure and using protective serums or oils can help prevent further damage. Regular trims are also essential to remove split ends and encourage healthy hair growth.

Dandruff, characterized by a flaky scalp, can be managed by using gentle, natural shampoos containing tea tree oil or neem, known for their antifungal and soothing properties. Maintaining a clean scalp and avoiding products that cause irritation or build-up is crucial for preventing dandruff.

Fungal nail infections require attention to hygiene, avoiding damp environments like public showers without protection, and using antifungal treatments. Supplements containing horsetail extract or silica can support nail strength and recovery from fungal damage.

For individuals experiencing these common hair and nail issues, a holistic approach that includes dietary adjustments, proper hydration, and the use of natural remedies can offer significant improvements. Ensuring a diet rich in vitamins, minerals, and antioxidants supports the body's ability to repair and maintain healthy hair and nails. Additionally, adopting gentle care practices, reducing exposure to harsh chemicals, and protecting hair and nails from environmental damage are key strategies for addressing these concerns effectively.

CHAPTER 2: NUTRITION FOR HAIR AND NAIL HEALTH

Ensuring the intake of essential nutrients is fundamental for maintaining the health of your hair and nails. These parts of our body often reflect our overall nutritional status, with deficiencies manifesting as brittle nails, hair loss, or lackluster hair. A balanced diet rich in vitamins, minerals, and other nutrients plays a critical role in supporting the structural integrity and growth of hair and nails.

Beneficial effects: A nutrient-rich diet can significantly improve the strength, growth, and appearance of hair and nails. By focusing on specific vitamins and minerals known to support hair and nail health, individuals can address common issues such as brittleness, splitting, and thinning hair.

Ingredients:

- Protein: Essential for hair and nail growth. Sources include chicken, turkey, fish, beans, and legumes.

- Omega-3 fatty acids: Promote healthy scalp and hair. Found in fatty fish, walnuts, flaxseeds, and chia seeds.

- Iron: Supports hair growth and strength. Rich sources include red meat, lentils, spinach, and iron-fortified cereals.

- Vitamin C: Aids in collagen production and iron absorption. Found in citrus fruits, strawberries, bell peppers, and broccoli.

- Biotin (Vitamin B7): Known for its role in hair and nail health. Sources include eggs, almonds, cauliflower, and cheese.

- Vitamin E: Protects hair and nails from oxidative stress. Sources include sunflower seeds, almonds, spinach, and avocados.

- Zinc: Essential for hair tissue growth and repair. Found in beef, pumpkin seeds, lentils, and chickpeas.

Instructions:

1. **Balanced Meal Plan**:

- Incorporate a variety of these foods into daily meals to ensure a balanced intake of the nutrients essential for hair and nail health. Aim for a mix of lean proteins, healthy fats, and colorful fruits and vegetables at each meal.

2. **Hydration**:

- Drink at least 8 glasses of water a day to help maintain the health of your hair and nails. Proper hydration helps to keep the hair shaft moisturized and supports the delivery of essential nutrients to the nail beds.

3. **Supplementation**:

- Consider supplementing your diet with a multivitamin or specific vitamins and minerals, after consulting with a healthcare provider, especially if you have dietary restrictions or suspect nutrient deficiencies.

Variations:

- Vegetarians and vegans can obtain omega-3 fatty acids from algae supplements and iron from plant-based sources like lentils and fortified cereals, paired with Vitamin C-rich foods to enhance absorption.

- For those with dietary restrictions or allergies, seek alternative sources of the same nutrients. For example, if allergic to nuts (a source of Vitamin E and biotin), opt for spinach and avocados for Vitamin E and eggs for biotin.

Storage tips:

- Keep nuts and seeds in airtight containers in the refrigerator to preserve their fatty acids.

- Store fresh fruits and vegetables in the crisper drawer of the refrigerator to maintain their vitamin content.

Tips for allergens:

- For those allergic to seafood (a primary source of omega-3s), flaxseeds and chia seeds are excellent plant-based alternatives.

- If dairy intolerant, biotin can also be found in high amounts in eggs, avocados, and nuts.

Scientific references:

- The role of omega-3 fatty acids in hair growth has been supported by a study in the "Journal of Cosmetic Dermatology," which found that supplements could improve hair density and diameter.

- Research in the "Journal of Nutritional Biochemistry" highlights the importance of iron and zinc in hair growth, indicating that deficiencies in these minerals can lead to hair loss.

- A study published in the "Archives of Dermatological Research" found that biotin supplementation could improve nail strength and thickness, supporting its role in nail health.

By focusing on a diet rich in these key nutrients, you can support the health and vitality of your hair and nails from the inside out. Remember, while nutrition plays a crucial role, overall health, and proper hair and nail care practices also contribute significantly to their condition.

PROTEIN AND BIOTIN FOR HAIR STRENGTH

Protein and biotin play pivotal roles in maintaining and enhancing hair strength, as both are fundamental building blocks for healthy hair growth. Hair is primarily made up of keratin, a type of protein, making adequate protein intake essential for its strength and resilience. Biotin, a B-vitamin, is equally crucial as it supports the body's keratin infrastructure, further aiding in the prevention of hair loss and promoting hair growth.

Beneficial effects: Incorporating protein and biotin into your diet can lead to stronger, healthier hair, reduce brittleness, and minimize hair loss. These nutrients help in repairing and strengthening hair follicles from within, ensuring the growth of stronger, thicker hair.

Ingredients:

- Lean meats (chicken, turkey, beef)
- Fish (salmon, mackerel, sardines)
- Eggs
- Legumes (beans, lentils)
- Nuts and seeds (almonds, walnuts, flaxseeds)
- Dairy products (milk, cheese, yogurt)
- Whole grains
- Avocado

Instructions:

1. **Protein-rich meal**: Combine grilled chicken or turkey, quinoa, and steamed broccoli for a balanced meal packed with protein.

2. **Biotin boost smoothie**: Blend 1 ripe banana, a handful of spinach, ¼ cup of Greek yogurt, 1 tablespoon of ground flaxseed, and 1 cup of almond milk.

3. **Snack on nuts and seeds**: Almonds, walnuts, and sunflower seeds are not only great sources of biotin but also omega-3 fatty acids, which support scalp health and hair shine.

4. **Incorporate eggs into your breakfast**: Eggs are rich in both protein and biotin, making them an ideal food for hair health. Enjoy them boiled, scrambled, or as part of an omelet.

Variations:

- Vegetarians can opt for legumes, nuts, and dairy products to meet their protein and biotin requirements.

- For a vegan option, rely on quinoa, lentils, and avocados, supplemented with biotin-rich nuts and seeds.

Storage tips:

- Keep nuts and seeds in a cool, dry place or refrigerate to maintain freshness.

- Store eggs and dairy products in the refrigerator.

Tips for allergens:

- For those allergic to nuts, focus on seeds, legumes, and whole grains as alternative sources of biotin and protein.

- Lactose-intolerant individuals can choose lactose-free dairy products or plant-based milk alternatives enriched with calcium and vitamin D.

Scientific references:

- Studies have shown that diets rich in protein and biotin can significantly improve hair strength and texture, reducing hair loss (Journal of Clinical and Aesthetic Dermatology, 2017).

SILICA AND ZINC FOR NAIL HEALTH

Silica and zinc are essential minerals that play a crucial role in maintaining nail health, promoting growth, and preventing brittleness. Silica, a trace mineral, strengthens nails by enhancing the connective tissue's health, including collagen, which is vital for nail strength and resilience. Zinc, on the other hand, is critical for protein synthesis and cell growth, processes fundamental for nail development. A deficiency in zinc can lead to weak nail structure, slow growth, and increased susceptibility to nail damage.

Beneficial effects: Incorporating silica and zinc into your diet can significantly improve nail strength, accelerate growth, and reduce breakage and splitting. These minerals support the underlying nail bed and matrix, ensuring the production of strong, healthy nails.

Ingredients:

- Silica sources: Bamboo extract, whole grains, green beans, bananas, and mineral water.

- Zinc sources: Pumpkin seeds, beef, spinach, oysters, lentils, and chickpeas.

Instructions:

1. **Daily Mineral Boost**:

- Start your day with a smoothie that includes bananas and a handful of spinach to kickstart your intake of silica and zinc.

2. **Snack on Seeds**:

- For a midday snack, opt for a mix of pumpkin seeds and chickpeas. Roast them for a crunchy treat that boosts your zinc levels.

3. **Silica-Rich Dinner**:

- Incorporate whole grains and green beans into your evening meal. A quinoa salad with green beans can be an excellent source of silica.

4. **Zinc-Enriched Meals**:

- Include beef or lentils in your diet several times a week to ensure adequate zinc intake, vital for nail health.

Variations:

- Vegetarians can focus on lentils and chickpeas for zinc and bananas and green beans for silica.

- For those who prefer not to consume beef, oysters are an excellent alternative zinc source.

Storage tips:

- Store grains and seeds in airtight containers in a cool, dry place to preserve their mineral content.

- Keep green beans and bananas in the refrigerator or a cool pantry to maintain freshness.

Tips for allergens:

- Individuals allergic to nuts or legumes can opt for mineral water and whole grains as alternative silica sources and oysters for zinc without compromising their nail health.

Scientific references:

- Research has shown that silica supplements can improve nail quality and strength (Journal of the American College of Nutrition, 2007).

- Studies indicate that zinc plays a vital role in nail health by supporting protein synthesis and cell growth (Dermatologic Therapy, 2010).

HYDRATION AND ITS IMPACT ON HAIR AND NAILS

Hydration plays a pivotal role in maintaining the health and vitality of hair and nails, acting as a crucial component for their growth and strength. Water, the essence of life, is not only vital for survival but also for sustaining the beauty and health of our hair and nails. Adequate hydration ensures that the hair remains moisturized from the inside out, preventing dryness, brittleness, and breakage. Similarly, for nails, proper hydration prevents them from becoming brittle and susceptible to cracking and splitting.

Beneficial effects: Proper hydration supports the delivery of essential nutrients to hair follicles and nail beds, promoting healthy growth and preventing common issues like dry scalp, dandruff, and brittle nails. It helps in maintaining the elasticity of hair, making it less prone to breakage, and ensures that nails are strong and resilient.

Ingredients:

- Water: The primary and most crucial ingredient for hydration.

- Cucumber: High in water content and provides silica for hair and nail strength.

- Watermelon: Rich in water and vitamins A, B6, and C, which support hair health.

- Coconut water: A natural hydration boost with electrolytes to support nutrient absorption.

- Green tea: Contains antioxidants that promote healthy hair growth and shine.

Instructions:

1. **Increase Daily Water Intake**:

- Aim to drink at least 8-10 glasses of water a day to maintain optimal hydration levels for supporting hair and nail health.

2. **Cucumber Water Infusion**:

- Slice one cucumber and add it to a pitcher of water. Let it infuse overnight and drink throughout the next day for added hydration and silica intake.

3. **Watermelon Smoothie**:

- Blend 2 cups of cubed watermelon with a half cup of coconut water and ice. Enjoy this hydrating smoothie, especially during warmer months.

4. **Daily Green Tea**:

- Replace one of your daily beverages with green tea to benefit from its antioxidant properties, supporting overall hair and nail health.

5. **Hydration Reminder**:

- Set reminders on your phone or use a hydration tracking app to ensure you're meeting your daily water intake goals.

Variations:

- Infuse water with other fruits like berries, lemon, or lime for variety and added vitamins.

- For those who find it challenging to consume enough water, herbal teas and natural fruit juices (without added sugar) can also contribute to daily fluid intake.

Storage tips:

- Keep infused waters in the refrigerator to maintain freshness and encourage consumption of cool, refreshing beverages.

- Store cut fruits like watermelon in the refrigerator to preserve their hydration benefits.

Tips for allergens:

- For individuals sensitive to caffeine in green tea, herbal teas such as chamomile or peppermint are excellent alternatives that also support hydration.

Scientific references:

- Studies have highlighted the importance of adequate water intake for maintaining skin hydration, which extends to scalp health, directly impacting hair quality (Journal of Clinical, Cosmetic and Investigational Dermatology, 2015).

- Research indicates that silica, found in high-water-content vegetables like cucumber, plays a vital role in hair and nail strength (Archives of Dermatological Research, 2007).

Maintaining adequate hydration is a simple yet effective strategy for enhancing the health and appearance of hair and nails. It's a foundational aspect of a holistic approach to beauty, emphasizing that true health starts from within.

FOODS TO AVOID FOR HAIR AND NAIL WELLNESS

Maintaining the health of your hair and nails is not just about what you should include in your diet but also about what foods to limit or avoid. Certain foods can negatively impact the strength, growth, and appearance of your hair and nails, contributing to issues such as brittleness, thinning, and slow growth. To support the wellness of your hair and nails, consider reducing or eliminating the following from your diet:

1. **High-Sugar Foods**: Excessive sugar intake can lead to inflammation and disrupt hormonal balance, affecting the health of your hair and nails. Foods high in sugar can also lead to glycation, where sugars attach

to proteins in the bloodstream, forming harmful molecules that can damage collagen and keratin, essential for hair and nail strength.

2. **Alcohol**: Alcohol consumption can lead to dehydration, impacting the hydration levels necessary for maintaining healthy hair and nails. It can also affect the levels of zinc in your body, a mineral crucial for hair growth and nail strength.

3. **High-Sodium Foods**: Foods that are high in salt can contribute to dehydration, similarly affecting the hydration needed for healthy hair and nails. Excessive salt intake can also lead to swelling, which may impact the circulation of nutrients to hair follicles and nail beds.

4. **Refined Carbohydrates**: Foods made with white flour and processed grains can spike blood sugar levels, leading to inflammation and potentially impacting hair growth. These foods often lack the fiber and nutrients found in whole grains, which support overall health, including that of your hair and nails.

5. **Fried and Processed Foods**: These foods are often high in unhealthy fats and chemicals that can lead to oxidative stress and inflammation, negatively affecting hair and nail health. Trans fats, in particular, can interfere with the body's ability to absorb nutrients like omega-3 fatty acids, which are essential for hair and nail wellness.

6. **Dairy Products**: For some individuals, dairy can trigger hormonal imbalances due to the presence of hormones and growth factors in milk. These imbalances can exacerbate conditions like acne and may also impact hair growth and nail health.

7. **Caffeine**: In excessive amounts, caffeine can contribute to dehydration, affecting the moisture levels in your hair and nails. It can also interfere with the absorption of essential nutrients such as iron and magnesium, important for hair and nail health.

By being mindful of these dietary choices and limiting the intake of foods that can harm your hair and nails, you can support their health and appearance from within. Remember, a balanced diet rich in vitamins, minerals, and hydration plays a crucial role in maintaining the wellness of your hair and nails.

CHAPTER 3: HAIR AND NAIL NATURAL CARE

Beneficial effects: The natural remedies provided here aim to nourish and strengthen hair and nails, reduce breakage, enhance growth, and improve overall health. By utilizing herbs, essential oils, and dietary changes, these treatments support the body's natural ability to regenerate and maintain healthy hair and nails.

Ingredients for Hair Health:

- Rosemary essential oil: Stimulates hair follicles for growth.

- Lavender essential oil: Soothes the scalp and reduces stress.

- Castor oil: Rich in ricinoleic acid, enhances hair thickness.

- Coconut oil: Moisturizes and protects hair from protein loss.

- Apple cider vinegar: Balances scalp pH and adds shine.

Instructions for Hair Health:

1. **Rosemary Scalp Treatment**:

- Mix 5 drops of rosemary essential oil with 2 tablespoons of coconut oil.

- Massage into the scalp and leave for at least 30 minutes before washing out.

2. **Lavender Hair Mask**:

- Combine 3 drops of lavender essential oil with 1 tablespoon of castor oil and 1 tablespoon of coconut oil.

- Apply to hair, focusing on ends, and leave on overnight with a shower cap. Wash out in the morning.

3. **Apple Cider Vinegar Rinse**:

- Mix 1 part apple cider vinegar with 4 parts water.

- Use as a final rinse after shampooing to remove buildup and close cuticles.

Ingredients for Nail Health:

- Horsetail: Silica-rich, strengthens nails.

- Biotin: Supports nail growth and strength.

- Flaxseed oil: Omega-3 fatty acids nourish nail beds.

- Lemon juice: Natural whitener for nail tips.

- Olive oil: Moisturizes and repairs nail and cuticle damage.

Instructions for Nail Health:

1. **Horsetail Soak**:

- Steep 2 teaspoons of dried horsetail in 1 cup of boiling water for 10 minutes. Cool and soak nails for 15 minutes.

2. **Biotin Supplement**:

- Consider taking a biotin supplement as directed by a healthcare provider to support nail strength.

3. **Flaxseed Oil Rub**:

- Massage flaxseed oil into nails and cuticles nightly to moisturize and strengthen.

4. **Lemon and Olive Oil Nail Treatment**:

- Mix 1 tablespoon of olive oil with a few drops of lemon juice. Soak nails for 10 minutes to whiten and strengthen.

Variations:

- For those allergic to nuts, replace coconut oil with jojoba or olive oil in hair treatments.

- If sensitive to lemon, omit from the nail treatment and use plain olive oil.

Storage tips:

- Store essential oils and carrier oils in a cool, dark place to maintain their potency.

- Keep dried horsetail in an airtight container away from direct sunlight.

Tips for allergens:

- Always perform a patch test on the skin before using essential oils to ensure no allergic reaction.

- Consult with a healthcare provider before starting any supplement, including biotin.

Scientific references:

- A study in the *Journal of Cosmetic Dermatology* found that rosemary oil was as effective as minoxidil for hair growth with less scalp itching.

- Research in the *Journal of Dermatological Treatment* highlighted the benefits of lavender oil for hair growth in mice, suggesting potential benefits for humans.

- A study published in the *International Journal of Trichology* showed that apple cider vinegar could improve the scalp health, leading to shinier and smoother hair.

- The *Journal of Dietary Supplements* reported on the effectiveness of biotin in improving nail strength and thickness in individuals with brittle nails.

By incorporating these natural remedies into your care routine, you can support the health and vitality of your hair and nails, leveraging the power of nature to enhance your beauty from the inside out. Remember, consistency and patience are key to seeing the benefits of these treatments.

CHAPTER 4: HERBAL HAIR AND NAIL CARE RECIPES

HORSETAIL AND NETTLE HAIR RINSE

Beneficial effects

The Horsetail and Nettle Hair Rinse leverages the natural strength of horsetail and nettle to enhance hair and scalp health. Horsetail, rich in silica, can help improve hair texture, promote growth, and strengthen hair strands, reducing breakage and split ends. Nettle is known for its ability to stimulate the scalp, improve circulation, and support hair growth. Together, they create a potent rinse that nourishes the scalp, reduces dandruff, and leaves hair looking vibrant and healthy.

Ingredients

- 1/4 cup dried horsetail
- 1/4 cup dried nettle leaves
- 4 cups water

Instructions

1. Bring 4 cups of water to a boil in a large pot.

2. Add the dried horsetail and nettle leaves to the boiling water.

3. Reduce the heat and allow the mixture to simmer for 20 to 30 minutes.

4. Remove the pot from the heat and let the infusion cool to room temperature.

5. Strain the mixture, discarding the leaves, and collect the liquid in a clean container.

6. After shampooing, pour the horsetail and nettle hair rinse through your hair as a final rinse. Do not rinse out with water.

7. Gently towel dry your hair and style as usual.

Variations

- For added shine and scalp health, include a tablespoon of apple cider vinegar to the rinse.

- To enhance the moisturizing properties, add a few drops of lavender or rosemary essential oil to the cooled mixture.

- For those with dry hair, mixing in a teaspoon of honey to the cooled rinse can provide extra hydration.

Storage tips

Store any unused portion of the Horsetail and Nettle Hair Rinse in the refrigerator for up to 1 week. Ensure the container is sealed properly to maintain freshness.

Tips for allergens

Individuals with sensitivities to horsetail or nettle should perform a patch test on the skin before applying the rinse to the scalp. For those allergic to any added essential oils, omit these from the recipe or substitute with another oil that is safe for you.

Scientific references

- "Efficacy of a cosmetic phyto-caffeine shampoo in female androgenetic alopecia," published in Skin Pharmacology and Physiology, highlights the benefits of natural ingredients like nettle in promoting hair growth.

- "Silicon and Plant-Based Diets" in the Journal of Nutrition, Health & Aging discusses the role of silica, found abundantly in horsetail, in hair and nail health.

ROSEMARY AND LAVENDER HAIR OIL

Beneficial effects

Rosemary and Lavender Hair Oil is a natural remedy designed to promote hair health, stimulate growth, and soothe the scalp. Rosemary oil is renowned for its ability to enhance circulation to the scalp, which can promote hair growth and prevent hair loss. Lavender oil adds to the benefits by providing anti-inflammatory and antimicrobial properties, helping to combat dandruff and scalp irritations. Together, they create a potent hair oil that not only nurtures the scalp and hair follicles but also leaves the hair smelling pleasantly aromatic.

Ingredients

- 2 tablespoons of rosemary essential oil
- 2 tablespoons of lavender essential oil
- 1/2 cup of carrier oil (such as coconut oil, jojoba oil, or almond oil)

Instructions

1. In a clean glass bottle or jar, combine the rosemary and lavender essential oils with the carrier oil of your choice.

2. Close the bottle or jar tightly and shake well to ensure the essential oils are thoroughly mixed with the carrier oil.

3. To use, apply a small amount of the oil mixture to your scalp and hair. Massage gently, focusing on the roots and scalp for several minutes to enhance blood circulation.

4. Leave the oil in your hair for at least 30 minutes or overnight for deeper conditioning. Cover your hair with a shower cap to avoid staining your pillow.

5. Wash your hair thoroughly with shampoo and condition as usual.

6. For best results, use the hair oil treatment 1-2 times a week.

Variations

- For an extra moisturizing effect, add a tablespoon of vitamin E oil to the mixture. Vitamin E can help repair damaged hair follicles and encourage healthy hair growth.

- If you have dry hair, consider using coconut oil as your carrier oil for its deep moisturizing properties.

- For oily hair, jojoba oil is an excellent carrier oil choice as it closely mimics the scalp's natural oils.

Storage tips

Store the Rosemary and Lavender Hair Oil in a cool, dark place to preserve the potency of the essential oils. If stored properly, the hair oil can last for up to 6 months.

Tips for allergens

Individuals with sensitivities to rosemary or lavender should perform a patch test on a small area of the skin before applying the oil to the scalp. For those allergic to nuts, avoid using almond oil as a carrier and opt for coconut or jojoba oil instead.

Scientific references

- "Randomized Trial of Aromatherapy: Successful Treatment for Alopecia Areata" in the Archives of Dermatology, 1998. This study supports the effectiveness of essential oils, including rosemary, in promoting hair growth.

- "Antimicrobial activity of lavender oil against Clostridium difficile" in the Journal of Medical Microbiology, 2013. This research highlights the antimicrobial properties of lavender oil, beneficial for maintaining a healthy scalp.

ALOE VERA AND PEPPERMINT SCALP TREATMENT

Beneficial effects

Aloe Vera and Peppermint Scalp Treatment is designed to soothe the scalp, reduce dandruff, and stimulate hair growth. Aloe vera, with its moisturizing and healing properties, helps to alleviate dryness and irritation, promoting a healthy scalp environment. Peppermint oil stimulates circulation to the scalp, which can encourage hair growth and provide a refreshing, cooling sensation. This treatment can also help to balance oil production, leaving hair feeling refreshed and revitalized.

Ingredients

- 1/2 cup pure aloe vera gel

- 10 drops peppermint essential oil

- 2 tablespoons coconut oil (melted)

- 1 teaspoon vitamin E oil (optional, for added nourishment)

Instructions

1. In a clean bowl, mix the pure aloe vera gel with the melted coconut oil until well combined.

2. Add the peppermint essential oil to the mixture. If using, incorporate the vitamin E oil at this stage.

3. Stir all the ingredients thoroughly to ensure they are evenly distributed.

4. Apply the mixture directly to the scalp, using gentle circular motions to massage it in.

5. Leave the treatment on the scalp for at least 30 minutes, or for an enhanced effect, leave it overnight.

6. Rinse the treatment out with a mild shampoo and follow with your regular hair care routine.

Variations

- For an extra soothing effect, add 5 drops of lavender essential oil to the mixture, which can help to further soothe the scalp and reduce inflammation.

- Incorporate 1 tablespoon of honey for its humectant properties, which can add moisture to the scalp and hair.

- For a thinner consistency, add a small amount of distilled water to the mixture.

Storage tips

Store any unused portion of the Aloe Vera and Peppermint Scalp Treatment in an airtight container in the refrigerator for up to one week. Ensure the mixture is brought to room temperature before application.

Tips for allergens

Individuals with sensitivities to peppermint or coconut oil should perform a patch test before applying the treatment to the scalp. For those allergic to aloe vera, a gentle scalp serum based on jojoba oil can be used as an alternative base for the treatment.

Scientific references

- "Aloe vera: a short review of its clinical and nutritional uses" published in the Journal of Dietary Supplements, highlights the moisturizing and healing effects of aloe vera on skin and scalp conditions.

- "Peppermint Oil Promotes Hair Growth without Toxic Signs" in Toxicological Research, discusses the stimulating effects of peppermint oil on hair growth and its potential as a treatment for hair loss.

BURDOCK ROOT AND HORSETAIL NAIL STRENGTHENER

Beneficial effects

Burdock Root and Horsetail Nail Strengthener leverages the rich silica content of horsetail and the purifying properties of burdock root to fortify nails and enhance their growth. Silica, a vital nutrient for nail health, contributes to the strength and resilience of nails, preventing breakage and brittleness. Burdock root supports overall nail health by promoting better nutrient absorption and circulation. This natural remedy is ideal for those seeking to improve the appearance and condition of their nails, ensuring they are strong, healthy, and less prone to damage.

Ingredients

- 1 tablespoon dried burdock root

- 1 tablespoon dried horsetail

- 2 cups water

- 1 teaspoon olive oil or coconut oil (optional, for moisturizing)

Instructions

1. Combine the dried burdock root and horsetail with 2 cups of water in a small saucepan.

2. Bring the mixture to a boil, then reduce the heat and simmer for about 20 minutes. This process extracts the beneficial compounds from the herbs.

3. Strain the mixture, discarding the solids, and allow the liquid to cool to room temperature.

4. If using, add 1 teaspoon of olive oil or coconut oil to the cooled herbal infusion for added moisturizing benefits.

5. Transfer the nail strengthener to a clean bottle or container for easy application.

6. To use, soak cotton balls in the solution and apply to the nails. Leave on for at least 15 minutes, then rinse with warm water. For best results, apply daily.

Variations

- For an enhanced soothing effect, add a few drops of lavender essential oil to the mixture after it has cooled.

- Incorporate a teaspoon of lemon juice to the final solution for its nail-whitening properties.

- For a more concentrated treatment, reduce the water to 1 cup for a stronger infusion.

Storage tips

Store the Burdock Root and Horsetail Nail Strengthener in the refrigerator in a sealed container for up to one week. Shake well before each use to ensure the ingredients are well combined.

Tips for allergens

Individuals with sensitivities to burdock root or horsetail should perform a patch test on a small area of the skin before applying the solution to their nails. Olive oil or coconut oil can be omitted or replaced with another carrier oil that is better tolerated.

Scientific references

- "Silica in dermatology and cosmetology: a review," published in Dermatologic Therapy, highlights the importance of silica, found in horsetail, for nail and skin health.

- "Burdock (Arctium lappa L.): A review on phytochemistry and pharmacological effects," in BioMed Research International, discusses the detoxifying and health-promoting properties of burdock root, supporting its use in enhancing nail health.

NETTLE AND HORSETAIL HAIR MASK

Beneficial effects

The Nettle and Horsetail Hair Mask leverages the potent natural properties of nettle and horsetail to promote hair and scalp health. Nettle is rich in vitamins A, C, and K, along with minerals like iron and magnesium that nourish the hair follicles, encourage growth, and can reduce dandruff. Horsetail, being a silica-rich herb, strengthens hair strands, enhances shine, and improves elasticity, reducing breakage. This mask is an excellent remedy for those looking to support healthy hair growth, restore vitality to dull hair, and improve overall hair texture.

Ingredients

- 1/4 cup dried nettle leaves
- 1/4 cup dried horsetail leaves
- 1 cup boiling water
- 2 tablespoons coconut oil
- 1 tablespoon aloe vera gel

Instructions

1. Place the dried nettle and horsetail leaves in a heat-resistant bowl.

2. Pour 1 cup of boiling water over the herbs and let them steep for 20-30 minutes to create a strong herbal infusion.

3. Strain the infusion, pressing the herbs to extract as much liquid as possible.

4. While the herbal infusion is still warm, mix in the coconut oil and aloe vera gel until you achieve a consistent paste.

5. Apply the mask evenly to damp hair and scalp, massaging gently.

6. Cover your hair with a shower cap and let the mask sit for at least 30 minutes.

7. Rinse the mask out thoroughly with warm water, followed by your regular shampoo and conditioner routine.

Variations

- For added moisture, include 1 tablespoon of honey to the mask mixture.

- To address scalp issues like itchiness or dandruff, add a few drops of tea tree oil for its antimicrobial properties.

- For an extra protein boost, mix in 1 egg yolk with the herbal infusion before adding the coconut oil and aloe vera gel.

Storage tips

It's best to use the Nettle and Horsetail Hair Mask fresh. However, any unused herbal infusion can be stored in the refrigerator for up to 2 days. Ensure it's brought to room temperature before use.

Tips for allergens

Individuals with sensitivity to aloe vera or coconut oil can substitute the aloe vera gel with olive oil and omit the coconut oil. Always conduct a patch test on the skin before applying the mask to the scalp and hair to ensure there are no adverse reactions.

Scientific references

- "Urtica dioica L., Urticaceae: A stinging nettle" in the International Journal of Pharmaceutical and Biomedical Research, highlighting the nutritional and medicinal properties of nettle that benefit hair health.

- "Silica in cosmetics and personal care products" in the Wiley Online Library, discussing the benefits of silica, found abundantly in horsetail, for hair strength and elasticity.

PART 22: MANAGING ALLERGIES AND IMMUNE RESPONSES

Allergies and immune responses are critical areas where the holistic health approach can offer significant benefits. Allergies, a manifestation of an overreactive immune system, can range from mild to life-threatening. Understanding how to manage these through natural means can empower individuals to lead healthier, more comfortable lives.

Beneficial effects of managing allergies and immune responses naturally include reduced dependency on medications, fewer side effects, and improved overall health. By strengthening the immune system and reducing inflammation, one can mitigate allergic reactions and enhance the body's ability to protect itself.

For those seeking to manage allergies and immune responses, incorporating specific foods, herbs, and lifestyle practices can be incredibly beneficial. Foods rich in vitamin C, such as oranges, strawberries, and bell peppers, can bolster the immune system.

Omega-3 fatty acids found in flaxseeds, chia seeds, and fatty fish reduce inflammation, which is a key component of allergic reactions. Incorporating quercetin-rich foods like apples, onions, and berries can help stabilize mast cells and prevent them from releasing histamine, the compound responsible for many allergy symptoms.

Herbal remedies also play a crucial role in managing allergies and immune responses. Nettle tea, known for its natural antihistamine properties, can alleviate sneezing, itching, and congestion. Butterbur extract, another potent herb, has been shown to be effective in reducing symptoms of hay fever without the drowsiness associated with many over-the-counter allergy medications.

Instructions for a simple nettle tea are as follows:

1. Boil 1 cup of water.

2. Add 1 tablespoon of dried nettle leaves to the boiling water.

3. Steep for 10-15 minutes.

4. Strain and enjoy. You can drink this tea 2-3 times a day during allergy season for best results.

Variations of this tea can include adding honey for sweetness or mixing nettle with peppermint leaves for an additional soothing effect.

Storage tips for herbs include keeping them in a cool, dark place in airtight containers to preserve their potency.

For those with specific allergens, it's crucial to find alternatives that don't trigger allergic reactions. For example, if you're allergic to chamomile, which is often recommended for its calming and anti-inflammatory properties, you might try lavender instead.

Scientific references supporting the health benefits of these natural remedies include studies published in the Journal of Phytotherapy Research, which have demonstrated the efficacy of nettle in managing allergic rhinitis, and research in the BMJ highlighting butterbur's potential as an effective herbal treatment for hay fever.

By adopting these holistic practices, individuals can achieve a more balanced immune response, reduce the frequency and severity of allergic reactions, and enhance their overall well-being.

CHAPTER 1: ALLERGIES AND IMMUNE BASICS

Allergies and immune responses are the body's natural defense mechanisms against substances it perceives as threats, even if they are harmless to most people. These substances, known as allergens, can trigger reactions ranging from mild to severe and impact the quality of life. Understanding the immune system's role in allergies is crucial for managing and potentially reducing allergic reactions through natural and holistic approaches.

The immune system is designed to protect the body from invaders such as bacteria, viruses, and toxins. In the case of allergies, the immune system mistakenly identifies a benign substance as harmful and mounts an attack against it. This response involves the production of antibodies called Immunoglobulin E (IgE), which bind to the allergen. Upon subsequent exposures, these IgE molecules signal immune cells to release histamine and other chemicals, leading to the symptoms commonly associated with allergies, such as sneezing, itching, swelling, and in severe cases, anaphylaxis.

Several factors can influence the likelihood of developing allergies, including genetics, environmental exposure, and lifestyle choices. For instance, a family history of allergies increases the risk, while early exposure to diverse microorganisms may decrease it. Diet, stress levels, and exposure to pollutants also play significant roles in immune system function and its response to allergens.

To manage allergies and strengthen the immune response naturally, consider incorporating foods rich in antioxidants, vitamins, and minerals that support immune health. Vitamin C, found in citrus fruits and leafy greens, can help reduce histamine levels and alleviate symptoms. Omega-3 fatty acids, present in flaxseeds and fatty fish, are known for their anti-inflammatory properties and can help modulate the immune response. Probiotics, found in yogurt and fermented foods, can promote a healthy gut microbiome, which is essential for a robust immune system.

Herbal remedies can also be beneficial in managing allergies. For example, quercetin, a natural compound found in apples, berries, and onions, has antihistamine and anti-inflammatory properties. Stinging nettle, taken as a supplement or tea, may help reduce hay fever symptoms by blocking histamine receptors and inhibiting inflammation.

Lifestyle modifications can further enhance the body's ability to handle allergens. Regular exercise boosts overall immune function, while stress-reduction techniques such as meditation and yoga can help prevent the overactivation of the immune response. Ensuring adequate sleep and hydration are also vital, as they allow the body to repair and maintain a balanced immune system.

In summary, allergies are the result of an overactive immune response to harmless substances. By understanding the underlying immune mechanisms and incorporating natural dietary and lifestyle changes, individuals can support their body's defenses and mitigate allergic reactions. While these strategies can be effective, it's important to consult with a healthcare provider for severe allergies or before starting any new health regimen.

CHAPTER 2: NUTRITION FOR ALLERGY CARE

Foods rich in certain nutrients can provide significant support for managing allergies by bolstering the immune system and reducing inflammation. A diet that emphasizes these nutrients can help mitigate allergic reactions and improve overall health.

Vitamin C is a powerful antioxidant that not only supports the immune system but also acts as a natural antihistamine, reducing the severity of allergic reactions. Foods high in vitamin C include citrus fruits like oranges and grapefruits, strawberries, bell peppers, and broccoli. Incorporating these foods into daily meals can help keep the immune system strong and more capable of warding off allergens.

Omega-3 fatty acids, found in flaxseeds, chia seeds, walnuts, and fatty fish such as salmon and mackerel, are known for their anti-inflammatory properties.

Regular consumption of these foods can help reduce the inflammatory response associated with allergic reactions.

Quercetin, a flavonoid present in apples, berries, onions, and parsley, has been shown to stabilize mast cells and prevent them from releasing histamine. Histamine is the compound that triggers many of the symptoms associated with allergies, such as sneezing, itching, and swelling. Including quercetin-rich foods in the diet can provide a natural way to manage allergy symptoms.

Probiotics play a crucial role in maintaining gut health, which is directly linked to the immune system. Foods rich in probiotics, such as yogurt, kefir, sauerkraut, and other fermented foods, can help balance the gut microbiome, enhancing the body's ability to fight allergens.

Magnesium-rich foods like spinach, pumpkin seeds, and dark chocolate can also support allergy management. Magnesium has been shown to relax airways and improve breathing, which can be particularly beneficial for those suffering from respiratory allergies.

Instructions for incorporating these nutrients into a daily diet include:

1. Start the day with a smoothie made with berries, citrus fruits, and a handful of spinach to boost vitamin C and magnesium intake.

2. Add flaxseeds or chia seeds to oatmeal, yogurt, or salads to increase omega-3 fatty acid consumption.

3. Include a serving of fatty fish, such as salmon or mackerel, in meals at least twice a week.

4. Snack on apples and nuts to get a healthy dose of quercetin throughout the day.

5. Incorporate fermented foods into meals, such as adding sauerkraut to sandwiches or enjoying a serving of kefir.

Variations for those with specific dietary preferences or restrictions can include using vitamin C-rich vegetables instead of fruits for those on a low-sugar diet or substituting fish with algae-based omega-3 supplements for vegetarians.

Storage tips for these foods include keeping berries and leafy greens in the refrigerator's crisper to maintain freshness, storing nuts and seeds in airtight containers in a cool, dark place to prevent rancidity, and keeping fermented foods refrigerated to preserve probiotic content.

For individuals with allergies to specific foods, alternatives that provide similar nutritional benefits can be used. For example, if allergic to citrus fruits, vitamin C can be obtained from bell peppers and strawberries. If dairy products are problematic, probiotic needs can be met with dairy-free fermented foods like kimchi.

Scientific references support the benefits of these nutrients for allergy management. Studies published in the Journal of Allergy and Clinical Immunology and the European Journal of Clinical Nutrition have highlighted the role of vitamin C, omega-3 fatty acids, quercetin, and probiotics in reducing allergic reactions and supporting immune health.

VITAMIN C AND QUERCETIN FOR IMMUNE SUPPORT

Vitamin C and quercetin stand out as formidable allies in the quest for immune support, particularly in managing allergies and bolstering the body's defense mechanisms. Vitamin C, a potent antioxidant, plays a pivotal role in the immune system's ability to fend off pathogens and recover from infections. It aids in the production of white blood cells, which are crucial for fighting infections, and protects these cells from damage by potentially harmful molecules, such as free radicals. Quercetin, a flavonoid found in many fruits and vegetables, works synergistically with vitamin C, enhancing its antioxidant activity. Moreover, quercetin has been shown to stabilize mast cells, reducing the release of histamine, a chemical that contributes to allergy symptoms.

Beneficial effects of vitamin C and quercetin include not only their immune-boosting properties but also their ability to alleviate allergic reactions, making them especially valuable during allergy seasons. Their combined action can help reduce inflammation, sneezing, itching, and other discomforts associated with allergic responses.

To harness these benefits, consider incorporating the following ingredients into your diet:

- Citrus fruits (rich in Vitamin C)

- Berries (sources of both Vitamin C and Quercetin)

- Apples (a good source of Quercetin)

- Onions (rich in Quercetin)

- Parsley (contains Quercetin)

- Bell peppers (high in Vitamin C)

- Dark leafy greens (sources of Vitamin C)

Instructions for a simple dietary addition that combines these ingredients could be a daily smoothie or salad.

For a smoothie, blend together:

1. 1 cup of mixed berries

2. 1 orange, peeled

3. 1 apple, cored and sliced

4. A handful of parsley

5. Water or ice as needed for desired consistency

For a salad, mix:

1. Sliced apples

2. Chopped parsley

3. Thinly sliced red onions

4. Bell peppers

5. Your choice of dark leafy greens

6. A dressing made from lemon juice (another source of Vitamin C) and olive oil

Variations of these recipes can include adding other fruits and vegetables rich in Vitamin C and Quercetin, such as grapefruits, kiwis, or broccoli. Adjusting the ingredients based on seasonal availability and personal taste preferences can keep these dietary additions exciting and flavorful.

Storage tips for the ingredients include keeping berries, leafy greens, and bell peppers in the refrigerator to maintain freshness. Apples, citrus fruits, and onions can be stored in a cool, dry place.

For those with allergies to any of the suggested ingredients, alternatives can be easily substituted. For example, if allergic to citrus fruits, consider using kiwi or strawberries as a Vitamin C source. If sensitive to onions, omit them from recipes or use a small amount of onion powder for flavor without the bulk of the vegetable.

Scientific references supporting the health benefits of Vitamin C and Quercetin include studies published in the "Journal of Allergy and Clinical Immunology" and "Nutrients" journal, which have highlighted their roles in immune function and allergy relief. These studies underscore the potential of dietary interventions in managing immune responses and providing natural allergy relief.

FOODS TO AVOID DURING ALLERGY SEASON

During allergy season, certain foods can exacerbate symptoms or trigger histamine responses in the body, making it crucial to be mindful of dietary choices. Foods that are high in histamines or that can trigger histamine release should be limited or avoided to help manage allergy symptoms more effectively. These include aged cheeses, processed meats like sausages and deli meats, smoked fish, and fermented foods such as sauerkraut, kombucha, and certain types of yogurt.

These foods contain higher levels of histamines, which can intensify symptoms such as sneezing, itching, and nasal congestion for those with allergies.

Additionally, alcohol, particularly red wine, beer, and champagne, can increase histamine levels in the body and impair the enzyme that breaks down histamine, potentially worsening allergy symptoms. Alcohol can also lead to dehydration, which may make mucus thicker and more difficult to clear from the nasal passages, further aggravating allergy symptoms.

Certain fruits, vegetables, and nuts, including bananas, tomatoes, avocados, eggplants, spinach, and cashews, are known as histamine liberators. Even though they may not be high in histamines themselves, they can trigger the body to release its own histamines, contributing to an increase in allergy symptoms. It's also advisable to avoid or limit consumption of artificial additives and preservatives found in many processed foods, as these can trigger allergic reactions in sensitive individuals.

Caffeinated beverages, such as coffee and certain types of tea, can also exacerbate allergy symptoms by stimulating the release of histamine. Switching to herbal teas or decaffeinated options can help reduce this effect.

During allergy season, focusing on a diet rich in fresh, whole foods with anti-inflammatory properties can support overall health and help manage allergy symptoms. Incorporating foods high in omega-3 fatty acids, antioxidants, and vitamins, such as leafy green vegetables, berries, and fatty fish, can be beneficial. Drinking plenty of water to stay hydrated and support the body's natural detoxification processes is also crucial.

For those with specific food allergies, it's essential to read labels carefully and be aware of potential cross-contamination issues. Consulting with a healthcare provider or a dietitian can provide personalized advice and help in identifying and avoiding trigger foods during allergy season.

By being mindful of these dietary considerations, individuals can take proactive steps to minimize allergy symptoms and support their overall well-being during challenging allergy seasons.

HYDRATION'S ROLE IN REDUCING ALLERGIC REACTIONS

Hydration plays a crucial role in maintaining the body's natural defenses against allergens and in reducing the severity of allergic reactions. Adequate water intake helps to thin the mucus in the nasal passages, making it easier for the body to clear out allergens and irritants that can cause symptoms such as sneezing, congestion, and itching. Furthermore, staying well-hydrated supports the overall function of the immune system, enabling it to respond more effectively to potential threats.

Beneficial effects of proper hydration include not only the dilution and removal of irritants from the respiratory system but also the prevention of dehydration, which can exacerbate allergy symptoms and lead to increased histamine production. Histamine is a compound that the body releases in response to an allergen, and it plays a key role in allergic reactions. By keeping the body hydrated, one can help regulate histamine levels and thus reduce the intensity of allergic responses.

To ensure adequate hydration, it is recommended to drink at least 8-10 glasses of water per day, more if you are active or live in a hot climate. This can include water, herbal teas, and other non-caffeinated beverages that do not contain high levels of sugar or artificial additives. Incorporating foods with high water content, such as cucumbers, celery, watermelon, and strawberries, can also contribute to overall fluid intake.

Instructions for maintaining hydration to manage allergies effectively include:

1. Start your day with a glass of water to kickstart hydration after a night's sleep.

2. Keep a reusable water bottle with you throughout the day to ensure that you have easy access to water at all times.

3. Set reminders on your phone or computer to drink water at regular intervals.

4. Drink a glass of water before and after each meal to aid digestion and absorption of nutrients, which are essential for immune health.

5. Opt for herbal teas such as chamomile or peppermint, which can soothe allergic reactions and provide hydration without caffeine.

Variations to enhance your hydration routine might include adding slices of lemon, lime, cucumber, or berries to your water for added flavor without artificial sweeteners. Herbal infusions and decaffeinated green tea are also excellent choices for increasing water intake while benefiting from the anti-inflammatory and antioxidant properties of these beverages.

Storage tips for ensuring you always have fresh, appealing options for hydration include keeping a pitcher of water with added fruits or herbs in the refrigerator. This not only makes the water more enticing to drink but also infuses it with additional nutrients.

For individuals with allergies to specific fruits or herbs, it's important to choose hydration options that do not trigger allergic responses. For example, if you are allergic to citrus fruits, infuse your water with cucumber or mint instead.

Scientific references underscore the importance of hydration in managing allergies. Studies have shown that dehydration can trigger histamine production as the body's way of conserving water, which can worsen allergy symptoms. Ensuring proper hydration is a simple yet effective strategy to support the body's natural ability to cope with allergens and reduce the occurrence of allergic reactions.

CHAPTER 3: NATURAL REMEDIES FOR ALLERGY RELIEF

B eneficial effects of natural remedies for allergy relief include reducing inflammation, stabilizing mast cells to prevent histamine release, and supporting the immune system to mitigate allergic reactions. These remedies offer a holistic approach to managing allergies, focusing on natural ingredients that provide relief without the side effects often associated with conventional medications.

Natural remedies for allergy relief work in harmony with the body to provide long-lasting benefits. By addressing the root causes of allergic reactions rather than merely suppressing symptoms, these remedies offer a gentle yet effective approach to healing. The key benefits include reducing inflammation, stabilizing mast cells, and supporting the immune system, which are essential for restoring balance and preventing future allergic flare-ups.

1. **Reducing Inflammation**: Inflammation is the body's natural response to allergens, but chronic inflammation can lead to discomfort and a weakened immune system. Herbal anti-inflammatories such as **turmeric** (Curcuma longa) and **quercetin** help calm the body's inflammatory response without the side effects associated with synthetic medications. These plant-based compounds work by inhibiting inflammatory pathways, allowing the body to heal naturally.

2. **Stabilizing Mast Cells**: Mast cells play a crucial role in allergic reactions, as they release histamine and other chemicals that trigger symptoms like itching, sneezing, and swelling. Natural remedies like **butterbur** (Petasites hybridus) and **stinging nettle** (Urtica dioica) have been shown to stabilize mast cells, reducing the release of histamine and thereby preventing allergic symptoms at their source.

3. **Supporting the Immune System**: Allergic reactions are often a sign of an imbalanced immune system. Strengthening the immune response is vital for long-term allergy management. Remedies such as **echinacea** (Echinacea purpurea) and **elderberry** (Sambucus nigra) support immune health by enhancing the body's natural defenses. This immune-boosting effect not only helps reduce the severity of allergic reactions but also promotes overall wellness.

Ingredients for a Ginger and Turmeric Anti-Inflammatory Drink:

- 1 inch fresh ginger root, peeled and sliced

- 1 inch fresh turmeric root, peeled and sliced (or 1 teaspoon turmeric powder)

- 1 tablespoon raw honey (optional, for sweetness)

- 2 cups water

- Juice of half a lemon

Instructions:

1. Bring the water to a boil in a small saucepan.

2. Add the sliced ginger and turmeric to the boiling water. Reduce the heat and simmer for 10-15 minutes.

3. Remove from heat and let it cool slightly. Strain the mixture into a cup.

4. Add the lemon juice and raw honey to the strained liquid. Stir well until the honey is dissolved.

5. Drink this mixture once or twice daily, especially during allergy season, for best results.

Variations:

- For an extra immune boost, add a pinch of black pepper. This enhances the absorption of curcumin, the active compound in turmeric.

- Incorporate a cinnamon stick during the simmering process for additional anti-inflammatory benefits and flavor.

Storage tips:

- The ginger and turmeric anti-inflammatory drink can be stored in the refrigerator for up to 2 days. Warm slightly before drinking for best taste and efficacy.

- Fresh ginger and turmeric roots should be stored in the refrigerator to maintain their freshness and potency.

Tips for allergens:

- If you are allergic to any of the ingredients listed, such as honey, you can substitute it with maple syrup or simply omit it from the recipe.

- For those with a citrus allergy, omit the lemon juice or replace it with a splash of apple cider vinegar for a similar zesty flavor.

Scientific references:

- Studies published in the "Journal of Allergy and Clinical Immunology" have demonstrated the anti-inflammatory properties of ginger and turmeric, highlighting their potential to alleviate allergic reactions.

- Research in the "International Journal of Preventive Medicine" supports the use of turmeric (curcumin) and ginger in reducing symptoms of allergic rhinitis and improving the quality of life for those with allergies.

By incorporating these natural remedies into your routine, you can take a proactive step towards managing allergies in a more holistic and health-conscious manner.

CHAPTER 4: 5 HERBAL RECIPES FOR ALLERGY RELIEF

NETTLE AND QUERCETIN TEA

Beneficial effects

Nettle and Quercetin Tea is a powerful blend designed to alleviate allergy symptoms naturally. Nettle is known for its anti-inflammatory properties, which can help reduce the severity of allergic reactions, such as sneezing, itching, and nasal congestion. Quercetin, a flavonoid found in many plants and foods, has been shown to stabilize mast cells, reducing the release of histamine, which is responsible for allergy symptoms. Together, they create a synergistic effect that can help manage seasonal allergies, improve respiratory health, and support the immune system.

Portions

2 servings

Preparation time

10 minutes

Cooking time

5 minutes

Ingredients

- 2 tablespoons dried nettle leaves
- 1 teaspoon quercetin powder
- 2 cups boiling water
- Honey or lemon to taste (optional)

Instructions

1. Place the dried nettle leaves and quercetin powder in a tea infuser or directly into a heat-resistant teapot.
2. Pour 2 cups of boiling water over the nettle leaves and quercetin powder.
3. Cover and let the tea steep for about 5 to 10 minutes.
4. Remove the tea infuser or strain the tea to remove the nettle leaves and any undissolved quercetin powder.
5. Optional: Add honey or lemon to taste for flavor enhancement.
6. Serve the tea warm, ideally in the morning to help manage allergy symptoms throughout the day.

Variations

- For added immune support, include a slice of fresh ginger or a cinnamon stick in the tea while it steeps.
- Combine with peppermint leaves during the steeping process for a refreshing flavor and additional nasal congestion relief.
- To make a cold beverage, allow the tea to cool and serve over ice for a refreshing allergy relief drink.

Storage tips

Store any leftover Nettle and Quercetin Tea in a sealed container in the refrigerator for up to 2 days. Enjoy chilled or gently reheat on the stove.

Tips for allergens

Individuals with sensitivities to nettle should start with a smaller amount to ensure no adverse reactions. For those avoiding honey due to dietary restrictions, substitute with maple syrup or simply omit the sweetener.

Scientific references

- "The effects of Urtica dioica (stinging nettle) on the severity of hay fever symptoms: a randomized, double-blind, placebo-controlled study" in Phytotherapy Research, 2009. This study supports the efficacy of nettle in reducing allergy symptoms.

- "Quercetin, Inflammation and Immunity" in Nutrients, 2016. This review highlights quercetin's role in modulating immune response and stabilizing mast cells, making it beneficial for allergy relief.

BUTTERBUR TINCTURE

Beneficial effects

Butterbur Tincture is recognized for its ability to provide relief from allergy symptoms such as sneezing, itchy eyes, and congestion. The active compounds in butterbur, petasins, are known to inhibit leukotrienes and histamines, which are substances in the body that cause allergic reactions. This makes butterbur a natural and effective option for managing seasonal allergies and hay fever without the drowsiness often associated with over-the-counter antihistamines.

Ingredients

- 1/4 cup dried butterbur leaves
- 1 cup high-proof alcohol (such as vodka or brandy)
- A clean glass jar with a tight-fitting lid

Instructions

1. Place the dried butterbur leaves into the clean glass jar.

2. Pour the high-proof alcohol over the leaves, ensuring they are completely submerged. Leave about an inch of space at the top of the jar.

3. Seal the jar tightly with the lid and label it with the date and contents.

4. Store the jar in a cool, dark place for 4 to 6 weeks. Shake the jar gently every few days to mix the contents and promote extraction.

5. After the infusion period, strain the tincture through a fine mesh sieve or cheesecloth into another clean, dark glass bottle. Press or squeeze the butterbur leaves to extract as much liquid as possible.

6. Label the bottle with the date and contents.

Variations

- For individuals sensitive to alcohol, the tincture can be evaporated slightly to reduce the alcohol content, or a glycerin-based tincture can be made as an alternative.

- Adding a few drops of peppermint oil to the finished tincture can enhance its flavor and add additional anti-inflammatory benefits.

Storage tips

Store the Butterbur Tincture in a cool, dark place. When stored properly in an airtight container, it can last for up to a year.

Tips for allergens

Individuals with allergies to ragweed, chrysanthemums, marigolds, or daisies should proceed with caution when using butterbur, as it may cause allergic reactions in sensitive individuals. Always consult with a healthcare provider before starting any new herbal remedy, especially if you are pregnant, nursing, or taking medications.

Scientific references

- "Randomized controlled trial of butterbur and cetirizine for treating seasonal allergic rhinitis" published in BMJ, 2002. This study supports the efficacy of butterbur in the treatment of allergic rhinitis.

- "Safety and efficacy of butterbur nasal spray in children with seasonal allergic rhinitis" in Pediatric Allergy and Immunology, 2005. This research highlights the safety and effectiveness of butterbur in managing allergy symptoms in children.

STINGING NETTLE SMOOTHIE

Beneficial effects

The Stinging Nettle Smoothie is designed to offer relief from allergy symptoms by leveraging the natural antihistamine properties of stinging nettle. This herbal remedy can help reduce inflammation, ease nasal congestion, and soothe irritation associated with allergic reactions. Stinging nettle is rich in nutrients and has been traditionally used to support the body's defense against seasonal allergies, providing a natural way to manage symptoms without the side effects often associated with over-the-counter medications.

Portions

2 servings

Preparation time

10 minutes

Ingredients

- 1 cup fresh stinging nettle leaves (use gloves when handling) or 2 tablespoons dried nettle leaves

- 1 ripe banana

- 1/2 cup pineapple chunks

- 1 cup almond milk

- 1 tablespoon honey (optional, for sweetness)

- Ice cubes (optional)

Instructions

1. If using fresh stinging nettle leaves, blanch them first by pouring boiling water over the leaves and then immediately rinsing them in cold water. This process removes the stinging chemicals from the leaves.

2. Place the blanched or dried nettle leaves, banana, pineapple, almond milk, and honey (if using) into a blender.

3. Add ice cubes if a colder smoothie is preferred.

4. Blend on high until the mixture is smooth and creamy.

5. Pour the smoothie into glasses and serve immediately to enjoy its allergy-relieving benefits.

Variations

- For an extra immune-boosting effect, add a teaspoon of spirulina powder to the smoothie.

- Substitute almond milk with coconut water for a lighter version that's still hydrating and flavorful.

- Add a handful of spinach to increase the smoothie's vitamin and mineral content without significantly altering the taste.

Storage tips

It's best to consume the Stinging Nettle Smoothie immediately after preparation to ensure maximum potency of the allergy-relieving properties. However, if necessary, it can be stored in an airtight container in the refrigerator for up to 24 hours.

Tips for allergens

Individuals with allergies to nuts should substitute almond milk with a non-nut milk alternative like oat milk or rice milk. For those with a honey allergy or following a vegan diet, substitute honey with maple syrup or omit it altogether.

Scientific references

- "Stinging nettle: An overview of the research on its health properties" published in the Journal of Ethnopharmacology, 2016. This study highlights the anti-inflammatory and antihistamine effects of stinging nettle, supporting its use in allergy relief.

- "The effect of stinging nettle on allergic rhinitis" in Phytotherapy Research, 2009. This research supports the efficacy of stinging nettle in reducing symptoms of allergic rhinitis, providing a natural alternative for allergy management.

TURMERIC AND GINGER ANTI-INFLAMMATORY DRINK

Beneficial effects

The Turmeric and Ginger Anti-Inflammatory Drink is a powerful concoction designed to reduce inflammation, boost the immune system, and improve digestion. Turmeric, with its active compound curcumin, offers potent anti-inflammatory and antioxidant properties, helping to alleviate symptoms of arthritis and other inflammatory conditions. Ginger complements turmeric by providing additional anti-inflammatory benefits, soothing nausea, and enhancing digestive health. This drink is an excellent choice for those looking to naturally manage inflammation and support overall wellness.

Portions

2 servings

Preparation time

5 minutes

Cooking time

10 minutes

Ingredients

- 1 inch fresh turmeric root, grated (or 1 teaspoon turmeric powder)

- 1 inch fresh ginger root, grated

- 4 cups of water

- Juice of 1 lemon

- Honey to taste (optional)

Instructions

1. In a small pot, bring 4 cups of water to a boil.

2. Add the grated turmeric and ginger to the boiling water.

3. Reduce the heat and simmer for about 10 minutes to allow the roots to infuse their properties into the water.

4. Remove the pot from the heat and let the mixture cool slightly.

5. Strain the drink to remove the turmeric and ginger pieces.

6. Stir in the lemon juice. Add honey to taste, if desired.

7. Serve the drink warm or allow it to cool and enjoy it as a refreshing cold beverage.

Variations

- For an extra immune boost, add a pinch of black pepper to the drink. Black pepper increases the bioavailability of curcumin, enhancing its benefits.

- Mix in a cinnamon stick during the simmering process for added flavor and blood sugar regulation benefits.

- For a cold version, chill the drink in the refrigerator and serve over ice with a sprig of mint for a refreshing twist.

Storage tips

Store any leftover Turmeric and Ginger Anti-Inflammatory Drink in a sealed container in the refrigerator for up to 2 days. Enjoy it chilled, or gently reheat on the stove.

Tips for allergens

Individuals with allergies to turmeric or ginger should proceed with caution and may consider consulting with a healthcare provider before consumption. For those avoiding honey due to dietary restrictions, substitute with maple syrup or simply omit the sweetener.

Scientific references

- "Curcumin: A Review of Its' Effects on Human Health," published in Foods, 2017. This review discusses the wide-ranging health benefits of curcumin, including its anti-inflammatory and antioxidant effects.

- "Ginger on Human Health: A Comprehensive Systematic Review of 109 Randomized Controlled Trials," in Nutrients, 2020. This systematic review highlights ginger's health benefits, particularly its anti-inflammatory properties and effectiveness in digestive health support.

PEPPERMINT AND EUCALYPTUS STEAM INHALATION

Beneficial effects

Peppermint and Eucalyptus Steam Inhalation offers immediate relief for congested airways, making it an effective natural remedy for those suffering from colds, sinusitis, or respiratory allergies. The menthol in peppermint acts as a natural decongestant, helping to break down mucus and clear the nasal passages, while eucalyptus oil contains eucalyptol, a compound known for its anti-inflammatory and antibacterial properties, which can soothe irritated respiratory tracts and kill pathogens causing congestion. This combination not only aids in breathing more comfortably but also promotes relaxation and reduces stress, contributing to overall well-being during illness.

Ingredients

- 3 to 4 cups of boiling water
- 5 to 10 drops of eucalyptus essential oil
- 5 drops of peppermint essential oil

Instructions

1. Boil 3 to 4 cups of water and pour it into a large heat-proof bowl.

2. Carefully add 5 to 10 drops of eucalyptus essential oil and 5 drops of peppermint essential oil to the hot water.

3. Lean over the bowl, keeping a safe distance to avoid burns, and drape a large towel over your head and the bowl to trap the steam.

4. Close your eyes and deeply inhale the steam for 5 to 10 minutes, or as long as it's comfortable. Take breaks as needed if the heat becomes too intense.

5. After the inhalation session, gently pat your face dry with a towel.

Variations

- For additional antibacterial benefits, add 2 drops of tea tree oil to the steam inhalation mixture.

- If suffering from a headache in addition to congestion, include a drop of lavender essential oil for its calming and pain-relieving properties.

- To enhance the soothing effect on the respiratory system, add a tablespoon of dried thyme to the boiling water before adding the essential oils.

Storage tips

Essential oils should be stored in a cool, dark place in tightly sealed bottles to maintain their potency and prevent oxidation.

Tips for allergens

Individuals with asthma or allergies to eucalyptus or peppermint should proceed with caution and may want to consult with a healthcare provider before trying this steam inhalation. For those sensitive to strong scents, start with fewer drops of essential oil and adjust as tolerated.

Scientific references

- "Eucalyptus essential oil as a natural remedy in the treatment of respiratory tract infections," published in the Laryngoscope Investigative Otolaryngology, 2019. This study highlights the antimicrobial and anti-inflammatory effects of eucalyptus oil on the respiratory system.

- "Menthol: Effects on nasal sensation of airflow and the drive to breathe," published in Current Allergy and Asthma Reports, 2003. This research supports the decongestant properties of menthol, found in peppermint, making it effective for clearing congestion and improving breathing.

PART 23: PAIN MANAGEMENT AND INFLAMMATION

Managing pain and inflammation naturally is a cornerstone of holistic health, focusing on the body's ability to heal itself through diet, lifestyle changes, and the use of herbal remedies. Chronic inflammation is often the root cause of many diseases and conditions, and by addressing this underlying issue, we can significantly improve our overall health and well-being. One of the first steps in managing pain and inflammation is understanding the foods that can either contribute to or alleviate these conditions. Foods high in omega-3 fatty acids, such as salmon, flaxseeds, and walnuts, are known for their anti-inflammatory properties. Incorporating these into your diet can help reduce the levels of inflammation in your body. On the other hand, processed foods, sugars, and trans fats can increase inflammation and should be consumed minimally.

Herbal remedies also play a crucial role in managing pain and inflammation. Turmeric, with its active compound curcumin, has been widely recognized for its potent anti-inflammatory effects and ability to reduce pain. Ginger, another powerful herb, not only combats inflammation but can also provide relief from pain due to its analgesic properties. Both of these herbs can be easily incorporated into your daily diet through cooking or as supplements.

Another important aspect of managing pain and inflammation is maintaining an active lifestyle. Regular exercise helps to strengthen the body, improve circulation, and reduce inflammation. Even gentle forms of exercise, such as walking or yoga, can have significant benefits. It's also crucial to ensure adequate rest and recovery, as sleep plays a vital role in the body's healing processes.

Hydration is another key factor in managing inflammation. Drinking plenty of water helps to flush toxins from the body, supports kidney function, and can reduce the buildup of inflammatory substances. Adding lemon to your water not only makes it more palatable but can also provide additional anti-inflammatory benefits due to its vitamin C content.

For those experiencing chronic pain and inflammation, stress management techniques such as meditation, deep breathing exercises, and mindfulness can be incredibly beneficial. Stress is known to exacerbate inflammation and pain, so finding effective ways to manage stress is crucial for long-term relief.

Incorporating these strategies into your daily routine can significantly impact your ability to manage pain and inflammation naturally. By focusing on a diet rich in anti-inflammatory foods, utilizing herbal remedies, staying active, ensuring adequate rest, and managing stress, you can support your body's natural healing processes and improve your quality of life.

In addition to dietary changes and lifestyle adjustments, specific supplements can further aid in the natural management of pain and inflammation. Omega-3 supplements, for example, can provide a concentrated dose of anti-inflammatory fatty acids, especially for those who might not consume enough fatty fish or seeds. Magnesium is another supplement that plays a crucial role in muscle relaxation and nerve function, potentially reducing pain and discomfort associated with muscle tension and nerve issues.

The application of heat and cold can also be an effective, immediate way to manage pain and inflammation. Heat therapy, through warm baths or heating pads, can increase blood flow and relax sore muscles, providing relief from pain. Cold therapy, on the other hand, can reduce inflammation and numb the surrounding area of a painful spot, offering a temporary reprieve from discomfort. Alternating between heat and cold therapy can be particularly beneficial for certain conditions like arthritis.

Essential oils offer another avenue for managing pain and inflammation naturally. Lavender oil is renowned for its calming and anti-inflammatory properties, making it an excellent choice for stress-related tension and pain. Peppermint oil, with its cooling effect, can alleviate headaches and muscle pain. Eucalyptus oil is another powerful option that can help reduce swelling and pain with its anti-inflammatory properties. These oils can be used in aromatherapy, added to baths, or diluted with a carrier oil for massage.

Practicing mindfulness and body awareness can also play a significant role in pain management. Techniques such as progressive muscle relaxation, guided imagery, and mindful meditation can help individuals become more aware of their bodies and manage pain through relaxation and stress reduction. These practices not only help in the short term but can also contribute to long-term wellness and pain management strategies.

Finally, consulting with a healthcare professional who understands holistic health can provide personalized strategies for managing pain and inflammation. This may include acupuncture, chiropractic care, or other forms of therapy that address the root cause of pain rather than just treating symptoms. Such therapies can complement the natural remedies and lifestyle changes, offering a comprehensive approach to managing pain and inflammation.

By integrating these natural remedies and practices into a holistic health regimen, individuals can find relief from pain and inflammation while supporting their body's overall health and well-being. It's important to remember that while these methods can be effective, they should be part of a broader health strategy that may include conventional medical treatments when necessary. The key is to create a balanced approach that prioritizes the body's natural healing capabilities while addressing specific health concerns in a thoughtful and informed manner.

CHAPTER 1: UNDERSTANDING PAIN AND INFLAMMATION

Pain and inflammation are the body's natural responses to injury or disease, serving as signals that something is wrong. When we experience pain, it's often the result of complex interactions within our nervous system, while inflammation is a critical part of the immune system's response to injury and infection. Understanding these processes is essential for managing them effectively and fostering a holistic approach to health.

At the core of pain perception is the nervous system, which includes the brain, spinal cord, and numerous nerves that traverse the entire body. Pain can be acute, serving as an immediate reaction to a threat to the body, or chronic, where pain persists long-term and may not be linked to an obvious cause. Chronic pain, in particular, can be debilitating and significantly impact quality of life, making its management a key focus for those seeking to improve their overall well-being.

Inflammation, on the other hand, is the body's defense mechanism against infection and injury. It aims to remove harmful stimuli, including damaged cells, irritants, or pathogens, and initiate the healing process. The classic signs of acute inflammation include redness, heat, swelling, pain, and loss of function.

However, like pain, inflammation can become chronic, contributing to a host of diseases, including heart disease, diabetes, and arthritis, by continually damaging healthy tissue.

The relationship between pain and inflammation is intricate, as they can both exacerbate each other. For instance, chronic inflammation can lead to increased sensitivity to pain by affecting nerve cells. Similarly, persistent pain can lead to increased stress levels, which may trigger an inflammatory response. This cycle highlights the importance of addressing both pain and inflammation to break this feedback loop and promote healing.

Diet plays a pivotal role in managing both pain and inflammation.

Foods rich in omega-3 fatty acids, such as salmon and flaxseeds, have been shown to reduce inflammation, while antioxidants found in fruits and vegetables can help protect the body from the oxidative stress that contributes to chronic inflammation and pain. Conversely, processed foods, sugars, and certain fats can exacerbate inflammatory responses and pain perception.

Herbal remedies also offer potential benefits for managing pain and inflammation. Turmeric, for example, contains curcumin, a compound with strong anti-inflammatory and antioxidant properties. Ginger, another potent herb, has been shown to reduce inflammation and act as a natural pain reliever. These natural approaches can complement traditional medical treatments, offering a holistic strategy for pain and inflammation management.

Regular physical activity is another crucial component of managing pain and inflammation. Exercise not only strengthens the body and improves flexibility but also triggers the release of endorphins, the body's natural painkillers. However, it's important to choose the right type and amount of exercise to avoid exacerbating pain or injury.

Hydration and stress management are additional factors that can influence pain and inflammation. Adequate hydration ensures that nutrients are efficiently transported throughout the body, waste products are removed, and tissues are well-hydrated and less prone to irritation. Stress, known to affect both pain perception and inflammatory responses, can be managed through techniques such as meditation, deep breathing, and yoga, which promote relaxation and well-being.

Understanding the mechanisms behind pain and inflammation is the first step towards effective management. By adopting a holistic approach that includes diet, exercise, herbal remedies, hydration, and stress management, individuals can mitigate the impact of pain and inflammation on their lives, promoting healing and enhancing their overall health and wellness.

Adopting a holistic approach to managing pain and inflammation involves not only addressing the physical aspects but also considering emotional and environmental factors that could be contributing to the condition. Mindfulness and emotional well-being play a significant role in this process, as chronic pain can often be intertwined with emotional stress, anxiety, and depression.

Techniques such as mindfulness-based stress reduction (MBSR) and cognitive-behavioral therapy (CBT) have shown promise in helping individuals cope with the emotional aspects of chronic pain, potentially reducing the intensity of pain experienced.

Environmental factors, including exposure to toxins and pollutants, can also exacerbate inflammation and pain. Reducing exposure to these harmful substances by opting for natural, non-toxic household cleaners, personal care products, and organic foods when possible can help minimize their impact on the body's inflammatory response.

Additionally, ensuring a healthy indoor environment free from mold and excessive dust can also contribute to reducing episodes of inflammation and pain.

Sleep is another critical component of managing pain and inflammation. Poor sleep quality and sleep deprivation can heighten pain sensitivity and increase stress, which in turn can worsen inflammatory conditions. Establishing a regular sleep routine, creating a comfortable sleep environment, and avoiding stimulants before bedtime can help improve sleep quality, thereby supporting the body's natural healing processes.

The role of supplements in managing pain and inflammation should not be overlooked.

Omega-3 fatty acids, magnesium, vitamin D, and probiotics are among the supplements that have been shown to provide anti-inflammatory benefits and support overall health.

However, it's important to consult with a healthcare provider before starting any new supplement regimen, especially for individuals with existing health conditions or those taking prescription medications.

Integrating complementary therapies such as acupuncture, massage therapy, and chiropractic care can offer additional relief from pain and inflammation.

These therapies can help improve circulation, reduce muscle tension, and promote relaxation, further supporting the body's healing process. While these therapies can be beneficial, selecting qualified practitioners and discussing these approaches with a healthcare provider is essential to ensure they complement existing treatment plans safely.

Personalized health strategies are paramount in the management of pain and inflammation. What works for one individual may not work for another, highlighting the importance of tailoring approaches based on personal health history, lifestyle, and preferences.

Working closely with healthcare professionals to develop a comprehensive, individualized plan can optimize outcomes and enhance quality of life.

In conclusion, managing pain and inflammation holistically requires a multifaceted approach that addresses dietary, lifestyle, emotional, and environmental factors.

By embracing a comprehensive strategy that includes proper nutrition, physical activity, stress management, sleep hygiene, and complementary therapies, individuals can effectively manage pain and inflammation, leading to improved health and well-being. This approach underscores the interconnectedness of the body and mind, emphasizing the importance of nurturing both to achieve optimal health.

CHAPTER 2: NUTRITIONAL SUPPORT FOR PAIN RELIEF

Foods rich in anti-inflammatory properties and essential nutrients offer a natural pathway to managing pain, complementing the holistic approach to health and wellness. Chronic pain, a pervasive issue affecting millions, can often be alleviated or managed through dietary choices that target inflammation and bolster the body's pain defense mechanisms. Incorporating a variety of nutrient-dense foods into one's diet can significantly impact one's ability to manage pain, offering a natural and sustainable method of pain relief.

Beneficial effects: Anti-inflammatory foods and those rich in omega-3 fatty acids, antioxidants, and phytochemicals can reduce inflammation, a common cause of pain. Foods high in magnesium and calcium are known for their muscle-relaxing properties, while vitamins C and E play crucial roles in repairing tissue and reducing pain perception. By focusing on a diet that supports pain relief, individuals can experience reduced inflammation, enhanced healing, and a strengthened immune system, contributing to overall pain reduction and improved quality of life.

Ingredients:

1. Omega-3 rich foods such as salmon, flaxseeds, and walnuts to reduce inflammation.

2. Leafy greens like spinach and kale, high in magnesium, for muscle relaxation.

3. Berries (blueberries, strawberries, raspberries) for their antioxidants and anti-inflammatory properties.

4. Ginger and turmeric, known for their anti-inflammatory effects.

5. Olive oil, a healthy fat that contains oleocanthal, which has properties similar to non-steroidal, anti-inflammatory drugs.

6. Tart cherries, which have been shown to reduce muscle pain and inflammation.

7. Whole grains to improve digestion and reduce inflammation.

8. Nuts and seeds, including almonds and chia seeds, for their anti-inflammatory fats.

9. Peppers and tomatoes, rich in antioxidants and vitamin C.

10. Dark chocolate (at least 70% cocoa) for antioxidants and mood-enhancing properties.

Instructions:

1. Start your day with a smoothie that includes flaxseeds or chia seeds blended with berries and spinach to kickstart your body with anti-inflammatory nutrients.

2. Incorporate whole grains like quinoa or brown rice into your lunch and dinner to ensure a steady supply of fiber and reduce inflammation.

3. Snack on a small handful of nuts or seeds to keep inflammation at bay throughout the day.

4. Include a source of omega-3 fatty acids in your meals, such as salmon or walnuts, to target inflammation directly associated with pain.

5. Add ginger and turmeric to your cooking or teas for their potent anti-inflammatory effects.

6. Opt for salads dressed with olive oil and a variety of colorful vegetables to maximize your intake of anti-inflammatory compounds.

7. For dessert or a treat, choose dark chocolate to satisfy cravings and provide your body with antioxidants.

8. Drink tart cherry juice after workouts or physical activities to reduce muscle soreness and inflammation.

Variations:

- For vegetarians or vegans, substitute fish with flaxseed oil or algae supplements to ensure adequate omega-3 intake.

- Use a variety of spices and herbs in cooking to find flavors that you enjoy and that contribute to reducing inflammation.

Storage tips:

- Store nuts and seeds in a cool, dry place or refrigerate to maintain freshness.

- Keep leafy greens and berries in the refrigerator to preserve their nutritional content.

- Whole grains should be stored in airtight containers in a cool, dry place to prevent spoilage.

Tips for allergens:

- For those allergic to nuts, focus on seeds such as pumpkin or sunflower seeds as alternatives.

- If gluten-sensitive, ensure that whole grains chosen are certified gluten-free.

Scientific references:

- Studies have shown that omega-3 fatty acids can significantly reduce the production of molecules and substances linked to inflammation, such as inflammatory eicosanoids and cytokines (Source: Calder, P.C. "Omega-3 fatty acids and inflammatory processes." Nutrients, 2010).

- Research on ginger and turmeric has demonstrated their effectiveness in reducing pain and inflammation in conditions such as osteoarthritis (Source: Daily, J.W., Yang, M., & Park, S. "Efficacy of Turmeric Extracts and Curcumin for Alleviating the Symptoms of Joint Arthritis: A Systematic Review and Meta-Analysis of Randomized Clinical Trials." Journal of Medicinal Food, 2016).

By integrating these foods into your diet, you can support your body's natural pain management systems, reduce inflammation, and promote healing, all of which are essential components of a holistic approach to health.

CHAPTER 3: NATURAL REMEDIES FOR PAIN RELIEF

Harnessing the power of nature, we delve into the realm of herbal remedies that offer relief from pain, a common ailment that affects many. These natural solutions not only aim to alleviate pain but also target the underlying causes, such as inflammation, without the side effects often associated with conventional medications. By integrating these remedies into your wellness routine, you can embrace a more holistic approach to managing pain.

Beneficial effects: The selected herbs and natural compounds are renowned for their analgesic (pain-relieving) and anti-inflammatory properties. They work synergistically to reduce pain, combat inflammation, and promote healing. These remedies are particularly beneficial for those suffering from joint pain, muscle aches, headaches, and chronic conditions like arthritis.

Ingredients:

- Willow Bark: Often referred to as "nature's aspirin," willow bark contains salicin, which the body converts into salicylic acid, providing pain relief and anti-inflammatory benefits.

- Arnica: Applied topically, arnica can significantly reduce pain and swelling associated with bruises, aches, and sprains.

- Capsaicin: Derived from chili peppers, capsaicin cream temporarily desensitizes nerve receptors called C-fibers, which are responsible for pain sensations.

- Turmeric: Curcumin, the active compound in turmeric, is a potent anti-inflammatory that can relieve pain, particularly in the joints.

- Peppermint Oil: Applied topically, peppermint oil creates a cooling sensation that can temporarily relieve muscle and joint pain.

- Lavender Oil: Known for its calming and anti-inflammatory properties, lavender oil can help ease headache and migraine pain when inhaled or applied topically.

Instructions:

1. For willow bark, prepare a tea by simmering 1 to 2 teaspoons of the dried bark in 8 ounces of water for 10 to 15 minutes. Drink this tea up to twice daily.

2. Apply arnica gel or cream to the affected area, but avoid broken skin or open wounds. Use up to four times daily.

3. Gradually introduce capsaicin cream by applying a small amount to the painful area, allowing your body to adjust to the heat. Use up to four times daily.

4. Incorporate turmeric into your diet by adding it to meals or taking a supplement as directed by a healthcare provider. For a direct remedy, mix 1 teaspoon of turmeric with a glass of warm milk or water and drink once daily.

5. Mix a few drops of peppermint oil with a carrier oil and massage onto sore muscles or joints. Avoid broken skin.

6. For headaches, add a few drops of lavender oil to a diffuser or apply diluted oil to temples.

Variations:

- Combine turmeric with black pepper to enhance absorption and effectiveness.

- For a soothing bath, add Epsom salts and a few drops of lavender or peppermint oil to warm water.

Storage tips:

- Store dried herbs in a cool, dark place in airtight containers.

- Keep essential oils in dark glass bottles away from direct sunlight.

Tips for allergens:

- Patch test topical remedies to ensure no allergic reaction.

- Consult a healthcare provider before consuming herbal supplements, especially if pregnant, nursing, or on medication.

Scientific references:

- A study published in the "Journal of Ethnopharmacology" supports the use of willow bark for pain relief and anti-inflammatory effects.

- Research in the "International Journal of Rheumatic Diseases" found that curcumin in turmeric effectively reduces joint pain in arthritis patients.

- The "Journal of Alternative and Complementary Medicine" published findings on the analgesic effects of peppermint oil and lavender oil in headache treatment.

By embracing these natural remedies for pain relief, individuals can explore the benefits of a holistic approach to health, utilizing the healing powers of plants to address pain and inflammation.

CHAPTER 4: 5 HERBAL RECIPES FOR PAIN MANAGEMENT

WHITE WILLOW BARK AND TURMERIC PAIN RELIEF TEA

Beneficial effects

White Willow Bark and Turmeric Pain Relief Tea combines the anti-inflammatory properties of turmeric with the natural pain-relieving qualities of white willow bark. This herbal blend is designed to reduce pain, inflammation, and discomfort associated with conditions like arthritis, headaches, and muscle pain. Turmeric contains curcumin, a compound known for its potent anti-inflammatory effects, while white willow bark acts as a natural aspirin, providing relief from pain without the side effects of synthetic drugs.

Portions

2 servings

Preparation time

5 minutes

Cooking time

15 minutes

Ingredients

- 1 teaspoon of dried white willow bark

- 1 teaspoon of turmeric powder

- 4 cups of water

- Honey or lemon to taste (optional)

Instructions

1. Bring 4 cups of water to a boil in a medium-sized pot.

2. Add the dried white willow bark and turmeric powder to the boiling water.

3. Reduce the heat and simmer for about 15 minutes to allow the herbs to infuse their properties into the water.

4. After simmering, remove the pot from the heat and let the tea cool slightly.

5. Strain the tea into cups, discarding the solids.

6. Optional: Add honey or lemon to taste for flavor enhancement.

7. Serve the tea warm to enjoy its pain-relieving benefits.

Variations

- For added anti-inflammatory benefits, include a slice of fresh ginger or a cinnamon stick in the tea while it simmers.

- Mix in a teaspoon of green tea leaves during the last 5 minutes of simmering for an antioxidant boost.

- For a cold beverage, allow the tea to cool and serve over ice for a refreshing pain relief drink.

Storage tips

Store any leftover White Willow Bark and Turmeric Pain Relief Tea in a sealed container in the refrigerator for up to 2 days. Enjoy it chilled, or gently reheat on the stove.

Tips for allergens

Individuals with allergies to salicylates (found in aspirin) should proceed with caution when using white willow bark. For those avoiding honey due to dietary restrictions, substitute with maple syrup or simply omit the sweetener.

Scientific references

- "Anti-inflammatory properties of curcumin, a major constituent of Curcuma longa: A review of preclinical and clinical research" published in Alternative Medicine Review, highlights turmeric's curcumin as an effective anti-inflammatory agent.

- "Willow bark extract: the contribution of polyphenols to the overall effect" in the journal Wiener Medizinische Wochenschrift discusses the pain-relieving effects of white willow bark, supporting its use in natural pain management.

DEVIL'S CLAW AND GINGER PAIN RELIEF TONIC

Beneficial effects

Devil's Claw and Ginger Pain Relief Tonic is designed to alleviate pain and reduce inflammation naturally. Devil's Claw, known for its anti-inflammatory properties, can help relieve symptoms of arthritis, back pain, and other musculoskeletal conditions. Ginger, with its potent anti-inflammatory and antioxidant effects, further enhances the tonic's ability to reduce pain and stiffness in joints and muscles. Together, they create a powerful remedy that supports pain management and promotes overall joint health.

Portions

2 servings

Preparation time

10 minutes

Ingredients

- 2 teaspoons of dried Devil's Claw root

- 1 inch of fresh ginger root, thinly sliced

- 4 cups of water

- Honey or lemon to taste (optional)

Instructions

1. Bring 4 cups of water to a boil in a medium-sized pot.

2. Add the dried Devil's Claw root and sliced ginger to the boiling water.

3. Reduce the heat and simmer for about 20 minutes to allow the herbs to infuse their properties into the water.

4. After simmering, remove the pot from the heat and allow the tonic to cool slightly.

5. Strain the tonic to remove the Devil's Claw and ginger pieces.

6. Optional: Add honey or lemon to taste for flavor enhancement.

7. Serve the tonic warm, ideally in the morning and evening, to help manage pain and inflammation.

Variations

- For an added boost of anti-inflammatory properties, include a teaspoon of turmeric powder during the simmering process.

- To enhance the tonic's soothing effects, add a chamomile tea bag in the last 5 minutes of simmering.

- For those preferring a cold beverage, chill the tonic in the refrigerator and serve over ice with a sprig of mint for a refreshing twist.

Storage tips

Store any leftover Devil's Claw and Ginger Pain Relief Tonic in a sealed container in the refrigerator for up to 48 hours. Enjoy chilled or gently reheat on the stove.

Tips for allergens

Individuals with sensitivities to Devil's Claw or ginger should start with a smaller dose to ensure no adverse reactions. For those avoiding honey due to dietary restrictions, substitute with maple syrup or simply omit the sweetener.

Scientific references

- "A randomized, double-blind, placebo-controlled trial of Devil's Claw for the treatment of arthritis," published in the Journal of Rheumatology, highlights the efficacy of Devil's Claw in reducing arthritis pain.

- "Ginger—An Herbal Medicinal Product with Broad Anti-Inflammatory Actions," in the Journal of Medicinal Food, discusses ginger's role in reducing inflammation and its potential as a pain relief agent.

BOSWELLIA AND FRANKINCENSE PAIN RELIEF BALM

Beneficial effects

The Boswellia and Frankincense Pain Relief Balm combines the anti-inflammatory and analgesic properties of Boswellia serrata and Frankincense essential oil to create a potent natural remedy for pain management. Boswellia serrata, also known as Indian frankincense, has been shown to reduce inflammation and pain in conditions such as osteoarthritis and rheumatoid arthritis. Frankincense essential oil complements these effects by further reducing inflammation and supporting joint health. Together, they offer a synergistic approach to relieving pain, improving mobility, and enhancing the quality of life for individuals suffering from chronic pain conditions.

Ingredients

- 1/4 cup coconut oil

- 1/4 cup beeswax pellets

- 2 tablespoons Boswellia serrata extract powder

- 20 drops Frankincense essential oil

- 10 drops Lavender essential oil (for additional pain relief and soothing properties)

- 1 tablespoon Olive oil (as a carrier oil)

Instructions

1. In a double boiler, melt the coconut oil and beeswax pellets together over medium heat until completely liquid.

2. Reduce the heat to low and stir in the Boswellia serrata extract powder until it is fully dissolved.

3. Remove the mixture from heat and allow it to cool slightly before adding the Frankincense and Lavender essential oils. Stir well to ensure the essential oils are evenly distributed.

4. Quickly stir in the olive oil to the mixture.

5. Pour the mixture into small jars or tins before it begins to harden. Allow the balm to cool and solidify completely at room temperature.

6. Once solidified, close the jars or tins with lids to store.

Variations

- For a vegan version, substitute beeswax with candelilla wax, using half the amount as it is denser than beeswax.

- Add a few drops of Peppermint essential oil for a cooling effect that can further soothe sore muscles and joints.

- For those with sensitive skin, reduce the amount of essential oil or perform a patch test prior to application.

Storage tips

Store the Boswellia and Frankincense Pain Relief Balm in a cool, dry place away from direct sunlight. If stored properly, the balm can last for up to a year.

Tips for allergens

Individuals with allergies to beeswax or coconut oil can substitute beeswax with soy wax and coconut oil with shea butter or another preferred carrier oil. Always ensure to use high-quality, pure essential oils to minimize the risk of skin irritation.

Scientific references

- "Boswellia serrata, a potential antiinflammatory agent: an overview" published in the Indian Journal of Pharmaceutical Sciences, highlights the anti-inflammatory properties of Boswellia serrata.

- "Frankincense: systematic review" in the British Medical Journal discusses the analgesic and anti-inflammatory effects of Frankincense essential oil, supporting its use in pain management.

ARNICA AND ST. JOHN'S WORT PAIN RELIEF OIL

Beneficial effects

Arnica and St. John's Wort Pain Relief Oil combines the potent anti-inflammatory properties of Arnica montana with the nerve-soothing benefits of St. John's Wort (Hypericum perforatum), making it an effective natural remedy for reducing pain, swelling, and bruising. This oil can be particularly beneficial for those suffering from arthritis, muscle soreness, and injuries. Arnica is known for its ability to alleviate pain and reduce inflammation, while St. John's Wort is recognized for its nerve-regenerative properties, helping to soothe nerve pain and heal damaged tissues.

Ingredients

- 1/4 cup dried Arnica montana flowers
- 1/4 cup dried St. John's Wort flowers
- 1 cup carrier oil (such as olive oil or almond oil)

Instructions

1. Combine the dried Arnica montana and St. John's Wort flowers in a clean, dry glass jar.

2. Pour the carrier oil over the flowers, ensuring they are completely submerged.

3. Seal the jar tightly and place it in a warm, sunny spot for 4 to 6 weeks, shaking the jar gently every few days to mix the contents.

4. After the infusion period, strain the oil through a fine mesh sieve or cheesecloth into another clean, dry glass bottle, squeezing out as much oil as possible from the flowers.

5. Label the bottle with the contents and date of production.

Variations

- For added pain relief, include a few drops of lavender essential oil or peppermint essential oil to the strained oil for their additional anti-inflammatory and soothing properties.

- To accelerate the infusion process, gently heat the oil and herbs in a double boiler over low heat for 2 to 3 hours instead of the solar infusion method.

Storage tips

Store the Arnica and St. John's Wort Pain Relief Oil in a cool, dark place. When stored properly, the oil can last for up to a year. Ensure the bottle is tightly sealed to maintain potency.

Tips for allergens

Individuals with sensitivity to Arnica montana, St. John's Wort, or the chosen carrier oil should perform a patch test before widespread use. For those allergic to nuts, ensure to select a nut-free carrier oil like olive oil.

Scientific references

- "Arnica montana L. – a plant of healing: review" published in the Journal of Pharmacy and Pharmacology, 2017. This study discusses the anti-inflammatory and healing properties of Arnica montana, supporting its use in topical applications for muscle soreness and bruises.

- "Hypericum perforatum L. (St John's wort) for depression – a systematic review" in the Cochrane Database of Systematic Reviews, highlighting the nerve-regenerative properties of St. John's Wort, which can be beneficial in soothing nerve pain and enhancing tissue healing.

CAYENNE AND PEPPERMINT PAIN RELIEF CREAM

Beneficial effects

Cayenne and Peppermint Pain Relief Cream combines the powerful analgesic properties of cayenne pepper with the cooling, soothing effects of peppermint oil to create an effective topical remedy for relieving pain. Cayenne pepper contains capsaicin, which is known to reduce pain sensations when applied to the skin. Peppermint oil provides a cooling sensation that can distract from pain and reduce discomfort. This cream is particularly beneficial for those suffering from muscle aches, joint pain, and nerve pain, offering a natural alternative to over-the-counter pain relief creams.

Ingredients

- 1/4 cup coconut oil
- 2 tablespoons beeswax pellets
- 1 teaspoon cayenne pepper powder
- 10 drops peppermint essential oil
- 1/2 teaspoon turmeric powder (optional, for added anti-inflammatory benefits)
- 1/4 cup shea butter (for added moisture)

Instructions

1. In a double boiler, melt the coconut oil and beeswax pellets together over low heat.

2. Once melted, remove from heat and allow the mixture to cool slightly.

3. Carefully stir in the cayenne pepper powder and turmeric powder, if using, until fully incorporated.

4. Add the peppermint essential oil and stir again to ensure even distribution.

5. Finally, mix in the shea butter until the mixture is smooth and uniform.

6. Pour the cream into a clean jar and allow it to solidify at room temperature or in the refrigerator for faster setting.

7. To use, apply a small amount of the cream to the affected area, gently massaging into the skin. Avoid contact with eyes and mucous membranes.

Variations

- For a vegan version, substitute beeswax with candelilla wax.

- Add a few drops of lavender essential oil for additional pain relief and a calming scent.

- For those with sensitive skin, reduce the amount of cayenne pepper powder and increase the shea butter to dilute the capsaicin's intensity.

Storage tips

Store the Cayenne and Peppermint Pain Relief Cream in a cool, dark place. If stored properly in an airtight container, the cream can last for up to 6 months.

Tips for allergens

Individuals with allergies to capsaicin, peppermint, or other ingredients should perform a patch test on a small area of the skin before widespread use. For those allergic to coconut oil, substitute with another carrier oil such as almond oil or olive oil.

Scientific references

- "Capsaicin: Current Understanding of Its Mechanisms and Therapy of Pain and Other Pre-Clinical and Clinical Uses," in Molecules, 2016. This study discusses the pain-relieving mechanisms of capsaicin found in cayenne pepper.

- "Peppermint Oil: Clinical Uses in the Treatment of Gastrointestinal Diseases," in JSM Gastroenterology and Hepatology, 2015. While focusing on gastrointestinal uses, this article highlights the soothing and analgesic properties of peppermint oil that are applicable to topical pain relief.

PART 24: MANAGING CHRONIC DISEASES NATURALLY

Managing chronic diseases naturally involves a holistic approach that focuses on lifestyle modifications, dietary changes, and the use of herbal remedies to support the body's healing processes and mitigate symptoms. Chronic diseases such as diabetes, heart disease, arthritis, and autoimmune conditions can often be managed effectively with a comprehensive plan that addresses the root causes of the disease rather than just treating symptoms. A key component of this approach is the emphasis on nutrition as a foundational element for health. A diet rich in whole, unprocessed foods provides the body with essential nutrients that support immune function, reduce inflammation, and promote overall well-being.

Incorporating anti-inflammatory foods such as leafy greens, berries, nuts, seeds, and fatty fish can make a significant difference in managing chronic conditions.

In addition to dietary changes, physical activity is another crucial aspect of managing chronic diseases naturally. Regular exercise helps to improve cardiovascular health, maintain a healthy weight, reduce inflammation, and enhance mood.

Activities such as walking, yoga, swimming, and cycling can be adapted to fit the individual's fitness level and preferences, making it easier to incorporate into daily life.

Stress management techniques such as meditation, deep breathing exercises, and mindfulness can also play a significant role in managing chronic diseases. Chronic stress has been linked to a variety of health issues, including exacerbating symptoms of chronic diseases. By finding effective ways to manage stress, individuals can improve their quality of life and potentially reduce the impact of chronic conditions.

Herbal remedies offer natural support for managing chronic diseases, providing therapeutic benefits without the side effects often associated with conventional medications. Herbs such as turmeric, ginger, and cinnamon have been shown to have anti-inflammatory and antioxidant properties, which can be beneficial for individuals with chronic conditions.

However, it's important to consult with a healthcare provider before starting any herbal supplement, especially for those with existing health conditions or those taking prescription medications, to avoid potential interactions.

Hydration is another key element in the natural management of chronic diseases. Adequate water intake supports detoxification, aids digestion, and helps maintain cellular health.

Often overlooked, hydration plays a vital role in the body's overall function and can impact the management of chronic conditions.

Sleep is an often underestimated but critical component of managing chronic diseases naturally. Quality sleep supports healing, reduces stress, and helps regulate hormones that control appetite and metabolism. Establishing a regular sleep routine, creating a restful environment, and addressing any sleep disorders can significantly contribute to the management of chronic diseases.

By adopting a holistic approach that includes these components, individuals with chronic diseases can empower themselves to manage their conditions more effectively, improving their quality of life and potentially reducing their reliance on conventional medications.

This approach requires a commitment to lifestyle changes and a willingness to explore various strategies to find what works best for the individual.

Embracing a holistic approach to managing chronic diseases naturally extends beyond diet and exercise into the realms of environmental and personal care products. The chemicals found in everyday cleaning agents, beauty products, and even in our water supply can contribute to the body's toxic burden, exacerbating chronic conditions. Opting for natural, non-toxic products helps reduce exposure to harmful chemicals and supports the body's healing processes.

This shift towards greener alternatives is not only beneficial for personal health but also for the environment, aligning with the principles of a holistic lifestyle that respects and nurtures both human health and the planet.

Personal relationships and social support networks play a significant role in managing chronic diseases. The emotional and psychological support from friends, family, and community resources can provide comfort, reduce stress, and encourage positive lifestyle changes. Engaging in support groups, whether in person or online, offers the opportunity to share experiences, strategies, and encouragement with others facing similar challenges. This sense of community and belonging is crucial for mental and emotional well-being, which in turn impacts physical health.

Detoxification practices such as dry brushing, sauna use, and lymphatic drainage massages can further support the body's natural healing processes.

These practices enhance circulation, promote the elimination of toxins, and support immune function, complementing the dietary and lifestyle changes aimed at managing chronic diseases. While these methods are beneficial, it's important to approach detoxification gently and with guidance from a healthcare professional, especially for individuals with chronic conditions.

The role of supplements in managing chronic diseases cannot be overlooked. While a whole-foods-based diet is foundational, certain nutrients may be difficult to obtain in adequate amounts through diet alone. Supplements such as omega-3 fatty acids, vitamin D, probiotics, and magnesium can fill nutritional gaps and support overall health.

However, it's crucial to choose high-quality supplements and to consult with a healthcare provider to ensure they are appropriate for your specific health needs and conditions.

Finally, embracing a holistic approach to managing chronic diseases naturally is an ongoing journey rather than a destination. It involves continuous learning, experimentation, and adjustment to find the balance that works best for each individual.

This path encourages a deeper connection with one's body, leading to greater self-awareness and self-care. By integrating these principles into daily life, individuals with chronic diseases can enhance their well-being, reduce symptoms, and potentially minimize their reliance on conventional medical treatments. This holistic perspective empowers individuals to take control of their health, advocating for a balanced and integrated approach to wellness that honors the interconnectedness of the mind, body, and spirit.

CHAPTER 1: UNDERSTANDING CHRONIC DISEASES

Chronic diseases, often long-term and progressive, are becoming increasingly prevalent in today's society, affecting millions worldwide. These conditions, such as heart disease, diabetes, arthritis, and autoimmune diseases, have complex causes that include genetics, environmental factors, lifestyle choices, and diet. The management of chronic diseases requires a comprehensive approach that goes beyond conventional medicine's focus on symptoms, aiming instead to address the root causes and promote overall well-being.

At the heart of managing chronic diseases naturally is the understanding that the body is an interconnected system where physical, emotional, and environmental factors all play a critical role. A diet rich in whole, unprocessed foods provides essential nutrients that can support the body's immune function, reduce inflammation, and promote healing.

Foods high in antioxidants, fiber, healthy fats, and phytonutrients can help counteract the oxidative stress and inflammation that are common in many chronic conditions.

Physical activity is another cornerstone of natural chronic disease management. Regular exercise not only helps in maintaining a healthy weight but also improves insulin sensitivity, reduces blood pressure, and enhances cardiovascular health. It can also boost mood and reduce symptoms of anxiety and depression, which are often associated with chronic illnesses. The type and intensity of exercise should be tailored to the individual's capabilities and preferences, emphasizing the importance of finding enjoyable activities that can be sustained long-term.

Stress management is equally crucial in the holistic approach to chronic disease. Chronic stress can exacerbate many health conditions by triggering inflammation and hormonal imbalances. Techniques such as meditation, yoga, deep breathing exercises, and mindfulness can help mitigate stress's negative effects on the body.

These practices not only promote relaxation but also enhance the body's resilience to stress, improving overall health and well-being.

Herbal remedies and supplements offer additional support in managing chronic diseases. Many herbs have been used for centuries for their medicinal properties, offering natural ways to support the body's healing processes.

Turmeric, for example, contains curcumin, a compound with potent anti-inflammatory and antioxidant properties, making it beneficial for conditions like arthritis and heart disease. Similarly, omega-3 supplements can reduce inflammation and are beneficial for heart health. However, it's essential to consult with a healthcare provider before starting any new supplement, especially for individuals with existing health conditions or those taking prescription medications.

Hydration plays a vital role in the body's overall function and can impact the management of chronic conditions.

Adequate water intake supports detoxification, aids digestion, and helps maintain cellular health. Similarly, ensuring quality sleep is critical for healing and recovery. Poor sleep can exacerbate chronic pain, affect mental health, and impair immune function. Establishing a regular sleep routine and creating a restful environment can help improve sleep quality, contributing to better management of chronic diseases.

The holistic approach to managing chronic diseases emphasizes the importance of a balanced lifestyle that incorporates dietary changes, physical activity, stress management, and natural remedies. This approach recognizes the individual as a whole, considering the intricate interplay between various factors that influence health. By adopting a comprehensive strategy that addresses these diverse aspects, individuals with chronic diseases can improve their quality of life and potentially reduce their reliance on conventional medical treatments.

Environmental factors also play a significant role in the natural management of chronic diseases. Exposure to pollutants, chemicals, and toxins can exacerbate symptoms and contribute to the progression of these conditions. Embracing a lifestyle that minimizes exposure to harmful substances is crucial. This can include using natural cleaning products, eating organic foods to reduce pesticide intake, and avoiding plastic containers to decrease exposure to endocrine-disrupting chemicals. Making these changes can help reduce the body's toxic burden and support overall health.

Personal care is another aspect that requires attention. The skin, being the largest organ, absorbs a significant amount of what we apply to it. Switching to natural, non-toxic personal care products can decrease the exposure to synthetic chemicals that may interfere with hormone balance and contribute to chronic health issues. This shift not only benefits personal health but also supports environmental sustainability.

The importance of a supportive community and positive relationships cannot be overstated in managing chronic diseases. Social support can provide emotional comfort, reduce stress, and encourage healthy lifestyle changes. Engaging in community activities, joining support groups, or even participating in online forums can offer valuable connections, advice, and encouragement. These social interactions can enhance mental health, which is intrinsically linked to physical health, creating a positive feedback loop that supports overall well-being.

Detoxification practices, while often overlooked, can be a valuable component of a holistic approach to chronic disease management. Techniques such as dry brushing, sauna use, and lymphatic drainage massages can enhance the body's natural detoxification processes, helping to eliminate toxins and reduce inflammation. These practices, coupled with a diet rich in detoxifying foods, can support the liver and kidneys, the body's primary detox organs, and contribute to improved health.

The role of supplements in filling nutritional gaps and supporting the body's healing processes is also significant. For instance, vitamin D deficiency is common in many chronic conditions and supplementing with vitamin D can support immune function, bone health, and reduce inflammation. Magnesium, known for its muscle-relaxing and nerve-function benefits, can help manage pain and improve sleep. Probiotics can support gut health, which is crucial for immune function and nutrient absorption. It's essential to choose high-quality supplements and consult with a healthcare provider to ensure they are appropriate and safe.

Finally, adopting a holistic approach to managing chronic diseases requires a commitment to continuous learning and self-care. It involves being proactive about health, staying informed about the latest research, and being willing to adjust lifestyle choices as needed. This approach empowers individuals to take control of their health, making informed decisions that support their well-being. It's a journey that acknowledges the complexity of chronic diseases and respects the body's capacity for healing and resilience. By integrating these principles, individuals can navigate their health challenges with greater confidence and improve their quality of life, demonstrating the power of a holistic, natural approach to health.

CHAPTER 2: NUTRITION FOR CHRONIC DISEASE MANAGEMENT

Adopting nutritional strategies for managing chronic diseases focuses on a diet that supports the body's natural healing processes, reduces inflammation, and provides essential nutrients to mitigate symptoms and potentially reverse disease progression. The foundation of this approach is a whole-food, plant-based diet rich in fruits, vegetables, whole grains, nuts, seeds, and legumes. These foods are packed with phytonutrients, antioxidants, fiber, and healthy fats that work together to support immune function, decrease inflammation, and promote overall health.

Fruits and vegetables, the cornerstone of a nutrient-dense diet, offer a wide array of vitamins, minerals, and antioxidants that protect the body from oxidative stress, a key factor in the development and progression of many chronic diseases. Incorporating a variety of colorful fruits and vegetables ensures a broad spectrum of these protective compounds. For instance, leafy greens are high in vitamin K, essential for bone health, while berries provide antioxidants that support brain function and reduce the risk of heart disease.

Whole grains contribute essential fibers, B vitamins, and minerals like iron, magnesium, and selenium. The fiber in whole grains not only aids digestion but also helps regulate blood sugar levels, crucial for managing diabetes and supporting cardiovascular health. Opting for whole grains over refined grains enhances nutrient intake and provides sustained energy throughout the day.

Nuts and seeds are excellent sources of healthy fats, including omega-3 fatty acids, which have anti-inflammatory properties beneficial for heart health and autoimmune conditions. They also supply protein, fiber, and essential nutrients like vitamin E, magnesium, and zinc. Incorporating a small portion of nuts and seeds into daily meals can improve lipid profiles and support brain health.

Legumes, including beans, lentils, and chickpeas, are rich in protein, fiber, iron, and folate. They are particularly beneficial for heart health, weight management, and diabetes control due to their low glycemic index and ability to improve cholesterol levels. Regular consumption of legumes can also support gut health by providing prebiotic fibers that nourish beneficial gut bacteria.

Healthy fats, particularly those from plant sources like avocados, olive oil, and flaxseeds, play a crucial role in managing chronic diseases. These fats are essential for absorbing fat-soluble vitamins, reducing inflammation, and maintaining cell membrane integrity. Choosing unsaturated fats over saturated and trans fats can help reduce the risk of heart disease and improve overall health.

Hydration is another key aspect of nutritional strategies for chronic disease management. Adequate water intake supports every cellular function, aids in detoxification, and helps maintain blood volume and pressure. It's essential to drink enough water throughout the day and to limit intake of sugary beverages, which can contribute to obesity, diabetes, and other health issues.

In addition to these dietary foundations, specific foods and nutrients may have targeted benefits for certain chronic conditions. For example, incorporating turmeric, known for its curcumin content, can provide anti-inflammatory benefits useful in conditions like arthritis and heart disease. Similarly, foods high in calcium and vitamin D are important for bone health, particularly in preventing and managing osteoporosis.

As dietary needs and responses to foods can vary widely among individuals, especially those with chronic diseases, it's important to personalize nutrition plans. Working with a healthcare provider or a dietitian can help tailor dietary choices to meet individual health needs, preferences, and goals. This personalized approach ensures that nutritional strategies not only help manage chronic diseases but also contribute to overall well-being and quality of life.

Monitoring portion sizes and meal timing plays a significant role in managing chronic diseases effectively. Eating smaller, balanced meals throughout the day can help stabilize blood sugar levels, manage weight, and reduce the risk of cardiovascular diseases. It's crucial for individuals, especially those with diabetes or metabolic syndrome, to understand the impact of meal timing and portion control on their health outcomes. Incorporating a variety of foods in the right proportions ensures that the body receives a balanced mix of nutrients without excessive calories that can lead to weight gain and exacerbate chronic conditions.

Spices and herbs, beyond adding flavor to meals, offer significant health benefits and can be powerful allies in managing chronic diseases. For instance, cinnamon has been shown to improve insulin sensitivity and lower blood sugar levels, making it beneficial for people with type 2 diabetes. Garlic has been found to have cardiovascular benefits, including lowering blood pressure and cholesterol levels. Incorporating these natural flavor enhancers not only enriches the diet but also contributes to disease management and prevention.

Fermented foods such as yogurt, kefir, sauerkraut, and kimchi are rich in probiotics, which are beneficial for gut health. A healthy gut microbiome is linked to improved digestion, enhanced immune function, and a reduced risk of several chronic diseases. By promoting a healthy balance of gut bacteria, fermented foods can play a role in managing autoimmune diseases, obesity, and even mental health conditions through the gut-brain axis.

Antioxidant-rich beverages like green tea and herbal teas offer hydration with the added benefit of polyphenols, which may protect against chronic diseases by reducing inflammation and oxidative stress. Swapping sugary drinks for these healthier options can contribute to better blood sugar control, weight management, and overall health.

Physical activity, in conjunction with a balanced diet, amplifies the benefits of nutritional strategies for chronic disease management. Regular exercise improves cardiovascular health, aids in weight management, enhances insulin sensitivity, and boosts mood and energy levels. Even moderate activities, such as walking or yoga, can have profound health benefits when incorporated into a daily routine.

Stress reduction techniques, including mindfulness, deep breathing, and adequate sleep, complement nutritional strategies by mitigating the impact of stress on chronic diseases. Chronic stress can lead to poor dietary choices, weight gain, and a host of metabolic disturbances. By addressing stress, individuals can improve their capacity to make healthier food choices and adhere to a nutritional plan that supports disease management.

Finally, ongoing education and support are essential for sustaining dietary changes over the long term. Engaging with support groups, seeking information from credible sources, and regular consultations with healthcare professionals can provide the motivation and knowledge needed to navigate the complexities of managing chronic diseases through diet.

By integrating these comprehensive strategies, individuals can harness the power of nutrition to support their health and well-being, demonstrating the critical role of diet in the prevention, management, and potential reversal of chronic diseases. This holistic approach, focusing on whole foods, balanced nutrients, and a healthy lifestyle, empowers individuals to take control of their health and improve their quality of life amidst chronic conditions.

CHAPTER 3: NATURAL REMEDIES FOR CHRONIC DISEASES

Chronic diseases, characterized by their long-term impact and often complex etiology, can benefit significantly from the targeted use of specific natural compounds known for their healing properties.

Turmeric, a spice renowned for its curcumin content, stands out for its potent anti-inflammatory and antioxidant effects. Regular incorporation of turmeric into the diet or as a supplement can help reduce inflammation, a common underlying factor in many chronic conditions such as arthritis, heart disease, and certain forms of cancer. The beneficial effects of turmeric are maximized when combined with black pepper, which contains piperine, a compound that enhances the absorption of curcumin by the body.

Ginger, another spice with a long history of medicinal use, offers remarkable anti-inflammatory and analgesic properties. It works by inhibiting the synthesis of pro-inflammatory compounds and has been shown to be effective in reducing pain and stiffness in osteoarthritis and rheumatoid arthritis. Ginger can be consumed fresh, dried, or as an extract, making it a versatile addition to the natural remedy toolkit.

Omega-3 fatty acids, found abundantly in fish oil, flaxseeds, and walnuts, are crucial for managing inflammation and supporting cardiovascular health. These essential fats have been shown to lower levels of triglycerides and reduce the risk of heart disease. For individuals with chronic diseases, supplementing with omega-3 fatty acids can be a strategic move to counteract inflammation and protect heart health.

Adaptogenic herbs like ashwagandha, rhodiola, and holy basil play a unique role in managing chronic diseases by helping the body resist stressors of all kinds, whether physical, chemical, or biological. These herbs have been used traditionally to improve energy levels, reduce stress-induced damage, and support overall vitality.

Their ability to modulate the immune system and enhance stress resilience makes them particularly valuable in the holistic management of chronic conditions.

Probiotics, beneficial bacteria found in fermented foods like yogurt, kefir, and sauerkraut, contribute to gut health, which is pivotal in the management of chronic diseases.

A healthy gut microbiome can influence the body's immune response, reduce inflammation, and even impact mental health through the gut-brain axis. Incorporating probiotic-rich foods into the diet or taking a high-quality probiotic supplement can support digestive health and by extension, overall well-being.

Antioxidant-rich foods such as berries, nuts, dark leafy greens, and green tea contain compounds that protect the body from oxidative stress, a condition linked to chronic disease progression.

By neutralizing free radicals, antioxidants can prevent cellular damage and support the body's natural repair mechanisms. A diet rich in these nutrients supports the management of chronic diseases by bolstering the body's defenses against oxidative stress.

In addition to these specific remedies, maintaining adequate hydration is essential for overall health and the effective management of chronic diseases.

Water supports every cellular function, aids in the elimination of toxins, and helps to transport nutrients throughout the body. Ensuring a sufficient intake of water can enhance the efficacy of natural remedies by facilitating their absorption and distribution.

As we continue to explore the realm of natural remedies for chronic disease management, it's important to remember that these strategies should complement, not replace, conventional medical treatments. Working in tandem with healthcare providers to integrate natural remedies into a comprehensive care plan can offer a holistic approach to managing chronic diseases, emphasizing the body's inherent capacity for healing and the powerful role of nature in supporting health and wellness.

Magnesium, an essential mineral, plays a crucial role in over 300 enzymatic reactions in the human body, including those involved in the regulation of blood pressure, muscle and nerve function, and blood sugar control. Its anti-inflammatory properties make it particularly beneficial for individuals with chronic diseases such as heart disease and diabetes. Magnesium can be found in foods like almonds, spinach, black beans, and whole grains, or taken as a supplement to ensure adequate daily intake. This mineral not only supports the body's physiological functions but also aids in the mitigation of chronic disease symptoms, particularly those related to muscle and nerve discomfort.

Vitamin D, often referred to as the "sunshine vitamin," is another critical nutrient for chronic disease management. Its role in bone health is well-known, but its importance extends to immune function and inflammation reduction. Vitamin D deficiency has been linked to an increased risk of chronic diseases, including cardiovascular diseases, diabetes, and certain cancers. Adequate levels can be maintained through regular sun exposure, dietary sources like fatty fish and fortified foods, or supplementation as advised by a healthcare provider.

Herbal teas, such as green tea, chamomile, and hibiscus, offer therapeutic benefits beyond hydration. Green tea is rich in catechins, antioxidants that protect against cellular damage and support heart health. Chamomile has a long history of use for its calming effects and potential to support digestive health, while hibiscus tea has been shown to lower blood pressure and offer liver protective benefits. Incorporating these teas into daily routines can provide a comforting, healing ritual that supports chronic disease management.

Essential oils, including frankincense and myrrh, have been used for centuries for their medicinal properties. Frankincense oil has been researched for its anti-inflammatory and analgesic properties, making it beneficial for individuals with arthritis and other inflammatory conditions. Myrrh oil is recognized for its antioxidant and antimicrobial benefits, supporting immune health and wound healing. Used in aromatherapy or topically with a carrier oil, these essential oils can be a valuable addition to a natural chronic disease management plan.

Selenium, a trace mineral, plays a pivotal role in the maintenance of immune function and antioxidant defense systems. Its intake is associated with reduced risk of certain cancers and heart disease. Selenium's protective effects are attributed to its role in the production of glutathione peroxidase, an enzyme that helps reduce oxidative stress. Foods rich in selenium include Brazil nuts, seafood, and eggs, making them beneficial additions to a diet focused on managing chronic diseases.

In conclusion, managing chronic diseases naturally encompasses a broad spectrum of strategies, including the use of specific nutrients, herbs, and other natural remedies. These approaches aim to support the body's healing processes, reduce symptoms, and improve quality of life. While natural remedies offer significant benefits, they should be used in conjunction with conventional medical treatments and under the guidance of healthcare professionals. By adopting a holistic approach to health, individuals with chronic diseases can harness the power of natural remedies to support their journey towards wellness and vitality.

CHAPTER 4: HERBAL REMEDIES FOR CHRONIC DISEASES

ASHWAGANDHA AND HOLY BASIL ADAPTOGEN TEA

Beneficial effects

Ashwagandha and Holy Basil Adaptogen Tea is crafted to combat stress, enhance mental clarity, and improve overall well-being. Ashwagandha, known for its stress-reducing properties, helps to lower cortisol levels and combat the effects of stress on the body. Holy Basil, or Tulsi, complements Ashwagandha with its own adaptogenic properties, promoting mental balance and reducing anxiety. Together, they create a powerful tea that supports the body's natural resilience to stress and fosters a sense of calm and focus.

Portions

2 servings

Preparation time

5 minutes

Cooking time

10 minutes

Ingredients

- 1 teaspoon dried Ashwagandha root
- 1 teaspoon dried Holy Basil (Tulsi) leaves
- 2 cups of water
- Honey or lemon to taste (optional)

Instructions

1. Bring 2 cups of water to a boil in a small pot.

2. Add the dried Ashwagandha root and Holy Basil leaves to the boiling water.

3. Reduce the heat and simmer for about 10 minutes, allowing the herbs to infuse their properties into the water.

4. After simmering, remove the pot from the heat and allow the tea to cool for a few minutes.

5. Strain the tea into cups, discarding the Ashwagandha and Holy Basil.

6. Optional: Add honey or lemon to taste for flavor enhancement.

7. Serve the tea warm to enjoy its adaptogenic benefits.

Variations

- For a cooling summer drink, allow the tea to cool completely, then refrigerate and serve over ice.
- Mix in a cinnamon stick during simmering for added flavor and potential blood sugar regulation benefits.
- Combine with green tea during the last 5 minutes of simmering for an added antioxidant boost.

Storage tips

Store any leftover Ashwagandha and Holy Basil Adaptogen Tea in a sealed container in the refrigerator for up to 2 days. Enjoy chilled or gently reheat on the stove.

Tips for allergens

Individuals with sensitivities to Ashwagandha or Holy Basil should consult with a healthcare provider before consumption. For those avoiding honey due to dietary restrictions, substitute with maple syrup or simply omit the sweetener.

Scientific references

- "An Overview on Ashwagandha: A Rasayana (Rejuvenator) of Ayurveda" published in the African Journal of Traditional, Complementary and Alternative Medicines, discusses the adaptogenic and stress-relief properties of ashwagandha.

- "Tulsi - Ocimum sanctum: A herb for all reasons" in the Journal of Ayurveda and Integrative Medicine, highlights the stress-reducing and cognitive-enhancing effects of Holy Basil.

TURMERIC AND BOSWELLIA JOINT RELIEF SMOOTHIE

Beneficial effects

The Turmeric and Boswellia Joint Relief Smoothie is specifically formulated to support joint health and alleviate inflammation associated with conditions like arthritis. Turmeric contains curcumin, a compound known for its potent anti-inflammatory and antioxidant properties, which can help reduce pain and stiffness in the joints. Boswellia, also known as Indian frankincense, has been shown to inhibit the production of pro-inflammatory enzymes, further supporting joint health and mobility. This smoothie is an excellent way to incorporate these powerful herbs into your diet for their synergistic effects on reducing inflammation and promoting overall joint comfort.

Portions

2 servings

Preparation time

10 minutes

Ingredients

- 1 cup almond milk

- 1/2 banana, frozen

- 1/2 cup pineapple, chopped and frozen

- 1 teaspoon turmeric powder

- 1 teaspoon Boswellia powder

- 1 tablespoon flaxseed meal

- Honey to taste (optional)

- Ice cubes (optional)

Instructions

1. Place the almond milk, frozen banana, and frozen pineapple into a blender.

2. Add the turmeric powder, Boswellia powder, and flaxseed meal to the blender.

3. Blend on high until the mixture is smooth and creamy. If the smoothie is too thick, add a little more almond milk to achieve the desired consistency.

4. Taste the smoothie and add honey if a sweeter taste is preferred. Blend again briefly to mix.

5. If a colder smoothie is desired, add ice cubes and blend until smooth.

6. Pour the smoothie into glasses and serve immediately for the best flavor and nutrient content.

Variations

- For an extra protein boost, add a scoop of your favorite protein powder to the blender before mixing.

- Substitute almond milk with coconut water for a lighter version that's still hydrating and flavorful.

- Add a pinch of black pepper to enhance the absorption of curcumin from turmeric.

Storage tips

It's best to consume the Turmeric and Boswellia Joint Relief Smoothie immediately after preparation to enjoy its full benefits. However, if necessary, it can be stored in an airtight container in the refrigerator for up to 24 hours. Stir well before consuming if separation occurs.

Tips for allergens

Individuals with allergies to nuts should substitute almond milk with a non-nut milk alternative like oat milk or rice milk. For those with a honey allergy or following a vegan diet, substitute honey with maple syrup or omit it altogether.

Scientific references

- "Curcumin: A Review of Its' Effects on Human Health," published in Foods, 2017. This review discusses the wide-ranging health benefits of curcumin, including its anti-inflammatory and antioxidant effects, which support its use for joint health.

- "Boswellia serrata, A potential antiinflammatory agent: An overview," published in the Indian Journal of Pharmaceutical Sciences, 2011. This study highlights the anti-inflammatory properties of Boswellia serrata, supporting its effectiveness in managing arthritis and joint pain.

GINGER AND GARLIC ANTI-INFLAMMATORY SOUP

Beneficial effects

Ginger and Garlic Anti-Inflammatory Soup is designed to combat inflammation and boost the immune system. Ginger contains gingerol, a substance with powerful anti-inflammatory and antioxidant properties, while garlic is known for its immune-boosting effects. This soup can help alleviate symptoms of chronic diseases such as arthritis, improve digestion, and promote overall health.

Portions

4 servings

Preparation time

15 minutes

Cooking time

45 minutes

Ingredients

- 4 cups vegetable broth

- 1 cup water

- 2 inches fresh ginger, peeled and minced

- 4 cloves garlic, minced

- 1 medium onion, chopped

- 2 carrots, peeled and sliced

- 2 stalks celery, sliced
- 1 cup chopped kale
- 1 tablespoon olive oil
- Salt and pepper to taste
- Juice of 1 lemon

Instructions

1. In a large pot, heat the olive oil over medium heat. Add the onion, garlic, and ginger, sautéing until the onion is translucent, about 5 minutes.

2. Add the carrots and celery to the pot, cooking for another 5 minutes until they begin to soften.

3. Pour in the vegetable broth and water, bringing the mixture to a boil.

4. Reduce the heat to a simmer, cover, and let cook for 30 minutes.

5. Add the chopped kale to the pot and cook for an additional 10 minutes.

6. Season the soup with salt and pepper to taste.

7. Remove from heat and stir in the lemon juice before serving.

Variations

- For added protein, include a cup of cooked chickpeas or shredded chicken.
- Spice it up with a teaspoon of turmeric or cayenne pepper for extra anti-inflammatory benefits.
- Replace kale with spinach or any other leafy green of your choice.

Storage tips

Store any leftover soup in an airtight container in the refrigerator for up to 3 days. The soup can also be frozen for up to 1 month. Thaw in the refrigerator overnight and reheat on the stove over medium heat until warm.

Tips for allergens

For those with allergies to specific vegetables used in this recipe, feel free to substitute or omit as necessary. Olive oil can be replaced with any other cooking oil that you're not allergic to.

Scientific references

- "Anti-Oxidative and Anti-Inflammatory Effects of Ginger in Health and Physical Activity: Review of Current Evidence," published in the International Journal of Preventive Medicine, highlights ginger's health benefits.
- "The immunomodulation and anti-inflammatory effects of garlic organosulfur compounds in cancer chemoprevention," published in Anti-Cancer Agents in Medicinal Chemistry, discusses garlic's role in immune support.

REISHI MUSHROOM AND ASTRAGALUS IMMUNE BOOST ELIXIR

Beneficial effects

The Reishi Mushroom and Astragalus Immune Boost Elixir is designed to strengthen the immune system, enhance the body's resistance to stress, and promote overall wellness. Reishi mushroom, often referred to as the "mushroom of immortality," is known for its immune-modulating properties, helping to increase the activity of white blood cells and reduce inflammation. Astragalus, a staple in traditional Chinese medicine, is recognized for its ability to boost the body's defense against viruses and bacteria, as well as support energy and vitality. Together, these ingredients create a powerful elixir that can help protect the body against illness and support a healthy immune response.

Portions

2 servings

Preparation time

15 minutes

Cooking time

N/A

Ingredients

- 1 teaspoon Reishi mushroom powder

- 1 teaspoon Astragalus root powder

- 2 cups of hot water

- 1 tablespoon honey (optional, for sweetness)

- Juice of half a lemon (optional, for added vitamin C and flavor)

Instructions

1. In a heat-resistant teapot or jar, combine the Reishi mushroom powder and Astragalus root powder.

2. Pour 2 cups of hot water over the powders, ensuring they are fully submerged.

3. Stir the mixture well to ensure the powders are dissolved in the water.

4. Cover and allow the mixture to steep for about 10 minutes.

5. Strain the elixir into mugs or glasses to remove any undissolved particles.

6. If desired, stir in honey and lemon juice to each mug for added flavor and health benefits.

7. Serve the elixir warm, ideally in the morning or early evening to support the immune system.

Variations

- For a cold version, allow the elixir to cool to room temperature, then refrigerate. Serve over ice for a refreshing immune-boosting drink.

- Add a slice of fresh ginger during the steeping process for additional anti-inflammatory and warming properties.

- Mix in a pinch of cinnamon or turmeric powder for extra flavor and health benefits.

Storage tips

Store any leftover Reishi Mushroom and Astragalus Immune Boost Elixir in a sealed container in the refrigerator for up to 48 hours. Gently reheat or enjoy cold.

Tips for allergens

Individuals with allergies to mushrooms or plants in the legume family (to which Astragalus belongs) should proceed with caution and may consider consulting with a healthcare provider before consumption. For those avoiding honey due to dietary restrictions, substitute with maple syrup or simply omit the sweetener.

Scientific references

- "Immunomodulating Effects of Reishi: A Systematic Review," published in the Journal of Alternative and Complementary Medicine, highlights the immune-enhancing properties of Reishi mushroom.

- "Astragalus membranaceus: A Review of its Protection Against Inflammation and Gastrointestinal Cancers," in the American Journal of Chinese Medicine, discusses Astragalus root's role in boosting the immune system and its potential anti-cancer properties.

MILK THISTLE AND DANDELION LIVER SUPPORT TEA

Beneficial effects

Milk Thistle and Dandelion Liver Support Tea is specifically formulated to enhance liver function and detoxification. Milk Thistle contains silymarin, a compound known to protect liver cells from damage and promote liver regeneration. Dandelion root aids in liver detoxification processes and improves bile flow, which is essential for fat metabolism and the body's natural detox pathways. Together, these herbs offer a synergistic effect that supports overall liver health, aids in the elimination of toxins, and can help in managing conditions such as fatty liver disease, hepatitis, and liver cirrhosis.

Portions

2 servings

Preparation time

5 minutes

Cooking time

10 minutes

Ingredients

- 1 tablespoon dried milk thistle seeds
- 1 tablespoon dried dandelion root
- 4 cups of water
- Honey or lemon to taste (optional)

Instructions

1. Crush the milk thistle seeds slightly to release their active compounds.

2. Combine the crushed milk thistle seeds and dried dandelion root in a medium saucepan.

3. Add 4 cups of water to the saucepan and bring the mixture to a boil.

4. Once boiling, reduce the heat and simmer for about 10 minutes.

5. Remove the saucepan from the heat and allow the tea to cool slightly.

6. Strain the tea into cups or a large pitcher, discarding the solids.

7. Optional: Add honey or lemon to taste for flavor enhancement.

8. Serve the tea warm, or allow it to cool and enjoy it chilled.

Variations

- For an added detox boost, include a slice of fresh ginger or a teaspoon of turmeric powder to the tea while it simmers.

- Mix in a cinnamon stick during the simmering process for additional flavor and blood sugar regulation benefits.

- For those preferring a cold beverage, chill the tea in the refrigerator and serve over ice with a sprig of mint for a refreshing detox drink.

Storage tips

Store any leftover Milk Thistle and Dandelion Liver Support Tea in a sealed container in the refrigerator for up to 48 hours. Enjoy it chilled, or gently reheat on the stove.

Tips for allergens

Individuals with allergies to plants in the Asteraceae family, such as dandelion, should proceed with caution and may consider consulting with a healthcare provider before consumption. For those avoiding honey due to dietary restrictions, substitute with maple syrup or simply omit the sweetener.

Scientific references

- "Silymarin, the antioxidant component and Silybum marianum extracts prevent liver damage," in the Food and Chemical Toxicology journal, highlights the liver-protective effects of milk thistle.

- "The diuretic effect in human subjects of an extract of Taraxacum officinale folium over a single day," published in the Journal of Alternative and Complementary Medicine, supports the use of dandelion root in promoting liver health and detoxification.

PART 25: SEASONAL HEALTH AND WELLNESS

Seasonal health and wellness are crucial for adapting to the changing environmental conditions and ensuring our bodies can withstand the variations in weather, daylight, and available foods. Each season brings its unique set of health challenges and opportunities, making it essential to adjust our lifestyle, diet, and wellness practices accordingly. By aligning our habits with the rhythms of nature, we can enhance our body's resilience, support immune function, and maintain a state of balance throughout the year.

Beneficial effects: Tailoring health and wellness practices to the seasons can help prevent seasonal affective disorder, boost immunity during cold and flu season, optimize energy levels, and ensure adequate nutrition year-round. Seasonal foods provide the nutrients our bodies need at specific times of the year, while outdoor activities aligned with the weather conditions can support physical and mental health.

Spring:

Ingredients: Leafy greens, strawberries, asparagus, radishes, peas

- Instructions:

1. Incorporate leafy greens like spinach and kale into salads and smoothies to detoxify the body after winter and provide a boost of vitamins and minerals.

2. Enjoy strawberries and other seasonal fruits rich in vitamin C to support immune function and skin health.

3. Add asparagus and radishes to meals for their detoxifying properties and to support liver health.

4. Use fresh peas in cooking for a healthy dose of protein and fiber, supporting digestion and energy levels.

Summer:

Ingredients: Berries, tomatoes, cucumbers, zucchini, peaches

- Instructions:

1. Snack on a variety of berries to take advantage of their antioxidant properties, which can protect the skin from sun damage.

2. Incorporate tomatoes into your diet for their lycopene content, beneficial for heart health and sun protection.

3. Stay hydrated with cucumbers and zucchini, which have high water content and can help maintain hydration during hot months.

4. Enjoy peaches and other stone fruits for their vitamins, minerals, and fiber, supporting overall health and wellness.

Fall:

Ingredients: Apples, pumpkins, sweet potatoes, Brussels sprouts, pears

- Instructions:

1. Use apples in recipes for their fiber and vitamin C content, supporting immune health and digestion.

2. Cook with pumpkins and sweet potatoes to benefit from their beta-carotene, enhancing eye health and immunity.

3. Add Brussels sprouts to meals for their high levels of vitamins K and C, supporting bone health and immune function.

4. Snack on pears for a healthy dose of fiber and to support heart health.

Winter:

Ingredients: Citrus fruits, root vegetables, nuts, seeds, leafy greens

- **Instructions**:

1. Increase intake of citrus fruits like oranges and grapefruits for vitamin C, crucial for immune support during the cold and flu season.

2. Rely on root vegetables such as carrots, beets, and turnips for their nutrient density and to add warmth and comfort to meals.

3. Incorporate nuts and seeds into your diet for healthy fats, protein, and to support energy levels and mood during shorter, darker days.

4. Continue to eat leafy greens, such as kale and Swiss chard, for their nutrient content and to support overall health.

Variations: For each season, explore local and organic options to maximize nutrient intake and support sustainable farming practices. Experiment with herbs and spices typical of each season to enhance flavor and nutritional value.

Storage tips: Store seasonal produce in a cool, dry place or refrigerate as necessary to preserve freshness and nutrient content. Use airtight containers for cut fruits and vegetables to maintain their quality and extend shelf life.

Tips for allergens: Individuals with specific food allergies can substitute allergenic ingredients with suitable alternatives. For example, those allergic to nuts can opt for seeds as a source of healthy fats and protein.

Scientific references:

- Studies have shown that consuming fruits and vegetables in season can provide higher nutrient levels compared to out-of-season produce (Source: "Seasonal variations in the nutrient content of fruits and vegetables," Journal of Agricultural and Food Chemistry).

- Research supports the benefits of vitamin D supplementation, especially in winter months, for immune health and mood regulation (Source: "Vitamin D and the immune system," Journal of Investigative Medicine).

By embracing the principles of seasonal health and wellness, we can live in harmony with nature's cycles, optimizing our health and well-being throughout the year. This approach encourages us to be mindful of our body's needs, adapt to the changing seasons, and make conscious choices that support our health and the environment.

CHAPTER 1: UNDERSTANDING SEASONAL HEALTH

Seasonal health recognizes the impact of changing seasons on our physical and mental well-being, emphasizing the importance of adjusting our lifestyle, diet, and wellness practices to align with these changes. As the environment around us shifts, so do our body's needs. The variations in temperature, daylight hours, and available foods can significantly influence our immune system, mood, energy levels, and overall health. Adapting to these changes by modifying our habits can enhance resilience, support immune function, and maintain a state of balance.

With each season, our body signals the need for different types of nourishment and care. In spring, the focus is on detoxification and renewal as we move away from the heavier foods and slower pace of winter. This is a time for incorporating more leafy greens, sprouts, and fresh fruits into our diet to help cleanse the body and boost vitality. Physical activity can increase with longer daylight hours, supporting the body's natural detoxification processes through sweat and movement.

Summer calls for hydration and protection from the sun.

The abundance of fresh fruits and vegetables helps keep our bodies hydrated and provides essential vitamins and antioxidants that protect skin from UV damage. Lighter meals and increased fluid intake are crucial to staying cool and energized. Outdoor activities and exercise should be timed to avoid the peak sun hours, reducing the risk of heat exhaustion.

Fall signals a transition to grounding and nourishment in preparation for winter.

The harvest brings a bounty of root vegetables, squashes, and grains that provide the nutrients needed to support immune health. As the temperature drops, incorporating warming spices and foods that are rich in beta-carotene and vitamin C can help strengthen the immune system in anticipation of cold and flu season.

Winter focuses on sustaining energy and warmth while supporting the immune system through the colder, darker months. Foods rich in healthy fats, proteins, and complex carbohydrates are essential for maintaining energy levels and warmth. Vitamin D supplementation becomes crucial due to reduced sunlight exposure. Staying active indoors and ensuring adequate rest and relaxation can help combat seasonal affective disorder and maintain mental health.

Beneficial effects: Tailoring our health and wellness practices to the rhythm of the seasons supports the body's natural functions, enhances our ability to adapt to environmental changes, and promotes a holistic approach to health. It encourages us to listen to our bodies and respond with appropriate nutritional and lifestyle adjustments, leading to improved immunity, energy, and mood regulation throughout the year.

Variations: Each individual's response to seasonal changes can vary, making it important to personalize practices based on personal health needs, preferences, and local climate conditions. For example, someone in a colder climate may need to focus more on indoor physical activities and vitamin D supplementation during winter, while someone in a warmer climate might prioritize hydration and sun protection year-round.

Storage tips: To make the most of seasonal foods, proper storage is key. Root vegetables can be stored in a cool, dark place, while leafy greens last longer in the refrigerator's crisper drawer. Fruits should be stored at room temperature until ripe and then moved to the refrigerator if not consumed immediately to extend freshness.

Tips for allergens: For those with food allergies, seasonal eating still offers a variety of options. Alternatives can be found among the wide range of fruits, vegetables, and grains available throughout the year. For example, someone allergic to nuts can enjoy seeds as a source of healthy fats and proteins, and gluten-free grains can replace traditional wheat products for those with gluten sensitivities.

By understanding and embracing seasonal health, we can optimize our well-being by living in harmony with the natural cycles of our environment. This approach not only benefits our physical and mental health but also connects us more deeply with the natural world, enhancing our appreciation for the rhythms of life.

DR. BARBARA'S APPROACH TO SEASONAL WELLNESS

Dr. Barbara's approach to seasonal wellness emphasizes the importance of adapting our health practices to the rhythm of nature's cycles. She believes that by aligning our lifestyle, diet, and wellness routines with the specific needs of each season, we can enhance our body's natural resilience, optimize our health, and live in greater harmony with our environment. This holistic perspective recognizes that as the seasons change, so too do the demands on our bodies, requiring us to adjust our habits accordingly to maintain balance and wellness.

For spring, a time of renewal and growth, Dr. Barbara suggests a focus on detoxifying the body and embracing fresh, nutrient-rich foods that awaken and energize us after the winter months. She recommends incorporating leafy greens such as spinach and arugula, which are high in vitamins and minerals, to help cleanse the liver and boost vitality. Additionally, engaging in outdoor activities and exercises that increase blood circulation and lymphatic drainage supports the body's natural detoxification processes.

Summer, with its abundance of sunlight and warmth, calls for hydration and protection from the elements. Dr. Barbara advises increasing the intake of water and hydrating foods like cucumbers, melons, and berries, which also provide essential vitamins and antioxidants to protect the skin from UV damage. She emphasizes the importance of moderate sun exposure for vitamin D synthesis while advocating for natural sunscreens and protective clothing to guard against sunburn and heatstroke.

As we transition into fall, the focus shifts to strengthening the immune system in preparation for the colder months. Dr. Barbara recommends a diet rich in vitamin C and zinc, found in pumpkins, squash, and cruciferous vegetables like broccoli and Brussels sprouts, to enhance immune function. Incorporating warming spices such as ginger, turmeric, and cinnamon can also support digestion and circulation, helping the body to adjust to cooler temperatures.

Winter wellness, according to Dr. Barbara, revolves around nourishing and warming the body while supporting mental health during shorter, darker days. Foods high in healthy fats and proteins, such as nuts, seeds, and fatty fish, provide sustained energy and mood support. She also highlights the importance of maintaining a regular exercise routine indoors and practicing stress-reduction techniques like meditation and deep breathing to combat seasonal affective disorder.

Throughout each season, Dr. Barbara underscores the significance of listening to our bodies and making conscious choices that support our health and well-being. This includes staying hydrated, getting adequate rest, and choosing organic, locally sourced foods whenever possible to maximize nutritional benefits and support environmental sustainability.

By following Dr. Barbara's approach to seasonal wellness, we can harness the power of natural cycles to improve our health, adapt more easily to environmental changes, and cultivate a deeper connection with the world around us. This holistic strategy not only enhances our physical well-being but also promotes a sense of balance and harmony within ourselves and with nature.

CHAPTER 2: NUTRITION FOR SEASONAL HEALTH

Adapting our nutrition to the shifting seasons is a powerful way to live in sync with nature's rhythm, ensuring our bodies receive the right balance of nutrients to thrive throughout the year. Each season brings its unique set of environmental conditions and challenges, influencing the availability of certain foods and our body's nutritional needs. By choosing seasonal foods, we not only enjoy fresher, tastier, and more nutritious meals but also support our body's health requirements for that time of year.

Spring marks a period of renewal and rejuvenation, making it the perfect time to focus on detoxifying foods that help clear out winter's heaviness.

Foods like leafy greens, including spinach, kale, and dandelion greens, are abundant and packed with vitamins, minerals, and fiber that support liver health and detoxification. Incorporating fresh herbs such as parsley, cilantro, and mint can also aid in cleansing the body. Spring fruits like strawberries, apricots, and cherries provide antioxidants and vital nutrients, rejuvenating the body and preparing it for the more active months ahead.

Summer emphasizes hydration and cooling foods to combat the heat and support active lifestyles. Cucumbers, watermelon, peaches, and tomatoes are high in water content and can help keep the body hydrated.

Berries, rich in antioxidants and vitamins, offer protection against sun damage.

Lighter meals consisting of salads, smoothies, and cold soups can keep you nourished without feeling heavy. Incorporating a variety of fresh, colorful fruits and vegetables ensures a broad intake of nutrients essential for maintaining energy levels and supporting the body's natural cooling mechanisms.

Fall transitions into a time for boosting the immune system as temperatures begin to drop. Foods rich in vitamin C, such as oranges, kiwis, and bell peppers, support immune health. Root vegetables like sweet potatoes, carrots, and beets are harvested in abundance and provide beta-carotene, fiber, and vitamins to strengthen the body's defenses.

Incorporating warming spices like ginger, turmeric, and cinnamon not only adds flavor but also offers anti-inflammatory and immune-boosting benefits. Whole grains and nuts, rich in B vitamins and minerals, support energy levels and prepare the body for the colder months.

Winter calls for nourishing, warming foods to sustain energy and warmth. Soups and stews made with legumes, lean meats, and root vegetables offer comfort and nutrition. Foods high in healthy fats, such as avocados, nuts, and seeds, along with fatty fish like salmon and mackerel, provide omega-3 fatty acids crucial for mood regulation and combating seasonal affective disorder.

Citrus fruits, packed with vitamin C, and dark leafy greens, rich in iron and folate, help combat fatigue and support overall well-being during the shorter, darker days.

Throughout the year, staying hydrated is essential, regardless of the season. Water, herbal teas, and hydrating foods play a crucial role in maintaining health. Additionally, adapting portion sizes and meal composition to match seasonal activity levels can help manage weight and energy. By embracing the diversity of foods each season offers, we can create a diet that not only tastes good but also profoundly supports our health, aligning our bodies with the natural world's cycles.

THE IMPORTANCE OF VITAMIN D IN WINTER

The importance of Vitamin D during the winter months cannot be overstated, especially considering the challenges posed by reduced daylight hours and the inclination for individuals to spend more time indoors. Known as the "sunshine vitamin," Vitamin D plays a crucial role in maintaining bone health by facilitating the absorption of calcium and phosphorus from the diet. Beyond its skeletal benefits, Vitamin D is also essential for immune function, reducing inflammation, and supporting muscle health. During winter, the body's ability to produce Vitamin D naturally decreases due to less exposure to sunlight, making it imperative to seek alternative sources to meet the daily recommended intake.

Beneficial effects of maintaining adequate Vitamin D levels in winter include enhanced immune response, a decrease in the risk of seasonal affective disorder (SAD), improved bone health, and a reduction in the likelihood of Vitamin D deficiency-related diseases. To compensate for the lack of natural sunlight exposure, individuals can turn to dietary sources and supplements to maintain adequate Vitamin D levels.

Ingredients:

- Fatty fish such as salmon, mackerel, and tuna (rich in Vitamin D)

- Egg yolks (small amounts of Vitamin D)

- Fortified foods such as milk, orange juice, and cereals (Vitamin D added)

- Vitamin D supplements (check labels for dosage)

Instructions:

1. Aim to include fatty fish in your diet 2-3 times per week to boost Vitamin D intake.

2. Incorporate fortified foods into your daily meals. For example, start your day with a bowl of Vitamin D-fortified cereal or oatmeal.

3. Use fortified milk or orange juice in smoothies or cooking to add an extra dose of Vitamin D.

4. For egg lovers, incorporating egg yolks into meals can provide a natural source of Vitamin D.

5. Consider taking a Vitamin D supplement, especially if dietary sources are limited or if you're at higher risk for deficiency. The recommended daily amount for most adults is 600-800 IU, but your healthcare provider may recommend higher doses if you are deficient or at risk.

Variations:

- Vegetarians or those who do not consume fish can rely more heavily on fortified foods and consider a Vitamin D supplement.

- Individuals with dietary restrictions or allergies can consult with a healthcare provider for the best ways to ensure adequate Vitamin D intake, considering potential allergens.

Storage tips:

- Keep fortified and perishable Vitamin D sources like milk and eggs refrigerated to maintain freshness.

- Store supplements in a cool, dry place, away from direct sunlight.

Tips for allergens:

- For those allergic to fish, fortified foods and supplements can provide a safe alternative source of Vitamin D.

- Always check labels on fortified foods for potential allergens and choose products that meet your dietary needs.

Maintaining adequate Vitamin D levels during winter is essential for overall health and well-being. By incorporating a mix of dietary sources and considering supplementation if necessary, individuals can ensure they receive an adequate amount of this vital nutrient even during the colder months.

FOODS TO AVOID DURING SEASONAL TRANSITIONS

As we navigate through the changing seasons, our bodies undergo adjustments that can be supported or hindered by our dietary choices. During these transitional periods, certain foods can exacerbate seasonal sensitivities, disrupt digestion, and impede our body's natural adaptation processes. Recognizing and reducing consumption of these foods can enhance our well-being and facilitate a smoother transition between seasons.

Highly processed and sugary foods are among the primary culprits to avoid. These foods can cause inflammation, weaken the immune system, and lead to energy spikes followed by crashes, making it harder for the body to adjust to new seasonal rhythms. Instead of reaching for packaged snacks or sugary treats, opt for whole, nutrient-dense foods that support steady energy levels and immune function.

Dairy products, for some individuals, can contribute to congestion and exacerbate allergies, particularly during times when our bodies are more susceptible to seasonal changes. If you notice increased mucus production or digestive discomfort after consuming dairy, consider reducing your intake or exploring plant-based alternatives like almond milk or coconut yogurt.

Caffeine and alcohol are other substances to moderate during seasonal transitions. Both can dehydrate the body, disrupt sleep patterns, and stress the adrenal glands. As our bodies work to adapt to new environmental conditions, ensuring adequate hydration and rest is crucial. Opt for herbal teas and water-rich foods to maintain hydration and support natural energy levels.

Fatty and fried foods can also be challenging during seasonal shifts. These foods are harder to digest, can strain the liver, and may contribute to feelings of sluggishness as the body diverts energy to digestion rather than adaptation to changing temperatures and light conditions. Emphasizing lightly cooked, easily digestible foods can aid in maintaining vitality and wellness during these times.

Lastly, overly spicy foods might disrupt the body's internal temperature regulation. While some spices can support digestion and circulation, excessive spicy food consumption during a seasonal transition might lead to imbalances. It's beneficial to strike a balance, using spices to support health without overwhelming the body.

By being mindful of these dietary choices during seasonal transitions, we can support our body's natural ability to adapt, maintain balance, and thrive throughout the year. This approach aligns with the holistic perspective of nurturing our bodies with care and attentiveness, recognizing the impact of our dietary choices on our overall health and well-being.

CHAPTER 3: SEASONAL HEALTH NATURAL REMEDIES

To combat seasonal health issues effectively, a holistic approach incorporating natural remedies can provide significant relief and support the body's adaptation to changing environmental conditions. Each season presents unique health challenges, from colds and flu in winter to allergies in spring. By utilizing natural ingredients and practices, we can enhance our resilience and maintain optimal health throughout the year.

Elderberry Syrup for Immune Support

Beneficial effects: Elderberry is renowned for its immune-boosting properties, making it an excellent remedy for preventing and easing cold and flu symptoms. Its high antioxidant content helps to reduce inflammation and protect against viruses and bacteria.

- **Portions**: Makes approximately 2 cups

- **Preparation time**: 15 minutes

- **Cooking time**: 45 minutes

Ingredients:

- 3/4 cup dried elderberries

- 3 cups water

- 1 teaspoon dried ginger

- 1 cinnamon stick

- 1/2 cup raw honey

- **Instructions**:

1. Combine elderberries, water, ginger, and cinnamon in a saucepan. Bring to a boil, then cover and reduce to a simmer for about 45 minutes, or until the liquid has reduced by half.

2. Remove from heat and let cool. Mash the berries to release any remaining juice and strain the mixture.

3. Stir in the raw honey until well combined.

4. Transfer the syrup to a clean, airtight jar and store in the refrigerator.

- **Variations:** Add cloves or star anise for additional flavor and benefits.

- **Storage tips:** Keep refrigerated and use within two months for best quality.

- **Tips for allergens:** For those allergic to honey, substitute with maple syrup or agave nectar.

Nettle Tea for Allergy Relief

Beneficial effects: Nettle is a natural antihistamine, which can help alleviate symptoms of seasonal allergies such as sneezing, nasal congestion, and itching.

- **Portions**: 1 serving

- **Preparation time**: 10 minutes

Ingredients:

- 1 tablespoon dried nettle leaves

- 1 cup boiling water

- **Instructions**:

1. Place nettle leaves in a tea infuser or directly in a mug.

2. Pour boiling water over the leaves and steep for 5-10 minutes.

3. Strain (if needed) and enjoy. Can be drunk up to three times daily during allergy season.

- **Variations:** Add honey or lemon for flavor, or mix with peppermint leaves to enhance the soothing effect on the respiratory system.

- **Storage tips:** Store dried nettle leaves in a cool, dry place away from direct sunlight.

- **Tips for allergens:** Ensure to source nettle from a reputable supplier to avoid cross-contamination with allergens.

Ginger Turmeric Tea for Inflammation

Beneficial effects: Both ginger and turmeric possess strong anti-inflammatory properties, making this tea an excellent remedy for reducing inflammation-related discomforts, such as joint pain that can flare up in colder weather.

- **Portions**: 1 serving

- **Preparation time**: 5 minutes

- **Cooking time**: 10 minutes

Ingredients:

- 1 inch fresh ginger root, thinly sliced

- 1 teaspoon turmeric powder or 1 inch turmeric root, thinly sliced

- 1 cup water

- Honey to taste (optional)

- **Instructions**:

1. Combine ginger, turmeric, and water in a small saucepan and bring to a boil.

2. Reduce heat and simmer for about 10 minutes.

3. Strain the tea into a mug, add honey if desired, and enjoy.

- **Variations:** Add a pinch of black pepper to enhance the absorption of turmeric's active compound, curcumin.

- **Storage tips:** Fresh ginger and turmeric root can be stored in the refrigerator. Keep dried turmeric powder in a cool, dry cupboard.

- **Tips for allergens:** This recipe is generally safe for most, but always consult with a healthcare provider if you have concerns about potential reactions.

By incorporating these natural remedies into your seasonal health care routine, you can support your body's ability to withstand the challenges each season brings. Remember, while these remedies can provide relief and support, they should complement a balanced diet, regular exercise, and adequate rest for overall health and well-being.

CHAPTER 4: 5 HERBAL RECIPES FOR SEASONAL WELLNESS

ELDERFLOWER CORDIAL

Beneficial effects

Elderflower cordial is renowned for its delightful flavor and its potential health benefits. Rich in antioxidants, elderflowers can help in boosting the immune system, reducing symptoms of colds and flu, and promoting skin health. The cordial, with its soothing properties, can also aid in alleviating allergies and inflammation, making it a refreshing choice for seasonal wellness.

Portions

Makes about 1 liter

Preparation time

15 minutes

Cooking time

24 hours for infusion

Ingredients

- 20 fresh elderflower heads, gently rinsed

- 1.5 liters of water

- 2 lemons, sliced

- 1 small orange, sliced (optional)

- 700g granulated sugar

- 50g citric acid

Instructions

1. In a large bowl, combine the elderflower heads, lemon slices, and orange slices if using.

2. In a saucepan, bring the water to a boil and dissolve the granulated sugar into it to create a syrup.

3. Pour the hot syrup over the elderflower and citrus mixture, ensuring all the flowers are submerged.

4. Stir in the citric acid until fully dissolved.

5. Cover the bowl with a clean cloth and allow the mixture to infuse for 24 hours at room temperature.

6. After infusion, strain the cordial through a fine mesh sieve or cheesecloth into a clean, sterilized bottle. Press the solids to extract maximum flavor.

7. Seal the bottle and store in the refrigerator.

Variations

- For a herbal twist, add a few sprigs of fresh mint or rosemary to the infusion.

- Replace granulated sugar with honey for a naturally sweetened version, adjusting the quantity to taste.

- Add a vanilla pod to the syrup while boiling for an aromatic flavor profile.

Storage tips

The elderflower cordial can be stored in the refrigerator for up to 6 weeks. For longer preservation, the cordial can be frozen in ice cube trays and used as needed.

Tips for allergens

Individuals with pollen allergies should proceed with caution when handling and consuming elderflowers. For those with citrus allergies, omit the lemon and orange slices and consider adding non-citrus flavorings like vanilla or herbs.

Scientific references

- "Antioxidant activities of elderflower extracts" in Food Chemistry, highlighting the antioxidant capacity of elderflower and its potential health benefits.

- "The use of elderflower (Sambucus nigra L.) in food and medicine: Tradition and current perspectives" in the Journal of Ethnopharmacology, discussing the traditional and contemporary uses of elderflower in promoting health and wellness.

NETTLE SOUP

Beneficial effects

Nettle Soup is a nourishing and detoxifying dish that supports seasonal wellness by harnessing the natural benefits of nettles. Rich in vitamins A, C, iron, potassium, manganese, and calcium, nettle soup can help boost the immune system, reduce inflammation, and alleviate allergy symptoms. Its high nutrient content also supports joint health, aids in detoxification, and promotes healthy skin.

Portions

4 servings

Preparation time

15 minutes

Cooking time

30 minutes

Ingredients

- 2 tablespoons olive oil

- 1 large onion, chopped

- 2 cloves garlic, minced

- 1 carrot, chopped

- 1 potato, diced

- 4 cups vegetable broth

- 4 cups fresh nettle leaves, carefully washed and stems removed

- Salt and pepper to taste

- Juice of 1/2 lemon

Instructions

1. In a large pot, heat the olive oil over medium heat. Add the onion and garlic, sautéing until soft and translucent.

2. Add the carrot and potato to the pot, cooking for an additional 5 minutes.

3. Pour in the vegetable broth and bring the mixture to a boil.

4. Reduce the heat to a simmer and add the nettle leaves. Cook for about 15 minutes, or until the vegetables are tender.

5. Using an immersion blender, blend the soup until smooth. Alternatively, carefully transfer the soup to a blender and blend in batches.

6. Season the soup with salt and pepper to taste. Stir in the lemon juice before serving.

7. Serve warm, garnished with a dollop of yogurt or a sprinkle of herbs if desired.

Variations

- For a creamier texture, add a splash of coconut milk or cream before blending.

- Incorporate other seasonal greens such as spinach or kale for added nutritional benefits.

- Add a pinch of nutmeg or cayenne pepper for a warming spice.

Storage tips

Store leftover Nettle Soup in an airtight container in the refrigerator for up to 3 days. The soup can also be frozen for up to 2 months. Thaw overnight in the refrigerator and reheat gently on the stove.

Tips for allergens

Individuals with sensitivities to nettles should handle them with gloves and may need to start with a smaller amount to ensure no adverse reactions. For those avoiding dairy, substitute yogurt garnish with a dairy-free alternative or omit it altogether.

Scientific references

- "Stinging nettle: extraordinary vegetable medicine," Journal of Herbal Medicine and Toxicology, 2008. This study discusses the anti-inflammatory and diuretic properties of nettle, highlighting its potential in supporting seasonal health and wellness.

- "The diuretic effect in human subjects of an extract of Taraxacum officinale folium over a single day," Journal of Alternative and Complementary Medicine, 2009. While focusing on dandelion, this study supports the use of diuretic herbs, like nettle, in promoting the elimination of toxins.

YARROW TEA

Beneficial effects

Yarrow Tea is known for its ability to enhance seasonal wellness by promoting digestion, reducing inflammation, and supporting the immune system. Its active compounds, including flavonoids and sesquiterpene lactones, contribute to its therapeutic properties, making it an excellent herbal remedy for colds, fevers, and minor digestive issues. Yarrow's diaphoretic action helps in managing fevers by inducing sweating, while its anti-inflammatory effects can alleviate symptoms associated with colds and flu, such as sore throats and nasal congestion.

Ingredients

- 2 teaspoons of dried yarrow flowers

- 2 cups of boiling water

- Honey or lemon to taste (optional)

Instructions

1. Place the dried yarrow flowers in a tea infuser or directly into a heat-resistant teapot.

2. Pour 2 cups of boiling water over the yarrow flowers.

3. Cover and let the tea steep for about 10 to 15 minutes.

4. Remove the tea infuser or strain the tea to remove the flowers.

5. Optional: Add honey or lemon to taste for flavor enhancement.

6. Serve the tea warm, ideally before bedtime or when experiencing the first signs of a cold or flu.

Variations

- To enhance the respiratory benefits, add a teaspoon of dried peppermint leaves to the steeping process for added menthol, which can help clear nasal passages.

- For additional immune support, mix in a slice of fresh ginger during the steeping process for its antiviral properties.

- Create a soothing blend for sore throats by combining yarrow tea with chamomile and a tablespoon of honey.

Storage tips

Store any leftover Yarrow Tea in a sealed container in the refrigerator for up to 2 days. Enjoy it chilled, or gently reheat on the stove.

Tips for allergens

Individuals with allergies to plants in the Asteraceae family, such as yarrow, should proceed with caution and may consider consulting with a healthcare provider before consumption. For those avoiding honey due to dietary restrictions, substitute with maple syrup or simply omit the sweetener.

Scientific references

- "Yarrow (Achillea millefolium L.): A neglected panacea? A review of its phytochemistry, pharmacology, and medicinal properties" in the Journal of Ethnopharmacology, 2011. This comprehensive review supports yarrow's use in traditional medicine for its wide range of health benefits, including its role in fever management and immune support.

- "Anti-inflammatory and skin barrier repair effects of topical application of some plant oils" in the International Journal of Molecular Sciences, 2017. This article discusses the anti-inflammatory properties of various plant oils, including yarrow, supporting its use for alleviating symptoms of colds and flu.

ECHINACEA TINCTURE

Beneficial effects

Echinacea Tincture is renowned for its immune-boosting properties, making it an effective remedy for preventing and alleviating the symptoms of colds, flu, and other respiratory infections. Its active compounds, including alkamides, polysaccharides, and glycoproteins, have been shown to enhance the body's immune response, reducing the duration and severity of symptoms. Additionally, Echinacea has anti-inflammatory properties that can help soothe sore throats and reduce inflammation, contributing to overall respiratory health and wellness.

Ingredients

- 1/4 cup dried Echinacea purpurea roots and leaves
- 1/2 cup high-proof alcohol (such as vodka or brandy)
- 1/2 cup water

Instructions

1. Finely chop or grind the dried Echinacea roots and leaves to increase their surface area.

2. Combine the Echinacea with the high-proof alcohol and water in a clean, dry glass jar.

3. Seal the jar tightly with a lid and shake well to mix the contents.

4. Store the jar in a cool, dark place for 4 to 6 weeks, shaking it gently every few days to promote extraction.

5. After the infusion period, strain the tincture through a fine mesh sieve or cheesecloth into another clean, dark glass bottle, pressing or squeezing the Echinacea to extract as much liquid as possible.

6. Label the bottle with the date and contents.

Variations

- For those sensitive to alcohol, the tincture can be evaporated by placing the desired amount in a wide, open container and allowing it to sit at room temperature until the alcohol has evaporated. Add the concentrated extract to warm water before consumption.

- Add a teaspoon of raw honey to each dose of the tincture when consuming to enhance the flavor and provide additional soothing properties for the throat.

- Combine with ginger or elderberry tincture for added immune support and flavor complexity.

Storage tips

Store the Echinacea Tincture in a cool, dark place, such as a cupboard or pantry. When stored properly in an airtight container, it can last for up to 2 years. Ensure the bottle is tightly sealed to maintain potency.

Tips for allergens

Individuals with allergies to plants in the daisy family, including Echinacea, should proceed with caution and may consider consulting with a healthcare provider before use. For those avoiding alcohol, ensure to evaporate the alcohol as described in the variations or seek alcohol-free commercial alternatives.

Scientific references

- "Immunomodulatory Activity of Echinacea purpurea Extract" in the Journal of Medicinal Food, which discusses the immune-enhancing effects of Echinacea.

- "Anti-inflammatory properties of Echinacea: A review of its potential use in the treatment of respiratory conditions" published in Phytotherapy Research, highlighting Echinacea's role in reducing inflammation and supporting respiratory health.

LEMON BALM SYRUP

Beneficial effects

Lemon Balm Syrup is known for its calming and soothing properties, making it an excellent remedy for reducing stress, anxiety, and promoting a sense of relaxation. The soothing properties of lemon balm can also help improve sleep quality and enhance cognitive function by easing nervous tension and irritability.

Portions

Approximately 2 cups

Preparation time

10 minutes

Cooking time

20 minutes

Ingredients

- 1 cup fresh lemon balm leaves, tightly packed

- 2 cups water

- 1 cup honey

Instructions

1. Rinse the lemon balm leaves thoroughly under cold water.

2. In a medium saucepan, bring 2 cups of water to a boil.

3. Add the lemon balm leaves to the boiling water and reduce the heat.

4. Simmer for about 15 minutes, allowing the leaves to infuse the water.

5. Strain the mixture through a fine mesh sieve, pressing the leaves to extract as much liquid as possible. Discard the leaves.

6. Return the infused water to the saucepan and add 1 cup of honey.

7. Heat the mixture over low heat, stirring constantly until the honey is completely dissolved.

8. Allow the syrup to cool before transferring it to a clean, airtight bottle or jar.

Variations

- For added flavor and health benefits, include a few slices of ginger or a cinnamon stick during the simmering process.

- Substitute honey with maple syrup for a vegan-friendly version.

- Add a squeeze of fresh lemon juice to the finished syrup for a refreshing twist.

Storage tips

Store the Lemon Balm Syrup in the refrigerator in an airtight container for up to 2 weeks. For longer storage, the syrup can be frozen in an ice cube tray and used as needed.

Tips for allergens

Individuals with allergies to honey can substitute it with maple syrup or agave nectar to avoid potential allergic reactions. Always ensure that lemon balm and any additional herbs used are sourced from reputable suppliers to avoid contamination with allergens.

Scientific references

- "Melissa officinalis L. – A Review of its Traditional Uses, Phytochemistry, and Pharmacology," published in the Journal of Ethnopharmacology, 2015. This review highlights the calming and cognitive-enhancing effects of lemon balm, supporting its use for stress relief and mental health.

PART 26: SLEEP AND RESTORATIVE HEALTH

Sleep and restorative health are foundational elements in maintaining and enhancing holistic well-being. Adequate sleep is not only essential for physical recovery but also plays a critical role in mental and emotional health. It's during sleep that the body undergoes repair and detoxification processes, the brain consolidates memories, and the immune system strengthens. To support restorative sleep, incorporating herbal remedies can be a powerful, natural approach to improving sleep quality and duration.

Sleep is not merely a passive state; it is a dynamic process that serves as the cornerstone of holistic well-being. Restorative sleep is essential for maintaining balance in both the body and mind, providing the foundation for physical, mental, and emotional health. From an integrative perspective, quality sleep is a non-negotiable pillar for achieving overall wellness, as it allows the body to heal, detoxify, and rejuvenate on multiple levels.

1. **Physical Recovery and Detoxification**: During sleep, the body enters a phase of deep rest, which is crucial for physical repair. Cells undergo regeneration, muscles recover from daily stress, and organs such as the liver engage in detoxification. This natural detox process is vital for eliminating toxins that accumulate throughout the day, helping the body maintain optimal functioning. **Sleep is the body's most profound healer**, and ensuring a regular sleep cycle can prevent the buildup of toxins that contribute to chronic conditions. Integrating **herbal adaptogens** like **ashwagandha** (Withania somnifera) and **reishi mushroom** (Ganoderma lucidum) can further support the body's ability to detoxify and heal during sleep.

2. **Mental and Emotional Restoration**: Sleep is essential for mental clarity and emotional resilience. It is during sleep, particularly in the REM stage, that the brain processes and consolidates memories, regulates mood, and resets neural pathways. Inadequate sleep can lead to emotional imbalances, anxiety, and cognitive decline. By ensuring restorative sleep, we nurture mental wellness and emotional equilibrium, which are crucial for facing daily challenges with a calm and focused mind. **Chamomile** (Matricaria chamomilla) and **lavender** (Lavandula angustifolia) are soothing herbs that calm the nervous system, promoting deep relaxation and easing the transition into restful sleep.

3. **Strengthening the Immune System**: A strong immune system is a reflection of the body's ability to maintain homeostasis, and sleep plays a pivotal role in immune regulation. During deep sleep, the body produces cytokines, proteins that help fight infection and inflammation. Chronic sleep deprivation can weaken the immune system, leaving the body more susceptible to illness. By prioritizing restorative sleep, we empower the immune system to perform optimally, enhancing the body's natural defense mechanisms. **Elderberry** (Sambucus nigra) and **echinacea** (Echinacea purpurea) are herbs that can support immune function, especially when combined with adequate sleep.

4. **Herbal Support for Restorative Sleep**: Herbal remedies have long been used in holistic practices to support healthy sleep patterns. These remedies work synergistically with the body to promote relaxation, balance hormones like cortisol and melatonin, and ease the mind into a state of tranquility. For instance, **valerian root** (Valeriana officinalis) is a powerful herbal sedative that helps reduce anxiety and promote deeper sleep, while **passionflower** (Passiflora incarnata) gently soothes the mind and alleviates insomnia. When incorporated into a nightly routine, these herbs can significantly improve both the quality and duration of sleep.

5. **Creating a Sacred Sleep Environment**: Holistic well-being emphasizes not only what we put into our bodies but also the environment in which we live. Creating a sacred space for sleep is an integral part of enhancing restorative rest. This can include reducing artificial light exposure, ensuring the bedroom is free from electromagnetic pollution, and incorporating calming rituals such as diffusing essential oils like **frankincense** (Boswellia carterii) or **cedarwood** (Cedrus atlantica) to promote a peaceful ambiance. Establishing a bedtime routine that honors the body's need for rest and reflection can transform sleep from a mundane activity into a sacred ritual of renewal.

Lavender Sleep Tea

Beneficial effects: Lavender is widely recognized for its calming and relaxing properties, which can help ease insomnia and improve sleep quality.

- **Portions**: 1 serving
- **Preparation time**: 5 minutes

Ingredients:

- 1 tablespoon dried lavender flowers
- 1 cup boiling water
- **Instructions**:

1. Place dried lavender flowers in a tea infuser or directly in a mug.

2. Pour boiling water over the flowers and cover the mug. Let it steep for 5-10 minutes.

3. Remove the infuser or strain the tea to remove the flowers. Enjoy the tea 30 minutes before bedtime.

- **Variations:** Combine with chamomile or mint for additional sleep-promoting effects.
- **Storage tips:** Store dried lavender flowers in a cool, dry place away from direct sunlight to preserve their potency.

Valerian Root Sleep Tonic

Beneficial effects: Valerian root has been used for centuries as a natural sedative and sleep aid, helping to reduce the time it takes to fall asleep and promote deeper, more restful sleep.

- **Portions**: 1 serving
- **Preparation time**: 10 minutes

Ingredients:

- 1 teaspoon dried valerian root
- 1 cup water
- **Instructions**:

1. Bring water to a boil in a small saucepan.

2. Add the valerian root to the boiling water and reduce the heat. Simmer for 10 minutes.

3. Strain the tonic into a mug and drink it 30 minutes before going to bed.

- **Variations:** Add honey or lemon to taste, or mix with other calming herbs like lavender or lemon balm.
- **Storage tips:** Keep dried valerian root in an airtight container in a cool, dark place.

Hops and Chamomile Sleep Aid

Beneficial effects: Hops and chamomile both possess natural sedative qualities that can help relax the mind and body, making it easier to fall asleep and stay asleep.

- **Portions**: 1 serving
- **Preparation time**: 5 minutes

Ingredients:

- 1 tablespoon dried chamomile flowers
- 1 tablespoon dried hops
- 1 cup boiling water
- **Instructions**:

1. Combine chamomile and hops in a tea infuser or directly in a mug.

2. Pour boiling water over the herbs and let steep for 10 minutes.

3. Strain and enjoy the tea an hour before bedtime.

- **Variations:** Blend with lavender or valerian root for enhanced effects.
- **Storage tips:** Store both hops and chamomile in airtight containers in a cool, dark place to maintain their efficacy.

Passionflower Sleep Elixir

Beneficial effects: Passionflower is known for its ability to reduce anxiety and improve sleep quality, particularly in individuals with insomnia or sleep disturbances.

- **Portions**: 1 serving
- **Preparation time**: 5 minutes

Ingredients:

- 1 teaspoon dried passionflower
- 1 cup boiling water
- **Instructions**:

1. Place passionflower in a tea infuser or directly in a cup.

2. Pour boiling water over the herb and let steep for 10 minutes.

3. Strain and drink the elixir 30 minutes to an hour before bedtime.

- **Variations:** Mix with lemon balm or chamomile for a more potent sleep-inducing blend.
- **Storage tips:** Keep dried passionflower in an airtight container away from light and moisture.

Lemon Balm Sleep Infusion

Beneficial effects: Lemon balm can help reduce stress and anxiety, promoting a sense of calm and making it easier to fall asleep and enjoy a more restful night.

- **Portions**: 1 serving
- **Preparation time**: 5 minutes

Ingredients:

- 2 tablespoons fresh lemon balm leaves (or 1 tablespoon dried)

- 1 cup boiling water

- **Instructions**:

1. If using fresh leaves, gently bruise them to release the oils.

2. Place lemon balm in a tea infuser or directly in a mug.

3. Pour boiling water over the leaves and steep for 5-10 minutes.

4. Strain and enjoy the infusion before bedtime.

- **Variations:** Combine with mint or chamomile for additional relaxing benefits.

- **Storage tips:** Dry lemon balm leaves should be stored in an airtight container in a cool, dark place. Fresh leaves can be kept in the refrigerator wrapped in a damp paper towel and placed in a plastic bag.

Incorporating these herbal remedies into your nighttime routine can significantly enhance sleep quality and contribute to overall restorative health. Always consult with a healthcare provider before starting any new herbal regimen, especially if you are pregnant, nursing, or taking medication.

CHAPTER 1: DR. BARBARA'S SLEEP STRATEGIES

D r. Barbara emphasizes the critical role of sleep and rest in holistic health, recognizing them as pillars of well-being that support the body's natural healing processes, cognitive function, and emotional balance. She advocates for a natural and integrative approach to improving sleep quality, incorporating a variety of strategies that align with the body's natural rhythms and promote a restful state.

Creating a conducive sleep environment is paramount in Dr. Barbara's approach.

She suggests maintaining a cool, dark, and quiet bedroom, free from electronic devices, to signal the body that it's time to wind down. The use of essential oils such as lavender in a diffuser can further enhance the sleep atmosphere by providing a calming scent that has been shown to relax the nervous system and facilitate the onset of sleep.

Routine plays a significant role in signaling to the body when it's time to sleep and wake. Dr. Barbara recommends establishing a consistent sleep schedule, going to bed, and waking up at the same time every day, even on weekends.

This consistency reinforces the body's internal clock, or circadian rhythm, aiding in smoother transitions between wakefulness and sleep.

Dietary habits also influence sleep quality. Dr. Barbara advises against consuming caffeine and heavy meals close to bedtime, as they can disrupt sleep patterns. Instead, she suggests incorporating foods rich in magnesium and potassium, such as bananas, almonds, and leafy greens, in the evening meal or snack to support muscle relaxation and overall sleep quality.

Mind-body relaxation techniques are integral to Dr. Barbara's sleep strategy. Practices such as deep breathing exercises, progressive muscle relaxation, and gentle yoga stretches before bed can help release physical tension and quiet the mind. She also highlights the importance of mindfulness and meditation in addressing the mental chatter that can often prevent us from falling asleep.

Herbal remedies play a supportive role in enhancing sleep. Dr. Barbara incorporates herbs known for their sedative properties, such as chamomile, valerian root, and passionflower, into teas or tinctures as part of the bedtime routine.

These herbs have been traditionally used to calm the nervous system and improve sleep latency and quality.

Physical activity is recognized for its sleep-promoting benefits, with Dr. Barbara recommending regular, moderate exercise during the day. Exercise helps to regulate mood and decompress the mind, making it easier to fall asleep. However, she advises against vigorous exercise close to bedtime as it can have the opposite effect, energizing the body when it's time to wind down.

Finally, Dr. Barbara addresses the importance of managing stress as part of a comprehensive approach to improving sleep. Chronic stress can lead to disrupted sleep patterns, and by employing stress reduction techniques such as journaling, spending time in nature, and engaging in hobbies, individuals can mitigate the impact of stress on sleep.

By adopting these holistic strategies, Dr. Barbara's approach to sleep and rest aims to support the body's natural rhythms, enhance sleep quality, and improve overall health and well-being.

CHAPTER 2: NUTRITION FOR BETTER SLEEP

The connection between diet and sleep quality is profound, with certain foods and nutrients playing a pivotal role in promoting restful sleep. To harness the power of nutrition for better sleep, it's essential to focus on foods that naturally enhance the body's sleep mechanisms and encourage a state of relaxation before bedtime.

Magnesium-Rich Foods for Muscle Relaxation

Beneficial effects: Magnesium is a mineral known for its ability to relax muscles and nerves, which is crucial for calming the body and preparing it for sleep. A deficiency in magnesium can lead to difficulty sleeping.

Ingredients:

- Spinach and other leafy greens

- Pumpkin seeds

- Almonds and cashews

- Whole grains such as brown rice and quinoa

- **Instructions**:

1. Incorporate a serving of magnesium-rich foods into your dinner or as an evening snack. For example, a salad with spinach and pumpkin seeds or a serving of quinoa with almonds.

Tryptophan-Enriched Foods to Boost Melatonin

Beneficial effects: Tryptophan is an amino acid that the body uses to produce serotonin, which is then converted into the sleep hormone melatonin. Foods high in tryptophan can help increase melatonin levels naturally, aiding in sleep.

Ingredients:

- Turkey and chicken

- Eggs

- Dairy products like milk and cheese

- Nuts and seeds

- **Instructions**:

1. For those who consume dairy, a glass of warm milk before bed can be soothing and provide the tryptophan needed to boost melatonin. Alternatively, a small portion of turkey or a handful of nuts can serve as an effective evening snack.

Complex Carbohydrates for Serotonin Production

Beneficial effects: Consuming complex carbohydrates can help increase the availability of tryptophan in the brain, enhancing the production of serotonin and promoting a sense of calm.

Ingredients:

- Whole grains like oatmeal, barley, and whole-wheat bread

- Sweet potatoes

- Beans and lentils

- **Instructions**:

1. Include a serving of complex carbohydrates in your evening meal. A bowl of oatmeal or a sweet potato side dish can be particularly effective.

Herbal Teas for Relaxation

Beneficial effects: Certain herbal teas contain compounds that can help relax the body and mind, making it easier to fall asleep.

Ingredients:

- Chamomile tea

- Valerian root tea

- Lemon balm tea

- **Instructions**:

1. Brew a cup of herbal tea about an hour before bedtime. Chamomile is widely recognized for its calming properties, while valerian root and lemon balm are also effective for promoting sleep.

Omega-3 Fatty Acids to Reduce Stress

Beneficial effects: Omega-3 fatty acids have been shown to reduce stress levels and may help improve sleep quality by lowering anxiety.

Ingredients:

- Fatty fish such as salmon, mackerel, and sardines

- Flaxseeds and chia seeds

- Walnuts

- **Instructions**:

1. Aim to include omega-3 rich foods in your diet regularly. Consuming fatty fish for dinner or adding flaxseeds to your evening snack can provide the omega-3s needed to support restful sleep.

Tips for Allergens:

- For those with nut allergies, seeds such as pumpkin or sunflower seeds are a safe alternative source of magnesium and tryptophan.

- Lactose intolerant individuals can opt for lactose-free milk or fortified plant-based milk to obtain tryptophan.

Storage Tips:

- Store nuts and seeds in a cool, dry place to prevent rancidity.

- Keep leafy greens and other perishables in the refrigerator to maintain freshness.

Incorporating these foods into your diet can significantly impact your sleep quality. It's important to note that heavy meals close to bedtime may disrupt sleep, so focus on light, nutrient-dense snacks if you're hungry in the evening. By choosing foods that support the body's natural sleep processes, you can enjoy deeper, more restful sleep and improve your overall health and well-being.

CHAPTER 3: NATURAL REMEDIES FOR BETTER SLEEP

Lavender Sleep Tea

Beneficial effects: Lavender is widely recognized for its calming and relaxing properties, which can help ease insomnia and improve sleep quality.

- **Portions**: 1 serving

- **Preparation time**: 5 minutes

Ingredients:

- 1 tablespoon dried lavender flowers

- 1 cup boiling water

- **Instructions**:

1. Place dried lavender flowers in a tea infuser or directly in a mug.

2. Pour boiling water over the flowers and cover the mug. Let it steep for 5-10 minutes.

3. Remove the infuser or strain the tea to remove the flowers. Enjoy the tea 30 minutes before bedtime.

- **Variations:** Combine with chamomile or mint for additional sleep-promoting effects.

- **Storage tips:** Store dried lavender flowers in a cool, dry place away from direct sunlight to preserve their potency.

Valerian Root Sleep Tonic

Beneficial effects: Valerian root has been used for centuries as a natural sedative and sleep aid, helping to reduce the time it takes to fall asleep and promote deeper, more restful sleep.

- **Portions**: 1 serving

- **Preparation time**: 10 minutes

Ingredients:

- 1 teaspoon dried valerian root

- 1 cup water

- **Instructions**:

1. Bring water to a boil in a small saucepan.

2. Add the valerian root to the boiling water and reduce the heat. Simmer for 10 minutes.

3. Strain the tonic into a mug and drink it 30 minutes before going to bed.

- **Variations:** Add honey or lemon to taste, or mix with other calming herbs like lavender or lemon balm.

- **Storage tips:** Keep dried valerian root in an airtight container in a cool, dark place.

Hops and Chamomile Sleep Aid

Beneficial effects: Hops and chamomile both possess natural sedative qualities that can help relax the mind and body, making it easier to fall asleep and stay asleep.

- **Portions**: 1 serving

- **Preparation time**: 5 minutes

Ingredients:

- 1 tablespoon dried chamomile flowers

- 1 tablespoon dried hops

- 1 cup boiling water

- **Instructions**:

1. Combine chamomile and hops in a tea infuser or directly in a mug.

2. Pour boiling water over the herbs and let steep for 10 minutes.

3. Strain and enjoy the tea an hour before bedtime.

- **Variations:** Blend with lavender or valerian root for enhanced effects.

- **Storage tips:** Store both hops and chamomile in airtight containers in a cool, dark place to maintain their efficacy.

Passionflower Sleep Elixir

Beneficial effects: Passionflower is known for its ability to reduce anxiety and improve sleep quality, particularly in individuals with insomnia or sleep disturbances.

- **Portions**: 1 serving

- **Preparation time**: 5 minutes

Ingredients:

- 1 teaspoon dried passionflower

- 1 cup boiling water

- **Instructions**:

1. Place passionflower in a tea infuser or directly in a cup.

2. Pour boiling water over the herb and let steep for 10 minutes.

3. Strain and drink the elixir 30 minutes to an hour before bedtime.

- **Variations:** Mix with lemon balm or chamomile for a more potent sleep-inducing blend.

- **Storage tips:** Keep dried passionflower in an airtight container away from light and moisture.

Lemon Balm Sleep Infusion

Beneficial effects: Lemon balm can help reduce stress and anxiety, promoting a sense of calm and making it easier to fall asleep and enjoy a more restful night.

- **Portions**: 1 serving

- **Preparation time**: 5 minutes

Ingredients:

- 2 tablespoons fresh lemon balm leaves (or 1 tablespoon dried)

- 1 cup boiling water

- **Instructions**:

1. If using fresh leaves, gently bruise them to release the oils.

2. Place lemon balm in a tea infuser or directly in a mug.

3. Pour boiling water over the leaves and steep for 5-10 minutes.

4. Strain and enjoy the infusion before bedtime.

- **Variations:** Combine with mint or chamomile for additional relaxing benefits.

- **Storage tips:** Dry lemon balm leaves should be stored in an airtight container in a cool, dark place. Fresh leaves can be kept in the refrigerator wrapped in a damp paper towel and placed in a plastic bag.

Incorporating these herbal remedies into your nighttime routine can significantly enhance sleep quality and contribute to overall restorative health. Always consult with a healthcare provider before starting any new herbal regimen, especially if you are pregnant, nursing, or taking medication.

CHAPTER 4: 5 HERBAL RECIPES FOR RESTFUL SLEEP

LAVENDER SLEEP TEA

Beneficial effects

Lavender Sleep Tea harnesses the calming and soothing properties of lavender to promote relaxation and improve sleep quality. Lavender is widely recognized for its ability to reduce anxiety, ease insomnia, and enhance overall sleep patterns. Drinking lavender tea before bedtime can help calm the mind, relax the body, and prepare you for a restful night's sleep, making it an ideal natural remedy for those struggling with sleep disturbances.

Portions

2 servings

Preparation time

5 minutes

Cooking time

10 minutes

Ingredients

- 2 tablespoons dried lavender flowers

- 2 cups boiling water

- Honey or lemon to taste (optional)

Instructions

1. Place the dried lavender flowers in a tea infuser or directly into a heat-resistant teapot.

2. Pour 2 cups of boiling water over the lavender flowers.

3. Cover and let the tea steep for about 5 to 10 minutes, depending on the desired strength.

4. Remove the tea infuser or strain the tea to remove the flowers.

5. Optional: Add honey or lemon to taste for flavor enhancement.

6. Serve the tea warm, ideally 30 minutes before bedtime, to enjoy its sleep-promoting benefits.

Variations

- For added relaxation, mix in a teaspoon of chamomile flowers with the lavender for a soothing blend.

- Incorporate a cinnamon stick during the steeping process for a warming flavor and additional calming effects.

- To create a refreshing iced tea version, allow the tea to cool, then refrigerate and serve over ice.

Storage tips

Store any leftover Lavender Sleep Tea in a sealed container in the refrigerator for up to 2 days. Enjoy chilled or gently reheat on the stove.

Tips for allergens

Individuals with allergies to lavender should avoid this tea. For those avoiding honey due to dietary restrictions, substitute with maple syrup or simply omit the sweetener.

Scientific references

- "Lavender and the Nervous System," published in Evidence-Based Complementary and Alternative Medicine, 2013. This article discusses the anxiolytic (anxiety-reducing) and sedative effects of lavender, supporting its use for stress relief and sleep improvement.

- "An olfactory stimulus modifies nighttime sleep in young men and women," in Chronobiology International, 2005. This study highlights the positive impact of lavender scent on sleep quality, further emphasizing the benefits of lavender tea for restful sleep.

VALERIAN ROOT SLEEP TONIC

Beneficial effects

Valerian Root Sleep Tonic is designed to promote relaxation and improve sleep quality. Valerian root contains compounds that may help reduce anxiety and promote a sense of calm, making it easier to fall asleep and stay asleep throughout the night. This natural remedy can be particularly beneficial for individuals experiencing insomnia, restlessness, or stress-related sleep disturbances.

Portions

2 servings

Preparation time

10 minutes

Ingredients

- 2 teaspoons of dried valerian root

- 2 cups of water

- Honey or lemon to taste (optional)

Instructions

1. Bring 2 cups of water to a boil in a small pot.

2. Add the dried valerian root to the boiling water.

3. Reduce the heat and simmer for about 5 minutes.

4. Remove the pot from the heat and allow the tonic to steep for an additional 5 minutes.

5. Strain the tonic into mugs, discarding the valerian root.

6. Optional: Add honey or lemon to taste for flavor enhancement.

7. Drink the tonic 30 minutes before bedtime to aid sleep.

Variations

- For a more complex flavor, add a cinnamon stick or a few slices of fresh ginger to the water along with the valerian root.

- Combine with chamomile tea for additional sleep-promoting benefits.

- For those preferring a cold beverage, chill the tonic in the refrigerator and serve over ice.

Storage tips

Prepare the Valerian Root Sleep Tonic fresh each night for the best results, as the potency of the valerian root may decrease over time.

Tips for allergens

Individuals with allergies to valerian root should avoid this tonic. For those avoiding honey due to dietary restrictions, substitute with maple syrup or simply omit the sweetener.

Scientific references

- "Valerian for sleep: a systematic review and meta-analysis" in the American Journal of Medicine. This review analyzes multiple studies on valerian root's effectiveness in improving sleep quality, supporting its use for insomnia and sleep disturbances.

- "Effects of valerian on subjective sedation, field sobriety testing and driving simulator performance" in Accident Analysis & Prevention. This study highlights the sedative effects of valerian root without significantly impairing motor function or reaction time, making it a safe sleep aid.

HOPS AND CHAMOMILE SLEEP AID

Beneficial effects

The Hops and Chamomile Sleep Aid is a natural remedy designed to promote relaxation and improve sleep quality. Hops contain compounds that have sedative effects, which can help reduce the time it takes to fall asleep. Chamomile is widely recognized for its calming properties, helping to soothe the nervous system and ease anxiety. Together, these herbs create a powerful blend that supports restful sleep, making it ideal for those who experience insomnia or restless nights.

Ingredients

- 1 tablespoon dried hops
- 1 tablespoon dried chamomile flowers
- 2 cups boiling water
- Honey or lemon to taste (optional)

Instructions

1. Place the dried hops and chamomile flowers in a tea infuser or directly into a heat-resistant teapot.

2. Pour 2 cups of boiling water over the herbs.

3. Cover and let the mixture steep for 10 to 15 minutes.

4. Remove the tea infuser or strain the tea to remove the herbs.

5. Optional: Add honey or lemon to taste for flavor enhancement.

6. Serve the tea warm, ideally 30 minutes before bedtime, to enjoy its sleep-promoting benefits.

Variations

- For added relaxation, include a teaspoon of lavender flowers in the steeping process for their additional calming effects.

- Mix in a slice of fresh ginger during the steeping process for a warming flavor and additional digestive benefits.

- For a cold beverage option, allow the tea to cool and then refrigerate. Serve over ice for a refreshing sleep aid during warmer months.

Storage tips

Store any leftover Hops and Chamomile Sleep Aid in a sealed container in the refrigerator for up to 2 days. Enjoy chilled or gently reheat on the stove before consumption.

Tips for allergens

Individuals with allergies to plants in the Asteraceae family, such as chamomile, should proceed with caution and may consider consulting with a healthcare provider before consumption. For those avoiding honey due to dietary restrictions, substitute with maple syrup or simply omit the sweetener.

Scientific references

- "A review of the bioactivity and potential health benefits of chamomile tea (Matricaria recutita L.)" in Phytotherapy Research, highlighting chamomile's role in promoting sleep and reducing anxiety.

- "Hops (Humulus lupulus L.) and their components: Effects on sleep and anxiety" published in the journal Phytomedicine, discusses the sedative effects of hops and their potential benefits for improving sleep quality.

PASSIONFLOWER SLEEP ELIXIR

Beneficial effects

Passionflower Sleep Elixir harnesses the calming and sedative properties of passionflower to promote relaxation and improve sleep quality. Known for its ability to increase gamma-aminobutyric acid (GABA) in the brain, passionflower helps reduce anxiety and induces sleep, making it an effective natural remedy for insomnia and sleep disturbances.

Ingredients

- 2 teaspoons dried passionflower
- 1 cup boiling water
- 1 teaspoon honey (optional)
- A slice of lemon (optional)

Instructions

1. Place the dried passionflower in a tea infuser or directly into a heat-resistant cup.

2. Pour 1 cup of boiling water over the passionflower.

3. Cover and allow to steep for 10-15 minutes.

4. Remove the tea infuser or strain to remove the passionflower.

5. Optional: Add honey and a slice of lemon to enhance the flavor.

6. Drink the elixir 30 minutes before bedtime to promote restful sleep.

Variations

- For a more potent sleep aid, combine passionflower with chamomile or valerian root during the steeping process.

- To create a cold sleep elixir, allow the tea to cool, then refrigerate and serve over ice.

- Add a cinnamon stick during the steeping process for a warming, comforting flavor.

Storage tips

Store any unused passionflower in a cool, dry place away from direct sunlight to preserve its potency. The prepared elixir should be consumed fresh, but any leftovers can be stored in the refrigerator for up to 24 hours.

Tips for allergens

Individuals with allergies to passionflower should avoid this elixir. Honey can be substituted with maple syrup for those with honey allergies or following a vegan diet.

Scientific references

- "A double-blind, placebo-controlled investigation of the effects of Passiflora incarnata (passionflower) herbal tea on subjective sleep quality" in Phytotherapy Research, 2011. This study supports the efficacy of passionflower in improving sleep quality and reducing sleep disturbances.

- "Passiflora incarnata Linneaus as an anxiolytic before spinal anesthesia" in the Journal of Anesthesia, 2013. This research highlights passionflower's anxiolytic effects, further supporting its use in promoting relaxation and sleep.

LEMON BALM SLEEP INFUSION

Beneficial effects

Lemon Balm Sleep Infusion is designed to promote relaxation and improve sleep quality. Lemon balm, with its mild sedative properties, can help reduce anxiety and induce a state of calmness, making it easier to fall asleep and stay asleep throughout the night. Its ability to improve sleep is supported by its interaction with the brain's GABA receptors, which play a key role in promoting relaxation. This herbal infusion is an excellent choice for those seeking a natural remedy to enhance their sleep routine and overall well-being.

Portions

2 servings

Preparation time

10 minutes

Ingredients

- 2 tablespoons dried lemon balm leaves

- 2 cups boiling water

- Honey or lemon to taste (optional)

Instructions

1. Place the dried lemon balm leaves in a tea infuser or directly into a heat-resistant teapot.

2. Pour 2 cups of boiling water over the lemon balm leaves.

3. Cover and let the infusion steep for about 10 minutes.

4. Remove the tea infuser or strain the infusion to remove the leaves.

5. Optional: Add honey or lemon to taste for flavor enhancement.

6. Serve the infusion warm, ideally 30 minutes before bedtime, to enjoy its sleep-promoting benefits.

Variations

- For added relaxation, include a few lavender flowers to the steeping process for their calming effects.

- Mix in a teaspoon of chamomile flowers with the lemon balm for additional sleep-enhancing properties.

- For a cooler, refreshing bedtime drink, allow the infusion to cool and then refrigerate. Serve over ice if desired.

Storage tips

Store any leftover Lemon Balm Sleep Infusion in a sealed container in the refrigerator for up to 2 days. Enjoy chilled or gently reheat on the stove.

Tips for allergens

Individuals with allergies to lemon balm should consult with a healthcare provider before consumption. For those avoiding honey due to dietary restrictions, substitute with maple syrup or simply omit the sweetener.

Scientific references

- "A review of the bioactivity and potential health benefits of lemon balm" published in Phytotherapy Research, highlights the sedative and sleep-enhancing effects of lemon balm, supporting its use for improving sleep quality.

- "Melissa officinalis L. Extract – An Evidence-Based Systematic Review by the Natural Standard Research Collaboration" in the Journal of Herbal Pharmacotherapy, discusses the anxiety-reducing and cognitive function-improving effects of lemon balm, supporting its use for mental clarity and relaxation.

PART 27: SUPPORTING VISION AND EYE HEALTH

Supporting vision and eye health is paramount in maintaining not just the quality of our sight but also our overall quality of life. Vision, one of our most crucial senses, allows us to connect with our surroundings, enjoy the beauty of the world, and perform daily tasks efficiently. To support and enhance eye health, incorporating a diet rich in specific nutrients is essential. These nutrients include vitamins A, C, E, zinc, and omega-3 fatty acids, all known for their roles in maintaining eye health and potentially reducing the risk of age-related macular degeneration.

Beneficial effects: The beneficial effects of a nutrient-rich diet on eye health are numerous. Vitamins A, C, and E are potent antioxidants that help protect the eyes from harmful oxidative stress and inflammation. Zinc plays a critical role in transporting vitamin A from the liver to the retina, supporting the production of melanin, a protective pigment in the eyes. Omega-3 fatty acids are essential for cell membrane health, particularly in the retina, and have been shown to reduce the risk of dry eye syndrome and other eye diseases.

Ingredients:

- 1 cup of kale or spinach (rich in vitamins C, E, and beta-carotene)

- ½ cup of berries (blueberries, strawberries, or blackberries for vitamin C and antioxidants)

- 1 medium carrot (rich in beta-carotene and vitamin A)

- 1 tablespoon of flaxseeds or chia seeds (for omega-3 fatty acids)

- 1 small orange (for vitamin C)

- 1 ounce of almonds or sunflower seeds (for vitamin E)

- ¼ cup of cooked quinoa (for zinc)

- 1 cup of water or almond milk (as the liquid base)

Instructions:

1. Wash the kale or spinach thoroughly to remove any dirt or pesticides.

2. Peel the carrot and cut it into small pieces to ensure it blends smoothly.

3. Place the kale or spinach, carrot, and berries into a blender.

4. Add the flaxseeds or chia seeds, and almonds or sunflower seeds to the mixture.

5. Squeeze the juice of the orange into the blender, ensuring no seeds get into the mixture.

6. Add the cooked quinoa, which should be cooled to room temperature.

7. Pour in the water or almond milk to achieve the desired consistency.

8. Blend all ingredients on high until the mixture is smooth.

9. Taste and adjust the sweetness by adding a little honey or maple syrup if desired (optional).

Variations:

- For an extra boost of omega-3s, add a teaspoon of fish oil to the smoothie.

- If you prefer a colder smoothie, use frozen berries instead of fresh ones.

- For those allergic to nuts, omit the almonds or sunflower seeds and consider adding a tablespoon of hemp seeds for added nutrients without the allergen.

Storage tips: This smoothie is best enjoyed fresh, but if needed, it can be stored in an airtight container in the refrigerator for up to 24 hours. Shake well before drinking if it has been stored.

Tips for allergens: Always ensure that the ingredients used do not contain allergens specific to your dietary needs. For a nut-free version, ensure that the almond milk is replaced with another plant-based milk like oat milk, which is generally well-tolerated.

Scientific references:

- The Age-Related Eye Disease Study 2 (AREDS2), conducted by the National Eye Institute, supports the role of vitamins C and E, zinc, and omega-3 fatty acids in reducing the risk of age-related macular degeneration progression.

- A study published in the "Journal of Nutrition" highlights the importance of dietary omega-3 fatty acids in preventing dry eye syndrome.

By incorporating these nutrient-rich foods into your diet, you can support your vision and overall eye health, potentially reducing the risk of common eye diseases and conditions. Remember, a balanced diet combined with regular eye check-ups and protecting your eyes from excessive UV light exposure forms the foundation of good eye health.

CHAPTER 1: UNDERSTANDING EYE HEALTH AND VISION

Eye health and vision are critical components of overall well-being, deeply interconnected with the body's nutritional intake and lifestyle choices. The eyes, complex organs, require a range of specific nutrients to function optimally and maintain health over time. Understanding the anatomy of the eye and the role of nutrition can empower individuals to make choices that support their vision.

The human eye works much like a camera, capturing light and sending signals to the brain to create images. Key structures such as the cornea, lens, retina, and macula play specific roles in this process, each susceptible to damage from environmental factors, aging, and nutritional deficiencies.

For instance, the macula, responsible for central vision, relies heavily on antioxidants to protect against oxidative stress, a leading cause of age-related macular degeneration.

Antioxidants such as vitamins A, C, and E, alongside minerals like zinc and omega-3 fatty acids, are foundational for eye health. Vitamin A is crucial for the maintenance of good vision, especially in low-light conditions, and for keeping the eyes' surface tissues healthy.

Deficiencies in this vitamin can lead to night blindness and increase susceptibility to eye infections.

Vitamin C, found abundantly in fruits and vegetables, helps the body form and maintain connective tissue, including collagen found in the cornea of the eye.

Vitamin E protects eye cells from damage by neutralizing free radicals, which can break down healthy tissue and contribute to cataracts and age-related macular degeneration.

Zinc plays a vital role in transporting vitamin A from the liver to the retina, aiding in the production of melanin, a protective pigment in the eyes.

Omega-3 fatty acids, particularly DHA, are present in high concentrations in the retina and are essential for maintaining the integrity of the nervous system, including visual development and retinal function.

To support eye health through diet, incorporating a variety of colorful fruits and vegetables is key.

Leafy greens such as kale and spinach are rich in lutein and zeaxanthin, two types of carotenoids that are present in the macula and retina, acting as natural antioxidants that protect the eyes from harmful light waves. Eggs, almonds, and fatty fish like salmon and mackerel offer valuable sources of these essential nutrients.

Hydration also plays a crucial role in maintaining eye health.

Adequate fluid intake helps support the production of tears, essential for keeping the eyes moist, clean, and free from infection. Regular physical activity and protecting the eyes from excessive exposure to UV light by wearing sunglasses are additional lifestyle choices that contribute significantly to long-term eye health.

In summary, the health of our eyes and the clarity of our vision are deeply influenced by our dietary and lifestyle choices.

By understanding the nutritional needs of our eyes and incorporating a variety of nutrient-rich foods into our diet, we can take proactive steps toward maintaining our vision and overall eye health.

Regular eye check-ups are essential for early detection and management of potential eye conditions, ensuring that our eyes remain healthy and functional throughout our lives.

DR. BARBARA'S INSIGHTS ON MAINTAINING EYE HEALTH

Dr. Barbara emphasizes the importance of a proactive approach to maintaining eye health, highlighting the critical role of lifestyle choices, diet, and regular eye care. She points out that while genetics play a part in eye health, the choices we make every day significantly impact the long-term health of our eyes. Key to her insights is the understanding that the eyes are not isolated organs but are deeply connected to the body's overall health and well-being.

Therefore, a holistic approach to eye health is not only beneficial but essential.

First and foremost, Dr. Barbara advocates for a diet rich in antioxidants, vitamins, and minerals known to support eye health. She underscores the importance of nutrients such as lutein and zeaxanthin, found in green leafy vegetables, which help protect the eyes from the harmful effects of blue light and oxidative stress. Omega-3 fatty acids, particularly DHA found in fish, are crucial for maintaining the health of the retina and may help prevent dry eyes.

Vitamin A, vital for vision in low light conditions and eye surface maintenance, can be sourced from carrots, sweet potatoes, and leafy greens. Dr. Barbara also highlights the role of vitamin C and E in combating free radical damage and supporting the health of eye tissues.

Beyond diet, Dr. Barbara stresses the significance of protecting the eyes from excessive UV light exposure. Wearing sunglasses with 100% UVA and UVB protection is a simple yet effective strategy to reduce the risk of cataracts and macular degeneration.

She also discusses the importance of managing screen time to prevent digital eye strain, recommending regular breaks using the 20-20-20 rule: every 20 minutes, look at something 20 feet away for at least 20 seconds.

Regular physical activity is another cornerstone of Dr. Barbara's approach to eye health. Exercise improves blood circulation, which is beneficial for the eyes as it helps remove toxins and provide nutrients. She encourages incorporating activities that increase heart rate, such as brisk walking, cycling, or swimming, into daily routines.

Hydration is often overlooked in discussions about eye health, but Dr. Barbara points out that staying well-hydrated is essential for maintaining the moisture levels in the eyes. Adequate fluid intake supports tear production, which is vital for keeping the eyes clean and free from irritants.

Lastly, Dr. Barbara underscores the importance of regular eye examinations as a critical component of maintaining eye health.

These exams not only assess vision and need for correction but also provide an opportunity to detect early signs of eye conditions such as glaucoma, diabetic retinopathy, and macular degeneration before they progress. She advises making eye exams a regular part of health care, even if no eye problems are currently evident.

In essence, Dr. Barbara's insights into maintaining eye health revolve around a holistic approach that incorporates a nutrient-rich diet, lifestyle modifications, and preventive care. By adopting these practices, individuals can significantly contribute to the longevity and health of their vision, ensuring that their eyes remain a vibrant connection to the world around them.

CHAPTER 2: NUTRITIONAL SUPPORT FOR BETTER VISION

Ensuring optimal eye health through nutrition involves focusing on foods rich in specific vitamins, minerals, and antioxidants known to support vision and protect against common eye diseases. A balanced diet that includes a variety of fruits, vegetables, nuts, seeds, and fatty fish can provide the essential nutrients necessary for maintaining healthy eyes and good vision.

Beneficial effects: Consuming a diet rich in vitamins A, C, and E, zinc, and omega-3 fatty acids contributes significantly to eye health. These nutrients can help reduce the risk of chronic eye diseases, including age-related macular degeneration and cataracts, by protecting the eyes from oxidative stress, improving cellular health, and supporting the proper functioning of the visual system.

Ingredients:

- 2 cups of mixed leafy greens (spinach, kale, collards) for vitamins C, E, and beta-carotene

- 1 cup of mixed berries (blueberries, strawberries) for antioxidants and vitamin C

- 1 medium sweet potato for beta-carotene and vitamin E

- 2 tablespoons of ground flaxseed or chia seeds for omega-3 fatty acids

- 1/2 cup of walnuts or almonds for vitamin E and omega-3s

- 1/4 cup of pumpkin seeds for zinc

- 2 medium-sized bell peppers (red or yellow) for vitamin C

- 3 ounces of cooked salmon or tuna for omega-3 fatty acids and vitamin D

- 1/2 cup of cooked quinoa for protein and zinc

Instructions:

1. Begin by preparing the leafy greens. Wash them thoroughly and chop if necessary. These can be used raw in salads or lightly steamed.

2. Wash and slice the berries. Berries can be eaten fresh or added to a smoothie.

3. Bake or steam the sweet potato until tender. It can be consumed alone, added to salads, or mashed.

4. Grind the flaxseed or chia seeds if they are not already in ground form. These can be sprinkled over salads, incorporated into smoothies, or mixed into yogurt.

5. Chop the walnuts or almonds and toast them lightly to enhance their flavor. Add these to salads or have them as a snack.

6. Toast the pumpkin seeds lightly. These can be eaten alone or added to salads and dishes for a zinc boost.

7. Slice the bell peppers and consume them raw in salads or lightly sautéed in dishes.

8. Cook the salmon or tuna to your preference. It can be grilled, baked, or added to salads.

9. Prepare the quinoa according to package instructions. It can serve as a base for salads or a side dish.

Variations:

- Vegetarians or vegans can substitute salmon with flaxseed oil or algae-based omega-3 supplements to ensure adequate intake of omega-3 fatty acids.

- For a nut-free diet, seeds like pumpkin and sunflower can replace nuts to provide zinc and vitamin E.

Storage tips: Most of these ingredients are best consumed fresh. However, cooked dishes can be stored in an airtight container in the refrigerator for up to 3 days. Nuts and seeds should be kept in a cool, dry place or refrigerated to maintain their freshness.

Tips for allergens: For those with specific food allergies, always ensure substitutes align with dietary restrictions. For example, those allergic to fish can find omega-3 fatty acids in flaxseeds, chia seeds, and hemp seeds.

Scientific references:

- The Age-Related Eye Disease Study (AREDS and AREDS2), funded by the National Eye Institute, has shown that a combination of vitamins C and E, zinc, copper, lutein, and zeaxanthin can slow the progression of age-related macular degeneration.

- Research published in the "Journal of the American Medical Association" suggests that omega-3 fatty acids are beneficial in preventing dry eye syndrome and other ocular conditions.

By incorporating these nutrient-rich foods into your daily diet, you can support your vision and overall eye health, potentially reducing the risk of common eye diseases and conditions. Remember, a balanced diet combined with regular eye check-ups and protecting your eyes from excessive UV light exposure forms the foundation of good eye health.

CHAPTER 3: NATURAL REMEDIES FOR EYE HEALTH

These remedies, often derived from herbs, plants, and natural compounds, offer a gentle yet effective way to nourish and protect the eyes, potentially reducing the risk of common eye conditions and supporting overall vision. Below are several herbal recipes and natural treatments designed to bolster eye health, each leveraging the inherent properties of its ingredients to provide targeted benefits.

In holistic health, the eyes are considered a reflection of the body's overall well-being. Nourishing and protecting eye health through natural remedies aligns with the belief that our body has an inherent capacity to heal and maintain itself when provided with the right nutrients and care. **Herbs, plants, and natural compounds** offer a gentle yet potent way to support eye health, focusing on prevention, nourishment, and healing from the inside out. Below is a closer look at how specific natural remedies can support and enhance eye health, potentially reducing the risk of common eye conditions such as macular degeneration, cataracts, and dry eyes.

1. **Nourishing the Eyes from Within: Herbal and Nutritional Support**

   o **Bilberry (Vaccinium myrtillus)**: Known for its high concentration of **anthocyanins**, bilberry has long been used to support vision and eye health. These powerful antioxidants help improve circulation to the eyes, reduce inflammation, and protect against oxidative stress, which is a major contributor to age-related eye conditions like macular degeneration and cataracts. Incorporating bilberry into the diet, whether through herbal teas, supplements, or fresh berries, can provide ongoing nourishment for the eyes.

   o **Ginkgo Biloba**: Ginkgo biloba is renowned for improving blood flow and oxygenation, not just to the brain but also to the eyes. Enhanced circulation helps to maintain retinal health and prevent issues related to poor oxygen supply to the eye tissues. This herb can be taken as a tea, tincture, or supplement and is particularly beneficial for those experiencing early signs of eye strain or fatigue.

   o **Omega-3 Fatty Acids**: Found in flaxseed, chia seeds, and fish oils, omega-3s are essential for maintaining the moisture balance in the eyes. They help reduce inflammation and support the structure of cell membranes in the eyes, which is particularly beneficial for preventing or alleviating dry eyes. Omega-3s also play a role in preventing macular degeneration, making them a key component of any holistic eye health regimen.

2. **Topical Treatments: Soothing and Rejuvenating Eye Compresses**

   o **Chamomile (Matricaria chamomilla)**: Chamomile's anti-inflammatory and calming properties make it an ideal herb for soothing tired, irritated eyes. Chamomile tea bags can be cooled and applied as compresses over the eyes to reduce puffiness, redness, and irritation. This simple remedy helps to relax the muscles around the eyes, alleviating tension and promoting a sense of calm.

   o **Cucumber (Cucumis sativus)**: Long known for its cooling and hydrating properties, cucumber slices placed on the eyes can help refresh and rejuvenate tired eyes. Cucumbers contain antioxidants such as vitamin C and caffeic acid, which help reduce swelling and inflammation. This treatment is particularly useful for reducing puffiness and dark circles around the eyes.

- o **Rose Water**: Rose water is a gentle and hydrating treatment that can be used as an eye wash or compress to soothe and refresh the eyes. Its anti-inflammatory and antioxidant properties help reduce eye strain, redness, and dryness. Rose water is also known for its calming aroma, which can help promote relaxation and relieve stress—important factors for overall eye health.

3. **Prevention and Protection: Herbs to Safeguard Vision**

- o **Eyebright (Euphrasia officinalis)**: Eyebright is an herb traditionally used in holistic medicine to address various eye conditions, including conjunctivitis, eye strain, and sensitivity to light. It contains compounds that help reduce inflammation and protect the delicate tissues of the eyes. Eyebright can be used in the form of eye drops, herbal teas, or as a compress to maintain eye health and prevent infections.

- o **Carotenoid-Rich Foods**: Carotenoids, such as **lutein** and **zeaxanthin**, are pigments found in dark leafy greens, carrots, and other brightly colored vegetables. These compounds are known to concentrate in the retina and act as a natural defense against harmful blue light and oxidative stress. Consuming a diet rich in these carotenoids helps protect the eyes from age-related degeneration and supports long-term vision health.

- o **Turmeric (Curcuma longa)**: Turmeric's active compound, **curcumin**, is a powerful anti-inflammatory agent. By reducing systemic inflammation, turmeric can help protect against chronic eye conditions, including uveitis and cataracts. Turmeric can be integrated into the diet or taken as a supplement to bolster eye health over time.

4. **Lifestyle Practices for Eye Health**

- o **Eye Exercises and Rest**: Beyond herbal remedies, it's important to incorporate practices that support overall eye health. Regular breaks from screens and focusing on distant objects can reduce eye strain. Simple eye exercises, such as rolling the eyes, blinking frequently, and palming (covering the eyes with the palms of your hands to relax them), can also improve circulation and reduce tension in the eye muscles.

- o **Hydration**: Staying well-hydrated is crucial for maintaining moisture in the eyes, particularly for those prone to dry eyes. Proper hydration ensures that the tear ducts function optimally and helps prevent irritation caused by dryness.

5. **Creating a Holistic Eye Care Routine**

- o **Daily Rituals**: Incorporating these natural remedies into your daily routine can have profound effects on eye health over time. Start the day with a bilberry or chamomile tea, apply a soothing eye compress in the evening, and include eye-supportive foods like leafy greens and omega-3-rich seeds in your diet. Creating a ritual around eye care fosters mindfulness and reinforces the connection between self-care and long-term health.

Beneficial effects: These natural remedies aim to support eye health by providing antioxidants, reducing inflammation, and enhancing hydration, which are crucial for maintaining clear vision and preventing conditions such as dry eyes, macular degeneration, and cataracts. The ingredients selected are known for their rich nutrient profiles and have been traditionally used to support various aspects of eye health.

Bilberry Eye Tonic

Ingredients:

- 1 cup of fresh or frozen bilberries

- 2 cups of water

- Honey to taste (optional)

- **Instructions**:

1. Bring the water to a boil in a small saucepan.

2. Add the bilberries and reduce the heat. Simmer for 10 minutes.

3. Strain the mixture to remove the bilberry solids, preserving the liquid.

4. Allow the tonic to cool to a comfortable temperature. Add honey to taste, if desired.

5. Consume 1 cup of the bilberry tonic daily.

Eyebright Infusion

Ingredients:

- 1 teaspoon of dried eyebright herb

- 1 cup of boiling water

- **Instructions**:

1. Place the dried eyebright in a tea infuser or teapot.

2. Pour boiling water over the herb and cover.

3. Steep for 10 minutes.

4. Strain and drink the infusion. Enjoy 1 cup daily for best results.

Goji Berry Eye Elixir

Ingredients:

- ¼ cup of goji berries

- 1 cup of boiling water

- **Instructions**:

1. Add goji berries to a mug or heatproof glass.

2. Pour boiling water over the berries and let them steep for 20-30 minutes.

3. Strain the mixture, pressing the berries to extract the juice.

4. Drink the elixir once daily.

Saffron and Honey Eye Drops

Ingredients:

- A pinch of saffron threads

- 1 tablespoon of distilled water

- 1 teaspoon of honey

- **Instructions**:

1. Crush the saffron threads into a fine powder.

2. Mix the saffron powder with distilled water and honey in a small, sterilized bottle.

3. Shake well until the honey is fully dissolved.

4. Use as eye drops, applying 1-2 drops in each eye at bedtime. Shake well before each use.

Turmeric and Aloe Eye Gel

Ingredients:

- 1 tablespoon of aloe vera gel

- ¼ teaspoon of turmeric powder

- **Instructions**:

1. In a small bowl, mix the aloe vera gel and turmeric powder until well combined.

2. Apply a small amount of the gel around the eyes, being careful to avoid direct contact with the eyes.

3. Leave on for 20 minutes, then rinse with cool water.

4. Use 2-3 times a week for best results.

Variations: For those with sensitivities, the ingredients can be adjusted. For example, if honey is not suitable, it can be omitted from the saffron eye drops. Similarly, for a nut-free version of the goji berry elixir, ensure no cross-contamination with nuts during preparation.

Storage tips: Store any leftover bilberry tonic, eyebright infusion, and goji berry elixir in the refrigerator for up to 48 hours. The saffron and honey eye drops and turmeric and aloe eye gel should be used within a week and stored in the refrigerator to maintain freshness.

Tips for allergens: Always patch test topical remedies to ensure no adverse reactions. For those with specific allergies, consult with a healthcare provider before incorporating new remedies into your routine.

Scientific references: Studies have shown the antioxidant properties of bilberries can support vision health, while eyebright has been traditionally used for eye irritation and discomfort. Goji berries are rich in zeaxanthin and lutein, known to benefit eye health. Saffron has been studied for its potential to improve retinal function, and turmeric's anti-inflammatory properties may help reduce puffiness and irritation around the eyes.

By integrating these natural remedies into your eye care regimen, alongside a diet rich in eye-supporting nutrients and regular eye check-ups, you can support your vision and eye health in a holistic and nurturing way.

CHAPTER 4: 5 HERBAL RECIPES FOR EYE HEALTH

BILBERRY AND EYEBRIGHT EYE WASH

Beneficial effects

Bilberry and Eyebright Eye Wash is a natural remedy designed to enhance eye health and relieve symptoms of eye strain and irritation. Bilberries are rich in anthocyanins, powerful antioxidants that can improve night vision, reduce eye fatigue, and protect against eye diseases such as macular degeneration. Eyebright, traditionally used for eye care, contains anti-inflammatory compounds that can soothe irritated eyes and reduce redness. Together, this eye wash can promote clearer vision, soothe eye discomfort, and support overall eye health.

Ingredients

- 1 tablespoon dried bilberries
- 1 tablespoon dried eyebright herb
- 2 cups distilled water

Instructions

1. Boil 2 cups of distilled water in a small pot.

2. Add the dried bilberries and eyebright herb to the boiling water.

3. Reduce the heat and simmer for 10 minutes, allowing the herbs to infuse their properties into the water.

4. Remove the pot from the heat and allow the mixture to cool to room temperature.

5. Strain the mixture through a fine mesh sieve or cheesecloth to remove the herbs, collecting the liquid in a clean container.

6. To use, pour a small amount of the eye wash into a sterile eye cup or use a clean dropper to apply several drops into each eye. Blink several times to distribute the wash over the entire eye surface.

7. Use the eye wash 1-2 times daily, especially after prolonged reading, computer work, or exposure to irritants.

Variations

- For added antimicrobial properties, dissolve a pinch of salt into the eye wash during the cooling process.

- To enhance the soothing effect, add a teaspoon of aloe vera juice to the cooled mixture.

- For a refreshing and cooling sensation, store the eye wash in the refrigerator before use.

Storage tips

Store the Bilberry and Eyebright Eye Wash in a sealed glass container in the refrigerator for up to one week. Ensure the container is sterilized before use to maintain the solution's purity.

Tips for allergens

Individuals with sensitivities to bilberries or eyebright should perform a patch test on the skin before applying the eye wash to the eyes. Substitute with chamomile tea for a gentler alternative if necessary.

Scientific references

- "Anthocyanins in Health and Disease," published in Critical Reviews in Food Science and Nutrition, highlights the antioxidant properties of bilberries and their benefits for eye health.

- "Anti-inflammatory and anti-allergic effects of Euphrasia officinalis and its components," in the Journal of Ethnopharmacology, discusses the anti-inflammatory benefits of eyebright in eye care.

CARROT AND SPINACH EYE SMOOTHIE

Beneficial effects

The Carrot and Spinach Eye Smoothie is designed to support eye health and improve vision clarity. Carrots are rich in beta-carotene, a type of vitamin A that is crucial for good vision, eye health, and immune function. Spinach is loaded with lutein and zeaxanthin, antioxidants that are known to reduce the risk of chronic eye diseases, including age-related macular degeneration and cataracts. This smoothie is a natural way to nourish the body and support eye health through essential nutrients and antioxidants.

Portions

2 servings

Preparation time

10 minutes

Ingredients

- 2 medium carrots, peeled and chopped

- 2 cups fresh spinach leaves

- 1 ripe banana

- 1/2 cup orange juice

- 1/2 cup water

- Ice cubes (optional)

Instructions

1. Place the chopped carrots, spinach leaves, and ripe banana into a blender.

2. Add the orange juice and water to the blender.

3. Blend on high until the mixture is smooth and creamy. If the smoothie is too thick, add a little more water to achieve the desired consistency.

4. If a colder beverage is preferred, add ice cubes and blend again until smooth.

5. Pour the smoothie into glasses and serve immediately to enjoy its eye health benefits.

Variations

- For an added boost of omega-3 fatty acids, include a tablespoon of flaxseeds or chia seeds in the blend.

- Substitute orange juice with apple juice for a different flavor profile.

- Add a scoop of your favorite protein powder to make the smoothie a more filling, nutrient-rich meal replacement or snack.

Storage tips

It's best to consume the Carrot and Spinach Eye Smoothie immediately after preparation to ensure maximum nutrient retention and freshness. However, if necessary, it can be stored in an airtight container in the refrigerator for up to 24 hours.

Tips for allergens

Individuals with allergies to any of the ingredients should substitute or omit as necessary. For those with citrus allergies, apple juice or water can be used in place of orange juice without significantly affecting the smoothie's benefits for eye health.

Scientific references

- "Nutritional and health benefits of carrots and their seed extracts," in the Food and Nutrition Sciences journal, discusses the role of beta-carotene in supporting eye health.

- "Dietary carotenoids, vitamins C and E, and risk of cataract in women: a prospective study," published in the Archives of Ophthalmology, highlights the importance of lutein and zeaxanthin in reducing the risk of cataracts.

BLUEBERRY AND KALE EYE HEALTH JUICE

Beneficial effects

Blueberry and Kale Eye Health Juice is a nutrient-rich beverage designed to support and enhance eye health. Blueberries are packed with antioxidants, particularly anthocyanins, which can help protect the eyes from oxidative stress and reduce the risk of age-related macular degeneration. Kale is a superfood high in lutein and zeaxanthin, two nutrients known for their protective effects on the eyes, especially against light-induced damage. Together, this juice provides a powerful combination of vitamins, minerals, and antioxidants that promote overall eye health and vision clarity.

Portions

2 servings

Preparation time

10 minutes

Ingredients

- 1 cup fresh blueberries

- 2 cups chopped kale, stems removed

- 1 apple, cored and sliced

- 1/2 cucumber, sliced

- 1/2 lemon, juiced

- 1 inch piece of fresh ginger, peeled

- 1 cup water or coconut water

Instructions

1. Wash all fruits and vegetables thoroughly under running water.

2. Add the blueberries, chopped kale, apple slices, cucumber slices, lemon juice, and ginger to a blender.

3. Pour in 1 cup of water or coconut water to help blend the ingredients smoothly.

4. Blend on high until the mixture is completely smooth. If the juice is too thick, add more water or coconut water until you reach the desired consistency.

5. Strain the juice through a fine mesh sieve or cheesecloth to remove any pulp, if preferred.

6. Serve the juice immediately, or chill in the refrigerator for a refreshing cold drink.

Variations

- For added sweetness, include a tablespoon of honey or agave syrup in the blend.

- Boost the antioxidant content by adding a handful of spinach or a scoop of your favorite greens powder.
- To enhance hydration, replace water with coconut water for its electrolyte content.

Storage tips

If there are leftovers, store the Blueberry and Kale Eye Health Juice in a sealed container in the refrigerator for up to 24 hours. Shake well before serving if separation occurs.

Tips for allergens

For individuals with allergies to citrus, omit the lemon juice or replace it with a small amount of apple cider vinegar for a similar zesty flavor without the allergen.

Scientific references

- "Anthocyanins in Health and Disease," published in the journal Critical Reviews in Food Science and Nutrition, discusses the role of blueberry anthocyanins in protecting against oxidative stress.
- "Dietary Sources of Lutein and Zeaxanthin Carotenoids and Their Role in Eye Health," in the journal Nutrients, highlights the importance of kale and other leafy greens for eye health due to their high lutein and zeaxanthin content.

CHAMOMILE AND FENNEL EYE COMPRESS

Beneficial effects

Chamomile and Fennel Eye Compress offers a soothing and anti-inflammatory remedy for tired, irritated eyes. Chamomile is renowned for its calming and soothing properties, which can help reduce eye puffiness and redness. Fennel, on the other hand, is known for its anti-inflammatory and antibacterial benefits, aiding in the relief of eye strain and promoting eye health. Together, they create a gentle, natural treatment to refresh and soothe the eyes.

Ingredients

- 1 tablespoon dried chamomile flowers
- 1 tablespoon dried fennel seeds
- 2 cups boiling water

Instructions

1. In a heat-resistant bowl, combine the dried chamomile flowers and fennel seeds.
2. Pour 2 cups of boiling water over the chamomile and fennel.
3. Cover the bowl and allow the mixture to steep for 10 to 15 minutes.
4. Strain the mixture to remove the solids, reserving the liquid.
5. Soak a clean cloth or cotton pads in the warm liquid.
6. Gently place the soaked cloth or cotton pads over closed eyes and rest for 10 to 15 minutes.
7. Repeat as needed for soothing relief.

Variations

- For additional soothing effects, add a few drops of lavender essential oil to the mixture after straining.
- To enhance the compress for dry eyes, mix in a teaspoon of aloe vera gel to the cooled liquid before soaking the cloth or cotton pads.
- For a refreshing morning eye treatment, chill the strained liquid in the refrigerator before use.

Storage tips

The strained liquid from the Chamomile and Fennel Eye Compress can be stored in a sealed container in the refrigerator for up to 48 hours. Use cold for a refreshing eye treatment or warm gently before use for a soothing effect.

Tips for allergens

Individuals with allergies to chamomile, fennel, or lavender should proceed with caution and may consider testing a small amount of the liquid on the skin before applying to the eyes. For those sensitive to aloe vera, it can be omitted from the variations without affecting the compress's benefits.

Scientific references

- "Chamomile: A herbal medicine of the past with a bright future" published in Molecular Medicine Reports, discusses the anti-inflammatory and soothing effects of chamomile, supporting its use in eye care.

- "Fennel (Foeniculum vulgare) and its effects on health" in the journal Critical Reviews in Food Science and Nutrition, highlights the medicinal properties of fennel, including its anti-inflammatory benefits, which are beneficial for eye health.

ROSEMARY AND LAVENDER EYE SOOTHER

Beneficial effects

The Rosemary and Lavender Eye Soother leverages the calming and anti-inflammatory properties of both rosemary and lavender to provide relief for tired, strained eyes. Rosemary enhances circulation and reduces puffiness, while lavender soothes and reduces irritation. This natural remedy can help alleviate symptoms of eye strain from computer use, environmental irritants, or lack of sleep, promoting a sense of relaxation and rejuvenation for the eyes.

Ingredients

- 1 tablespoon dried rosemary leaves
- 1 tablespoon dried lavender flowers
- 2 cups boiling water
- Cotton pads or a clean cloth

Instructions

1. Place the dried rosemary leaves and lavender flowers in a heat-resistant bowl.

2. Pour 2 cups of boiling water over the herbs.

3. Cover the bowl and allow the herbs to steep for 15 to 20 minutes.

4. Strain the infusion, discarding the herbs, and allow the liquid to cool to a comfortable temperature.

5. Soak cotton pads or a clean cloth in the cooled infusion.

6. Apply the soaked pads or cloth over closed eyes and rest for 10 to 15 minutes.

Variations

- For additional soothing effects, add a teaspoon of chamomile flowers to the infusion.

- To enhance the cooling sensation, refrigerate the strained infusion for an hour before use.

- For a more concentrated solution, reduce the amount of water to 1 cup for steeping the herbs.

Storage tips

Store any unused Rosemary and Lavender Eye Soother infusion in a sealed container in the refrigerator for up to 48 hours. Ensure the infusion is at room temperature or slightly chilled before applying to the eyes.

Tips for allergens

Individuals sensitive to rosemary or lavender should perform a patch test on the skin before applying the infusion near the eyes. For those allergic to chamomile or other suggested variations, omit these ingredients or substitute with another gentle, non-irritating herb like cucumber slices.

Scientific references

- "Anti-inflammatory and skin barrier repair effects of topical application of some plant oils" in the International Journal of Molecular Sciences, 2017. This study supports the anti-inflammatory properties of lavender, beneficial for soothing eye irritation.

- "Rosmarinus officinalis L.: An update review of its phytochemistry and biological activity" in Future Science OA, 2018. This review highlights the circulatory benefits of rosemary, supporting its use in reducing puffiness around the eyes.

PART 28: HOLISTIC PAIN MANAGEMENT

Holistic pain management focuses on treating the whole person, recognizing that pain is not just a physical sensation but can also be influenced by emotional, social, and spiritual factors. This approach combines traditional medical treatments with alternative therapies to address pain's root causes and improve overall well-being. Effective holistic pain management strategies include a combination of dietary changes, physical activities, herbal remedies, and mindfulness practices, each tailored to the individual's unique needs and preferences.

Dietary Changes for Pain Management

Inflammation in the body can exacerbate pain. Adopting an anti-inflammatory diet can help reduce inflammation and, consequently, pain. Foods rich in omega-3 fatty acids, such as salmon, flaxseeds, and walnuts, have been shown to reduce inflammation. Incorporating a variety of fruits and vegetables, especially berries, leafy greens, and tomatoes, can also support inflammation reduction due to their high antioxidant content. Turmeric, ginger, and garlic are spices known for their anti-inflammatory properties and can be easily added to meals to enhance flavor and health benefits.

Physical Activities

Regular physical activity is crucial for managing pain. Exercise releases endorphins, the body's natural painkillers, and helps reduce inflammation. Activities such as walking, swimming, and yoga can be particularly beneficial. Yoga, for instance, not only improves physical strength and flexibility but also incorporates breathing exercises and meditation, which can help manage pain by reducing stress and improving mental focus.

Herbal Remedies

Several herbs have been traditionally used to manage pain and support overall health. Below are herbal recipes known for their pain-relieving properties:

White Willow Bark and Ginger Pain Relief Tea

Beneficial effects: White willow bark contains salicin, which the body converts into salicylic acid, providing pain relief and anti-inflammatory benefits. Ginger further enhances these effects by reducing inflammation and supporting circulation.

Ingredients:

- 1 teaspoon of dried white willow bark

- 1 teaspoon of grated fresh ginger

- 2 cups of water

- Honey to taste (optional)

- **Instructions**:

1. Boil water in a small saucepan.

2. Add white willow bark and ginger to the boiling water.

3. Reduce heat and simmer for 15 minutes.

4. Strain the tea into a cup and add honey if desired.

5. Drink once or twice daily to help manage pain.

Mindfulness and Relaxation Techniques

Mindfulness meditation and relaxation techniques can be powerful tools for managing pain. By focusing on the present moment and practicing deep breathing, individuals can alter their perception of pain. Techniques such as progressive muscle relaxation, guided imagery, and mindfulness-based stress reduction (MBSR) can help reduce the intensity of pain, improve emotional well-being, and enhance quality of life.

Acupuncture and Massage Therapy

Acupuncture involves the insertion of thin needles into specific points on the body to relieve pain and promote healing. Massage therapy can help reduce muscle tension, improve circulation, and alleviate pain. Both therapies can be integrated into a holistic pain management plan, offering additional avenues for relief and healing.

Scientific references:

- Studies have shown that omega-3 fatty acids can reduce the production of substances linked to inflammation, making them beneficial for managing conditions associated with chronic pain (Journal of Pain Research).

- Research on the efficacy of yoga for pain management suggests that it can significantly reduce pain and improve physical function in individuals with various chronic pain conditions (International Journal of Yoga).

By embracing a holistic approach to pain management, individuals can explore a wide range of strategies that address both the physical and emotional aspects of pain. This comprehensive approach not only seeks to alleviate pain but also aims to enhance overall health and well-being, empowering individuals to lead more fulfilling lives despite chronic pain conditions.

CHAPTER 1: NUTRITIONAL SUPPORT FOR PAIN RELIEF

dopting an anti-inflammatory diet is a cornerstone for managing pain through nutrition, focusing on foods that naturally reduce inflammation and thus, the body's pain response. Foods rich in omega-3 fatty acids, antioxidants, and phytochemicals play a pivotal role in this dietary approach.

Beneficial effects: An anti-inflammatory diet can significantly reduce the body's inflammatory markers, leading to decreased pain, especially for those suffering from chronic pain conditions such as arthritis, fibromyalgia, and inflammatory bowel disease. Incorporating specific nutrients can also aid in muscle recovery, reduce stiffness, and improve overall joint health.

Ingredients:

- Omega-3 fatty acids: Found in fatty fish like salmon, mackerel, and sardines, as well as in flaxseeds, chia seeds, and walnuts.

- Antioxidants: Berries, leafy greens, nuts, and seeds are excellent sources.

- Phytochemicals: Vegetables like tomatoes, bell peppers, and other brightly colored vegetables contain phytochemicals that reduce inflammation.

- Whole grains: Quinoa, brown rice, and oats help fight inflammation.

- Spices: Turmeric and ginger are known for their anti-inflammatory properties.

Instructions:

1. **Salmon with Turmeric and Ginger**:

- Season a salmon fillet with ground turmeric, ginger, salt, and pepper.

- Bake at 375°F for 20-25 minutes or until cooked through.

- Serve with a side of quinoa and steamed vegetables for a balanced, anti-inflammatory meal.

2. **Berry and Spinach Smoothie**:

- Blend 1 cup of mixed berries (blueberries, strawberries, raspberries), 1 cup of spinach, 1 tablespoon of chia seeds, and 1 cup of almond milk until smooth.

- Enjoy as a refreshing, anti-inflammatory drink, perfect for starting the day or as a post-workout snack.

3. **Walnut and Avocado Salad**:

- Combine mixed greens, sliced avocado, chopped walnuts, and cherry tomatoes in a bowl.

- Dress with a vinaigrette made from olive oil, lemon juice, salt, and pepper.

- This salad is rich in omega-3 fatty acids and antioxidants, promoting anti-inflammatory benefits.

4. **Ginger Tea**:

- Peel and slice fresh ginger root.

- Boil slices in water for 15-20 minutes.

- Strain and enjoy the tea, adding honey for sweetness if desired.

- Ginger tea can help reduce inflammation and soothe pain.

Variations:

- For a vegan option, replace salmon with tofu. Marinate tofu in turmeric, ginger, and olive oil before baking.

- Add a scoop of protein powder to the smoothie for an extra protein boost.

- For the salad, sprinkle with hemp seeds instead of walnuts for a different source of omega-3.

Storage tips:

- Cooked salmon should be consumed within 2 days when stored in the refrigerator.

- Smoothies are best enjoyed immediately but can be stored in the fridge for up to 24 hours.

- Salad ingredients can be prepped ahead and stored separately in the fridge for quick assembly.

Tips for allergens:

- For those allergic to nuts, omit walnuts from the salad and use seeds like pumpkin or sunflower seeds.

- Ensure any added protein powder in the smoothie is free from allergens specific to your dietary needs.

Scientific references:

- Studies have shown that omega-3 fatty acids can significantly reduce the production of molecules and substances linked to inflammation, such as inflammatory eicosanoids and cytokines (Source: "Journal of the American College of Nutrition").

- Research indicates that curcumin, the active ingredient in turmeric, has potent anti-inflammatory properties and is effective in treating symptoms of arthritis (Source: "Journal of Medicinal Food").

By incorporating these foods and recipes into your diet, you can harness the power of nutrition to support pain relief and improve your overall health.

CHAPTER 2: NATURAL REMEDIES FOR PAIN RELIEF

arnessing the power of nature, several herbs and natural compounds offer profound benefits for pain relief, acting as alternatives or complements to conventional treatments. These remedies can reduce inflammation, alleviate discomfort, and promote healing without the reliance on pharmaceuticals. Below are detailed recipes for creating effective herbal remedies for pain relief, each chosen for its proven efficacy and safety profile.

Devil's Claw and Ginger Pain Relief Tonic

Beneficial effects: Devil's Claw is renowned for its anti-inflammatory properties, making it beneficial for arthritis and lower back pain. Ginger, with its potent anti-inflammatory and antioxidant effects, complements Devil's Claw, enhancing pain relief and circulation.

Ingredients:

- 1 teaspoon of dried Devil's Claw root

- 1 teaspoon of grated fresh ginger

- 2 cups of water

- Honey or lemon to taste (optional)

- **Instructions**:

1. Combine water, Devil's Claw root, and grated ginger in a saucepan.

2. Bring to a boil, then simmer for 20 minutes.

3. Strain the mixture into a cup, removing the solids.

4. Add honey or lemon to taste, if desired.

5. Consume this tonic once daily to help manage pain.

Boswellia and Frankincense Pain Relief Balm

Beneficial effects: Boswellia, also known as Indian Frankincense, contains compounds that have strong anti-inflammatory effects and can reduce pain associated with arthritis and other inflammatory conditions. When applied topically, it can provide localized relief from muscle and joint pain.

Ingredients:

- ¼ cup of coconut oil

- ¼ cup of beeswax pellets

- 2 tablespoons of Boswellia serrata extract

- 10 drops of Frankincense essential oil

- **Instructions**:

1. Melt coconut oil and beeswax together in a double boiler over low heat.

2. Once melted, remove from heat and stir in the Boswellia extract and Frankincense essential oil.

3. Pour the mixture into a small container and let it cool until solid.

4. Apply the balm directly to painful areas as needed.

Arnica and St. John's Wort Pain Relief Oil

Beneficial effects: Arnica is widely used for its remarkable ability to reduce bruising and swelling, making it ideal for treating sprains, strains, and bruises. St. John's Wort has anti-inflammatory properties and can help soothe nerve pain.

Ingredients:

- ½ cup of Arnica flowers
- ½ cup of St. John's Wort flowers
- 1 cup of olive oil or almond oil
- **Instructions**:

1. Combine Arnica and St. John's Wort flowers in a glass jar.
2. Cover the flowers with olive oil or almond oil, ensuring they are completely submerged.
3. Seal the jar and place it in a sunny window for 4-6 weeks, shaking it daily.
4. After the infusion period, strain the oil through a cheesecloth into a clean jar.
5. Apply the oil to affected areas 2-3 times daily for pain relief.

Cayenne and Peppermint Pain Relief Cream

Beneficial effects: Cayenne pepper contains capsaicin, which depletes the body's supply of substance P, a chemical component of nerve cells that transmits pain signals to the brain. Peppermint offers a cooling sensation, providing relief from muscular aches and pains.

Ingredients:

- ¼ cup of coconut oil
- ¼ cup of shea butter
- 2 tablespoons of cayenne pepper powder
- 10 drops of peppermint essential oil
- **Instructions**:

1. Gently melt the coconut oil and shea butter in a double boiler over low heat.
2. Stir in the cayenne pepper powder until fully incorporated.
3. Remove from heat and let the mixture cool slightly before adding the peppermint essential oil.
4. Pour the cream into a container and allow it to solidify.
5. Apply to sore muscles and joints sparingly, and wash hands thoroughly after application.

Variations: For sensitive skin, reduce the amount of cayenne pepper or essential oils to prevent irritation. Always patch test a small area before widespread use.

Storage tips: Store these remedies in a cool, dark place. The shelf life of oils and balms is typically up to one year if stored properly.

Tips for allergens: For those with allergies to nuts, substitute almond oil with an alternative such as jojoba or grapeseed oil. Always check for allergies to specific herbs or essential oils before application.

Scientific references: Numerous studies validate the anti-inflammatory and pain-relieving properties of these natural ingredients. For instance, research published in the "Journal of Ethnopharmacology" supports the use of Devil's Claw for pain relief in arthritis, while a study in the "Journal of Rheumatology" highlights capsaicin's effectiveness in reducing pain.

By incorporating these natural remedies into your pain management strategy, you can leverage the healing power of herbs and natural compounds to alleviate discomfort and improve your quality of life.

CHAPTER 3: 10 HERBAL RECIPES FOR PAIN MANAGEMENT

WHITE WILLOW BARK AND GINGER PAIN RELIEF TEA

Beneficial effects

White Willow Bark and Ginger Pain Relief Tea combines the natural anti-inflammatory properties of white willow bark with the warming, soothing effects of ginger. This herbal tea is designed to alleviate pain, reduce inflammation, and provide relief from conditions such as arthritis, headaches, and menstrual cramps. White willow bark acts as a natural aspirin, offering pain relief without the side effects of synthetic drugs, while ginger enhances circulation and eases stomach discomfort, making this tea an all-around remedy for pain management.

Portions

2 servings

Preparation time

10 minutes

Cooking time

15 minutes

Ingredients

- 1 teaspoon white willow bark

- 1 inch piece of fresh ginger, peeled and sliced

- 2 cups water

- Honey or lemon to taste (optional)

Instructions

1. Bring 2 cups of water to a boil in a small pot.

2. Add the white willow bark and sliced ginger to the boiling water.

3. Reduce the heat and simmer for about 10 minutes, allowing the ingredients to infuse their properties into the water.

4. Remove the pot from the heat and let the tea steep for an additional 5 minutes.

5. Strain the tea into mugs, discarding the white willow bark and ginger slices.

6. Optional: Add honey or lemon to taste for flavor enhancement.

7. Serve the tea warm, ideally twice a day, to help manage pain and inflammation.

Variations

- For added anti-inflammatory benefits, include a teaspoon of turmeric powder during the simmering process.

- Mix in a cinnamon stick for additional flavor and potential blood sugar regulation benefits.

- For those preferring a cold beverage, allow the tea to cool and serve over ice for a refreshing pain relief drink.

Storage tips

Store any leftover White Willow Bark and Ginger Pain Relief Tea in a sealed container in the refrigerator for up to 2 days. Enjoy chilled or gently reheat on the stove.

Tips for allergens

Individuals with allergies to salicylates (found in aspirin) should proceed with caution when using white willow bark. For those avoiding honey due to dietary restrictions, substitute with maple syrup or simply omit the sweetener.

Scientific references

- "The analgesic and anti-inflammatory effects of Salix alba L. bark extract" in the Journal of Ethnopharmacology, 2009. This study highlights the effectiveness of white willow bark in treating pain and inflammation.

- "Ginger on Human Health: A Comprehensive Systematic Review of 109 Randomized Controlled Trials" in Nutrients, 2020. This systematic review highlights ginger's health benefits, particularly its anti-inflammatory properties and effectiveness in digestive health support.

DEVIL'S CLAW AND TURMERIC PAIN RELIEF TONIC

Beneficial effects

Devil's Claw and Turmeric Pain Relief Tonic is a natural remedy designed to alleviate pain and reduce inflammation. Devil's Claw is renowned for its anti-inflammatory properties, making it beneficial for conditions such as arthritis, back pain, and other forms of chronic pain. Turmeric, containing the active compound curcumin, further enhances the anti-inflammatory effects and provides antioxidant benefits. This tonic can help improve mobility, reduce stiffness, and support overall joint health.

Ingredients

- 1 teaspoon of dried Devil's Claw root
- 1 teaspoon of turmeric powder
- 2 cups of water
- Honey or lemon to taste (optional)

Instructions

1. Bring 2 cups of water to a boil in a small pot.

2. Add the dried Devil's Claw root and turmeric powder to the boiling water.

3. Reduce the heat and simmer for about 10 minutes.

4. Remove the pot from the heat and allow the tonic to steep for an additional 10 minutes.

5. Strain the tonic into a cup, discarding the solids.

6. Optional: Add honey or lemon to taste for flavor enhancement.

7. Drink the tonic warm, preferably in the morning and evening, to maximize its pain-relieving benefits.

Variations

- For added benefits, include a slice of fresh ginger during the simmering process to enhance the anti-inflammatory properties.

- Mix in a pinch of black pepper to increase the bioavailability of curcumin from turmeric.

- Replace water with green tea for an antioxidant-rich base that complements the anti-inflammatory effects.

Storage tips

Prepare the Devil's Claw and Turmeric Pain Relief Tonic fresh for each use to ensure potency. However, if you need to store it, keep the tonic in a sealed container in the refrigerator for up to 24 hours. Reheat gently before consuming.

Tips for allergens

Individuals with sensitivities to Devil's Claw or turmeric should start with a smaller dose to ensure no adverse reactions. For those avoiding honey due to dietary restrictions, substitute with maple syrup or simply omit the sweetener.

Scientific references

- "Efficacy and safety of Devil's Claw (Harpagophytum procumbens) in the treatment of osteoarthritis: a systematic review," published in the Journal of Alternative and Complementary Medicine, highlights the effectiveness of Devil's Claw in pain management and inflammation reduction.
- "Curcumin: A Review of Its' Effects on Human Health," published in Foods, discusses the wide-ranging health benefits of curcumin, including its anti-inflammatory and antioxidant effects, which support its use for joint health and pain relief.

BOSWELLIA AND GINGER PAIN RELIEF BALM

Beneficial effects

Boswellia and Ginger Pain Relief Balm offers a natural solution for managing pain and inflammation. Boswellia, known for its potent anti-inflammatory properties, can significantly reduce pain associated with conditions like arthritis and joint discomfort. Ginger complements Boswellia by providing additional anti-inflammatory and analgesic benefits, helping to soothe muscle soreness and reduce swelling. This balm is ideal for those seeking a holistic approach to pain management without the side effects of conventional medications.

Ingredients

- 1/4 cup coconut oil
- 2 tablespoons beeswax pellets
- 2 teaspoons Boswellia serrata extract powder
- 2 teaspoons ginger extract or finely grated ginger
- 10 drops lavender essential oil (for added pain relief and a calming scent)
- 1 tablespoon olive oil (to enhance the skin's absorption of the balm)

Instructions

1. In a double boiler, melt the coconut oil and beeswax pellets together over medium heat until completely liquid.

2. Reduce the heat to low and stir in the Boswellia serrata extract powder and ginger extract or grated ginger until fully incorporated.

3. Remove from heat and allow the mixture to cool slightly before adding the lavender essential oil. Stir well to ensure the essential oil is evenly distributed throughout the balm.

4. Mix in the olive oil to the slightly cooled mixture to help with absorption and skin hydration.

5. Pour the balm into small jars or tins and allow it to solidify at room temperature.

6. Once solidified, close the jars or tins with lids for storage.

Variations

- For those sensitive to lavender, substitute with peppermint essential oil for a refreshing scent and additional pain-relieving properties.

- Add a teaspoon of turmeric powder to the mixture for its anti-inflammatory benefits and to enhance the balm's effectiveness.

- For a vegan alternative, replace beeswax pellets with candelilla wax, using half the amount as it has a denser consistency.

Storage tips

Store the Boswellia and Ginger Pain Relief Balm in a cool, dry place away from direct sunlight. If stored properly in an airtight container, the balm can last for up to 6 months.

Tips for allergens

Individuals with allergies to coconut, beeswax, or any of the essential oils should substitute these ingredients with suitable alternatives or perform a patch test before applying the balm extensively. Olive oil can be replaced with another carrier oil like almond oil for those with specific sensitivities.

Scientific references

- "Boswellia serrata, A potential antiinflammatory agent: An overview" published in the Indian Journal of Pharmaceutical Sciences, highlights the anti-inflammatory properties of Boswellia serrata.

- "Ginger—An Herbal Medicinal Product with Broad Anti-Inflammatory Actions" in the Journal of Medicinal Food discusses ginger's role in reducing inflammation and its potential as a pain relief agent.

ARNICA AND LAVENDER PAIN RELIEF OIL

Beneficial effects

Arnica and Lavender Pain Relief Oil combines the anti-inflammatory properties of Arnica montana with the soothing effects of Lavender essential oil to create a potent remedy for relieving pain and inflammation. Arnica is widely recognized for its ability to reduce swelling and alleviate pain, making it particularly effective for treating bruises, sprains, and muscle soreness. Lavender, known for its calming and anti-inflammatory properties, further enhances the oil's effectiveness by promoting relaxation and reducing tension in the affected area. This synergistic blend is ideal for those seeking natural pain relief and a reduction in inflammation.

Ingredients

- 1/4 cup Arnica montana flowers (dried)

- 1 cup carrier oil (such as almond or olive oil)

- 15 drops Lavender essential oil

Instructions

1. Place the dried Arnica montana flowers in a clean, dry jar.

2. Pour the carrier oil over the flowers until they are completely submerged.

3. Seal the jar tightly and place it in a warm, sunny spot for 2-3 weeks, shaking it gently every few days.

4. After the infusion period, strain the oil through a fine mesh sieve or cheesecloth, discarding the Arnica flowers.

5. Add the Lavender essential oil to the infused Arnica oil and stir well to combine.

6. Transfer the final Arnica and Lavender Pain Relief Oil into a clean, dark glass bottle for storage.

Variations

- For added cooling and pain-relieving effects, include 10 drops of Peppermint essential oil to the blend.

- If a quicker preparation is desired, gently heat the carrier oil and Arnica flowers over a double boiler for 2-3 hours instead of the infusion method.

- Substitute almond oil with jojoba oil for a lighter texture that's suitable for sensitive skin.

Storage tips

Store the Arnica and Lavender Pain Relief Oil in a cool, dark place to preserve its potency. When stored properly, the oil can last up to a year. Ensure the bottle is tightly sealed to prevent oxidation.

Tips for allergens

Individuals with sensitivities to Arnica, Lavender, or the chosen carrier oil should perform a patch test before widespread use. For those allergic to nuts, ensure to select a nut-free carrier oil like olive oil.

Scientific references

- "Arnica montana L. – a plant of healing: review" published in the Journal of Pharmacy and Pharmacology, highlights the anti-inflammatory and pain-relieving properties of Arnica.

- "Lavender and the Nervous System" in Evidence-Based Complementary and Alternative Medicine, discusses the calming, anti-inflammatory, and analgesic effects of Lavender essential oil, supporting its use in pain management and inflammation reduction.

CAYENNE AND ST. JOHN'S WORT PAIN RELIEF CREAM

Beneficial effects

Cayenne and St. John's Wort Pain Relief Cream harnesses the analgesic properties of cayenne pepper and the soothing effects of St. John's Wort to create a powerful topical remedy for relieving pain. Cayenne pepper, containing capsaicin, is known to reduce pain sensations by decreasing substance P, a chemical that sends pain signals to the brain. St. John's Wort, with its anti-inflammatory properties, aids in soothing nerve pain and reducing inflammation. This combination makes the cream an effective treatment for joint pain, muscle aches, and nerve-related discomfort.

Ingredients

- 1/4 cup coconut oil
- 2 tablespoons beeswax pellets
- 1 teaspoon cayenne pepper powder
- 2 teaspoons St. John's Wort oil
- 10 drops lavender essential oil (for additional soothing properties)
- 1/2 teaspoon vitamin E oil (as a preservative and skin conditioner)

Instructions

1. In a double boiler, melt the coconut oil and beeswax pellets together over medium heat until fully dissolved.

2. Once melted, remove from heat and allow the mixture to cool slightly before adding the cayenne pepper powder. Stir well to ensure even distribution.

3. Add the St. John's Wort oil, lavender essential oil, and vitamin E oil to the mixture. Stir thoroughly to combine all ingredients.

4. Pour the mixture into a clean, small jar or tin and allow it to cool and solidify.

5. Once cooled, seal the container and label it with the date and contents.

Variations

- For sensitive skin, reduce the amount of cayenne pepper powder to lessen the warming sensation.

- Add a few drops of peppermint oil for a cooling effect that contrasts with the warmth of the cayenne.

- Substitute coconut oil with shea butter for a creamier texture and additional moisturizing benefits.

Storage tips

Store the Cayenne and St. John's Wort Pain Relief Cream in a cool, dark place to maintain its potency. If stored properly, the cream can last for up to 6 months. Avoid exposure to extreme temperatures to preserve the therapeutic properties of the ingredients.

Tips for allergens

Individuals with sensitivity to capsaicin (cayenne pepper) or any of the essential oils should perform a patch test before widespread use. For those allergic to coconut, shea butter or another hypoallergenic carrier oil can be used as an alternative base for the cream.

Scientific references

- "Capsaicin: Current Understanding of Its Mechanisms and Therapy of Pain and Other Pre-Clinical and Clinical Uses," published in Molecules, discusses the pain-relieving mechanisms of capsaicin found in cayenne pepper.

- "Hypericum perforatum (St John's Wort) in Depression: Pest or Blessing?" in the Journal of Clinical Psychiatry, highlights the anti-inflammatory and nerve-soothing properties of St. John's Wort, supporting its use in managing pain and inflammation.

ASHWAGANDHA AND TURMERIC JOINT RELIEF SMOOTHIE

Beneficial effects

The Ashwagandha and Turmeric Joint Relief Smoothie is designed to alleviate joint pain and inflammation, making it an excellent choice for individuals suffering from conditions like arthritis. Ashwagandha is known for its stress-reducing properties and its ability to improve the body's defense against disease, which can be particularly beneficial for inflammatory conditions. Turmeric, rich in curcumin, offers potent anti-inflammatory and antioxidant benefits that can help reduce pain and stiffness in the joints. Together, these ingredients create a powerful smoothie that supports joint health, reduces inflammation, and enhances overall well-being.

Portions

2 servings

Preparation time

10 minutes

Ingredients

- 1 cup almond milk

- 1/2 banana, frozen

- 1/2 cup pineapple, chopped and frozen

- 1 teaspoon turmeric powder

- 1 teaspoon Ashwagandha powder

- 1 tablespoon flaxseed meal

- Honey to taste (optional)

- Ice cubes (optional)

Instructions

1. Place the almond milk, frozen banana, and frozen pineapple into a blender.

2. Add the turmeric powder, Ashwagandha powder, and flaxseed meal to the blender.

3. Blend on high until the mixture is smooth and creamy. If the smoothie is too thick, add a little more almond milk to achieve the desired consistency.

4. Taste the smoothie and add honey if a sweeter taste is preferred. Blend again briefly to mix.

5. If a colder smoothie is desired, add ice cubes and blend until smooth.

6. Pour the smoothie into glasses and serve immediately for the best flavor and nutrient content.

Variations

- For an extra protein boost, add a scoop of your favorite protein powder to the blender before mixing.

- Substitute almond milk with coconut water for a lighter version that's still hydrating and flavorful.

- Add a pinch of black pepper to enhance the absorption of curcumin from turmeric.

Storage tips

It's best to consume the Ashwagandha and Turmeric Joint Relief Smoothie immediately after preparation to ensure maximum potency of the ingredients. However, if necessary, it can be stored in an airtight container in the refrigerator for up to 24 hours. Stir well before consuming if separation occurs.

Tips for allergens

Individuals with allergies to nuts should substitute almond milk with a non-nut milk alternative like oat milk or rice milk. For those with a honey allergy or following a vegan diet, substitute honey with maple syrup or omit it altogether.

Scientific references

- "Efficacy and safety of curcumin in major depressive disorder: a randomized controlled trial" in Phytotherapy Research, 2014. This study highlights the anti-inflammatory properties of turmeric and its benefits for mental health.

- "An Overview on Ashwagandha: A Rasayana (Rejuvenator) of Ayurveda" published in the African Journal of Traditional, Complementary and Alternative Medicines, discusses the adaptogenic and stress-relief properties of ashwagandha, supporting its use for joint health and inflammation reduction.

GINGER AND BOSWELLIA ANTI-INFLAMMATORY SOUP

Beneficial effects

Ginger and Boswellia Anti-Inflammatory Soup is crafted to alleviate inflammation and pain, particularly beneficial for individuals suffering from joint discomfort and arthritis. Ginger, with its potent anti-inflammatory compounds, can help reduce swelling and pain, while Boswellia is known for its ability to inhibit pro-inflammatory markers in the body. This combination not only aids in managing chronic pain but also supports overall joint health and mobility.

Portions

4 servings

Preparation time

15 minutes

Cooking time

40 minutes

Ingredients

- 1 tablespoon olive oil

- 1 large onion, chopped

- 2 cloves garlic, minced

- 2 inches fresh ginger, peeled and grated

- 1 teaspoon Boswellia powder

- 4 cups vegetable broth

- 2 large carrots, peeled and diced

- 1 cup red lentils, rinsed

- Salt and pepper to taste

- Juice of 1 lemon

Instructions

1. Heat olive oil in a large pot over medium heat. Add onion and garlic, sautéing until soft and translucent.

2. Stir in grated ginger and Boswellia powder, cooking for another 2 minutes.

3. Pour in vegetable broth and bring to a boil.

4. Add diced carrots and red lentils to the pot. Reduce heat, cover, and simmer for about 30 minutes, or until lentils and carrots are tender.

5. Season with salt and pepper to taste.

6. Remove from heat and stir in lemon juice.

7. Serve warm to enjoy its anti-inflammatory benefits.

Variations

- For an added protein boost, include diced chicken breast or tofu cubes.

- Incorporate spinach or kale during the last 5 minutes of cooking for extra nutrients.

- Add a pinch of turmeric for additional anti-inflammatory properties.

Storage tips

Store leftover soup in an airtight container in the refrigerator for up to 3 days. Reheat on the stove or in the microwave until thoroughly warm.

Tips for allergens

Individuals with sensitivities to Boswellia should start with a smaller dose to ensure no adverse reactions. For those avoiding garlic or onions due to FODMAP sensitivities, these can be omitted or replaced with garlic-infused olive oil and the green parts of spring onions.

Scientific references

- "Anti-Oxidative and Anti-Inflammatory Effects of Ginger in Health and Physical Activity: Review of Current Evidence," published in the International Journal of Preventive Medicine, highlights ginger's anti-inflammatory properties.

- "Boswellia serrata, A potential antiinflammatory agent: An overview," published in the Indian Journal of Pharmaceutical Sciences, discusses the anti-inflammatory and pain-relieving effects of Boswellia.

REISHI MUSHROOM AND GINGER IMMUNE BOOST ELIXIR

Beneficial effects

The Reishi Mushroom and Ginger Immune Boost Elixir combines the immune-enhancing properties of Reishi mushrooms with the warming, anti-inflammatory benefits of ginger. Reishi mushrooms are known for their ability to support the immune system by increasing the activity of white blood cells, which helps the body fight off infections and cancer. Ginger adds to this potent mix with its ability to reduce inflammation, soothe sore throats, and alleviate nausea. Together, they create a powerful elixir that not only boosts the immune system but also provides a comforting, warming sensation that can help ward off colds and flu.

Ingredients

- 1 teaspoon Reishi mushroom powder
- 1 inch fresh ginger, peeled and sliced
- 2 cups of water
- Honey to taste (optional)

Instructions

1. Bring 2 cups of water to a boil in a small pot.

2. Add the sliced ginger to the boiling water.

3. Reduce the heat and simmer for about 10 minutes to allow the ginger to infuse the water.

4. Stir in the Reishi mushroom powder and continue to simmer for another 5 minutes.

5. Remove the pot from the heat and let the elixir cool slightly.

6. Strain the elixir into a mug or glass, removing the ginger slices.

7. Add honey to taste, if desired, and stir until dissolved.

8. Enjoy the elixir warm, ideally in the morning or evening to boost the immune system.

Variations

- For an extra immune boost, add a slice of lemon or a dash of cayenne pepper to the elixir during the simmering process.

- Replace water with green tea for an added antioxidant boost.

- For those who prefer a sweeter taste without honey, try adding a few drops of stevia or a slice of apple during the simmering process for natural sweetness.

Storage tips

This elixir is best enjoyed fresh, but if needed, it can be stored in the refrigerator for up to 24 hours. Reheat gently on the stove or enjoy cold.

Tips for allergens

Individuals with allergies to mushrooms should avoid Reishi powder. For those who cannot consume honey, maple syrup serves as a great alternative sweetener.

Scientific references

- "Immunomodulating Effects of Fungal Metabolites" in the Journal of Medicinal Food discusses the immune-supporting properties of Reishi mushrooms.

- "Anti-Oxidative and Anti-Inflammatory Effects of Ginger in Health and Physical Activity: Review of Current Evidence" in the International Journal of Preventive Medicine highlights ginger's health benefits, including its role in immune support and inflammation reduction.

MILK THISTLE AND TURMERIC LIVER SUPPORT TEA

Beneficial effects

Milk Thistle and Turmeric Liver Support Tea is formulated to enhance liver function and detoxification processes. Milk Thistle, known for its liver-protecting silymarin content, aids in regenerating liver cells and protecting the liver from toxins. Turmeric, rich in curcumin, provides strong anti-inflammatory and antioxidant benefits that support liver health. This tea is beneficial for those looking to maintain liver health, support detoxification, and protect against liver diseases.

Ingredients

- 1 tablespoon dried milk thistle seeds
- 1 teaspoon turmeric powder
- 4 cups of water
- Honey or lemon to taste (optional)

Instructions

1. Crush the milk thistle seeds slightly to release their active compounds.

2. Bring 4 cups of water to a boil in a medium-sized pot.

3. Add the crushed milk thistle seeds and turmeric powder to the boiling water.

4. Reduce the heat and simmer for 10 minutes, allowing the herbs to infuse their properties into the water.

5. Remove the pot from the heat and allow the tea to cool slightly.

6. Strain the tea into cups or a large pitcher, discarding the solids.

7. Optional: Add honey or lemon to taste for flavor enhancement.

8. Serve the tea warm, or allow it to cool and enjoy it chilled.

Variations

- For added detoxification benefits, include a slice of fresh ginger or a dash of cayenne pepper to the tea while it simmers.

- Mix in a cinnamon stick during the simmering process for additional flavor and blood sugar regulation benefits.

- Substitute honey with maple syrup for a vegan-friendly sweetener option.

Storage tips

Store any leftover Milk Thistle and Turmeric Liver Support Tea in a sealed container in the refrigerator for up to 2 days. Enjoy it chilled, or gently reheat on the stove.

Tips for allergens

Individuals with allergies to milk thistle or turmeric should proceed with caution and may consider consulting with a healthcare provider before consumption. For those avoiding honey due to dietary restrictions, substitute with maple syrup or simply omit the sweetener.

Scientific references

- "Silymarin, the Antioxidant Component and Silybum marianum Extracts Prevent Liver Damage" in Food and Chemical Toxicology highlights the liver-protective effects of milk thistle.

- "Curcumin and Liver Disease: from Chemistry to Medicine" in Comprehensive Reviews in Food Science and Food Safety discusses the beneficial impact of turmeric on liver health, including its anti-inflammatory and antioxidant effects.

ELDERFLOWER AND GINGER CORDIAL

Beneficial effects

Elderflower and Ginger Cordial is a delightful, natural remedy known for its immune-boosting and anti-inflammatory properties. Elderflower is rich in antioxidants and has been traditionally used to alleviate cold and flu symptoms, while ginger adds digestive benefits and further enhances the cordial's anti-inflammatory effects. This combination makes the cordial not only a refreshing drink but also a supportive tonic for overall health and wellness.

Portions

Makes about 1 liter

Preparation time

15 minutes

Cooking time

24 hours for infusion

Ingredients

- 20 fresh elderflower heads, gently rinsed

- 1.5 liters of water

- 2 lemons, sliced

- 1 small orange, sliced (optional)

- 700g granulated sugar

- 50g citric acid

Instructions

1. In a large bowl, combine the elderflower heads, lemon slices, and orange slices if using.

2. In a saucepan, bring the water to a boil and dissolve the granulated sugar into it to create a syrup.

3. Pour the hot syrup over the elderflower and citrus mixture, ensuring all the flowers are submerged.

4. Stir in the citric acid until fully dissolved.

5. Cover the bowl with a clean cloth and allow the mixture to infuse for 24 hours at room temperature.

6. After infusion, strain the cordial through a fine mesh sieve or cheesecloth into a clean, sterilized bottle. Press the solids to extract maximum flavor.

7. Seal the bottle and store in the refrigerator.

Variations

- For a herbal twist, add a few sprigs of fresh mint or rosemary to the infusion.

- Replace granulated sugar with honey for a naturally sweetened version, adjusting the quantity to taste.

- Add a vanilla pod to the syrup while boiling for an aromatic flavor profile.

Storage tips

The elderflower cordial can be stored in the refrigerator for up to 6 weeks. For longer preservation, the cordial can be frozen in ice cube trays and used as needed.

Tips for allergens

Individuals with pollen allergies should proceed with caution when handling and consuming elderflowers. For those with citrus allergies, omit the lemon and orange slices and consider adding non-citrus flavorings like vanilla or herbs.

Scientific references

- "Antioxidant activities of elderflower extracts" in Food Chemistry, highlighting the antioxidant capacity of elderflower and its potential health benefits.

- "The use of elderflower (Sambucus nigra L.) in food and medicine: Tradition and current perspectives" in the Journal of Ethnopharmacology, discussing the traditional and contemporary uses of elderflower in promoting health and wellness.

CHAPTER 29: DR. BARBARA'S DETOX METHODS

Detoxification and cleansing are integral components of Dr. Barbara's holistic health approach, emphasizing the body's innate ability to heal and purify itself. Recognizing the modern lifestyle's challenges, including exposure to environmental toxins, processed foods, and stress, Dr. Barbara advocates for regular detoxification practices to support the body's natural detox systems: the liver, kidneys, digestive system, skin, and lungs. Her methods are grounded in the principle that a well-supported detoxification system can lead to improved energy levels, better digestion, clearer skin, and overall enhanced well-being.

One of Dr. Barbara's foundational detox methods involves incorporating a diet rich in whole, unprocessed foods. She emphasizes the importance of organic fruits and vegetables, particularly those high in antioxidants and fiber, to aid the body in eliminating toxins. Foods such as leafy greens, berries, beets, and seeds are staples in her detox diet plan.

These foods not only support the liver and kidneys, crucial organs in the detoxification process, but also promote a healthy gut microbiome, essential for efficient digestion and toxin removal.

Hydration is another cornerstone of Dr. Barbara's detoxification methods. Drinking ample amounts of filtered or spring water throughout the day is encouraged to facilitate the elimination of waste products through the kidneys. Additionally, herbal teas such as dandelion or green tea are recommended for their diuretic properties and their ability to support liver function.

Physical activity and sweating are also viewed as vital detoxification practices. Regular exercise boosts circulation and encourages the elimination of toxins through sweat. Dr. Barbara often suggests incorporating sauna sessions or steam baths as additional means to promote sweating and toxin release, always advising proper hydration before and after such practices to maintain electrolyte balance.

To further support the body's detox pathways, Dr. Barbara incorporates specific herbal supplements known for their cleansing properties. Milk thistle, for instance, is heralded for its liver-protective effects, aiding in the regeneration of liver cells and the stabilization of cell membranes.

Dandelion root is another herb frequently recommended for its ability to support both liver and kidney function, acting as a natural diuretic without depleting the body of essential minerals.

Mindfulness and stress reduction are also integral to Dr. Barbara's detoxification approach. Recognizing the impact of stress on the body's physiological processes, including its ability to detoxify effectively, she incorporates practices such as yoga, meditation, and deep breathing exercises.

These practices not only help in reducing the body's stress response but also enhance the overall detoxification process by promoting relaxation and facilitating a deeper connection with the body.

In addition to these foundational practices, Dr. Barbara emphasizes the importance of a supportive environment and community in the detoxification journey. She encourages the creation of a toxin-free living space by choosing natural cleaning products and personal care items, as well as fostering relationships that support healthy lifestyle choices.

Embracing seasonal detoxification rituals is a key aspect of Dr. Barbara's holistic health approach, aligning the body's cleansing processes with the natural rhythms of the earth.

She advocates for gentle seasonal cleanses during the spring and fall, times traditionally associated with renewal and letting go, respectively. These cleanses often involve a simplified diet focusing on seasonal fruits and vegetables, increased intake of fluids, and the incorporation of herbs that naturally support detoxification, such as nettle and burdock root.

The objective is not only to eliminate toxins but also to reset the digestive system, rejuvenate the body's energy, and prepare the body for the season ahead.

Sleep plays a crucial role in the body's natural detoxification processes, particularly in the brain. Dr. Barbara highlights the importance of quality sleep for the glymphatic system, a unique cleanup process in the brain that occurs during sleep.

This system removes waste products from the brain, which can include toxins associated with neurodegenerative diseases. Ensuring adequate and restful sleep, therefore, becomes essential in supporting the body's overall detox efforts.

Strategies to enhance sleep quality include establishing a regular sleep schedule, creating a restful environment free of electronic devices, and possibly incorporating herbal teas like chamomile or valerian root that promote relaxation and sleep.

Emotional and spiritual detoxification is another dimension of Dr. Barbara's comprehensive detox methods. She believes that emotional wellbeing and physical health are deeply interconnected, and holding onto negative emotions can impede the body's ability to detoxify fully.

Practices such as journaling, spending time in nature, and engaging in community or spiritual gatherings can facilitate emotional release and healing.

These practices not only support mental and emotional health but also enhance the physical detoxification process by reducing stress and promoting a sense of peace and well-being.

Incorporating fasting or intermittent fasting as part of a detoxification strategy can also be beneficial, under proper guidance.

Dr. Barbara suggests that short periods of fasting can help rest the digestive system, promote cellular autophagy (the body's way of cleaning out damaged cells), and improve metabolic functions.

It's important, however, to approach fasting with care, ensuring it's done in a way that supports the body's needs and in consultation with a healthcare professional, especially for individuals with specific health conditions.

Finally, Dr. Barbara underscores the significance of listening to the body's signals during any detoxification process. She encourages a mindful approach to detox, paying attention to how the body responds to different foods, activities, and practices.

This mindfulness can guide individuals in making adjustments that best support their unique detoxification needs, leading to enhanced vitality, improved health, and a deeper connection with their body's natural rhythms and capabilities.

By weaving together these various strands of detoxification—dietary, physical, emotional, and spiritual—Dr. Barbara presents a holistic blueprint for cleansing that can lead to profound health benefits.

Her methods emphasize the body's inherent wisdom and capacity for self-healing, advocating for a gentle, supportive approach to detoxification that nurtures the body, mind, and spirit.

CHAPTER 1: THE ROLE OF DETOXIFICATION IN HEALTH

Detoxification plays a pivotal role in maintaining optimal health, acting as the body's natural mechanism for cleansing and renewing itself. This process involves the elimination of toxins from the body, which can accumulate due to environmental pollutants, processed foods, and lifestyle choices that may not support health. The liver, kidneys, digestive system, skin, and lungs all work in concert to ensure these unwanted substances are effectively removed from the body. When these systems function optimally, they can more efficiently process and eliminate toxins, leading to improved health outcomes.

A diet rich in whole, unprocessed foods is fundamental to supporting the body's detoxification pathways. Foods that are high in antioxidants, such as berries, nuts, and leafy greens, play a crucial role in neutralizing free radicals and supporting the liver, one of the primary detoxification organs. Similarly, foods high in fiber, such as whole grains and legumes, aid in maintaining a healthy digestive system, which is essential for the elimination of toxins through waste.

Hydration is another key element in the detoxification process. Water not only supports kidney function but also helps in the transportation of nutrients and the removal of waste products from the body. Herbal teas, rich in compounds that support liver and kidney health, offer an additional benefit by providing hydration while also delivering antioxidants and other phytonutrients that aid in detoxification.

Engaging in regular physical activity stimulates the circulatory and lymphatic systems, enhancing the body's ability to detoxify by increasing blood flow and promoting the elimination of toxins through sweat. Exercise also supports the health of the lungs, encouraging deeper breathing which in turn facilitates the removal of carbon dioxide and other gaseous wastes from the body.

Incorporating specific herbal supplements into one's routine can further support detoxification. Milk thistle, for example, is renowned for its liver-protective properties, helping to shield the liver from damage and support its regenerative capacity. Dandelion root acts as a natural diuretic, supporting the kidneys in flushing out waste. These herbs, among others, can be integrated into the diet through teas, capsules, or tinctures, offering a natural way to enhance the body's detoxification processes.

Stress reduction is an often-overlooked aspect of detoxification. Chronic stress can negatively impact the body's ability to detoxify by affecting the digestive system and altering the balance of gut bacteria. Practices such as yoga, meditation, and deep breathing exercises not only help in managing stress but also improve the body's resilience, supporting overall detoxification and well-being.

The environment one lives in can also influence the body's detoxification process. Reducing exposure to toxins by choosing natural cleaning products, avoiding processed foods, and minimizing the use of synthetic personal care items can significantly decrease the body's toxic burden. Creating a living space that supports health and well-being can make a substantial difference in the effectiveness of the body's natural detoxification efforts.

As we delve deeper into the role of detoxification in health, it becomes clear that a multifaceted approach, encompassing diet, lifestyle, and environmental factors, is essential for supporting the body's natural detoxification pathways. This holistic view not only emphasizes the importance of removing toxins from the body but also highlights the need for nurturing practices that support overall health and well-being.

Adopting a holistic approach to detoxification extends beyond diet and exercise, encompassing the need for emotional and spiritual cleansing as well. Emotional well-being plays a critical role in the body's ability to detoxify, as negative emotions and stress can lead to physical manifestations, including the inhibition of natural detox processes. Engaging in activities that foster emotional release and balance, such as journaling, art therapy, and spending time in nature, can significantly enhance the body's detoxification capabilities by reducing stress and promoting mental clarity.

Spiritual practices, including meditation, mindfulness, and prayer, contribute to a sense of inner peace and well-being, further supporting the body's detoxification pathways. These practices help in aligning the body and mind, creating a conducive environment for healing and renewal. By fostering a deeper connection with oneself and the surrounding world, individuals can enhance their capacity for self-care and detoxification.

The quality of sleep is another vital component of effective detoxification. During sleep, the body undergoes numerous restorative processes, including the removal of toxins and the repair of cellular damage. Ensuring a restful and uninterrupted sleep cycle supports these natural processes, allowing the body to heal and rejuvenate. Creating a sleep-conducive environment, free from electronic distractions and rich in comfort, can help in achieving deep, restorative sleep.

The use of specific detoxifying herbs and supplements should be tailored to individual needs and conditions, with consideration for potential interactions and contraindications. Consulting with a healthcare professional before beginning any new supplement regimen is essential to ensure safety and efficacy. Herbs such as cilantro, known for its heavy metal chelating properties, and turmeric, with its potent anti-inflammatory and antioxidant effects, can be incorporated into the diet to support detoxification. However, their use should be personalized and monitored.

Seasonal detoxification practices, aligned with the body's natural rhythms and the changing seasons, offer an opportunity to reset and rejuvenate the body's systems. These practices may include short-term dietary modifications, increased fluid intake, and the use of seasonal herbs. Embracing these rituals can help in maintaining optimal health and supporting the body's innate detoxification processes.

Incorporating fasting or intermittent fasting can stimulate autophagy, the body's mechanism for cleaning out damaged cells and regenerating new ones, offering profound detoxification and health benefits. However, it's crucial to approach fasting with mindfulness, listening to the body's cues, and ensuring that any fasting practice is undertaken in a healthy and supportive manner.

The journey of detoxification is deeply personal and should be approached with patience and self-compassion. Recognizing that detoxification is not a one-size-fits-all process but rather a personalized journey that can vary greatly from one individual to another is key. By listening to the body and responding to its needs, individuals can navigate their detoxification path with awareness and intention.

Ultimately, the goal of detoxification is to support the body's natural healing processes, promoting vitality, wellness, and a balanced state of health. By embracing a comprehensive approach that includes dietary, physical, emotional, and spiritual practices, individuals can enhance their body's ability to detoxify and achieve a greater sense of well-being. This holistic perspective not only supports the removal of toxins but also nurtures the body, mind, and spirit, leading to a healthier, more vibrant life.

CHAPTER 2: FOODS THAT PROMOTE DETOXIFICATION

Foods that promote detoxification are integral to flushing out toxins from the body, supporting liver function, and enhancing overall health. These foods are rich in antioxidants, vitamins, minerals, and fibers, which are essential for the body's natural detoxification processes. Including a variety of these foods in your diet can help in the elimination of harmful substances and the promotion of optimal health.

Leafy greens like kale, spinach, and Swiss chard are powerhouse foods for detoxification. They are high in chlorophyll, which aids in purifying the blood, protecting the liver, and removing chemicals and heavy metals from the body. Incorporating these greens into your diet through salads, smoothies, or as a cooked side dish can significantly enhance your body's detoxification efforts.

Cruciferous vegetables such as broccoli, Brussels sprouts, and cauliflower contain glucosinolates, sulfur-containing compounds that help the liver produce enzymes for detoxification. These vegetables also provide a substantial amount of fiber, which is crucial for cleansing the digestive tract and ensuring the regular elimination of toxins through bowel movements.

Beets are another excellent food for detoxification. They are high in antioxidants and nutrients, including betaine, which helps the liver cells eliminate toxins; pectin, a fiber that clears the toxins that have been removed from the liver so they don't reincorporate back into the body; and betalains, pigments with high anti-inflammatory properties to encourage the detoxification process.

Eating beets raw in salads, juiced, or roasted can help boost your detoxification efforts.

Garlic, with its high sulfur content, activates liver enzymes that help your body flush out toxins.

Garlic also has significant amounts of allicin and selenium, two natural compounds that aid in liver cleansing. Incorporating garlic into your meals not only adds flavor but also enhances the detoxifying benefits of your diet.

Green tea is rich in antioxidants called catechins, a compound known to assist in liver function and enhance detoxification.

Drinking green tea daily can provide a gentle detox and improve your overall health by protecting the liver from toxic substances, including alcohol and other environmental pollutants.

Citrus fruits, particularly lemons, limes, and grapefruits, are high in vitamin C, which aids the body in transforming toxins into digestible material. Starting your day with a warm glass of lemon water can stimulate the liver and hydrate the body, providing a simple yet effective daily detox.

Apples are high in pectin, a type of fiber that binds to heavy metals in the body (especially in the colon) and assists with their excretion. This reduces the load on the liver and helps eliminate toxins. Consuming an apple a day can support natural detoxification pathways.

Turmeric, used in cooking or as a supplement, supports the detoxification process by assisting enzymes that actively flush out dietary carcinogens. The main compound in turmeric, curcumin, is known for its anti-inflammatory and antioxidant properties, which further aid in detoxification.

Ginger aids digestion and stimulates the metabolism, which contributes to the excretion of toxins. It also has powerful antioxidant effects. Adding ginger to your diet can enhance the cleansing process by promoting the elimination of toxins through sweat and supporting liver health.

Incorporating these foods into your diet can significantly support your body's natural detoxification processes. It's important to consume a variety of these detoxifying foods to ensure a broad spectrum of nutrients and antioxidants that aid in the elimination of toxins. Remember, the key to effective detoxification is not just the consumption of these foods but also maintaining a balanced diet, staying hydrated, and engaging in regular physical activity to support overall health and well-being.

CHAPTER 3: NATURAL DETOX PRACTICES

Dry brushing is a traditional practice that supports the lymphatic system, a crucial part of the body's detoxification process. By stimulating the lymph nodes, dry brushing aids in the elimination of toxins and strengthens the immune system. The beneficial effects include improved skin texture, removal of dead skin cells, and enhanced blood circulation.

Materials:

- A natural bristle brush

- Essential oils (optional for aftercare)

Preparation:

1. Choose a comfortable, warm place where you can stand or sit naked for the brushing process.

2. If you're new to dry brushing, start with a softer brush to accustom your skin to the sensation.

Instructions:

1. Begin with your feet and move upwards towards your heart using long, smooth strokes. The direction towards the heart is crucial as it aligns with the lymphatic flow.

2. Use circular motions around your joints (ankles, knees, and elbows) and long strokes on long bone areas (shins, thighs, forearms, and upper arms).

3. When reaching your stomach and chest, continue the gentle, circular motions. For women, avoid direct brushing over the breasts.

4. Spend extra time on areas where lymph nodes are concentrated, such as the armpits and groin.

5. After brushing, take a shower to wash away dead skin cells and impurities. Alternate between warm and cold water to further stimulate blood circulation.

6. After showering, consider applying a natural oil like coconut or jojoba to moisturize the skin.

Safety tips:

- Avoid brushing over cuts, wounds, or rashes.

- Do not brush too hard; the goal is to stimulate, not irritate the skin.

- People with sensitive skin should be especially cautious and may want to consult with a dermatologist first.

Maintenance:

- Clean your brush with soap and water once a week. Dry it in a clean, sunny spot to prevent mold.

- Replace your brush every 6-12 months, as the bristles will eventually wear down.

Difficulty rating: ★☆☆☆☆

Variations:

- Add a few drops of essential oils to your brush before starting to add a therapeutic aroma to the experience.

- For those with highly sensitive skin, a loofah or a soft towel can be used as an alternative to a brush.

Storage tips:

- Keep your brush in a dry, airy space to avoid moisture buildup.

- Do not store the brush in the shower or any damp area.

Scientific references:

While scientific studies on dry brushing specifically are limited, research on the lymphatic system and skin exfoliation supports the practice's benefits for health and well-being. Studies on manual lymphatic drainage techniques, which share similarities with dry brushing, indicate positive effects on the immune system and toxin elimination.

Incorporating dry brushing into your daily or weekly routine can be a simple, yet effective way to support your body's natural detoxification processes, complementing other detox practices like healthy eating, hydration, and exercise.

CHAPTER 4: 5 HERBAL RECIPES FOR DETOXIFICATION

BURDOCK AND RED CLOVER DETOX TEA

Beneficial effects

Burdock and Red Clover Detox Tea is designed to support the body's natural detoxification processes, promoting liver health and purifying the blood. Burdock root is known for its blood-cleansing properties and ability to remove toxins from the bloodstream, while red clover acts as a powerful detoxifier and supports overall lymphatic health. This tea can help improve skin clarity, reduce inflammation, and enhance the body's ability to fight off infections by supporting the elimination of toxins.

Portions

2 servings

Preparation time

10 minutes

Ingredients

- 1 tablespoon dried burdock root

- 1 tablespoon dried red clover blossoms

- 4 cups of water

Instructions

1. Bring 4 cups of water to a boil in a medium-sized pot.

2. Add the dried burdock root and red clover blossoms to the boiling water.

3. Reduce the heat and simmer for about 10 minutes, allowing the herbs to infuse their properties into the water.

4. After simmering, remove the pot from the heat and let the tea steep for an additional 10 minutes.

5. Strain the tea into cups or a large pitcher, discarding the herbs.

6. Serve the tea warm, or allow it to cool and enjoy it chilled.

Variations

- For added flavor and detoxification benefits, include a slice of fresh lemon or a teaspoon of honey to the tea while it steeps.

- Mix in a cinnamon stick during the simmering process for a warming, spicy flavor.

- For a more potent detox effect, add a few slices of fresh ginger to the boiling water along with the burdock root and red clover.

Storage tips

Store any leftover Burdock and Red Clover Detox Tea in a sealed container in the refrigerator for up to 2 days. Enjoy it chilled, or gently reheat on the stove.

Tips for allergens

Individuals with sensitivities to burdock or red clover should start with a smaller dose to ensure no adverse reactions. For those avoiding honey due to dietary restrictions, substitute with maple syrup or simply omit the sweetener.

Scientific references

- "The role of burdock in the treatment of chronic diseases" in the Journal of Pharmaceutical Biology, which discusses burdock root's detoxification properties and its role in chronic disease management.

- "Red clover (Trifolium pratense) monograph: A clinical decision support tool" in the Journal of Herbal Medicine, highlighting red clover's use in detoxification and its potential health benefits.

PARSLEY AND DANDELION DETOX SMOOTHIE

Beneficial effects

The Parsley and Dandelion Detox Smoothie is designed to support the body's natural detoxification processes, leveraging the diuretic properties of parsley and dandelion. These herbs are known for their ability to cleanse the liver and kidneys, remove toxins from the bloodstream, and improve overall digestion. Rich in vitamins and minerals, this smoothie can also boost the immune system, provide anti-inflammatory benefits, and contribute to increased energy levels and clearer skin.

Portions

2 servings

Preparation time

10 minutes

Ingredients

- 1 cup fresh parsley, tightly packed
- 1 cup fresh dandelion greens, tightly packed
- 1 ripe banana
- 1 apple, cored and sliced
- 1 tablespoon lemon juice
- 1 cup water or coconut water
- Ice cubes (optional)

Instructions

1. Wash the parsley and dandelion greens thoroughly to remove any dirt or impurities.

2. Place the parsley, dandelion greens, banana, and apple slices into a blender.

3. Add the lemon juice and water or coconut water to the blender.

4. Blend on high until the mixture is smooth and creamy. If the smoothie is too thick, add a little more water or coconut water to achieve the desired consistency.

5. If a colder beverage is preferred, add ice cubes and blend again until smooth.

6. Pour the smoothie into glasses and serve immediately to enjoy its detoxifying benefits.

Variations

- For added sweetness, include a tablespoon of honey or agave syrup in the blend.

- To enhance the smoothie's detoxifying properties, add a small piece of ginger or a teaspoon of turmeric powder.

- Substitute water or coconut water with almond milk for a creamier texture and added nutrients.

Storage tips

It's best to consume the Parsley and Dandelion Detox Smoothie immediately after preparation to ensure maximum freshness and potency of the detoxifying ingredients. However, if necessary, it can be stored in an airtight container in the refrigerator for up to 24 hours. Stir well before consuming if separation occurs.

Tips for allergens

Individuals with allergies to any of the ingredients should substitute or omit as necessary. For those with allergies to citrus, omit the lemon juice or replace it with a small amount of apple cider vinegar for a similar zesty flavor without the allergen.

Scientific references

- "The diuretic effect in human subjects of an extract of Taraxacum officinale folium over a single day," published in the Journal of Alternative and Complementary Medicine, supports the use of dandelion in promoting the elimination of toxins.

- "Parsley: a review of ethnopharmacology, phytochemistry and biological activities" in the Journal of Traditional and Complementary Medicine discusses parsley's role in detoxification and its health benefits.

ACTIVATED CHARCOAL AND LEMON DETOX DRINK

Beneficial effects

The Activated Charcoal and Lemon Detox Drink is designed to cleanse the body by absorbing toxins and chemicals in the gut, aiding their removal from the body. This can help reduce bloating, prevent hangovers, and support overall digestive health. Additionally, the lemon juice in the recipe provides a healthy dose of vitamin C, promoting immune function and skin health.

Ingredients

- 2 tablespoons of activated charcoal powder (from coconut shells)
- Juice of 2 lemons
- 2 tablespoons of organic honey or maple syrup
- 4 cups of filtered water
- Ice cubes (optional)

Instructions

1. In a large pitcher, combine the lemon juice and honey or maple syrup. Stir well until the honey or syrup is fully dissolved in the lemon juice.

2. Add the activated charcoal powder to the pitcher. Stir vigorously to ensure the charcoal is evenly distributed and no clumps remain.

3. Add the filtered water to the pitcher and stir well to combine all the ingredients.

4. Serve the lemonade over ice cubes in glasses, if desired.

Variations

- For a sparkling version, replace half of the filtered water with carbonated water for a fizzy twist.
- Add a pinch of Himalayan pink salt to replenish electrolytes, making it a great post-workout drink.
- Infuse the lemonade with fresh mint leaves or a slice of ginger for additional digestive and flavor benefits.

Storage tips

This Activated Charcoal and Lemon Detox Drink is best enjoyed fresh. However, if you need to store it, keep it in a sealed container in the refrigerator for up to 24 hours. Shake well before drinking if separation occurs.

Tips for allergens

For individuals with sensitivities to honey, maple syrup serves as an excellent vegan alternative. Ensure the activated charcoal used is food-grade and derived from coconut shells to avoid potential allergens found in other types of activated charcoal.

Scientific references

- "Adsorption of Gastrointestinal Toxicants by Activated Charcoal" - American Journal of Emergency Medicine, 1986. This study outlines the effectiveness of activated charcoal in adsorbing toxins, supporting its use in detoxification.

- "Vitamin C in Disease Prevention and Cure: An Overview" - Indian Journal of Clinical Biochemistry, 2013. This article highlights the health benefits of vitamin C, found in lemon juice, including its role in immune function and skin health.

MILK THISTLE AND GINGER DETOX ELIXIR

Beneficial effects

The Milk Thistle and Ginger Detox Elixir is designed to support liver detoxification and overall digestive health. Milk Thistle is renowned for its liver-protective qualities, primarily due to silymarin, a group of compounds said to have antioxidant and anti-inflammatory properties that help repair liver cells damaged by toxins. Ginger adds to this detoxifying effect with its ability to improve digestion, reduce nausea, and help combat inflammation, making this elixir a potent aid in cleansing the body and promoting liver health.

Portions

2 servings

Preparation time

10 minutes

Ingredients

- 1 tablespoon milk thistle seeds, crushed
- 1 inch fresh ginger, peeled and sliced
- 2 cups boiling water
- Honey or lemon to taste (optional)

Instructions

1. Place the crushed milk thistle seeds and sliced ginger in a heat-resistant teapot or jar.

2. Pour 2 cups of boiling water over the milk thistle and ginger.

3. Cover and allow the mixture to steep for about 10 minutes.

4. Strain the elixir into cups, removing the milk thistle seeds and ginger slices.

5. Optional: Add honey or lemon to taste for flavor enhancement.

6. Serve the elixir warm, or allow it to cool and enjoy it chilled.

Variations

- For an added immune boost, include a teaspoon of turmeric powder to the elixir during the steeping process.
- Mix in a cinnamon stick with the milk thistle and ginger for additional anti-inflammatory benefits and a warming flavor.

- For a cold beverage option, refrigerate the strained elixir and serve over ice with a sprig of mint for a refreshing detox drink.

Storage tips

Store any leftover Milk Thistle and Ginger Detox Elixir in a sealed container in the refrigerator for up to 48 hours. Enjoy chilled or gently reheat on the stove.

Tips for allergens

Individuals with allergies to milk thistle or ginger should consult with a healthcare provider before consumption. For those avoiding honey due to dietary restrictions, substitute with maple syrup or simply omit the sweetener.

Scientific references

- "Silymarin, the Antioxidant Component and Silybum marianum Extracts Prevent Liver Damage," in Food and Chemical Toxicology, highlights the liver-protective effects of milk thistle.
- "Ginger in gastrointestinal disorders: A systematic review of clinical trials," in Food Science & Nutrition, 2019. This review supports ginger's benefits in improving digestion and its anti-inflammatory properties.

CILANTRO AND CHLORELLA DETOX JUICE

Beneficial effects

Cilantro and Chlorella Detox Juice is designed to support the body's natural detoxification processes, particularly in removing heavy metals and other toxins. Cilantro, also known as coriander, has been shown to bind to heavy metals, facilitating their removal from the body. Chlorella, a type of green algae, is rich in chlorophyll and other nutrients that support detoxification and enhance immune function. Together, they create a potent detoxifying drink that can help improve energy levels, reduce inflammation, and promote overall health.

Portions

2 servings

Preparation time

10 minutes

Ingredients

- 1 cup fresh cilantro leaves
- 1 teaspoon chlorella powder
- 1 apple, cored and sliced
- 1 lemon, juiced
- 1 cucumber, sliced
- 1 cup water or coconut water

Instructions

1. Wash the cilantro leaves thoroughly to remove any dirt or debris.

2. Place the cilantro leaves, chlorella powder, sliced apple, lemon juice, sliced cucumber, and water or coconut water into a blender.

3. Blend on high until the mixture is smooth.

4. If desired, strain the juice through a fine mesh sieve or cheesecloth to remove any pulp for a smoother texture.

5. Serve the detox juice immediately, or chill in the refrigerator for a refreshing cold drink.

Variations

- For added sweetness, include a tablespoon of honey or agave syrup in the blend.

- To boost the detoxifying effects, add a piece of ginger or a pinch of cayenne pepper.

- Substitute apple with pear for a different flavor profile.

Storage tips

The Cilantro and Chlorella Detox Juice is best consumed fresh but can be stored in a sealed container in the refrigerator for up to 24 hours. Shake well before serving if separation occurs.

Tips for allergens

Individuals with sensitivities to chlorella or cilantro should start with a smaller amount to ensure no adverse reactions. For those avoiding honey due to dietary restrictions, maple syrup can be used as a sweetener alternative.

Scientific references

- "Chlorella vulgaris: A Multifunctional Dietary Supplement with Diverse Medicinal Properties" in the Journal of Medicinal Food, highlights chlorella's role in detoxification and immune support.

- "Effect of Coriandrum sativum (coriander) on lead-induced oxidative stress in rats" in the journal Food and Chemical Toxicology, discusses cilantro's potential in heavy metal detoxification.

CHAPTER 30: HOLISTIC LIVING WITH DR. BARBARA

Embracing a holistic lifestyle is about integrating natural practices for holistic well-being into every aspect of life, fostering a deep connection with oneself, the community, and the environment. This approach is rooted in the understanding that health is not merely the absence of disease but a state of complete physical, mental, and social well-being. Dr. Barbara's methods emphasize the importance of nutrition as the foundation of a holistic lifestyle, recognizing that the foods we consume play a crucial role in shaping our health, energy levels, and overall vitality.

Holistic living, as embraced by Dr. Barbara, is a comprehensive approach to well-being that integrates natural practices into every facet of life. It's grounded in the understanding that true health transcends the mere absence of illness, encompassing a state of complete physical, mental, and social wellness.

This perspective sees health as a dynamic and interconnected state, where each aspect of life influences the whole person.

Dr. Barbara's methods highlight the importance of nutrition as a cornerstone of a holistic lifestyle.

The foods we eat are not just sources of energy but also critical components in shaping our overall health, vitality, and energy levels. By focusing on a diet rich in natural, nutrient-dense foods, Dr. Barbara aims to support and enhance the body's intrinsic ability to maintain balance and prevent illness.

The beneficial effects of embracing a holistic lifestyle can be profound. They include:

1. **Improved Physical Health**: A balanced diet, combined with regular physical activity and mindful practices, can lead to better physical health, including a stronger immune system, improved digestion, and enhanced energy levels.

2. **Enhanced Mental Clarity and Emotional Stability**: Holistic living promotes practices that support mental health, such as stress management techniques, mindfulness, and adequate rest. These practices can improve cognitive function and emotional resilience.

3. **Strengthened Social Connections**: By fostering a sense of community and encouraging meaningful social interactions, holistic living helps build supportive relationships and a sense of belonging.

4. **Greater Environmental Awareness**: Embracing holistic principles often involves a commitment to sustainable practices that protect and respect the environment. This not only benefits personal health but also contributes to the well-being of the planet.

5. **Overall Vitality and Well-being**: Integrating these practices into daily life can lead to a greater sense of overall vitality, satisfaction, and balance, making it easier to navigate life's challenges with a positive and resilient mindset.

Beneficial effects of adopting a holistic lifestyle include improved physical health, enhanced mental clarity, increased energy, better stress management, and a deeper sense of inner peace.

By prioritizing natural practices and mindful living, individuals can support their body's natural healing processes, reduce their environmental impact, and cultivate a life of wellness and fulfillment.

Lemon Balm and Lavender Relaxation Elixir

- **Portions:** Makes about 2 cups

- **Preparation time:** 10 minutes

Ingredients:

- 2 tablespoons dried lemon balm leaves

- 2 tablespoons dried lavender flowers

- 4 cups boiling water

- Honey or sweetener of choice, to taste (optional)

- **Instructions:**

1. Place the lemon balm and lavender flowers in a large teapot or heatproof jar.

2. Pour the boiling water over the herbs and cover.

3. Let the mixture steep for 5-7 minutes, depending on desired strength.

4. Strain the elixir into cups, discarding the herbs.

5. Sweeten with honey or your choice of sweetener if desired.

6. Enjoy this elixir in the evening to promote relaxation and a restful night's sleep.

- **Variations:** For a refreshing twist, add a slice of lemon or a few fresh mint leaves to each cup.

- **Storage tips:** Refrigerate any leftover elixir and consume within 24 hours for best quality.

- **Tips for allergens:** Ensure all ingredients are free from contaminants and processed in an allergen-free facility if allergies are a concern.

Holy Basil and Lemon Verbena Stress Relief Tea

- **Portions:** Makes about 2 cups

- **Preparation time:** 5 minutes

Ingredients:

- 1 tablespoon dried holy basil leaves

- 1 tablespoon dried lemon verbena leaves

- 4 cups boiling water

- **Instructions:**

1. Combine the holy basil and lemon verbena leaves in a teapot or heatproof jar.

2. Add the boiling water and cover to steep.

3. Allow the tea to infuse for about 5 minutes.

4. Strain the tea into cups and enjoy hot.

5. Drink this tea during times of stress or anxiety to help calm the mind and soothe the nerves.

- **Variations:** Add a cinnamon stick or a few slices of fresh ginger for additional flavor and benefits.

- **Storage tips:** This tea is best enjoyed fresh but can be stored in the refrigerator for up to 24 hours.

- **Tips for allergens:** Check the source of herbs for potential cross-contamination with allergens.

Incorporating these recipes into a holistic lifestyle not only provides the body with natural, healing compounds but also encourages taking time for oneself, fostering mindfulness and relaxation. Alongside these practices, Dr. Barbara advocates for regular physical activity, adequate rest, and engaging in activities that nourish the spirit, such as spending time in nature, practicing yoga or meditation, and cultivating meaningful relationships.

By adopting these holistic practices, individuals can create a balanced and harmonious lifestyle that supports their health and well-being on all levels.

CHAPTER 1: NUTRITION IN HOLISTIC LIVING

Nutrition plays a pivotal role in the foundation of a holistic lifestyle, emphasizing the profound impact that food has on our physical health, mental clarity, and overall vitality. The choices we make at the dining table transcend mere caloric intake; they are deeply interwoven with our well-being, influencing everything from our energy levels to our emotional state. A diet centered around whole, unprocessed foods is not just a pathway to better health but a cornerstone of a life lived in harmony with nature's rhythms and balances.

Whole foods, rich in vitamins, minerals, and antioxidants, serve as the body's fuel, providing the necessary nutrients for optimal functioning. These foods, including fruits, vegetables, whole grains, nuts, and seeds, are the building blocks of a diet that supports the body's natural healing processes.

They are packed with phytonutrients that combat inflammation, bolster the immune system, and protect against chronic diseases. By prioritizing these nutrient-dense foods, individuals can create a dietary pattern that not only nourishes the body but also supports mental and emotional well-being.

The concept of bioindividuality is crucial in understanding the role of nutrition in a holistic lifestyle. Recognizing that each person has unique nutritional needs allows for a more personalized approach to diet. What nourishes one individual may not have the same effect on another, underscoring the importance of listening to the body's signals and adjusting dietary choices accordingly.

This personalized approach fosters a deeper connection with one's own body, encouraging a mindful eating practice that is attuned to the body's natural hunger and fullness cues.

Hydration, often overlooked, is another fundamental aspect of nutrition in a holistic lifestyle. Water is essential for every cellular function in the body, from aiding digestion to flushing toxins and facilitating nutrient absorption.

Incorporating herbal teas and natural hydrating foods like cucumbers and watermelon can add variety and additional nutrients to one's hydration practices.

The role of nutrition extends beyond the physical to influence the mental and emotional realms. Foods high in omega-3 fatty acids, for example, are known to support brain health and mood regulation.

Similarly, complex carbohydrates can help stabilize blood sugar levels, impacting energy and mood. Understanding the connection between food and mood is vital in crafting a diet that supports not just physical health but also mental and emotional balance.

Sustainability and mindfulness in food choices play a significant role in holistic nutrition. Choosing organic, locally sourced foods not only reduces the environmental impact but also supports local communities and ensures that the food is of the highest quality.

Mindful eating practices, such as taking the time to savor each bite and being fully present during meals, enhance the nutritional experience, turning it into an opportunity for gratitude and reflection.

Incorporating a variety of foods into the diet ensures a broad spectrum of nutrients, promoting balance and preventing nutritional deficiencies.

Experimenting with different cuisines and flavors can make healthy eating enjoyable and exciting, encouraging a lifelong commitment to nourishment.

As we delve deeper into the intricacies of nutrition as the foundation of a holistic lifestyle, it becomes clear that our dietary choices are a powerful tool for shaping our health and well-being. By embracing the principles of whole foods nutrition, bioindividuality, hydration, and mindful eating, individuals can embark on a journey toward a more balanced, vibrant life.

Embracing seasonal eating is a natural extension of a holistic lifestyle, aligning our diets with the cycles of nature. This practice not only ensures that we consume fruits and vegetables at their peak nutritional value but also fosters a deeper connection with the environment.

Seasonal foods tend to be fresher and tastier, enhancing the joy and satisfaction derived from meals. Additionally, this approach supports the body's nutritional needs throughout the year, such as the demand for more vitamin C-rich foods during cold months to bolster the immune system.

The concept of food as medicine is central to holistic nutrition, emphasizing the therapeutic properties of certain foods and herbs.

Incorporating anti-inflammatory foods like turmeric, ginger, and berries can help mitigate chronic inflammation, a root cause of many diseases. Similarly, adaptogenic herbs such as ashwagandha and holy basil can be used to support the body's stress response, illustrating how diet can be tailored to address specific health concerns and promote healing.

Understanding the gut-brain connection highlights the importance of nutrition in mental health. A diet rich in probiotics and prebiotics supports a healthy gut microbiome, which in turn influences mood and cognitive function. Fermented foods like yogurt, kefir, and sauerkraut are excellent sources of probiotics, while prebiotic foods include garlic, onions, and bananas.

Nurturing gut health through diet can have profound effects on overall well-being, underscoring the interconnectedness of physical and mental health in a holistic lifestyle.

The avoidance of processed foods and artificial additives is crucial in maintaining the integrity of a holistic diet. These substances can disrupt the body's natural processes and contribute to health issues. Instead, focusing on whole, unprocessed foods ensures that the diet remains clean and conducive to health. This principle extends to the preparation of meals, where gentle cooking methods like steaming and sautéing preserve the nutritional content of foods.

Finally, the practice of gratitude and intentionality in eating rituals enriches the holistic nutrition experience. Taking a moment to express gratitude for the nourishment provided, acknowledging the journey of the food from farm to table, and eating with intention can transform mealtime into a meditative practice.

This mindful approach to nutrition not only enhances the digestive process but also cultivates a sense of peace and fulfillment.

In conclusion, nutrition as the foundation of a holistic lifestyle encompasses much more than the mere act of eating. It involves a comprehensive understanding of the intricate relationship between food, the body, and the mind. By honoring the principles of whole foods nutrition, seasonal and therapeutic eating, gut health, and mindful consumption, we can nurture our bodies, support our mental and emotional well-being, and live in greater harmony with the natural world.

This holistic approach to nutrition empowers individuals to take control of their health and embark on a transformative journey toward vitality and wellness.

CHAPTER 2: HOLISTIC WELL-BEING PRACTICES

Holistic well-being encompasses a broad spectrum of practices that aim to balance and nourish the physical, mental, and spiritual aspects of an individual's life. These practices are designed to foster a deep sense of connection with oneself and the surrounding world, promoting health, happiness, and harmony. By integrating these natural practices into daily life, individuals can enhance their overall well-being and navigate life's challenges with greater resilience and peace. Dr. Barbara's perspective on holistic well-being emphasizes a comprehensive approach that integrates practices designed to harmonize and nourish the multiple dimensions of a person's life. According to Dr. Barbara, achieving holistic well-being involves a balance of physical, mental, and spiritual elements, creating a cohesive and supportive framework for a fulfilling and healthy life.

Here's a deeper dive into each aspect of holistic well-being according to Dr. Barbara:

1. Physical Nourishment

Dr. Barbara asserts that physical health is foundational to holistic well-being. This encompasses:

- **Nutrition**: A diet rich in whole, natural foods—such as fruits, vegetables, lean proteins, and whole grains—provides the necessary nutrients that support bodily functions and energy levels.
- **Exercise**: Regular physical activity not only strengthens the body but also boosts mood and cognitive function. Dr. Barbara advocates for a variety of exercises, including aerobic activities, strength training, and flexibility exercises.
- **Rest and Recovery**: Adequate sleep and rest are crucial for physical repair and overall health. Dr. Barbara emphasizes the importance of quality sleep and restorative practices like yoga or meditation.

2. Mental Clarity

Mental well-being is equally important in Dr. Barbara's holistic approach:

- **Mindfulness and Meditation**: These practices help to center the mind, reduce stress, and improve focus. Dr. Barbara encourages regular mindfulness practices to foster mental clarity and emotional balance.
- **Stress Management**: Techniques such as deep breathing, progressive muscle relaxation, and time management are key to managing stress effectively.
- **Cognitive Engagement**: Engaging in intellectually stimulating activities, such as reading, puzzles, or learning new skills, helps to keep the mind sharp and engaged.

3. Spiritual Connection

Spiritual well-being involves a sense of purpose and connection beyond the self:

- **Personal Reflection**: Regular self-reflection and introspection can help individuals understand their values, beliefs, and goals. Dr. Barbara supports practices like journaling and spiritual exploration to foster a deeper connection with oneself.
- **Community and Belonging**: Building strong, supportive relationships and engaging in community activities can enhance feelings of belonging and purpose.
- **Purpose and Fulfillment**: Aligning daily actions with personal values and goals helps individuals find meaning and satisfaction in their lives.

4. Integration and Harmony

Dr. Barbara stresses that holistic well-being is achieved by integrating these practices into daily life:

- **Routine Practices**: Incorporating physical, mental, and spiritual practices into a daily routine helps create consistency and balance. Dr. Barbara advocates for setting aside time each day for activities that support holistic health.
- **Resilience**: By maintaining a balanced approach to life, individuals can better navigate challenges and adapt to changes with resilience and peace. Dr. Barbara believes that holistic practices build a strong foundation that supports well-being through life's ups and downs.

Daily Meditation and Mindfulness

Beneficial effects: Reduces stress, enhances focus and clarity, improves emotional balance, and supports overall mental health.

- **Instructions:**

1. Find a quiet, comfortable space where you can sit or lie down without interruptions.

2. Set a timer for the desired length of your meditation, starting with 5 to 10 minutes.

3. Close your eyes and take a few deep breaths, allowing your body to relax with each exhale.

4. Focus your attention on your breath, observing the sensations of inhaling and exhaling without trying to change them.

5. If your mind wanders, gently acknowledge the thoughts and return your focus to your breath.

6. Continue this practice until the timer ends, then slowly open your eyes and take a moment to notice how you feel.

- **Variations:** Incorporate guided meditations, use mindfulness apps, or focus on a mantra or positive affirmation.

Regular Physical Activity

Beneficial effects: Boosts physical health, improves mood, increases energy levels, and reduces the risk of chronic diseases.

- **Instructions:**

1. Choose an activity you enjoy, such as walking, yoga, dancing, or cycling.

2. Aim for at least 30 minutes of moderate activity most days of the week.

3. Incorporate variety to engage different muscle groups and prevent boredom.

4. Listen to your body and adjust the intensity and duration of your activities to match your current fitness level.

- **Variations:** Try outdoor activities to connect with nature, join group classes for social interaction, or explore new sports for fun and challenge.

Balanced Nutrition

Beneficial effects: Supports physical health, enhances mental clarity, and provides the energy needed for daily activities.

Ingredients: A variety of whole foods including fruits, vegetables, whole grains, lean proteins, and healthy fats.

- **Instructions:**

1. Fill half your plate with colorful fruits and vegetables at each meal.

2. Choose whole grains over refined grains for added fiber and nutrients.

3. Include a source of lean protein to support muscle health and satiety.

4. Add healthy fats, such as avocados, nuts, and olive oil, for flavor and heart health.

5. Stay hydrated by drinking water throughout the day, and limit sugary beverages.

- **Variations:** Experiment with plant-based meals, explore international cuisines for variety, or try meal prepping for convenience.

Quality Sleep

Beneficial effects: Essential for physical health, cognitive function, and emotional well-being.

- **Instructions:**

1. Establish a consistent sleep schedule by going to bed and waking up at the same time every day.

2. Create a relaxing bedtime routine to signal your body it's time to wind down.

3. Keep your bedroom cool, dark, and quiet to promote restful sleep.

4. Limit exposure to screens and bright lights in the evening.

5. Avoid caffeine and heavy meals close to bedtime.

- **Variations:** Use aromatherapy with lavender or chamomile for relaxation, practice gentle yoga or stretching before bed, or listen to calming music or white noise.

Connection with Nature

Beneficial effects: Reduces stress, improves mood, and enhances physical well-being.

- **Instructions:**

1. Spend time outdoors daily, whether it's a walk in the park, gardening, or simply sitting in a natural setting.

2. Practice mindfulness while in nature by paying attention to the sights, sounds, and smells around you.

3. Engage in outdoor activities such as hiking, kayaking, or bird-watching to deepen your connection with the natural world.

4. Use natural elements in your home decor, such as plants or natural materials, to bring the outdoors in.

- **Variations:** Plan regular trips to different natural environments, such as forests, mountains, or beaches, to experience the diverse beauty of nature.

Integrating these natural practices for holistic well-being into daily life can lead to profound improvements in health, happiness, and harmony. By taking a holistic approach, individuals can cultivate a lifestyle that supports their highest potential for well-being.

CHAPTER 3: HERBAL RECIPES FOR HOLISTIC LIVING

LEMON BALM AND LAVENDER RELAXATION ELIXIR

Beneficial effects

The Lemon Balm and Lavender Relaxation Elixir combines the soothing properties of lemon balm and lavender, known for their ability to reduce stress, anxiety, and promote a sense of calm and relaxation. Lemon balm, with its mild sedative effects, can help ease the mind and improve sleep quality, while lavender's calming scent is widely recognized for its relaxation benefits. This elixir is perfect for unwinding after a long day, easing into a restful night's sleep, or simply finding a moment of peace and tranquility.

Portions

2 servings

Preparation time

10 minutes

Ingredients

- 2 tablespoons dried lemon balm leaves

- 2 tablespoons dried lavender flowers

- 4 cups of boiling water

- Honey or lemon to taste (optional)

Instructions

1. Place the dried lemon balm leaves and lavender flowers in a heat-resistant teapot or jar.

2. Pour 4 cups of boiling water over the herbs.

3. Cover and allow the mixture to steep for about 10 minutes.

4. Strain the elixir into cups or a large pitcher, discarding the herbs.

5. Optional: Add honey or lemon to taste for flavor enhancement.

6. Serve the elixir warm to enjoy its relaxing benefits.

Variations

- For a cooling, refreshing drink during warmer months, allow the elixir to cool to room temperature, then refrigerate and serve over ice.

- Mix in a teaspoon of chamomile flowers with the lemon balm and lavender for additional sleep-promoting properties.

- Add a slice of fresh ginger during the steeping process for a warming flavor and additional digestive benefits.

Storage tips

Store any leftover Lemon Balm and Lavender Relaxation Elixir in a sealed container in the refrigerator for up to 2 days. Enjoy chilled or gently reheat on the stove.

Tips for allergens

Individuals with sensitivities to lemon balm or lavender should consult with a healthcare provider before consumption. For those avoiding honey due to dietary restrictions, substitute with maple syrup or simply omit the sweetener.

Scientific references

- "A review of the bioactivity and potential health benefits of lemon balm" published in Phytotherapy Research, highlights the sedative and sleep-enhancing effects of lemon balm, supporting its use for improving sleep quality.

- "Lavender and the Nervous System" in Evidence-Based Complementary and Alternative Medicine, discusses the anxiolytic (anxiety-reducing) and sedative effects of lavender, supporting its use for stress relief and relaxation.

HOLY BASIL AND LEMON VERBENA STRESS RELIEF TEA

Beneficial effects

Holy Basil and Lemon Verbena Stress Relief Tea harnesses the calming and soothing properties of both herbs to combat stress, reduce anxiety, and promote relaxation. Holy Basil, also known as Tulsi, is revered for its adaptogenic properties, helping the body to manage and adapt to stress more effectively. Lemon Verbena adds a gentle, soothing effect, aiding in relaxation and improving sleep quality. Together, they create a harmonious blend that not only soothes the mind but also uplifts the spirit, making it an ideal beverage for those seeking to maintain a balanced and holistic lifestyle.

Portions

2 servings

Preparation time

10 minutes

Ingredients

- 1 tablespoon dried Holy Basil leaves

- 1 tablespoon dried Lemon Verbena leaves

- 2 cups boiling water

- Honey or lemon to taste (optional)

Instructions

1. Place the dried Holy Basil and Lemon Verbena leaves in a tea infuser or directly into a heat-resistant teapot.

2. Pour 2 cups of boiling water over the herbs.

3. Cover and let the tea steep for about 10 minutes to allow the flavors and beneficial properties to infuse.

4. Remove the tea infuser or strain the tea to remove the leaves.

5. Optional: Add honey or lemon to taste for flavor enhancement.

6. Serve the tea warm, ideally in the evening or whenever stress relief is needed.

Variations

- For a refreshing twist, serve the tea chilled over ice, garnished with a slice of lemon or a sprig of fresh Holy Basil.

- Add a slice of fresh ginger during the steeping process for an additional warming and digestive aid.

- Combine with a teaspoon of chamomile flowers for enhanced relaxation and sleep support.

Storage tips

Store any leftover Holy Basil and Lemon Verbena Stress Relief Tea in a sealed container in the refrigerator for up to 2 days. Enjoy chilled or gently reheat on the stove.

Tips for allergens

Individuals with sensitivities to Holy Basil or Lemon Verbena should consult with a healthcare provider before consumption. For those avoiding honey due to dietary restrictions, substitute with maple syrup or simply omit the sweetener.

Scientific references

- "Adaptogenic effects of Ocimum sanctum (Tulsi) in a physical stress model" in the International Journal of Ayurveda Research, which discusses the stress-relieving properties of Holy Basil.
- "Lemon verbena: A promising herb with health benefits" in the Journal of Functional Foods, highlighting Lemon Verbena's soothing effects on the nervous system and its potential in promoting relaxation and reducing anxiety.

GINGER AND LEMON IMMUNE BOOST TONIC

Beneficial effects

Ginger and Lemon Immune Boost Tonic is designed to enhance the immune system, promote digestion, and provide anti-inflammatory benefits. Ginger, with its potent anti-inflammatory compounds, helps in reducing inflammation and boosting immunity. Lemon, rich in Vitamin C, aids in increasing the body's resistance to infections. Together, they create a powerful tonic that supports overall health and wellness, particularly during cold and flu season.

Portions

2 servings

Preparation time

10 minutes

Ingredients

- 1 inch fresh ginger, peeled and sliced
- Juice of 2 lemons
- 2 cups of boiling water
- 1 tablespoon honey (optional)

Instructions

1. Place the sliced ginger in a heat-resistant pitcher or jar.

2. Squeeze the juice of 2 lemons and add it to the pitcher.

3. Pour 2 cups of boiling water over the ginger and lemon juice.

4. Allow the mixture to steep for about 5-10 minutes.

5. Strain the tonic to remove the ginger slices.

6. Add honey to the warm tonic and stir until it dissolves completely.

7. Serve the tonic warm or allow it to cool and enjoy it chilled.

Variations

- For an extra immune boost, add a pinch of cayenne pepper to the tonic during the steeping process.
- Incorporate a teaspoon of turmeric powder for additional anti-inflammatory and antioxidant benefits.
- Replace honey with maple syrup for a vegan-friendly sweetener option.

Storage tips

Store any leftover Ginger and Lemon Immune Boost Tonic in a sealed container in the refrigerator for up to 2 days. Reheat gently on the stove or enjoy cold.

Tips for allergens

Individuals with sensitivities to ginger or lemon should adjust the amount used according to their tolerance. For those avoiding honey due to allergies or dietary preferences, maple syrup serves as a suitable alternative.

Scientific references

- "Ginger in gastrointestinal disorders: A systematic review of clinical trials," published in Food Science & Nutrition, 2019. This review supports ginger's benefits in improving digestion and its anti-inflammatory properties.

- "The effects of dietary lemon peels on the immune system and gastrointestinal tract: A preliminary study," in the Journal of Nutrition & Intermediary Metabolism, 2016. This study highlights lemon's role in enhancing immune function and supporting digestive health.

TURMERIC AND GINGER ANTI-INFLAMMATORY SMOOTHIE

Beneficial effects

The Turmeric and Ginger Anti-Inflammatory Smoothie is designed to combat inflammation throughout the body, offering a natural remedy for those suffering from chronic inflammatory conditions such as arthritis, digestive disorders, and autoimmune diseases. Turmeric, with its active component curcumin, provides potent anti-inflammatory and antioxidant benefits, helping to alleviate pain and prevent oxidative stress. Ginger complements turmeric with its own anti-inflammatory properties, further enhancing the smoothie's effectiveness in reducing inflammation and promoting overall health.

Portions

2 servings

Preparation time

10 minutes

Ingredients

- 1 cup almond milk
- 1 ripe banana
- 1/2 cup frozen pineapple
- 1 tablespoon turmeric powder
- 1 tablespoon grated fresh ginger
- 1 teaspoon ground cinnamon
- 1 tablespoon flaxseed meal
- Honey or maple syrup to taste (optional)

Instructions

1. Place almond milk, ripe banana, frozen pineapple, turmeric powder, grated fresh ginger, ground cinnamon, and flaxseed meal into a blender.

2. Blend on high until smooth and creamy.

3. Taste and add honey or maple syrup if a sweeter smoothie is desired. Blend again to incorporate the sweetener.

4. Pour into glasses and serve immediately for optimal freshness and potency.

Variations

- For an extra protein boost, add a scoop of your favorite protein powder.

- To increase the anti-inflammatory effects, include a pinch of black pepper to enhance the absorption of curcumin from turmeric.

- Substitute almond milk with coconut water for a lighter, hydrating version, perfect for post-workout recovery.

Storage tips

For best results, consume the Turmeric and Ginger Anti-Inflammatory Smoothie immediately after preparation. If needed, it can be stored in an airtight container in the refrigerator for up to 24 hours. Shake well before serving if separation occurs.

Tips for allergens

Individuals with nut allergies can substitute almond milk with oat milk or any other non-nut milk alternative. For a vegan-friendly sweetener, opt for maple syrup instead of honey.

Scientific references

- "Curcumin: A Review of Its' Effects on Human Health," published in Foods, 2017. This review discusses the wide-ranging health benefits of curcumin, including its anti-inflammatory and antioxidant effects.

- "Ginger on Human Health: A Comprehensive Systematic Review of 109 Randomized Controlled Trials," in Nutrients, 2020. This systematic review highlights ginger's health benefits, particularly its anti-inflammatory properties and effectiveness in digestive health support.

PEPPERMINT AND CHAMOMILE DIGESTIVE AID

Beneficial effects

Peppermint and Chamomile Digestive Aid is a soothing remedy designed to alleviate digestive discomfort, reduce bloating, and promote a healthy digestive system. Peppermint is known for its ability to relax the muscles of the digestive tract, easing indigestion and reducing spasms. Chamomile, with its anti-inflammatory properties, can help soothe irritated stomach lining and reduce acid reflux symptoms. Together, they create a calming tea that supports digestive health and provides relief from gastrointestinal distress.

Portions

2 servings

Preparation time

5 minutes

Cooking time

10 minutes

Ingredients

- 1 tablespoon dried peppermint leaves

- 1 tablespoon dried chamomile flowers

- 2 cups of water

- Honey or lemon to taste (optional)

Instructions

1. Bring 2 cups of water to a boil in a small pot.

2. Add the dried peppermint leaves and chamomile flowers to the boiling water.

3. Reduce the heat and simmer for about 5 minutes.

4. Remove the pot from the heat and allow the tea to steep for an additional 5 minutes.

5. Strain the tea into mugs, discarding the peppermint and chamomile.

6. Optional: Add honey or lemon to taste for flavor enhancement.

7. Serve the tea warm, ideally after meals, to aid in digestion.

Variations

- For an added soothing effect, include a slice of fresh ginger during the simmering process.

- Mix in a teaspoon of fennel seeds with the peppermint and chamomile for additional digestive benefits.

- For a cold beverage option, allow the tea to cool and then refrigerate. Serve over ice for a refreshing digestive aid.

Storage tips

Store any leftover Peppermint and Chamomile Digestive Aid in a sealed container in the refrigerator for up to 2 days. Enjoy chilled or gently reheat on the stove.

Tips for allergens

Individuals with allergies to peppermint or chamomile should consult with a healthcare provider before consumption. For those avoiding honey due to dietary restrictions, substitute with maple syrup or simply omit the sweetener.

Scientific references

- "Peppermint oil for the treatment of irritable bowel syndrome: a systematic review and meta-analysis" in the Journal of Clinical Gastroenterology, highlighting peppermint's effectiveness in managing IBS symptoms.

- "Chamomile: A herbal medicine of the past with a bright future" in Molecular Medicine Reports, discusses the anti-inflammatory and gastrointestinal benefits of chamomile, supporting its use for digestive health.

Made in the USA
Columbia, SC
07 October 2024

43788751R00309